Cardiology
1987

Cardiology
1987

WILLIAM C. ROBERTS, MD, Editor
Chief, Pathology Branch
National Heart, Lung, and Blood Institute
National Institutes of Health, Bethesda, Maryland, and
Clinical Professor of Pathology and Medicine (Cardiology)
Georgetown University, Washington, D. C.
Editor-in-Chief, The American Journal of Cardiology

CHARLES E. RACKLEY, MD
Chairman, Department of Medicine
Anton and Margaret Fuisz
Professor of Medicine
Georgetown University Medical Center
Washington, D. C.

DEAN T. MASON, MD
Chairman, Department of
Cardiovascular Medicine
St. Mary's Hospital and Medical Center
San Francisco, California
Editor-in-Chief, American Heart Journal

JAMES T. WILLERSON, MD
Professor of Medicine
Chief, Division of Cardiology
Department of Medicine
University of Texas Health Science Center
Dallas, Texas

ALBERT D. PACIFICO, MD
Professor and Director
Division of Cardiothoracic Surgery
University of Alabama Medical Center
Birmingham, Alabama

THOMAS P. GRAHAM, JR, MD
Professor of Pediatrics
Chief, Division of Pediatric Cardiology
Department of Pediatrics
Vanderbilt University
Nashville, Tennessee

ROBERT B. KARP, MD
Chief, Cardiac Surgery Section
Department of Surgery
University of Chicago Medical Center
Chicago, Illinois

Cardiology: 1987

First Edition

International Standard Book Number: 0-914316-53-2

International Standard Serial Number: 0275-0066

Contents

3. Acute Myocardial Infarction and Its Consequences   127

6. Valvular Heart Disease 303

_____

Preface

Cardiology 1987 is the seventh book to be published in this series. It contains summaries of 858 articles, all published in 1986. A total of 25 medical journals (Table I) were examined and at least 1, and usually many articles, were summarized from each of these journals. The number of articles summarized by each of the 7 authors is summarized in Table II. All of Rackley's submissions were from *Circulation*; Mason's from *The American Heart Journal*, and Willerson's from *The Journal of American College of Cardiology*. Karp's and Pacifico's summaries were from articles published in surgical journals. The contributions of Graham and Roberts were from a variety of medical journals. The summaries from each contributor were submitted to me, organized into the various sections in each of the 10 chapters, and each summary was copyedited by me.

A book of this type is made possible because of unselfish contributions from several individuals, none of whom are rewarded by authorship. I am enormously grateful to Marjorie Hadsell for typing perfectly the 503 summaries contributed by me, to Richard M. Frederickson for organizing the figures

TABLE I. *Journals containing articles summarized in Cardiology 1987.*

1. American Heart Journal
2. American Journal of Cardiology
3. American Journal of Medicine
4. Annals of Internal Medicine
5. Annals of Thoracic Surgery
6. Archives of Internal Medicine
7. Archives of Pathology and Laboratory of Medicine
8. Atherosclerosis
9. British Heart Journal
10. British Medical Journal
11. Catheterization and Cardiovascular Diagnosis
12. Chest
13. Circulation
14. European Heart Journal
15. Human Pathology
16. Journal of American College of Cardiology
17. Journal of the American Medical Association
18. Journal of Arteriosclerosis
19. Journal of Thoracic & Cardiovascular Surgery
20. Lancet
21. Mayo Clinic Proceedings
22. Medicine
23. Morbidity and Mortality Weekly Report
24. New England Journal of Medicine
25. Progress in Cardiovascular Diseases

TABLE II.   *Contributions of the 7 Authors to CARDIOLOGY 1987*

AUTHOR	1	2	3	4	5	6	7	8	9	10	TOTALS
WCR	67	79	84	67	60	46	13	4	18	65	503 (58.62%)
CER	9	21	20	9	2	11	3	0	10	5	90 (10.49%)
DTM	5	18	16	20	6	4	4	3	3	3	82 (9.56%)
JTW	0	18	19	9	1	12	8	0	5	4	76 (8.86%)
ADP	0	0	0	0	0	0	0	41	0	0	41 (4.78%)
TPG, Jr	0	2	0	0	0	1	0	35	0	0	38 (4.43%)
RBK	0	7	3	1	0	11	0	0	0	6	28 (3.26%)
TOTALS	81	145	142	106	69	85	28	83	36	83	858 (100%)
Figures	23	28	30	9	12	17	6	8	9	11	153
Tables	17	5	0	4	10	11	1	3	1	2	54

and tables for photography, to Janet M. Rohrbaugh for typing the detailed table of contents, to Leslie Silvernail, Laurie Christian, Nancy Dickey, Joyce Phillips, Sue Long, Sue Scaletta, and Mary Sawallisch also for typing many summaries. Jennifer Granger managed to carry the 30-pound package of edited summaries, reference cards, figures and tables from Bethesda to New York. Herbert V. Paureiss, Jr., Judith Wagner, and Vicky Weisman efficiently coordinated the publishing of the book in New York.

William C. Roberts, MD
Editor

1

Factors Causing or Accelerating Coronary Arterial Atherosclerosis

---

The Low Risk Coronary Male

Henry Blackburn from Minneapolis, Minnesota, wrote the following piece[1]:

"Maybe you have heard this now classic satire by Gordon Myers of Boston on the "theoretical low coronary risk male":

An effeminate municipal worker or embalmer, completely lacking in physical and mental alertness and without drive, ambition or competitive spirit, who has never attempted to meet a deadline of any kind. A man with poor appetite, subsisting on fruits and vegetables laced with corn and whale oil; detesting tobacco, spurning ownership of radio, TV or motor car; with full head of hair and scrawny and unathletic in appearance yet constantly straining his puny muscles by exercise; low in income, blood pressure, blood sugar, uric acid, and cholesterol; who has been taking nicotinic acid, pyridoxine, and long-term anticoagulant therapy ever since his prophylactic castration.

In contrast, let me sketch the 'real low coronary risk male,' who is documented to live on the Isle of Crete:

He is a shepherd or small farmer, a beekeeper or fisherman, or a tender of olives or vines.

He walks to work daily and labors in the soft light of his Greek isle, midst the droning of crickets and the bray of distant donkeys, in the peace of his land.

At the end of the morning's work, he rests and socializes with cohorts at the local cafe under a grape trellis, celebrating the day with a cool glass of lemonade and a single, hand-rolled, hand-cured cigarette of long-leafed Macedonian tobacco.

He continues the siesta with a meal and nap at home, and returns refreshed to complete the day's work.

His midday, main meal is of eggplant, with large livery mushrooms, crisp vegetables and country bread dipped in the nectar that is golden Cretan olive oil.

Once a week there is a bit of lamb, naturally spiced from sheep grazing in thyme-filled pastures.

Once a week there is chicken.

Twice a week there is fish fresh from the sea.

Other meals are hot dishes of legumes seasoned with meats and condiments.

The main dish is followed by a tangy salad, then by dates, Turkish sweets, nuts or succulent fresh fruits.

A sharp local wine completes this varied and savory cuisine.

This living pattern, repeated six days a week, is climaxed by a happy Saturday evening.

The ritual family dinner is followed by relaxing fellowship with peers.

Festivity builds to a passionate midnight dance under the brilliant moon in the field circle where the grain of the region is winnowed.

Our Cretan, in the presence of admiring friends, is a man dignified in bearing, happy in countenance and graceful in the dance.

On Sunday he strolls to worship with his children and wife. In church he listens to good sense preached by the orthodox priest, a respected leader involved in turn, with his own family and his political and religious responsibilities.

Then our truly low risk male returns home for a quiet Sunday afternoon, chatting with family in the shade, cooled by the salubrious sea breeze gently perfumed by smoke from olive-wood charcoal grills, and fragrances wafted from the fields of herbs and fresh animal dung.

This man of Crete gazes on a severe but harmonious landscape.

He is secure in his niche in a long history from the Minoans and before, a human in the long line of humanity.

He relishes the natural rhythmic cycles and contrasts of his culture: work and rest, solitude and socialization, seriousness and laughter, routine and revelry.

In his elder years, he sits in the slanting bronze light of the Greek sun, enveloped in a rich lavender aura from the Aegean sea and sky.

He is handsome, rugged, kindly and virile.

His is the lowest heart attack risk, the lowest death rate and the greatest life expectancy in the Western world.

Finally, though healthy, he is prepared to die.

This, then, is a portrait of the man truly most free of coronary risk of all men on earth."

More data from the multiple risk factor intervention trial

The Multiple Risk Factor Intervention Trial (MRFIT)[2] was a randomized clinical study to test whether a special-intervention (SI) program aimed at reducing serum cholesterol levels, BP and cigarette smoking would prevent CAD in middle-aged men. The main endpoint reported here is the percentage of participants having first major CAD events (either nonfatal AMI or CAD death) during 7 years of follow-up. This outcome was slightly less frequent in the 6,428 SI men than in the 6,438 men assigned to their usual source of care (UC). However, the relative differences—either 1% or 8%, depending on how AMI was classified—was not statistically significant. Regression analyses within the SI and UC groups suggested that the cholesterol and cigarette smoking interventions reduced the number of first major CAD events: the associations between lowering the levels of these 2 factors and reductions in CAD rates were significant and of the anticipated magnitude. A similar analysis of antihypertensive treatment in the SI group revealed no favorable association between lowering BP and CAD rate, and other subgroup comparisons suggested that a mixture of beneficial and adverse effects may underlie this finding. Thus, the nonsignificant overall UC/SI contrast in CAD rates may reflect a combination of the expected beneficial effects of the cholesterol and smoking interventions with unexpected heterogeneous effects of the antihypertensive intervention. Seven of 8 other prespecified cardiovascular endpoints occurred less frequently among SI than among UC men, the difference being nominally significant for angina pectoris, CHF and peripheral arterial disease.

The 1982 report (JAMA 1982: 1465–1477) on the MRFIT results revealed 7% fewer CAD deaths in SI than in UC men. Three explanations for this statistically nonsignificant difference were proposed: "(1) the overall intervention program, under these circumstances, does not affect CAD mortality; (2) the intervention used does affect CAD mortality, but the benefit was not observed in this trial of 7 years' average duration, with lower-than-expected mortality and with considerable risk factor change in the UC group; and (3) the measures to reduce cigarette smoking and to lower blood cholesterol levels may have reduced CAD mortality within subgroups of the SI cohort, with a possibly unfavorable response to antihypertensive drug therapy in certain but not all hypertensive subjects."

The current report, while indicating a beneficial effect on several other cardiovascular endpoints, does not reveal a statistically significant difference in first major CAD events (nonfatal AMI and CAD death) experienced by SI and UC men. An effort to interpret this finding, based on analyses within the MRFIT and evidence from other studies, leads us to continue to favor the second and third of the explanations proposed in 1982.

The MRFIT evidence for a beneficial effect of cholesterol and smoking intervention is as follows: 1) Within-group analysis in both SI and UC groups reveals favorable associations between the change in serum cholesterol and cigarette smoking levels and the occurrence of CAD; men with greater reductions in these risk factors had lower CAD rates. 2) The magnitude of this benefit is nearly identical to that projected from analyzing the baseline risk factors as predictors of CAD, suggesting that intervention can remove most of the excess risk associated with these risk factors. The projected impact on the UC/SI percentage difference in CAD events is small—only 9%—because risk factor changes in the UC group attenuated the UC/SI differences in risk factor levels.

The MRFIT evidence suggesting unexpected effects of BP intervention is as follows: 1) Within-group analysis of the SI men reveals no favorable association between change in BP and the occurrence of CAD; there was a tendency for greater reduction in BP to be associated with an increase in the CAD rate of SI men. 2) Between-group analyses suggest the possibility that BP treatment had beneficial effects in some subgroups and adverse effects in others.

Crow and associates[3] from multiple centers examined the association between CAD risk factors and submaximal exercise performance among 12,866 men at high risk in MRFIT. Men were selected from a risk score based on serum cholesterol level, diastolic BP and number of cigarettes smoked per day. Multivariate analysis using exercise ST depression as the dependent variable showed that age, diastolic BP and serum cholesterol level were significant positive predictors of ST depression, and cigarettes per day, body mass index and heart rate at rest were significant negative predictors of ST depression. Similarly, multivariate analysis, using exercise duration as the dependent variable, revealed that age, cholesterol level, body mass index and heart rate at rest were significant negative predictors of exercise duration, whereas cigarettes per day and leisure-time physical activity were significant positive predictors. Some of these relations with exercise performance are consistent with established epidemiologic CAD risk factor associations and others are not. The MRFIT selection process, which resulted in smokers who were significantly younger and who had significantly lower levels of other CAD risk factors than nonsmokers, was partially responsible.

In a study carried out by Kannel and associates[4] from Boston, Massachusetts, Minneapolis, Minnesota, Chicago, Illinois and San Francisco, California, the influence of risk factors on CAD and all-cause mortality rates in 35- to 57-year-old men was examined by means of data on 325,348 white men who were screened for the MRFIT. This large data set permitted an unusually detailed analysis of factors associated with the 6,968 deaths, including 2,426 ascribed to CAD, that were detected in the Social Security Administration data set during 6 years of follow-up. Simple cross classification of the data confirmed the independent effect of serum cholesterol concentration, diastolic BP, and cigarette smoking as risk factors for CAD and all-cause mortality rates. A distinct escalation of risk was noted for combinations of these risk factors. The strength of the association of each of the risk factors with CAD and all-cause mortality rates diminished with increasing age, although the number of excess deaths attributable to the risk factors increased because of the higher death rates in older men. Comparison of these findings with those observed in the 5 populations studied in the Pooling Project revealed an overall similarity in the risk relations. It was estimated that elimination of these risk factors has the potential for reducing the CAD mortality rate by two-thirds in 35- to 45-year-old men, and by one-half in 46- to 57-year-old men.

Martin and associates[5] from San Francisco, California, Pittsburgh, Pennsylvania, and Minneapolis, Minnesota, determined the risks associated with various levels of serum total cholesterol by analysis of 6-year mortality in 361,662 men aged 35–57 years (Figs. 1-1, 1-2, 1-3). Above the 20th percentile for serum total cholesterol (>181 mg/dl, >4.68 mmol/liter), CAD mortality increased progressively; the relative risk was large (3.8) in the men with total cholesterol levels above the 85th percentile (>253 mg/dl, >6.54 mmol/liter). When men below the 29th cholesterol percentile were used as the baseline risk group, half of all CAD deaths were associated with raised serum cholesterol concentrations; half of these excess deaths were in men with cholesterol levels above the 85th percentile. For both CAD and total mortality, serum cholesterol was similar to diastolic BP in the shape of the risk curve and in the size of the high-risk group (Fig. 1-4). This new evidence supports the policy of a moderate fat intake for the general population and intensive treatment for those at high risk. There was a striking analogy between serum cholesterol and BP in the epidemiologic basis for identifying a large segment of the population (10–15%) for intensive treatment.

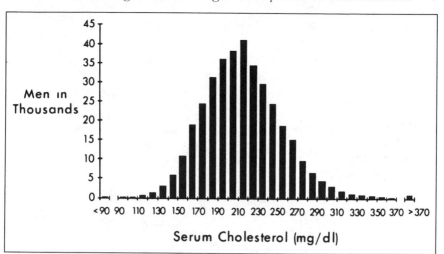

Fig. 1-1. Distribution of serum cholesterol concentrations in 361,662 men screened for MRFIT (1973–75). Reproduced with permission from Martin et al.[5]

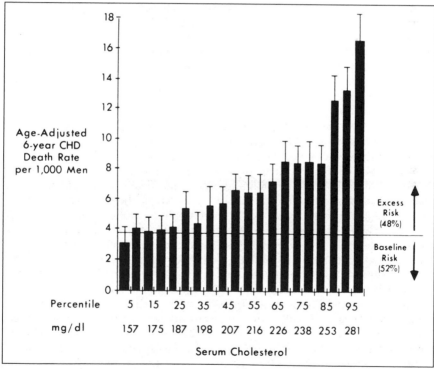

Fig. 1-2. Age-adjusted 6-year CHD death rate per 1000 men screened for MRFIT according to serum cholesterol percentile. Reproduced with permission from Martin et al.[5]

European collaborative trial of multifactorial prevention of coronary artery disease

In 1983 the initial report of the incidence and mortality results from the World Health Organization, European Collaborative Trial of Multifactorial Prevention of Coronary Heart Disease was reported. The initial analysis con-

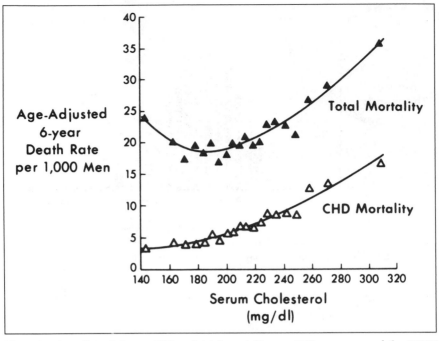

Fig. 1-3. Age-adjusted 6-year CHD and total mortality per 1000 men screened for MRFIT according to serum cholesterol. Reproduced with permission from Martin et al.[5]

sidered only the overall differences between the intervention and control groups to try to see what happened when an attempt was made to change a community's coronary risk factors. In the large Belgian center there was a 24% reduction in total incidents of CAD. Similar reductions in the Rome and Cracow centers did not individually reach significance. The absence of a positive result from the UK center reduced the overall benefit to a nonsignificant level. The present report[6] gives the complete results from all 4 centers (Belgium, Italy, Poland, and the UK) and analyzes them in an attempt to see what happens when the coronary risk factors in a community are changed. Thus, in the controlled randomized evaluation of multifactorial prevention of CAD among 60,881 men employed in 80 factories in the 4 countries, a 10.2% reduction in CAD occurred, a 6.9% reduction in fatal CAD, a 14.8% in nonfatal AMI, and a 5.2% in total death, with a neutral result for non-CAD deaths. Benefit was significantly related to the extent of risk-factor change. The observed reduction in total CAD was 62% of that predicted by means of a multiple logistic function summary of risk-factor changes. The ages of the 60,881 working men were 40 to 59 years when they entered the trial. One-half received preventive advice on cholesterol-lowering diet, control of cigarette smoking, overweight and BP, and regular exercise. The other half formed a control group, 10% of whom were screened at entry and at intervals during the trial to assess their risk factor levels; the other 90%, who were not examined during the trial, formed the at-risk population for incidents measurements. The WHO collaborative trial is the largest randomized trial of CAD prevention of death. These results compare favorably to 3 other randomized primary prevention trials, namely the Oslo Study, the MRFIT Study, and the Goteborg Trial.

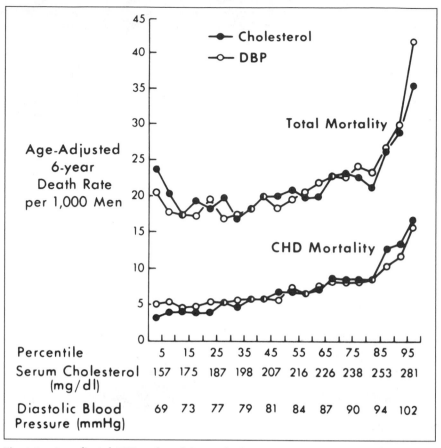

Fig. 1-4. Age-adjusted CHD and total 6-year death rate per 1000 men screened for MRFIT according to serum cholesterol or diastolic blood pressure percentiles. Reproduced with permission from Martin et al.[5]

For persons >62 years of age

Aronow and associates[7] from Bronx, New York, correlated a history of smoking 5–60 cigarettes per day, fasting total serum cholesterol ≥200 mg/dl, history of systolic (≥160 mmHg) or diastolic (≥90 mmHg) hypertension, diabetes mellitus (fasting venous plasma glucose ≥140 mg/dl) and obesity (≥20% than ideal body weight) in 138 men (mean age 82 ± 8 years) and 380 women (mean age 82 ± 8 years) with CAD in a long-term health care facility. CAD occurred in 43 of 138 men (31%) and in 103 of 380 women (27%), difference not significant. A history of smoking 5–60 cigarettes per day significantly correlated with CAD in men but not in women (Table 1-1). Hypercholesterolemia significantly correlated with CAD in both men and women. A history of systemic hypertension significantly correlated with CAD in women but not in men. Diabetes mellitus did not significantly correlate with CAD in men or women but weakly correlated with CAD in men plus women. Obesity did not significantly correlate with CAD in men or women. Hypercholesterolemia, a history of smoking 5–60 cigarettes per day, and a history of systemic hypertension were considered major risk factors. Having 2 or 3 major risk factors correlated with CAD significantly better than having no or 1 major risk factor in both elderly men and women.

TABLE 1-1. *Prevalence of history of smoking 5 to 60 cigarettes daily, hypercholesterolemia, history of systolic or diastolic hypertension, diabetes mellitus and obesity in elderly men and women*

RISK FACTOR	MEN		WOMEN	
	N	%	N	%
History of smoking 5–60 cigarettes/day	$\frac{28}{138}$	20	$\frac{23}{380}$	6
Serum cholesterol ≥200 mg/dl	$\frac{76}{138}$	55	$\frac{262}{380}$	69
History of hypertension	$\frac{37}{138}$	27	$\frac{141}{380}$	37
Diabetes mellitus	$\frac{19}{138}$	14	$\frac{76}{380}$	20
Weight ≥20% above ideal body weight	$\frac{6}{138}$	4	$\frac{25}{380}$	7

Effect of earthquake on risk factors

Trevisan and associates[8] from Naples, Italy, screened participants a few weeks after a major earthquake to see its effect on heart rate, serum cholesterol levels, and serum triglyceride levels compared to matched participants that were screened shortly before the catastrophic event (Table 1-2). The 2 groups of participants did not differ with regard to their characteristics at the baseline examination carried out 5 years previously. The lack of difference in BP between exposed and nonexposed participants could be explained by the lag-time between the earthquake and the BP measurements. The authors concluded that the acute stress associated with major disasters can influence risk factors for CAD.

BLOOD LIPIDS

Methods of measuring blood lipid levels

Blank and associates[9] from Bethesda, Maryland, compared the levels of total cholesterol derived from the Lipid Research Clinics (LRC) with those obtained from 2 commonly used clinical laboratory instruments. Both the

TABLE 1-2. *Serum cholesterol, triglycerides, and heart rate at 1980–1981 examination. Reproduced with permission from Trevisan et al.[8]*

CHARACTERISTIC	EXPOSED	NONEXPOSED
No. of subjects	96	96
Serum cholesterol (mg/dl)	213.92	201.61*
Serum triglycerides (mg/dl)	166.40	132.57*
Heart rate (bpm)	75.20	71.69*

* p <0.05. Values have been adjusted by the weight gain between the 1975–1976 and 1980–1981 examinations.

Technicon SMAC and the DuPont aca had positive bias compared with the LRC method (Table 1-3). Therefore, many patients with cholesterol concentrations >265 mg/dl (6.85 mmol/liter) as determined by these routinely used methods have markedly lower levels determined by LRC methods. These findings not only indicate that rigorous interlaboratory standardization is required to conform to LRC reference values, but also suggest that the clinician should be aware of these methodologic considerations when the decision to treat hypercholesterolemia is made.

Using data from over 10,000 men, women, and children who participated in the Lipid Research Clinics prevalence studies, DeLong and associates[10] from several centers in the USA examined the formula adopted by Friedewald and associates (Clinical Chemistry 1972; 18:499–502) for estimating plasma or serum concentrations of LDL cholesterol when (for economy, or in the absence of an ultracentrifuge) only fasting total cholesterol, HDL cholesterol, and triglyceride concentrations were measured in mg/liter, ie, LDL cholesterol = total cholesterol − (HDL cholesterol + 0.20 × triglyceride). Values for LDL cholesterol obtained by use of the Friedewald et al formula were compared with values derived from the Lipid Research Clinics ultracentrifugal procedure for LDL cholesterol, which was used as a reference. Participants who were pregnant, who had not fasted, or whose plasma contained chylomicrons or floating B-lipoproteins were excluded. The authors concluded that a better estimator for LDL cholesterol was provided by the equation LDL cholesterol = total cholesterol − (HDL cholesterol + 0.16 × triglyceride), since it produced an error (relative to the reference method) of lesser magnitude than the previous formula. The expression 0.16 × triglyceride (0.37 × triglyceride when measurements are reported in mmol/liter) also produced a more accurate estimate of very low density lipoprotein cholesterol relative to values obtained by the standard Lipid Research Clinics procedure for this component. The proposed formula is more precise for plasmas or sera with a triglyceride concentration within the normal range.

Superko and associates[11] from Stanford, California, and Baltimore, Maryland, reviewed a number of laboratories to determine the accuracy of HDL cholesterol measurements in them. These authors concluded that often plasma HDL cholesterol measurements lack sufficient accuracy to be of practical use in an individual clinical setting.

TABLE 1-3. *Comparison of lipid research clinics (LRC) and clinical laboratory values for selecting men and women at moderate and high risk requiring treatment.* Reproduced with permission from Blank et al.[9]*

AGE, y	MODERATE RISK: VALUES GREATER THAN			HIGH RISK: VALUES GREATER THAN		
	LRC RESULT	SMAC RESULT†	*aca* RESULT†	LRC RESULT	SMAC RESULT†	*aca* RESULT†
2–19	170 (4.40)	190 (4.91)	200 (5.17)	185 (4.78)	210 (5.43)	220 (5.69)
20–29	200 (5.17)	225 (5.82)	240 (6.21)	220 (5.69)	250 (6.47)	265 (6.85)
30–39	220 (5.69)	250 (6.47)	265 (6.85)	240 (6.21)	275 (7.11)	290 (7.50)
≥40	240 (6.21)	275 (7.11)	290 (7.50)	260 (6.72)	295 (7.63)	315 (8.15)

* Values, in milligrams per deciliter (millimoles per liter).
† Result rounded to nearest 5 mg/dL (0.13 mmol/L).

Population screening of cholesterol levels

Wynder and associates[12] from New York, New York, conducted a screening for plasma total cholesterol levels at 6 sites in the New York metropolitan area and involved hospitals, health professionals, paraprofessionals, media experts, and instruments that provided cholesterol levels rapidly. During the 5 days of testing, over 12,000 participants were screened. Because the program was limited to customary working hours and because of self-selection of participants, the subjects were probably an unusually health-conscious group as evidenced by the low prevalence of cigarette smokers (11%). Nevertheless, 12% were at moderate risk and 16% were at high risk for CAD (Table 1-4). Approximately half of the population reported never having had their cholesterol levels tested, and >40% had no idea what levels were optimal (Table 1-5). A subsample of patients at risk was screened by telephone survey. In most cases, when a patient's physician was consulted for advice, no action was recommended. The results demonstrate that a large population screening can be implemented, that at least certain segments of the public will respond to such a program, and that educational efforts must be directed at both the public at large and physicians.

Racial differences in lipid levels

To test the hypothesis that high levels of HDL cholesterol in black men than in white men may offer the former greater protection against CAD, Watkins and associates[13] from Augusta, Georgia, Minneapolis, Minnesota, and Pittsburgh, Pennsylvania, examined the relation between HDL cholesterol and 7-year incidence of CAD in the 5,792 white men and in the 465 black men assigned to the usual care group of the Multiple Risk Factor Intervention Trial. CAD events included nonfatal AMI diagnosed on the basis of serial electrocardiographic change or medical record review, and fatal CAD events including sudden coronary death, deaths attributed to AMI or CHF caused by CAD, and deaths associated with CABG. At baseline, mean dia-

TABLE 1-4. *Cholesterol levels. Reproduced with permission from Wynder et al.[12]*

AGE, y	SEX	N	AVERAGE CHOLESTEROL, MG/DL (MMOL/L)	CHOLESTEROL RANGES, MG/DL (MMOL/L)*				
				<180 (<4.65)	180–199 (4.65–5.15)	200–219 (5.17–5.66)	220–239 (5.69–6.18)	≥240 (≥6.21)
20–29	M	460	175 (4.53)	48.7	17.4	12.9	9.7	11.2
	F	277	176 (4.55)	60.6	20.6	11.2	3.3	4.3
30–39	M	573	193 (4.99)	35.7	18.9	17.7	14.5	13.2
	F	399	184 (4.76)	52.3	21.0	11.1	7.5	8.0
40–49	M	475	202 (5.22)	27.8	23.2	19.3	13.2	16.5
	F	457	196 (5.07)	34.8	24.3	14.8	11.8	14.3
50–59	M	627	213 (5.51)	19.8	19.7	20.1	16.7	23.7
	F	832	223 (5.77)	12.9	14.1	18.5	18.3	36.1
60–69	M	1056	209 (5.40)	21.2	19.5	21.4	16.3	21.5
	F	1564	228 (5.90)	9.8	14.6	18.4	19.6	37.6
70–98	M	771	201 (5.20)	30.5	18.8	19.4	15.4	15.8
	F	1242	228 (5.90)	10.4	14.1	18.7	18.8	38.0
Age and/or sex unknown	...	1424	210 (5.43)	25.6	17.1	18.9	15.3	23.1

* Values are percentages of the participants in each category.

TABLE 1-5. *Cholesterol knowledge. Reproduced with permission from Wynder et al.[12]*

	NO. (%) OF RESPONSES	
RESPONSE	MEN	WOMEN
Question: Have You Ever Had Your Cholesterol Levels Checked?*		
Yes	1420 (38)	2193 (39)
No	1700 (46)	2415 (44)
I don't know	605 (16)	967 (17)
Question: What Is the Ideal Serum Cholesterol Level?†		
Level, mg/dL (mmol/L)		
125–150 (3.23–3.88)	306 (8)	446 (8)
151–175 (3.90–4.53)	420 (11)	691 (12)
176–200 (4.55–5.17)	1080 (29)	1309 (24)
201–225 (5.20–5.28)	431 (12)	527 (10)
226–250 (5.84–6.47)	193 (5)	298 (5)
251–300 (6.49–7.76)	39 (1)	108 (2)
I don't know	1243 (34)	2178 (39)

* A total of 1200 subjects did not answer the question.
† A total of 1750 subjects did not answer the question.

stolic BP and prevalence of cigarette smoking were significantly higher in black men, but the reverse was true for serum cholesterol (246 -vs- 254 mg/dl). Mean HDL cholesterol was higher in black men than in white men (49.3 -vs- 41.6 mg/dl) (Fig. 1-5), but LDL cholesterol levels were similar (159 -vs- 160 mg/dl). An inverse association between HDL cholesterol and socioeconomic status was observed in black men, whereas a direct association was observed in white men. During follow-up, small reductions occurred in HDL cholesterol and LDL cholesterol in both groups. No black men died of stroke; 16 black and 404 white men sustained CAD events (5.1 -vs- 10.4/1,000 person-years risk). The black-white relative risk was 0.49. Cox regression analyses revealed an inverse association of HDL cholesterol with CAD events, which was not significantly different in black men from white men. After adjustment for age, diastolic BP, cigarettes per day, HDL cholesterol and LDL cholesterol, the black-white relative risk of CAD was 0.57 (0.35–0.95, 95% confidence interval). Although CAD incidence was lower in black men than in white men, different distributions of HDL cholesterol may not account for this difference.

As part of the Bogalusa Heart Study, Srinivasan and co-workers[14] in New Orleans, Louisiana, studied the cross-sectional relation of endogenous androgens (testosterone, androstenedione, and dehydroepiandrosterone sulfate [DHEA-S]), estrogen (estradiol) and progestin (progesterone) to serum levels of lipoprotein cholesterol (very low density [VLDL], LDL, and HDL) and apolipoproteins (apo A-I and apo B) in white (251) and black (258) adolescent boys, aged 11 to 17 years. Black boys had significantly higher levels of estradiol, HDL cholesterol, and apo A-I, and lower levels of androstenedione and VLDL cholesterol than white boys, independent of age and adiposity. Age correlated strongly with testosterone and androstenedione, and moderately with DHEA-S and estradiol levels in both races. Only in white boys was age consistently related to VLDL cholesterol (positively), HDL cholesterol (negatively), and apo A-I (negatively). Overall, testosterone was associated inversely with HDL cholesterol and apo A-I in white boys, while progesterone was related positively to apo A-I in both races after adjusting for age and

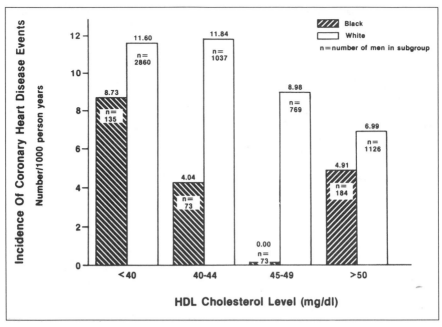

Fig. 1-5. Incidence of coronary heart disease events by race and level of high-density lipoprotein (HDL) cholesterol.

adiposity. These relations were found to differ with age. Partial correlations between levels of sex hormones and lipoproteins adjusted for age and adiposity showed no associations in the 11- and 12-year age group in boys of either race. A significant positive relation of testosterone to VLDL cholesterol, and inverse relations of testosterone to HDL cholesterol and apo A-I and DHEA-S to HDL cholesterol were apparent only in white boys in the 13- to 14-year age group. Among the older subjects (15–17 years old), the relations of testosterone to HDL cholesterol and androstenedione to apo A-I were positive only in black boys. In addition, a significant positive association between progesterone and apo A-I was noted for both races among boys in the older age group. That the sex hormone-lipoprotein associations vary among different age groups suggests the influence of sexual maturation-related hormonal makeup on lipoproteins. Inherent metabolic differences between the races may account for some of the divergent sex hormone-lipoprotein associations.

Maynard and colleagues[15] in Bethesda, Maryland, examined the relation between risk factors and angiographically determined CAD for blacks and whites enrolled in the Coronary Artery Surgery Study (CASS). Analysis of data from the CASS registry indicated that blacks had a higher incidence of systemic hypertension and current cigarette smoking than did whites in CASS and that chest pain was the major reason both blacks and whites underwent coronary angiography for suspected or proven CAD. The CASS data also revealed that, despite high levels of risk factors and chest pain, blacks had minimal or absent CAD. The results of this study raise several questions. First, to what extent are blacks in CASS representative of 1) blacks in the general population and 2) blacks undergoing coronary angiography? Additionally, are risk factors for CAD different for blacks than for whites? And finally, how does the physician effectively treat the black patient with high levels of risk factors and minimal CAD. Thus an understanding of the etiology of chest pain in blacks is required, and studies of predominantly black populations from different regions of the country are needed to clarify the findings from CASS and other large clinical trials.

Effects of genetics on blood lipid levels

Williams and associates[16] from Salt Lake City, Utah, screened 1,134 persons from 18 Utah pedigrees to study the genetic influence on serum cholesterol levels in early CAD. In most pedigrees, serum cholesterol appeared to be a purely polygenic trait with 54% heritability. In 4 pedigrees with dominant familial hypercholesterolemia, male heterozygotes had a mean serum total cholesterol level of 352 mg/dl, AMI at an average age of 42 years, and CAD death at an average age of 45 years. An informative pedigree structure allowed the identification of 4 ancestral males born before 1880 who carried this lethal gene and survived to ages 62, 68, 72, and 81 years. This finding suggests that some healthy life-style factors protected these men against the expression of a gene that had led to CAD by age 45 years in all of their heterozygous great-grandsons. One heterozygote showed a drop in serum total cholesterol level from 426–248 mg/dl, with strict adherence to a low-fat diet without drugs.

Lipid levels in children of parents who had an acute myocardial infarction

De Backer and associates[17] from Gent, Belgium, measured lipids and apoproteins and other coronary risk factors in offspring of patients who had AMI before the age of 50 years, and compared results with those of a control group matched for age and sex. Significant differences were observed in the apoprotein A-1 level, in the protein/fat ratios of HDL and LDL and in smoking habits. In a multivariate analysis, the offspring group was different from the control group in non–HDL cholesterol/apoprotein B ratio, HDL cholesterol/apoprotein A-1 ratio, smoking habits, apoprotein A-1, and apoprotein A-2. By means of these variables, 85% of all subjects could be correctly classified. It was concluded that as early as age 21 years the offspring of patients with premature CAD differ from matched control subjects in lipoprotein measurements and in smoking habits.

Freedman and associates[18] from New Orleans, Louisiana, assessed the association between levels of apolipoprotein B, apolipoprotein A-1, lipids and lipoprotein cholesterol in children and the reported histories of AMI in their parents in 2,416 black and white school-age children. Compared with children whose fathers did not report an AMI, those whose fathers reported having had an AMI had a lower mean level of apolipoprotein A-1 (137 -vs- 141 mg/dl) and a lower ratio of LDL cholesterol to apolipoprotein B (1.08 -vs- 1.11), along with a higher ratio of apolipoprotein B to apolipoprotein A-1 (0.64 -vs- 0.61). These associations existed independently of the children's race, sex, age, and history of obesity, smoking, alcohol intake, and use of oral contraceptives. Children whose mothers reported having had an AMI had no decrease in the ratio of LDL cholesterol to apolipoprotein B, but they tended to have an elevated ratio of apolipoprotein B to apolipoprotein A-1. In contrast, serum lipoprotein-cholesterol fractions in children were not related to AMI in either parent. These results provide further evidence that apolipoproteins are more strongly related to the risk of cardiovascular disease than are lipoprotein-cholesterol fractions.

Lipid levels in diabetes mellitus

Winocour and associates[19] from Manchester, UK, compared levels of serum cholesterol, triglycerides, LDL cholesterol, and HDL cholesterol in 57 men with insulin-dependent diabetes mellitus and in 81 nondiabetic control subjects. They found all of these 4 lipid levels to be similar in the diabetic patients and in the nondiabetic controls. They also found substantially lower serum levels of apolipoprotein B, the principal apolipoprotein of LDL, and a concomitant increase in the cholesterol-loading of apolipoprotein B in the diabetics compared with the nondiabetics. The likely changes in LDL density and particle size resulting from this compositional abnormality might lead to accelerated atherogenesis analogous to that seen in type III hyperlipoproteinemia. In addition, there was an increase in the concentration of cholesterol in the smaller, denser, HDL III subfraction of serum HDL in the diabetic patients.

Laakso and associates[20] from Kuopio, Finland, measured serum lipid and lipoprotein levels in 63 insulin-dependent diabetic patients (32 men and 32 women), in 63 nondiabetic control subjects (32 men and 32 women without CAD), in 19 insulin-dependent diabetic patients (11 men and 8 women), and in 18 nondiabetic subjects (8 men and 10 women) with CAD (Table 1-6). All diabetic patients had postglucagon C-peptide levels of >0.60 mmol/liter and none had signs of renal failure. Male insulin-dependent diabetic patients with CAD had higher levels of total cholesterol, LDL cholesterol, total triglycerides, VLDL triglycerides and lower levels of HDL cholesterol than male insulin-dependent diabetic patients without CAD. In female insulin-dependent diabetic patients, similar lipid and lipoprotein abnormalities were observed between the groups of diabetics with and without CAD except for total cholesterol, which was the same in both groups. A comparison between insulin-dependent diabetic patients without CAD and nondiabetic control subjects without CAD showed no difference in lipid and lipoprotein levels in males; female insulin-dependent diabetic patients without CAD showed even higher levels of HDL and HDL_2 cholesterol and lower levels of VLDL triglycerides than nondiabetic controls. These results indicate that in insulin-dependent diabetic patients without nephropathy and CAD, the lipid and lipoprotein levels do not differ from nondiabetic control subjects, but in insulin-dependent diabetic patients with CAD the lipid and lipoprotein pattern is similar to that known to be characteristic for nondiabetic patients with CAD.

Relation of lipid levels to frequency and severity of coronary artery disease

Newman and associates[21] from New Orleans, Louisiana, assessed the relation of risk factors for cardiovascular disease to early atherosclerotic lesions in aorta and coronary arteries in 35 patients (mean age at death, 18 years). Aortic involvement with fatty streaks was greater in blacks than in whites (37 -vs- 17%). However, aortic fatty streaks were strongly related to antemortem levels of both total and LDL cholesterol (Fig. 1-6), independently of race, sex, and age, and were inversely correlated with the ratio of HDL cholesterol to LDL plus VLDL cholesterol. Coronary-artery fatty streaks were correlated with VLDL cholesterol. This article was followed by an editorial by Glueck[22] from Cincinnati, Ohio. He simply reiterated the evidence reported by Newman et al relating risk factors for CAD in children to the development of early atherosclerotic lesions.

TABLE 1-6. *Serum lipids and lipoproteins in nondiabetic controls and in insulin-dependent diabetic patients with (CHD+) and without (CHD−) coronary heart disease by sex. Reproduced with permission from Laakso et al.*[20]

	Men				Women			
	Nondiabetic controls		Patients with IDD		Nondiabetic controls		Patients with IDD	
	CHD − (32)	CHD + (8)	CHD − (32)	CHD + (11)	CHD − (26)	CHD + (10)	CHD − (31)	CHD + (8)
Total-C	6.54 ± 0.22	7.22 ± 0.46	6.54 ± 0.23	7.51 ± 0.45* (p <0.05)	6.90 ± 0.22	8.79 ± 0.50‡	6.89 ± 0.19	7.31 ± 0.28
HDL-C	1.32 ± 0.07	1.31 ± 0.10	1.48 ± 0.08	1.19 ± 0.09* (p <0.05)	1.40 ± 0.06	1.36 ± 0.10	1.74 ± 0.06 (p <0.001)	1.45 ± 0.10*
HDL_2-C	0.91 ± 0.07	0.88 ± 0.08	1.05 ± 0.07	0.81 ± 0.08	0.97 ± 0.07	0.92 ± 0.11	1.39 ± 0.06 (p <0.001)	1.08 ± 0.10*
HDL_3-C	0.42 ± 0.02	0.43 ± 0.04	0.43 ± 0.02	0.38 ± 0.02	0.43 ± 0.02	0.44 ± 0.02	0.35 ± 0.02 (p <0.01)	0.36 ± 0.02
LDL-C	4.32 ± 0.19	4.80 ± 0.40	4.21 ± 0.18	5.17 ± 0.38* (p <0.05)	4.67 ± 0.19	6.29 ± 0.43‡	4.45 ± 0.17	4.69 ± 0.22
VLDL-C	0.90 ± 0.07	1.11 ± 0.10	0.86 ± 0.09	1.15 ± 0.16	0.82 ± 0.10	1.13 ± 0.12	0.70 ± 0.07	1.17 ± 0.15†
Total-TG	1.44 ± 0.11	1.51 ± 0.19	1.46 ± 0.16	2.01 ± 0.26* (p <0.05)	1.51 ± 0.16	1.72 ± 0.18	1.24 ± 0.08	1.84 ± 0.20†
HDL-TG	0.12 ± 0.01	0.11 ± 0.01	0.11 ± 0.01	0.13 ± 0.02	0.12 ± 0.01	0.15 ± 0.02	0.17 ± 0.01 (p <0.01)	0.19 ± 0.02
LDL-TG	0.29 ± 0.02	0.40 ± 0.07	0.32 ± 0.02	0.39 ± 0.06	0.31 ± 0.02	0.45 ± 0.05‡	0.32 ± 0.03	0.41 ± 0.05
VLDL-TG	1.00 ± 0.09	1.01 ± 0.16	1.03 ± 0.14	1.49 ± 0.20* (p <0.05)	1.09 ± 0.14	1.12 ± 0.14	0.75 ± 0.07 (p <0.05)	1.24 ± 0.16†
Total-C/HDL-C	5.19 ± 0.24	5.68 ± 0.46	4.68 ± 0.25	6.57 ± 0.52‡ (p <0.01)	5.16 ± 0.27	6.60 ± 0.38‡	4.08 ± 0.17 (p <0.01)	5.21 ± 0.39†
LDL-C/HDL-C	3.45 ± 0.20	3.81 ± 0.39	3.05 ± 0.19	4.61 ± 0.50‡ (p <0.05)	3.45 ± 0.16	4.72 ± 0.32‡	2.65 ± 0.14 (p <0.001)	3.36 ± 0.30*

C = cholesterol; TG = triglycerides; CHD = coronary heart disease; IDD = insulin-dependent diabetes.

* p <0.05; † p <0.01; ‡ p <0.001; Student's t test for independent samples; IDD patients with or without CHD vs nondiabetic controls without CHD.

To convert values for cholesterol to milligrams per deciliter, multiply by 38.7; for triglycerides, multiply by 88.0.

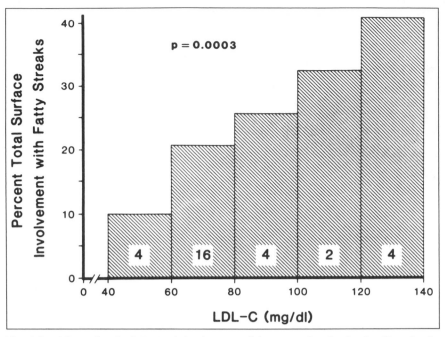

Fig. 1-6. Atherosclerotic fatty-streak involvement of the aorta related to levels of low-density lipoprotein cholesterol (LDL-C) in 30 young persons. Increasing LDL-C levels are significantly related to increasing amounts of aortic fatty streaks. To convert values for cholesterol to millimoles per liter, multiply by 0.026. Reproduced with permission from Newman et al.[21]

Rose and Shipley[23] from London, UK, examined the relation between initial plasma total cholesterol concentration and 10-year mortality from CAD in 17,718 men aged 40–64 years. The relative risk of death from CAD declined with age, but the absolute excess risk did not. The risk gradient was continuous over the whole range of total cholesterol concentrations, the lowest mortality being among men with concentrations below the lowest decile. It seems that, as with BP, the average total cholesterol concentration in the population is too high: lowest concentrations are prognostically the best. A quarter of all deaths from CAD related to cholesterol occurred among men with concentrations above the top decile, but 55% occurred among men with concentrations in the middle ⅗ of the distribution; this figure of 55% could be reduced only by a policy aimed at lowering concentrations in the whole population.

Hamsten and co-investigators[24] in Stockholm, Sweden, investigated the relation of serum lipoprotein and apolipoprotein concentrations to angiographically determined CAD in 105 consecutive male survivors of AMI younger than age 45 years. Concentrations and composition of lipoproteins, lipid indexes, and nonlipid risk factors (tobacco consumption, systemic hypertension, reduced glucose tolerance, and obesity) were related to a recently developed scoring system for semiquantitative estimation of diffuse CAD, and to the number of severity of significant coronary artery stenoses. The concentrations of cholesterol in VLDL, LDL, and HDL, in combination with serum triglyceride or VLDL triglyceride levels, comprised the best set of independent discriminatory lipid variables between patients and control subjects. LDL cholesterol and apolipoprotein B levels showed strong relation to the extent and severity of CAD but not to the number and severity of discrete coronary stenoses. HDL$_2$ cholesterol concentration correlated inversely with the CAD score, whereas other variables reflecting HDL concentration and composition of VLDL lipids were not independently related to any coronary scores. The LDL triglyceride level, an index of intermediate density lipoprotein (IDL) accumulation, was significantly correlated to the coronary atheromatosis score in univariate analysis. Nonlipid risk factors were correlated neither to CAD nor to severity of stenoses. Data from this investigation demonstrate the importance of elevated LDL cholesterol and apolipoprotein B concentrations for the development of CAD. The lack of correlation between the levels of lipoprotein lipids and serum apolipoproteins and the severity of CAD suggest that mechanisms other than disturbances of lipoprotein metabolism may be involved in the progression of more advanced coronary lesions.

Dahlen and co-workers[25] in Houston, Texas, examined the relation of CAD to plasma levels of lipoprotein Lp(a) and other lipoprotein variables in a study of 307 white patients who underwent coronary angiography. Lp(a) resembled LDL in several ways, but can be distinguished and quantified by electroimmunoassay. CAD was rated as present or absent and also was represented by a quantitative lesion score derived from estimates of stenosis in 4 major coronary arteries. Coronary lesion scores significantly correlated with Lp(a), total cholesterol, triglycerides, LDL cholesterol, and HDL cholesterol levels by univariate statistical analysis. By multivariate analysis, levels of Lp(a) were associated significantly and independently with the presence of CAD, and tended to correlate with lesion scores. Among subgroups Lp(a) level was associated with CAD in women in all ages and in men 55 years old or younger. An apparent threshold for coronary risk occurred at Lp(a) mass concentrations of 30–40 mg/dl, corresponding to Lp(a) cholesterol concentrations of approximately 10–13 mg/dl. Plasma Lp(a) in white patients appears to be a major coronary risk factor with an importance approaching that of the level of LDL or HDL cholesterol.

Stamler and associates[26] from the Multiple Risk Factor Intervention Trial (MRFIT) Research Group analyzed the 356,222 men aged 35–57 years, who were free of a history of hospitalization for AMI, and who were screened by the MRFIT in its recruitment effort; they found for each 5-year age group the relation between serum total cholesterol and CAD death rate to be continuous, graded, and strong (Table 1-7, 1-8, 1-9). For the entire group aged 35–57 years at entry, the age-adjusted risks of CAD death in total cholesterol quintiles 2 through 5 (182–202, 203–220, 221–244, and ≥245 mg/dl [4.71–5.22, 5.25–5.69, 5.72–6.31, and ≥6.34 mmol/liter]) relative to the lowest quintile

TABLE 1-7. *Quintiles of serum cholesterol and six-year CHD mortality for 356,222 primary screenees of MRFIT.* Reproduced with permission from Stamler et al.*[26]

		CHD MORTALITY BY AGE GROUP, NO. OF CHD DEATHS (6-y DEATH RATE PER 1000)					
QUIN-TILE	SERUM CHOLESTEROL, MG/DL (MMOL/L)	35–39 y (N = 74 077)	40–44 y (N = 78 578)	45–49 y (N = 84 319)	50–54 y (N = 82 544)	55–57 y (N = 36 704)	35–57 y (N = 356 222)†
1	≤181 (≤4.68)	12 (0.59)	21 (1.28)	43 (2.95)	72 (5.39)	48 (8.31)	196 (3.23)
2	182–202 (4.71–5.22)	11 (0.67)	37 (2.29)	62 (3.72)	108 (6.92)	70 (9.97)	288 (4.18)
3	203–220 (5.25–5.69)	19 (1.37)	52 (3.37)	88 (5.28)	129 (7.73)	107 (14.50)	395 (5.60)
4	221–244 (5.72–6.31)	18 (1.44)	73 (4.72)	123 (6.97)	190 (10.59)	129 (16.05)	533 (7.14)
5	≥245 (≥6.34)	51 (4.57)	112 (7.41)	215 (11.46)	299 (15.78)	169 (19.91)	846 (11.06)
Total		111 (1.50)	295 (3.75)	531 (6.30)	798 (9.67)	523 (14.25)	2258 (6.34)

* CHD indicates coronary heart disease; MRFIT, Multiple Risk Factor Intervention Trial. Analysis is age specific and age standardized.

† Age-standardized six-year death rate per 1000.

TABLE 1-8. *Quintiles of serum cholesterol and relative risk of 6-year CHD mortality for 356,222 primary screenees of MRFIT.* Reproduced with permission from Stamler et al.[26]*

QUINTILE	SERUM CHOLESTEROL, MG/DL (MMOL/L)	RELATIVE RISK OF CHD MORTALITY BY AGE GROUP					
		35–39 y	40–44 y	45–49 y	50–54 y	55–57 y	35–57 y
1	≤181 (≤4.68)	1.00	1.00	1.00	1.00	1.00	1.00
2	182–202 (4.71–5.22)	1.14	1.79	1.26	1.28	1.20	1.29
3	203–220 (5.25–5.69)	2.32	2.63	1.79	1.43	1.74	1.73
4	221–244 (5.72–6.31)	2.44	3.69	2.36	1.96	1.93	2.21
5	≥245 (≥6.34)	7.75	5.79	3.88	2.93	2.40	3.42

* CHD indicates coronary heart disease; MRFIT, Multiple Risk Factor Intervention Trial. Analysis is age specific and age standardized.

TABLE 1-9. *Deciles of serum cholesterol and 6-year CHD mortality for 356,222 primary screenees of MRFIT.* Reproduced with permission from Stamler et al.[26]*

DECILE	SERUM CHOLESTEROL, MG/DL (MMOL/L)	MEAN SERUM CHOLESTEROL, MG/DL (MMOL/L)	CHD MORTALITY		
			NO. OF DEATHS	RATE PER 1000	RELATIVE RISK
1	≤167 (≤4.32)	153.2 (3.962)	95	3.16	1.00
2	168–181 (4.34–4.68)	175.0 (4.526)	101	3.32	1.05
3	182–192 (4.71–4.97)	187.1 (4.838)	139	4.15	1.31
4	193–202 (4.99–5.22)	197.6 (5.110)	149	4.21	1.33
5	203–212 (5.25–5.48)	207.5 (5.366)	203	5.43	1.72
6	213–220 (5.51–5.69)	216.1 (5.588)	192	5.81	1.84
7	221–231 (5.72–5.97)	225.9 (5.842)	261	6.94	2.20
8	232–244 (6.00–6.31)	237.7 (6.147)	272	7.35	2.33
9	245–263 (6.34–6.80)	253.4 (6.553)	352	9.10	2.88
10	≥264 (≥6.83)	289.5 (7.486)	494	13.05	4.13

* CHD indicates coronary heart disease; MRFIT, Multiple Risk Factor Intervention Trial. Analysis is age standardized.

were 1.29, 1.73, 2.21, and 3.42. Of all CAD deaths, 46% were estimated to be excess deaths attributable to serum cholesterol levels ≥180 mg/dl (≥4.65 mmol/liter), with almost half the excess deaths in serum cholesterol quintiles 2 through 4. The pattern of a continuous, graded, strong relation between serum cholesterol and 6-year age-adjusted CAD death rate prevailed for nonhypertensive nonsmokers, nonhypertensive smokers, hypertensive non-smokers, and hypertensive smokers. These data of high precision show that the relation between serum cholesterol and CAD is not a threshold one, with increased risk confined to the 2 highest quintiles, but rather is a continuously graded one that powerfully affects risk for most middle-aged American men.

Pocock and associates[27] from London, UK, measured the total cholesterol, HDL cholesterol, and non-HDL cholesterol (total cholesterol minus HDL cholesterol) and the HDL cholesterol to total cholesterol ratio in 7,415 men aged 40–59 years living in 24 British towns. After an average follow-up of 4.2 years, 193 cases of major CAD occurred in the 7,415 men. The mean HDL cholesterol concentration was lower in the men with CAD compared with the men without clinical CAD, but the difference became small and nonsignificant after adjustment for age, body mass index, BP, number of cigarettes smoked daily, and concentration of non-HDL cholesterol. The higher mean concentration of non-HDL cholesterol remained higher in the CAD cases after adjustment for the other factors. Multivariant analysis showed that non-HDL cholesterol was a more powerful predicter of risk than the HDL to total cholesterol ratio (Fig. 1-7).

Castelli and associates[28] from Framingham, Massachusetts, had earlier found an inverse relation between HDL cholesterol and the incidence of CAD, and that earlier report was based on 4 years of surveillance. These participants, aged 49–82 years, have now been followed up for 12 years. The present report shows that the relation between the fasting HDL cholesterol level and subsequent incidence of CAD does not diminish appreciably with time (Fig. 1-8). Since a second measurement of HDL cholesterol is available 8 years after the initial determination, the relation of HDL cholesterol measurements on the same subjects at 2 points in time was examined. This second HDL cholesterol measurement also was used to a multivariate model that included cigarette smoking, relative weight, alcohol consumption, casual blood glucose, total cholesterol, and BP. It was concluded that even after these adjustments, nonfasting HDL cholesterol and total cholesterol levels were related to development of CAD in both men and women aged 49 years and older. Study participants at the 80th percentile of HDL cholesterol were found to have half the risk of CAD developing when compared with subjects at the 20th percentile of HDL cholesterol.

Gordon and colleagues[29] in Bethesda, Maryland, found that plasma levels of HDL cholesterol at entry and subsequent changes from these baseline levels were inversely predictive of CAD end points in hypercholesterolemic men followed 7–10 years in the Lipid Research Clinics Coronary Primary

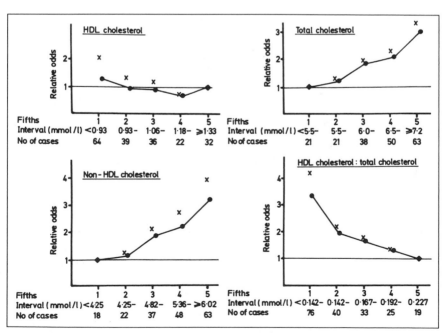

Fig. 1-7.   Relative odds for HDL cholesterol, non-HDL cholesterol, total cholesterol, and HDL cholesterol to total cholesterol ratio (by fifths of ranked distribution). (♦ = Base group. × = Unadjusted. ● = Adjusted for other risk factors.) *Conversion: SI to traditional units*— Cholesterol and HDL cholesterol: 1 mmol/l ≈ 38 · 6 mg/100 ml. Reproduced with permission from Pocock et al.[27]

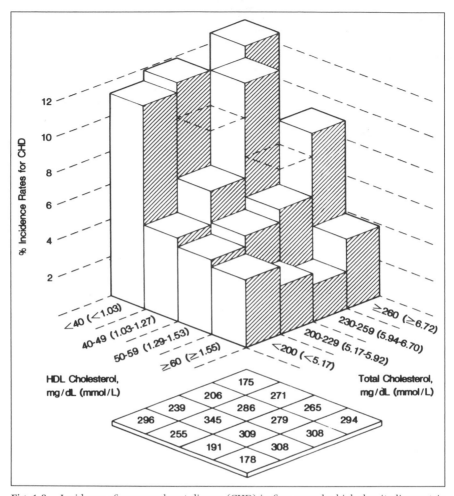

Fig. 1-8. Incidence of coronary heart disease (CHD) in four years by high-density lipoprotein cholesterol (HDL-C) and total plasma cholesterol level for men and women free of cardiovascular disease. Dashed lines indicate two bars that are hidden from view: HDL-C less than 40 mg/dL (<1.03 mmol/L), total cholesterol of 230 to 259 mg/dL (5.95 to 6.70 mmol/L), rate = 10.7%; HDL-C 40 to 49 mg/dL (1.03 to 1.27 mmol/L), total cholesterol greater than or equal to 260 mg/dL (6.72 mmol/L), rate = 6.6%. Diagram at bottom shows number of observations from combined sample that fell into each cell and were therefore at risk for CHD. Reproduced with permission from Castelli et al.[28]

Prevention Trial, especially in the 1,907 participants receiving cholestyramine. When the men in this cohort were compared, each 1-mg/dl increment in baseline HDL cholesterol was associated with a 5.5% decrement in risk of "definite" CAD death or AMI, and each 1 mg/dl increase from baseline HDL levels during the trial was associated with a 4.4% risk reduction. In the 1,899 participants receiving placebo, the corresponding risk decrements were 3.4% and 1.1%. Although the baseline HDL cholesterol level remained a significant risk predictor in the placebo cohort, increases in HDL were not significantly predictive of CAD unless "suspect" and "definite" end points were analyzed. When the associations between HDL (baseline plus change) and incidence of definite CAD end points within each treatment cohort were compared, their difference approached nominal significance. The results from this large study suggest a synergistic interaction, in which cholestyramine reduced CAD risk most substantially in men maintaining the highest HDL levels.

Kottke and associates[30] from Rochester, Minnesota, compared the relative utility of plasma levels of total cholesterol, triglycerides, HDL cholesterol, and apolipoproteins in identifying men with angiographically significant CAD in a combined sample of consecutive men undergoing coronary angiography (n = 304) and healthy, normal male control subjects (n = 135). The plasma apolipoprotein levels of apolipoprotein A-I, followed by those of apolipoproteins A-II and B, were better discriminators than plasma cholesterol, triglycerides, or HDL cholesterol levels for identifying those with CAD. In confirmation of previous findings, the presence of CAD resulted in lower levels of apolipoproteins A-I and A-II and HDL cholesterol and higher levels of apolipoprotein B, cholesterol, and triglycerides. Linear and quadratic discriminant function analysis demonstrated that by using the age of the patients and apolipoproteins A-I, A-II, and B levels, one could correctly classify patients either as being normal or as having angiographically significant CAD in >75% of the cases. Thus, plasma apolipoprotein levels (especially A-I and A-II) may be considerably better markers for CAD than traditional lipid determinations. This article was followed by an editorial by Ivan D. Frantz, Jr.,[31] entitled "Cardiovascular Risk—What Should be Measured?" Frantz concluded that further investigative studies must be conducted before measurement of apolipoproteins alone can replace other methods of identifying patients who have significant CAD or of predicting in whom it will develop. With the patients reported by Kottke and associates, even when age and apolipoproteins A-I, A-II, and B were all included, the sensitivity for prediction was only 81% and the specificity was 58%.

Sedlis and co-workers[32] in St. Louis, Missouri, correlated plasma levels of lipids, lipoproteins, and apoproteins in 281 patients undergoing cardiac catheterization with the frequency and severity of CAD to determine if measurements of apoprotein levels are more predictive of the presence and severity of CAD than the corresponding levels of lipoproteins in lipids. In 156 men with CAD among 194 men in the study, the only variable other than age that correlated with the severity of CAD, defined by the number of narrowings and percent stenosis, was the ratio of apoprotein A1 to apoprotein B. The ratio of apoprotein A1 to apoprotein B was a more accurate predictor of the severity of CAD than was the ratio of the corresponding HDL to LDL cholesterol levels. Multivariate analysis confirmed the independent effect of the ratio of apoprotein A1 to apoprotein B on the severity of CAD even after adjustments were made for lipid levels, age, presence of systemic hypertension of diabetes mellitus, and therapy with beta blockers or diuretics. Among men with total occlusion of a coronary artery, apoprotein E and apoprotein B levels were significantly higher than in control subjects with a similar extent of CAD. The lipid profiles of the 37 women with CAD were very different from those of men. In women, only total triglycerides and apoprotein B levels correlated with the severity of CAD. These results indicate that levels of certain apoproteins may be more accurate predictors of the severity of CAD than are the corresponding levels of lipoprotein lipids. Both lipids and apoproteins are weak predictors of the severity of narrowings and cannot be used in the diagnosis of CAD.

Aro and associates[33] from Kuopio and Helsinki, Finland, determined serum lipoprotein cholesterol and triglyceride and apoproteins A-I, A-II, and B in 71 consecutive men undergoing coronary angiography because of severe angina pectoris. Among the factors studied, apoprotein B, apoprotein B/A-I ratio, VLDL and LDL cholesterol showed the most consistent association with the severity of CAD as assessed by angiography, whereas serum HDL cholesterol and apoproteins A-I and A-II showed no correlation (Table 1-10). Subjects with stenosis of the LM coronary artery had higher serum HDL cholesterol and apoprotein A-I and B levels than the others. In this series, which comprised males with severe angina pectoris derived from a population with high prevalence of CAD, LDL was the best indicator of the severity of CAD.

Detection of familial hypercholesterolemia by assaying LDL receptors on lymphocytes

In familial hypercholesterolemia, structural and functional abnormalities of the receptor for LDL lead to hypercholesterolemia and premature atherosclerosis. Cuthbert and associates[34] from Dallas, Texas, developed a simplified method to identify LDL receptor defects in peripheral blood lymphocytes. When lymphocytes are cultured in lipoprotein-depleted medium and endogenous sterol biosynthesis is suppressed with mevinolin, mitogen-stimulated proliferation of lymphocytes is dependent on an exogenous source of cholesterol. Whereas a small concentration of supplemental LDL cholesterol (3–4 µg/ml) permits a maximal response in normal lymphocytes, even high concentrations (10–50 µg/ml) are unable to support the proliferation of lymphocytes from patients with homozygous familial hypercholesterolemia. Thus, functional LDL receptors are necessary to allow lymphocyte proliferation in these cultures. The response of lymphocytes from patients with hyperlipidemia not caused by defective LDL receptors was like that of normal cells. In contrast, the response of lymphocytes from patients with heterozygous familial hypercholesterolemia was intermediate between that of homozygotes and that of normal or hyperlipidemic controls. This method can be used to identify persons who are heterozygous for abnormalities of LDL receptors.

Lipid-lowering diets and drugs

Hoeg and associates[35] from Bethesda, Maryland, developed a systematic approach to the management of patients with hyperlipoproteinemia which may lead to normalization of plasma lipoprotein concentrations in most hyperlipoproteinemia patients (Table 1-11, 1-12). The accompanying algorithm illustrates the evaluation to be undertaken in the hyperlipidemic patient (Figs. 1-9–1-12).

TABLE 1-10. *Serum and lipoprotein cholesterol and triglyceride values (mean ± SEM) in male patients with angina pectoris, grouped according to the presence or severity of coronary artery disease (CAD) as assessed by coronary angiography. Reproduced with permission from Aro et al.[33]*

	NO CAD (N = 6)	MODERATE CAD (N = 22)	SEVERE CAD (N = 43)	ANOVA F	ANOVA P-VALUE
Serum cholesterol (mmol/l)	6.73 ± 0.23	6.46 ± 0.19	7.30 ± 0.24*	3.12	<0.05
VLDL cholesterol (mmol/l)[a]	0.60	1.09**	1.05**	5.22	<0.01
LDL cholesterol (mmol/l)	4.94 ± 0.28	4.39 ± 0.19	5.20 ± 0.21*	3.27	<0.05
HDL cholesterol (mmol/l)	1.14 ± 0.14	0.86 ± 0.06	0.95 ± 0.04	2.83	n.s.
LDL/HDL cholesterol ratio	4.79 ± 0.75	5.46 ± 0.36	5.71 ± 0.28	0.73	n.s.
Serum triglycerides (mmol/l)[a]	1.67	1.94	1.90	0.27	n.s.
VLDL triglycerides (mmol/l)[a]	1.19	1.45	1.34	0.39	n.s.
LDL triglycerides (mmol/l)	0.38 ± 0.04	0.38 ± 0.03	0.43 ± 0.02	1.10	n.s.
HDL triglycerides (mmol/l)	0.11 ± 0.03	0.13 ± 0.02	0.13 ± 0.01	0.18	n.s.

[a] Calculated after logarithmic transformation of individual values.
* p <0.05 indicating difference to moderate CAD.   ** p <0.01 indicating difference to no CAD.

TABLE 1-11. *Plasma cholesterol concentrations associated with increased risk of cardiovascular disease.* Reproduced with permission from Hoeg et al.*[35]

AGE, YR	TOTAL CHOLESTEROL,* MG/DL		LDL† CHOLESTEROL,* MG/DL		HDL† CHOLESTEROL,‡ MG/DL (INCREASED RISK)
	MODERATE RISK	HIGH RISK	MODERATE RISK	HIGH RISK	
Men					
0–14	173	190	106	120	38
15–19	165	183	109	123	30
20–29	194	216	128	148	30
30–39	218	244	149	171	29
40–49	231	254	160	180	29
≥50	230	258	166	188	29
Women					
0–14	174	170	113	126	36
15–19	173	195	115	135	35
20–29	184	208	127	148	35
30–39	202	220	143	163	35
40–49	223	246	155	177	34
≥50	252	281	170	195	36

* Values are adopted from the 75th percentile (moderate-risk) and 90th percentile (high-risk) values obtained by the Lipid Research Clinics.

† LDL indicates low-density lipoproteins; HDL, high-density lipoproteins.

‡ The HDL cholesterol values for the lower fifth percentile were taken from the Lipid Research Clinics.

TABLE 1-12. *Dietary management of hyperlipoproteinemia.* Reproduced with permission from Hoeg et al.*[35]

DIETARY PARAMETER	LIPOPROTEIN LEVELS INCREASED			
	VLDL CHOLESTEROL (VLDL >200) TYPES I, V	TG ÷ 5 (VLDL >200) TYPE IV	LDL CHOLESTEROL TYPE IIa	VLDL AND LDL CHOLESTEROL TYPES IIb, III
Attain and maintain ideal body weight	+	+	+	+
Total fat, % energy	10–20	20–30	25–30	20–30
Dietary cholesterol, mg/day	ND	<300	150–250	150–250
Polyunsaturated-saturated fatty acid ratio	ND	1–1.5	1.5–2.0	1.5–2.0
Alcohol, oz/day	0	≤1	ND	≤1
Carbohydrate, % energy	60–70†	50–60†	ND	50–60†
High-fiber intake	+	+	+	+

* VLDL indicates very low-density lipoproteins; LDL, low-density lipoproteins; and ND, that this parameter is not specifically defined for this phenotype.

† Limit monosaccharides and disaccharides to 25% of total carbohydrate intake (lactose, frustose, and sucrose).

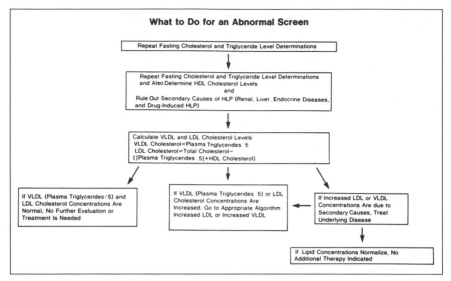

Fig. 1-9. Algorithm illustrating evaluation to be undertaken in hyperlipidemic patient. HLP indicates hyperlipoproteinemia. Reproduced with permission from Hoeg et al.[35]

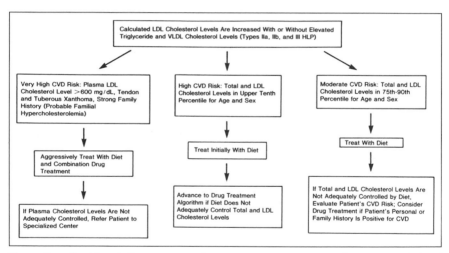

Fig. 1-10. Algorithm indicating approach to treatment of patient with elevated calculated low-density lipoprotein (LDL) cholesterol concentration. CVD indicates cardiovascular disease; HLP, hyperlipoproteinemia. Reproduced with permission from Hoeg et al.[35]

Connor and associates[36] from Portland, Oregon, calculated the contribution of cholesterol and saturated fats to develop a *cholesterol/saturated-fat index* (CSI) based on a modification of a regression equation computed from metabolic studies designed to lower plasma lipids (Table 1-13). A low CSI indicates low saturated fat and cholesterol content and low atherogenicity. The CSI may be used to compare different foods and recipes and to evaluate daily intake quickly and easily (Fig. 1-13).

To examine the effects of dietary fatty acids and carbohydrates on plasma lipids and lipoproteins, Grundy[37] from Dallas, Texas, studied 11 patients with a mean plasma total cholesterol level of 251 ± 10 mg/dl on a metabolic

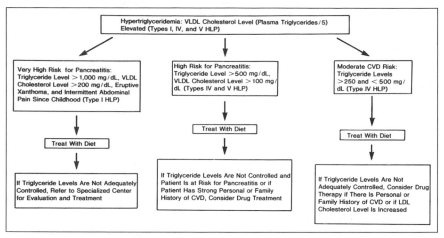

Fig. 1-11. Algorithm outlining treatment approach to patient with elevated very low-density lipoprotein (VLDL) level (types I, IV, and V hyperlipoproteinemia [HLP]). CVD indicates cardiovascular disease. Reproduced with permission from Hoeg et al.[35]

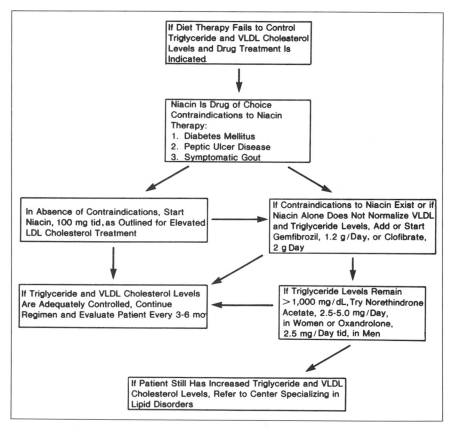

Fig. 1-12. Algorithm demonstrating approach to drug treatment of hypertriglyceridemia (types IV and V). VLDL indicates very low-density lipoprotein. Reproduced with permission from Hoeg et al.[35]

TABLE 1-13. *CSI and kcal content of selected foods. Reproduced with permission from Connor et al.[36]*

FOOD	CSI	kcal
Fish, poultry, red meat (100 g cooked):		
Whitefish (snapper, perch, sole, cod, halibut, & c), shellfish (clams,		
oysters, scallops), water-pack tuna	4	91
Salmon	5	149
Shellfish (shrimp, crab, lobster)	6	104
Poultry, no skin	6	171
Beef, pork, and lamb:		
10% fat (ground sirloin, flank steak)	9	214
15% fat (ground round)	10	258
20% fat (ground chuck, pot roasts)	13	286
30% fat (ground beef, pork and lamb-steaks, ribs, pork and		
lamb chops, roasts)	18	381
Cheeses (100 g):		
2% fat cheeses (low-fat cottage cheese, pot cheese), tofu		
(bean curd)	1	98
5–10% fat cheeses (cottage cheese, low-fat cheese slices)	6	139
25–30% fat cheeses*	6	317
11–20% fat cheeses (part skimmed milk)	12	256
32–38% fat cheeses (gruyere, cheddar, cream cheese)	26	386
Eggs:		
Whites (3)	0	51
Egg substitute (equivalent to 2 eggs)	1	91
Whole (2)	29	163
Fats (¼ cup, 4 tablespoons or 55 g):		
Peanut butter	5	353
Most vegetable oils	8	530
Mayonnaise	10	431
Soft vegetable margarines	10	432
Hard stick margarines	15	432
Soft shortenings	16	530
Bacon grease	23	541
Very hydrogenated shortenings	27	530
Butter	37	430
Coconut oil, palm oil, cocoa butter (chocolate)	47	530
Frozen desserts (1 cup):		
Water ices, sorbet (193 g)	0	245
Frozen yogurt, low-fat (166 g)	2	144
Sherbet (193 g)	2	218
Frozen yogurt† (166 g)	4	155
Ice milk (141 g)	6	214
Ice cream, 10% fat (141 g)	13	272
Rich ice cream, 16% fat (141 g)	18	349
Specialty ice cream, 22% fat (214 g)	34	684
Milk products (1 cup, 240 ml):		
Skimmed milk (0–1% fat) or skimmed milk yoghurt	<1	88
1% milk, buttermilk	2	115
2% milk or plain low-fat yoghurt	4	144
Whole milk (3–5% fat) or whole milk yoghurt	7	159
Sour cream	37	468
Imitation sour cream	43	499

* Cheeses made with skimmed milk and vegetable oils.
† Made with added cream.

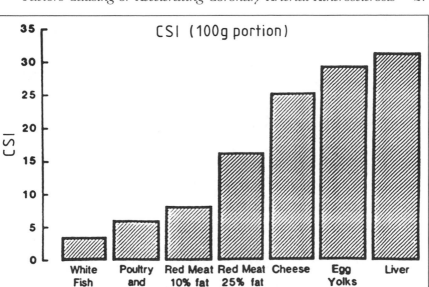

Fig. 1-13. The CSI of 100 g of fish, meat, cheese, egg yolk, and liver. Reproduced with permission from Connor et al.[36]

ward during 3 dietary periods, each lasting 4 weeks. A liquid diet rich in monounsaturated fatty acids ("High-Mono") and a diet low in fat ("Low-Fat") were compared with a diet high in saturated fatty acids ("High-Sat"). The High-Sat and High-Mono diets contained 40% of their total calories as fat and 43% as carbohydrate; the Low-Fat diet had 20% fat and 63% carbohydrate. Body weight was kept constant by adjusting total caloric intake. As compared with the High-Sat diet, both the High-Mono and Low-Fat diets lowered plasma total cholesterol (by 13% and 8%, respectively) and LDL cholesterol (by 21% and 15%, respectively). As compared with the High-Sat diet, the Low-Fat diet raised triglyceride levels and significantly reduced plasma HDL cholesterol. In contrast, the High-Mono diet had no effect on levels of triglycerides or HDL cholesterol. The ratio of LDL to HDL cholesterol was also significantly lower when the High-Mono diet rather than the Low-Fat diet was followed. Therefore, in short-term studies in which liquid diets are used and body weight is kept constant, a diet rich in monounsaturated fatty acids appears to be at least as effective in lowering plasma cholesterol as a diet low in fat and high in carbohydrate.

Saturated fatty acids and cholesterol in the diet raise the plasma cholesterol concentration, and reduction in these constituents is widely recommended. There is not general agreement, however, as to which nutrient should replace saturated fatty acids. Several different substitute nutrients are possible. Grundy and associates[38] from Dallas, Texas, compared 3 cholesterol-lowering diets in 9 men living in a domicile. On a typical American diet at baseline, cholesterol levels were in the normal range. One replacement diet was high in polyunsaturated fatty acids (High Poly): another had 30% fat and corresponded to the American Heart Association's (AHA) recommended diet for the general public (AHA phase I); the third diet had 20% fat, equivalent to the AHA phase III diet for treatment of hypercholesterolemia. Compared with baseline levels, all diets caused similar reductions in total cholesterol and LDL cholesterol levels, but the High Poly and AHA phase III diets lowered the HDL cholesterol level more than the AHA phase I diet. Thus, for the patients in this study, the diet recommended for the general public appeared as effective for lowering cholesterol levels as diets containing more polyunsaturates or more carbohydrates.

Sacks and associates[39] from Boston and Stoneham, Massachusetts, gave 20 normolipidemic nonvegetarians dietary instruction and supervision in a low-fat, semivegetarian diet for 3 months. Mean consumption of total fat, saturated fat, and cholesterol decreased, whereas intake of carbohydrate increased significantly on a low-fat diet. Plasma LDL levels decreased by 18% and HDL levels by 7% from prestudy baseline levels. The LDL/HDL ratio declined by 11%. Plasma triglyceride levels and body weight were unchanged. In individual subjects, the decrements in consumption of saturated fat and the increments in ingestion of polyunsaturated fat were each significantly correlated with decreases in LDL. One year after the subjects had returned to a self-selected diet, levels of dietary saturated fat and cholesterol and the plasma LDL/HDL ratio remained significantly below prestudy levels. This study and others suggest that a low-fat, high carbohydrate diet favorably affects the plasma LDL/HDL proportion by decreasing LDL on a percentage basis 2.5 to 3 times more than it decreases HDL.

Kuusisto and associates[40] from Helsinki, Finland, treated 7 patients with hypercholesterolemia for 4 weeks with an activated *charcoal mixture* in a suspension of water at a dose of 8 g 3 times daily followed by a 4-week nontreatment period. Plasma total cholesterol and LDL cholesterol decreased by 25% and 41%, respectively, and HDL cholesterol increased by 8% (Fig. 1-14). Adverse effects were negligible.

Hoeg and associates[41] from Bethesda, Maryland, compared the safety and efficacy of lovastatin (mevinolin) using a double-blind, randomized, crossover placebo-controlled trial in 24 patients with type II hyperlipoproteinemia with heterozygous familial hypercholesterolemia (FH) (n = 6) or without FH type II HLP (n = 18). Compared with placebo treatment, both apolipoprotein B and LDL cholesterol levels were reduced in both FH and non-FH patients by 28–34% with lovastatin treatment. In addition, HDL cholesterol levels were significantly increased in both patients with FH (16%) and those with non-FH type II HLP (14%). Patients had no serious or clinically significant adverse effects. Thus, lovastatin is a useful drug for treatment of most patients with elevated plasma LDL cholesterol concentrations.

The Lovastatin Study Group II[42] investigated *lovastatin*, a potent inhibitor of 3-hydroxy-3-methylglutaryl coenzyme A reductase in a double-blind, placebo-controlled multicenter study of 101 patients with nonfamilial primary hypercholesterolemia. Dosages varied from 10–80 mg/day in single or divided doses (Fig. 1-15, 1-16, 1-17). Patients receiving 40 mg twice a day had mean total and LDL cholesterol reductions of 32% and 39%, respectively. HDL levels tended to increase slightly and plasma triglyceride levels were moderately decreased. Adverse effects attributable to lovastatin were infrequent and no patient was withdrawn from therapy. Lovastatin was a well tolerated and effective agent for the treatment of nonfamilial hypercholesterolemia.

Patients with homozygous familial hypercholesterolemia produce no normal LDL receptors, and as a result, LDL accumulates in plasma, causing severe premature atherosclerosis. East and associates[43] from Dallas, Texas, performed hepatic transplantation in a child with homozygous familial hypercholesterolemia and the procedure restored LDL receptor activity to about 60% of normal and reduced the LDL cholesterol by 81%. However, the patient's lipoprotein levels remained significantly elevated for her age and sex. Treatment with *lovastatin* 1 year after transplantation produced a marked

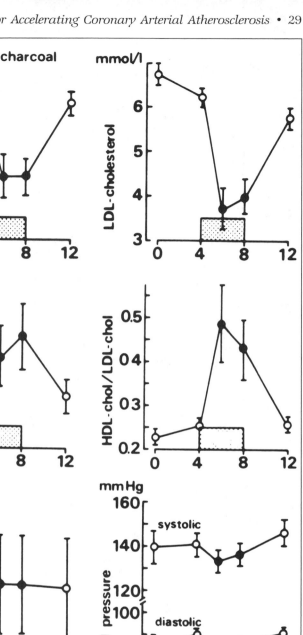

Fig. 1-14. Effect of 4 weeks' intake of activated charcoal (8 g three times a day) on serum cholesterol, body weight, and blood pressure in seven hypercholesterolemic patients. Reproduced with permission from Kuusisto et al.[40]

improvement in the patient's lipoprotein profile. The total and LDL cholesterol levels decreased 40% and 49%, respectively, to values within the normal range. The level of VLDL cholesterol decreased 41%, and the level of total triglycerides declined 28%. Whereas lovastatin therapy decreased the production rate of LDL by 35%, it did not affect the LDL fractional clearance rate.

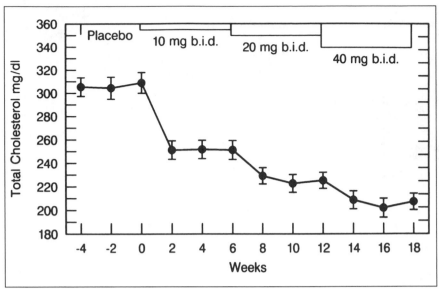

Fig. 1-15. Lovastatin nonfamilial hypercholesterolemia study total cholesterol levels (mean ± SE) in group 3 (N = 16–20 at each point). Abbreviation "b.i.d." indicates *bis in die* ("twice a day"). Reproduced with permission of the Lovastatin Study Group II.[42]

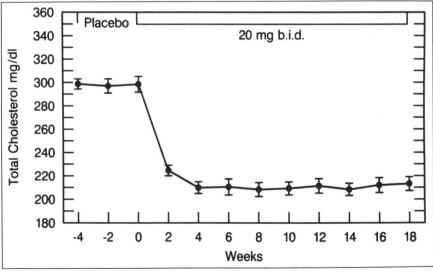

Fig. 1-16. Lovastatin nonfamilial hypercholesterolemia study total cholesterol levels (mean ± SE) in group 4 (N = 16–19 at each point). Abbreviation "b.i.d." indicates *bis in die* ("twice a day"). Reproduced with permission of the Lovastatin Study Group II.[42]

Thus, the combination of liver transplantation and lovastatin restored total and LDL cholesterol levels to normal in this patient with homozygous familial hypercholesterolemia.

Mol and associates[44] from Utrecht, Leiden, and Amsterdam, The Netherlands, investigated the effects of *synvinolin*, a competitive inhibitor of 3-hydroxy-3-methylglutaryl coenzyme A reductase, in 43 patients with heterozygous familial hypercholesterolemia in a double-blind, placebo-controlled, dose-finding study. Synvinolin was given in doses ranging from 2.5–80 mg/

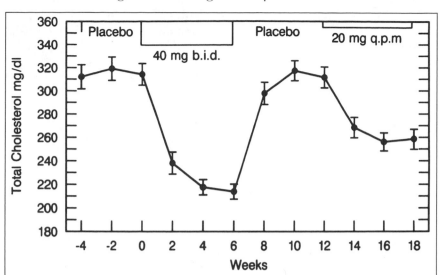

Fig. 1-17. Lovastatin nonfamilial hypercholesterolemia study total cholesterol levels (mean ± SE) in group 5 (N = 17–20 at each point). Abbreviation "b.i.d." indicates *bis in die* ("twice a day"); abbreviation "q.p.m." indicates *quaque post meridiem* ("once daily with the evening meal"). Reproduced with permission from the Lovastatin Study Group II.[42]

day for 4 weeks. Eight patients received placebo. LDL cholesterol decreased on average by 18% on 2.5 mg/day and 42% on 80 mg/day. The drug was as effective whether it was given once or twice daily. Serum HDL cholesterol tended to increase and serum triglycerides to decrease with the larger doses. The drug was tolerated well. Except for a slight increase in alanine aminotransferase in 3 patients no objective adverse effects were observed.

Synvinolin is a key enzyme in the biosynthesis of cholesterol, 3-hydroxy-3-methylglutaryl coenzyme A (HMG-CoA) reductase. The 2 prototype inhibitors, the fungal products compactin and lovastatin, reduced LDL cholesterol in familial hypercholesterolemia patients by about 30% with excellent tolerance. Synvinolin differs from compactin by 2 additional methyl groups and from lovastatin by 1. Because of the additional methyl groups in mevinolin, it has a greater inhibitory effect on HMG-COA reductase than compactin. Synvinolin is obtained by chemical synthesis from lovastatin. After oral ingestion it is rapidly absorbed from the intestine, reaching its peak plasma concentration after 2 hours in healthy volunteers. Approximately 4 hours after ingestion, the plasma concentrations have decreased by 50%.

Brown and associates[45] from 11 medical centers randomized 227 patients with type IIa or IIb hypercholesterolemia to double-blind treatment with either *fenofibrate* (100 mg 3 times daily) or matching placebo for 24 weeks. A group of 192 of these patients were studied for a further 24 weeks during which all received fenofibrate in open-label fashion. For the 92 type IIa patients receiving fenofibrate in the double-blind phase, there were significant reductions in total plasma cholesterol (−18%), LDL cholesterol (−20%), VLDL cholesterol (−38%) and total triglycerides (−38%). Mean plasma HDL cholesterol increased by 11%. With the exception of LDL, which was not high before treatment, similar changes were seen in the 24 fenofibrate-treated type IIb subjects. Lipid parameters of placebo-treated patients did not change significantly. This pattern of change was repeated in the open period for the 94 patients previously taking placebo, whereas the 98 who had been taking fenofibrate remained stable with small further reductions in total and

LDL cholesterol (−3.8% and −5.5%, respectively). Adverse effects were some allergic-type skin reactions early in treatment and an occasional increase in transaminases, blood urea nitrogen, or creatinine. The results were similar to those obtained in European open trials of fenofibrate and were better than the lipid changes seen at comparable times in the Lipid Research Clinics Coronary Primary Prevention Trial (LRC-CPPT) cholestyramine study (Table 1-14).

The Committee on Atherosclerosis and Hypertension in Childhood of the Council of Cardiovascular Disease in the Young and the Nutrition Committee of the American Heart Association[46] prepared a joint statement for physicians on *diagnosis and treatment of primary hyperlipidemia in childhood*. The enclosed tables are from that article and the original article is well worth the reading (Table 1-15, 1-16, 1-17).

In a superb review article which should be read by nearly all physicians, Grundy[47] from Dallas, Texas, reviewed the relation between cholesterol and CAD. Grundy's conclusion from his and other studies was the following: Evidence relating plasma cholesterol levels to atherosclerosis and CAD has become so strong as to leave little doubt of the etiologic connection. Mechanisms responsible for high concentrations of LDL are becoming well understood, and the LDL receptor is now recognized as the crucial element in the

TABLE 1-14. *Mean plasma lipid changes from baseline after 1 year of treatment with fenofibrate compared with values from LRC-CPPT study of cholestyramine. Reproduced with permission from Brown et al.[45]*

PLASMA LIPIDS	CHANGES FROM BASELINE VIS A VIS PLACEBO (%)	
	FENOFIBRATE (U.S. TRIAL)	CHOLESTYRAMINE (LRC-CPPT TRIAL)
Total cholesterol	−20	−12
LDL cholesterol	−22	−16
HDL cholesterol	+9	+3
Total triglycerides	−38	−4
HDL-C/total C	+36	+21

In the U.S. Trial, there were 85 male and female patients who received fenofibrate throughout both the double-blind (24-week) and open (24-week) periods of the study. In the LRC-CPPT Trial, there were 1,900 men at start of trial in the cholestyramine-treated group.

TABLE 1-15. *Normal plasma lipid and lipoprotein concentrations at birth. Reproduced with permission from the Committee on Atherosclerosis and Hypertension in Childhood.[46]*

LIPID	CONCENTRATION (MG/DL)
Cholesterol	
Total	74 (11)
HDL	37 (8)
LDL	31 (6)
VLDL	6 (4)
Triglycerides	
Total	37 (15)

Data are the mean (one standard deviation) from 36 normal, full-term newborns. The 95th percentiles (mg/dl) for total cholesterol, LDL cholesterol, and total triglycerides are 92, 41, and 67, respectively.

TABLE 1-16. *Normal plasma lipid concentrations in the first two decades of life (mg/dl). Reproduced with permission from the Committee on Atherosclerosis and Hypertension in Childhood.*[46]

AGE (YR)	NO.	CHOLESTEROL			TRIGLYCERIDES		
		5TH	MEAN	95TH	5TH	MEAN	95TH
0–4							
Males	238	114	155	203	29	56	99
Females	186	112	156	200	34	64	112
5–9							
Males	1253	121	160	203	30	56	101
Females	1118	126	164	205	32	60	105
10–14							
Males	2278	119	158	202	32	66	125
Females	2087	124	160	201	37	75	131
15–19							
Males	1980	113	150	197	37	78	148
Females	2079	120	158	203	39	75	132

Lipids were determined on plasma from 11,219 fasting, white subjects (5,749 males; 5,470 females) who were studied in seven North American Lipid Research Clinics using common protocols and laboratory methodology.

TABLE 1-17. *Normal plasma lipoprotein concentrations in the first two decades of life (mg/dl). Reproduced with permission from the Committee on Atherosclerosis and Hypertension in Childhood.*[46]

AGE (YR)	HDL CHOLESTEROL				LDL CHOLESTEROL				VLDL CHOLESTEROL			
	NO.	5TH	MEAN	95TH	NO.	5TH	MEAN	95TH	NO.	5TH	MEAN	95TH
5–9												
Males	145	38	56	75	132	63	93	129	132	0	8	18
Females	127	36	53	73	114	68	100	140	113	1	10	24
10–14												
Males	298	37	55	74	288	64	97	133	288	1	10	22
Females	248	37	52	70	245	68	97	136	245	2	11	23
15–19												
Males	300	30	46	63	298	62	94	130	297	2	13	26
Females	297	35	52	74	295	59	96	137	295	2	12	24

Lipoproteins were determined on plasma from 1,415 fasting, white subjects (743 males, 672 females) who were studied in seven North American Lipid Research Clinics, using common protocols and laboratory methodology.

control of the cholesterol level. The demonstration that lowering the plasma cholesterol level will reduce the risk of CHD provides a strong impetus to intervene in the "mass hypercholesterolemia" prevalent among Americans. Dietary modification for this purpose will likely remain the foundation of intervention, but the full impact of new drugs that will dramatically lower the plasma cholesterol level cannot be predicted with certainty at this time. The introduction of these drugs does, however, create a great urgency to determine the proper means of effectively reducing the plasma cholesterol level for the purpose of decreasing coronary risk. With little doubt, the next decade will see a massive effort to utilize these recent breakthroughs in cholesterol control for prevention of CAD.

A supplement was published to the January 1986 issue of *CIRCULATION* entitled "Dyslipoproteinemia in North America: The Lipid Research Clinics Program Prevalence Study." This symposium includes 14 articles summarizing observations on dyslipoproteinemias and their clinical correlates in the cross-sectional Lipid Research Clinics Prevalence Study[48-61].

Rifkind and Lenfant[62] from Bethesda, Maryland, initiated in 1985 the *National Cholesterol Education Program*. Many major US organizations involved in aspects of medicine pertinent to the diagnosis and treatment of high blood cholesterol are represented on its National Coordinating Committee. The major objectives of the program are to reduce coronary mortality and morbidity through the improved detection, diagnosis, and treatment of high blood cholesterol levels. The National High Blood Pressure Education Program, a predecessor and now a companion program of the National Cholesterol Education Program, has led to improved detection, diagnosis, and treatment of another major cardiovascular disease risk factor, high BP. It serves as a model for what can be achieved through such coordinated efforts. There is good reason to believe that focus on reducing high blood cholesterol levels is leading to similar improvements and should lead to further declines in morbidity and mortality from CHD.

CIGARETTE SMOKING

Smoking and health: A national status report

When the Comprehensive Smoking Education Act, Public Law 98-474, was signed into law in October 1984, it was the first major smoking and health legislation enacted by the Congress in over 15 years. The law required that all cigarette packages and advertising include 4 new health warnings and that these warnings be rotated quarterly. These new warnings replaced the single statement that had appeared on packs and in advertising since 1970. The legislation also required the Department of Health and Human Services to undertake significant new activities, including a biennial report to Congress. On November 29, 1986, the Department issued the first of these reports. "Smoking and Health: A National Status Report" provides significant new information on smoking and health at the national, state, and local levels.[63] A summary of key findings is presented below.

Smoking prevalence 1955–1985: By 1985, 21 years after the first report of the Surgeon General's Advisory Committee, smoking prevalence rates in the USA had declined to the lowest level observed in nearly 40 years. Only 30% of all persons >18 years of age now smoke cigarettes on a regular basis. This figure is down from nearly 45% at the time of the Advisory Committee's report in 1964. Smoking rates for men have declined more rapidly than smoking rates for women (Fig. 1-18). In the early 1960s, male cigarette-use rates were >50%. In 1985, male smoking prevalence had decreased to 33%— probably the lowest rate among men in this country at any time except before World War I. From the mid-1960s–1985, female smoking rates declined from 34%–18%. However, the gap between male and female smoking is narrowing. When life-time smoking prevalence is examined by birth cohort, it is clear that among contemporary age groups, there no longer exists a significant difference between men and women either in initiating smoking or in regular use of cigarettes.

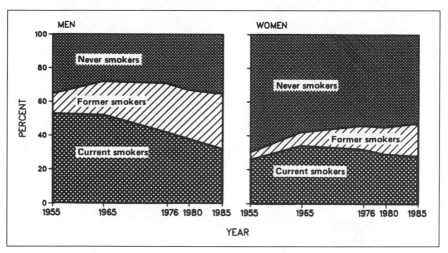

Fig. 1-18. Percentage of current, former, and never smokers, by sex and year, United States, 1955–1985. Reproduced with permission from Smoking and Health.[63]

Age of initiation of regular cigarette smoking: Data from the National Health Interview Survey shows a narrowing of the average age of initiation between men and women. Cigarette smoking among men began to increase around the turn of the century, and, by World War I, large numbers of men were smoking cigarettes. Women, however, did not begin to smoke in significant numbers until some 25 years later—just before and during World War II. In more recent birth cohorts, most men and women began smoking as teenagers. For the cohorts born from 1940–1949 and from 1950–1959, there is little difference in the proportion of men and women who began regular smoking before their 20th birthday (Fig. 1-19). For the cohort born from 1950 to 1959, 88% of male and 84% of female ever smokers had initiated their behavior before age 20. Few adults initiate and adopt the behavior on a regular basis after age 20. Reports of the Surgeon General and others have consistently noted a strong dose-response effect between smoking initiation at an early age and mortality from all the major smoking-related diseases, including cancer, cardiovascular disease, and chronic obstructive lung disease. The current report also states that the earlier a person begins to smoke as a teenager, the less likely that person is to quit smoking as an adult and the more likely that person is to be a heavy smoker.

State legislation on smoking and health: The new report contains a complete review of all state legislation on smoking and health. One of the major findings relates to sales and distribution of cigarettes and other tobacco products to minors. Thirty-eight states have enacted legislation restricting the sale or distribution of tobacco products to minors. However, 12 states have no such laws, and 14 states with restrictive legislation have set the minimum age for purchasing tobacco products at <18. The Secretary of Health and Human Services, Dr. Otis Bowen, in his letter transmitting the report to the Congress, strongly urged all jurisdictions to adopt 18 as the minimum age at which any person should be allowed to purchase tobacco products. Concerning laws that impede the sale or availability of tobacco products to minors, Dr. Bowen wrote, "Enactment and enforcement of such legislation could have a strong preventive effect on early uptake of cigarettes and other tobacco products."

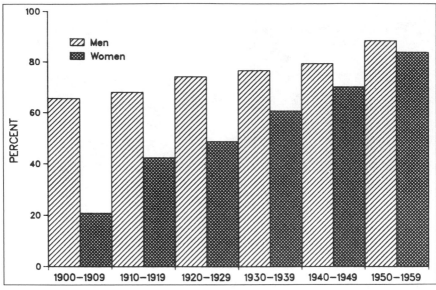

Fig. 1-19. Percentage of persons initiating smoking before age 20, by sex and 10-year birth cohorts, United States, 1900–1959. Reproduced with permission from Smoking and Health.[63]

Benefit of discontinuing cigarette smoking on risk of heart attack

In a prospective study of 7,735 middle-aged men, both current and ex-cigarette smokers, Cook and associates[64] from London, UK, found more than twice the risk of a major CAD event compared with men who had never smoked cigarettes; men who had given up smoking >20 years earlier still had an increased risk (Fig. 1-20). This excess risk among ex-smokers is only to a small extent explained by their higher BP, serum total cholesterol, and body-mass index. An increased prevalence of CAD in men who had recently given up smoking also made a small contribution to excess risk. In both current and former cigarette smokers, the number of years a man had smoked cigarettes ("smoking-years") was the clearest indicator of CAD risk due to cigarettes. The major benefit of giving up smoking may lie in halting the accumulation of smoking years.

Smoking-induced coronary vasoconstriction

In atherosclerotic CAD, cigarette smoking increases myocardial oxygen demand but may cause an inappropriate decrease in coronary blood flow and myocardial oxygen supply. Winniford and co-investigators[65] in Dallas, Texas, explored the mechanism of smoking-induced coronary vasoconstriction and determined if smoking causes an alpha-adrenergically-mediated increase in coronary artery tone. In 36 chronic smokers with CAD (27 men and 9 women), heart rate–systolic arterial BP double product and coronary sinus blood flow (by thermodilution) were measured before and during smoking both before and after 1) normal saline, 2) an alpha-adrenergic blocking agent, phentolamine 5 mg, 3) a beta-adrenergic blocking agent, propranolol 0.1 mg/kg, or 4) sodium nitroprusside, 0.4–0.8 μg/kg/min, given in a dose sufficient to diminish systolic arterial BP by 15%. During the initial smoking period, rate-BP product increased and coronary sinus blood flow

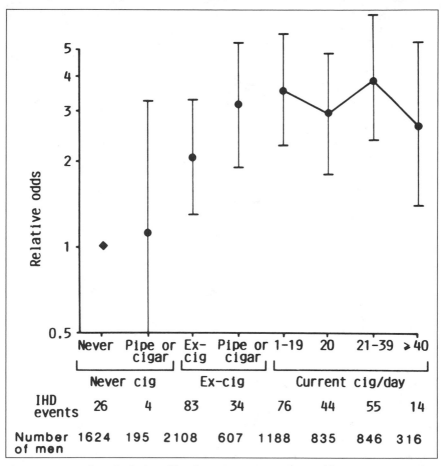

Fig. 1-20. Age-adjusted relative odds of a major IHD event by smoking status at screening.
◆ Base group; bars, 95% confidence limits. Reproduced with permission from Cook et al.[64]

was unchanged by smoking in all groups. After 30–75 minutes, saline, phentolamine, propranolol, or sodium nitroprusside was given, and measurements were repeated. In the control subjects, rate-BP product and coronary sinus blood flow responded in a similar manner to that observed previously. In those receiving phentolamine, rate-BP product was unchanged, but coronary sinus blood flow increased substantially with smoking. In the 12 patients who received propranolol, rate-BP product was unchanged, but coronary sinus blood flow decreased with smoking. In those who received sodium nitroprusside, rate-BP product decreased slightly, and coronary sinus blood flow responded in a similar manner to that observed previously. These hemodynamic measurements indicate that smoking-induced coronary vasoconstriction is due to an alpha-adrenergically-mediated increase in coronary artery tone.

PHYSICAL ACTIVITY AND FITNESS

Relation to risk of coronary artery disease

Paffenbarger and associates[66] from Stanford, California, and Boston, Massachusetts, examined the physical activity and other lifestyle characteristics of 16,936 Harvard alumni, aged 36–74 years, for relations to rates of mortality from all causes and for influences on length of life. A total of 1,413 alumni died during 12–16 years of follow-up (1962 to 1978). Exercise reported as walking, stair climbing, and sports play related inversely to total mortality, primarily to death due to cardiovascular or respiratory causes. Death rates declined steadily as energy expended on such activity increased from <500–3,500 kcal/week, beyond which rates increased slightly. Rates were one quarter to one third lower among alumni expending ≥2,000 kcal during exercise per week than among less active men. With or without consideration of systemic hypertension, cigarette smoking, extremes or gains in body weight, or early parental death, alumni mortality rates were significantly lower among the physically active. Relative risks of death for individuals were highest among cigarette smokers and men with hypertension, and attributable risks in the community were highest among smokers and sedentary men. By the age of 80, the amount of additional life attributable to adequate exercise, as compared with sedentariness, was 1 to >2 years.

Kannel and associates[67] from Boston, Massachusetts, investigated cardiovascular events over 24 years of surveillance in 1,166 men participating in the Framingham Study, classified by physical demands of their work and by a 24-hour index of physical activity. Findings were based on 303 noncardiovascular, 220 coronary, and 325 cardiovascular deaths in men aged 45–64 years at time of physical activity assessment. For level of physical activity over 24 hours, there was a clear trend of improved overall, cardiovascular, and coronary mortality with increased level of physical activity at all ages, including the elderly. The effect was sustained with a more pronounced effect with the passage of time, despite presumed decrease in level of activity. The mortality benefits applied to both those with and without intervening overt cardiovascular disease, making it unlikely that the physical inactivity-mortality relations reflected already existent myocardial damage. For physical demands of the job, there was only a suggestion of benefit for cardiovascular mortality including coronary deaths. In sharp contrast, noncardiovascular mortality was positively related to both physical demand of the job and 24-hour physical activity index.

Effects of change on cardiovascular risk

Jennings and colleagues[68] in Victoria, Australia, studied the effects of 4 levels of activity on heart rate, BP, cardiac index, total peripheral resistance (TPR) index, norepinephrine (NE) spillover rate, insulin sensitivity, and levels of lipids and some hormones in 12 normal subjects. The randomized periods were 4 weeks of below-sedentary activity, 4 weeks of sedentary activity, 4 weeks of 40 minutes of bicycling 3 times per week, and 4 weeks of similar bicycling 7 times per week. Exercise 3 times per week reduced resting BP by 10/7 mmHg, and it was reduced by 12/7 mmHg after exercise 7 times per week. This was associated with reduction in TPR index, an increase in cardiac index, and cardiac slowing. At the highest level of activity, NE spillover rate, an index of sympathetic activity, decreased to 35% of the sedentary value in 8 of 10 subjects. Metabolic changes included lowering of total cholesterol, but HDL level was unchanged. Insulin sensitivity increased 27% after exercise 3 times per week, but declined to sedentary levels with exercise performed 7 times per week. Maximal oxygen uptake increased linearly with activity. Exercise performed 3 times per week lowers BP and should reduce cardiovascular risk. The same exercise performed 7 times per week enhances physical performance with little further reduction in cardiovascular risk factors.

The *effect of exercise training on myocardial perfusion* was assessed using initial and 1-year thallium-201 exercise studies in 56 patients with stable CAD in a study by Sebrechts and associates[69] from San Diego and Long Beach, California. Subjects had been randomized into a trained group participating in supervised exercise 3 times per week and a control group. Indexes (nondimensional units) based on computer-analyzed circumferential count profile from 9 regions of the heart, assessed in 3 projections, were used to eliminate observer bias and more accurately quantitate thallium-201 distribution and 4-hour washout. There was serial improvement of the global distribution count profiles in 21 of 27 (78%) of the trained and in 9 of 29 (31%) of the control subjects. The mean interval change in global initial distribution over the year period was 5 ± 13 in the trained and −6 ± 14 in the control groups. The mean initial distribution of the trained group had improvement in all 9 regions (significant in 3), while the control group showed mean improvement in only 1 of 9 regions. Additionally, the trained group showed improvement in the mean washout in 5 of 9 regions (significant in 3), while no mean regional washout improvement occurred in the control group. Thus, in this group of patients with stable CAD, exercise training resulted in apparently improved cardiac perfusion evidenced by enhanced thallium-201 uptake and washout.

Cardiac rehabilitation after a coronary event

Fletcher and associates[70] from Atlanta, Georgia, evaluated phase II intensive monitored cardiac rehabilitation using a 6-level, 6-session protocol, involving 31 patients who were placed on a progressive 6-level exercise protocol with careful supervision and assessment of heart rate, rhythm, BP and perceived exertion. Duration after the cardiac event ranged from 12 days–8 years (median 10 months). Each exercise prescription was based on exercise testing with oxygen consumption determinations. Exercise activities were individually prescribed according to percentages of maximal MET level achieved on the exercise test. Each exercise session incorporated calisthenics, treadmill exercise, and bicycle and arm ergometry with progressively greater workloads on the various stations. All patients completed the 6 levels within 6 sessions of approximately 1 hour each, and achieved their designated 50–75% target heart rate with perceived exertion level ≤13. There were no critical cardiac events, i.e., high-grade ventricular arrhythmias or AMI. All completed the 6-level protocol and progressed to a nonmonitored exercise program with no difficulty. The results of this short-term method of telemetry-monitored rehabilitation suggest benefits of proper exercise instruction, successful achievement of the 50–75% exercise target heart rate, detection of minor new arrhythmias and alterations of BP response, adequate use of the perceived exertion scale, and a safe and effective transition to subsequent exercise programs.

To determine the incidence of major cardiovascular complications in outpatient cardiac rehabilitation programs, Van Camp and Peterson[71] from San Diego, California, obtained data from 167 randomly selected cardiac rehabilitation programs by way of mailed questionnaires and follow-up telephone calls. These 167 programs reported that 51,303 patients exercised 2,351,916 hours from January 1980 through December 1984: 21 cardiac arrests (18 in which the patient was successfully resuscitated and 3 fatal) and 8 nonfatal AMIs were reported. The incidence rates per million patient hours of exercise were 8.9 for cardiac arrests (1 per 111,996 patient-hours), 3.4 for AMI (1 per 293,990 patient-hours), and 1.3 for fatalities (1 per 783,972 patient-hours). There was no statistically significant difference in frequency of these events among programs of varying size or extent of electrocardiographic monitoring. These data indicate that current cardiac rehabilitation practice allows for prescribed supervised exercise by patients with cardiovascular disease to be performed at a low risk of major cardiovascular complications.

FEMALE SEX

A population-based survey, using data from the Framingham study, assessed sex-specific patterns of CAD occurring over a 26-year period of time, reported by Lerner and Kannel[72] of Boston, Massachusetts. Among persons aged 35–84 years, men have about twice the total incidence of morbidity and mortality of women. The sex gap in morbidity tends to diminish during the later years of the age range, mainly because of a surge in growth of female morbidity after age 45 years, whereas by that age, the growth in the male rate begins to taper off (Fig. 1-21). An approximate 10-year difference between the sexes persists in mortality rates throughout the life span. The relative health advantage that is possessed by women, however, is buffered by a case fatality rate from coronary attacks that exceeds the male rate (32% -vs- 27%). In addition, CAD manifestations differ between the sexes. AMI is more likely to be unrecognized in women than in men (34% -vs- 27%). Angina pectoris in women more frequently is uncomplicated (80%), whereas in men angina tends to evolve out of AMI (66%). Also, sudden death comprises a greater proportion of deaths in men than in women (50% -vs- 39%). Because women maintain a lesser probability of CAD than do men at any level of the major cardiovascular risk factors, distinctions in their risk factor profiles do not explain completely the observed disease patterns.

FAMILY HISTORY

A family history of heart attack is reported to be an independent predictor of cardiovascular death in men. In a 9-year follow-up of 4,014 adults

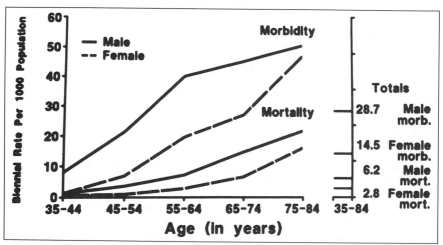

Fig. 1-21. Incidence of CHD, morbidity, and mortality by age and sex: 26-year follow-up, Framingham study.

from 40–79 years old in the Rancho Bernardo Study, men >60 years of age with a family history of "heart attack" were at 5-fold increased risk. Khaw and Barrett-Connor[73] in San Diego, California, sought to determine whether modifiable risk factors, i.e., BP, plasma cholesterol, obesity, and cigarette smoking, have a differential effect on cardiovascular risk in those with and without a family history of heart attack. For both sexes, cigarette smoking was a stronger predictor of cardiovascular disease in those with a family history of heart attack (relative risk of smokers vs nonsmokers was 2.5 for men and 14 for women) than in those with no family history (relative risk of smokers vs nonsmokers was 1.1 for men and 1.7 for women). Conversely, an increased risk of cardiovascular mortality in men with a family history of heart attack was present predominantly in smokers (relative risk related to positive family history was 1.2 in nonsmokers and 3.3 in smokers). An estimated 68% of the excess deaths in men with a family history of heart attack were attributable solely to the interaction of a family history with a smoking habit and were therefore potentially avoidable. Thus, in this study the risk of cardiovascular disease associated with an apparently inherited predisposition appears to be profoundly affected by modifiable behavior.

COFFEE DRINKING

LaCroix and associates[74] from Baltimore and Hyattsville, Maryland, conducted a prospective investigation of the effect of coffee consumption on CAD in 1,130 male medical students who were followed for 19–35 years. Changes in coffee consumption and cigarette smoking during follow-up were examined in relation to the incidence of clinically evident CAD in 3 measures of coffee intake—baseline, average, and most recent intake reported before the manifestation of CAD. Clinical evidence of CAD included AMI, angina, and sudden coronary death. In separate analyses for each measure of coffee intake, the relative risks for men drinking ≥5 cups of coffee per day, compared with nondrinkers, were approximately 2.8 for all 3 measures in the univariate analyses (maximal width of 95% confidence intervals, 1.3 to 6.5). After adjustment for age, current smoking, hypertension status, and baseline level of serum cholesterol, the estimated relative risk for men drinking ≥5 cups of coffee per day (using the most recent coffee intake measure), compared with those drinking none, was 2.49 (maximal width of 95% confidence interval, 1.1–5.8). The association between coffee and CAD was strongest when the time between the reports of coffee intake and the CAD was shortest. These findings support an independent, dose-responsive association of coffee consumption with clinically evident CAD, which is consistent with a 2- to 3-fold elevation of risk among heavy coffee drinkers.

CLOTTING FACTORS

Meade and associates[75] from Harrow, UK, investigated the thrombotic component of CAD by the inclusion of measures of hemostatic function. Among 1,511 white men aged 40–64 years at recruitment, 109 subsequently had a first major coronary event. High levels of factor VII coagulant activity and of plasma fibrinogen were associated with increased risk, especially for events occurring within 5 years of recruitment. These associations seemed to be stronger than for cholesterol, elevations of 1 standard deviation in factor

VII activity, fibrinogen, and cholesterol being associated with increases in the risk of an episode of CAD within 5 years of 62%, 84%, and 43%, respectively. Multiple regression analyses indicated independent associations between each of the clotting factor measures and CAD but not between the blood cholesterol level and CAD incidence. The risk of CAD in those with high fibrinogen levels was greater in younger than in older men. Much of the association between smoking and CAD may be mediated through the plasma fibrinogen level. The biochemical disturbance leading to CAD may lie at least as much in the coagulation system as in the metabolism of cholesterol.

COCAINE ABUSE

The increasingly widespread use of cocaine in the USA has been accompanied and perhaps exacerbated by the misconception that the drug is not associated with serious medical complications. In particular, the potential for cocaine to precipitate life-threatening cardiac events needs to be reemphasized. Isner and associates[76] from Boston, Massachusetts, Providence, Rhode Island, and Chicago, Illinois, reported clinical and morphologic findings in 7 persons in whom nonintravenous "recreational" use of cocaine was temporarily related to AMI, VT and VF, myocarditis, sudden death, or a combination of these events. These authors also reviewed data on 19 previously reported cases of cocaine-related cardiovascular disorders. Analysis of all 26 cases indicated the following findings: the cardiac consequences of cocaine abuse are not unique to parenteral use of the drug because nearly all the patients took the drug intranasally; underlying heart disease is not a prerequisite for cocaine-related cardiac disorders; seizure activity, a well-documented noncardiac complication of cocaine abuse, is neither a prerequisite for nor an accompanying feature of cardiac toxicity of cocaine; and the cardiac consequences of cocaine are not limited to massive doses of the drug. Although the pathogenesis of cardiac toxicity of cocaine remains incompletely defined, available circumstantial evidence suggests that cocaine has medical consequences that are equal in importance to its well-documented psychosocial consequences.

This article was followed by an editorial entitled "Medical Complications of Cocaine Abuse" by Cregler and Mark[77] from New York, New York.

DECLINE IN MORTALITY RATE FROM CORONARY ARTERY DISEASE

Explanations for the continuing decline in mortality from CAD are unclear. A combination of primary preventive measures and medical interventions appear to have contributed to the decline. The decline in mortality from CAD in Auckland, New Zealand, between 1974 and 1981 was assessed by Beaglehole[78] from Auckland, New Zealand, using data from several population-based studies. There were 126 fewer deaths from CAD in Auckland in 1981 than expected from the 1974 rates among people <70 years of age. The specific medical interventions probably accounted for about 51 (40%) of the 126 fewer deaths. Local data indicate that resuscitation before admission to hospital was responsible for 20 (16%) of the 126 fewer deaths. Projections based on local data and other trials suggest that up to 15 (12%) of the fewer deaths were due to the treatment of systemic hypertension. Coronary care units and the use of beta blockers after AMI were estimated to be responsible for 6 (5%) and 3 (2%) of the 126 fewer deaths, respectively. The impact of CABG was especially difficult to determine in the absence of appropriate randomized controlled trial data. Estimates of its contribution ranged from 7 to 23 (5% to 18%) of the 126 fewer deaths.

Thom et al[79] examined the death rates from heart disease (nonrheumatic heart disease and systemic hypertension) for 6 periods from 1950–1978 in 26 countries (Fig. 1-22). Their main purpose was to show national trends in mortality over time. Their study showed clearly the striking differences in the rates of heart disease between countries. One may loosely separate the countries into high, moderate, and low categories. Countries such as the USA, Finland, Australia, and Scotland have high mortality rates. England and Wales, Ireland, Israel, and Belgium are in the moderate category. Italy, Yugoslavia, and Portugal are in the low category. While the rate in Finland is decreasing, the other Scandanavian countries (Norway, Sweden, and Denmark) all show clear patterns of increasing mortality during this review period. During the war of 1939–1945, the mortality from "arteriosclerotic" heart disease (including CAD) declined sharply in Finland, Norway, and Sweden (Fig. 1-23). The decline was associated with a marked reduction in the consumption of meat, butter, eggs, and other food stuffs high in saturated fats and cholesterol. The decline was most marked in the urban population, which had little opportunity for obtaining food beyond the official rations. In the USA, where the food supplies were undiminished, the mortality rates from heart disease showed a progressive increase. In England and Wales, the mortality rates for heart disease leveled off during the war years but did not decline. They increased again rapidly in peacetime. Thus, to achieve the immediate and marked decline in heart disease mortality seen in the Scandanavian countries, a drastic change in diet was necessary[80].

Burch[81] from Leeds, UK, calculated the trends in mortality in England and Wales according to the 6th and 7th international classification of diseases for CAD from 1950 to 1967, and also for the revision of international classification of diseases for CAD from 1968 to 1978. Burch used the same age range as did Thom and associates in their article entitled Trends in Total

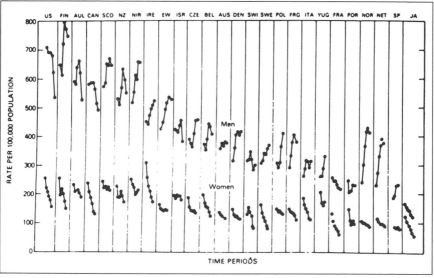

Fig. 1-22.   Death rates from heart disease in twenty-six countries 1950–1978. Reproduced with permission from Thom et al.[79]

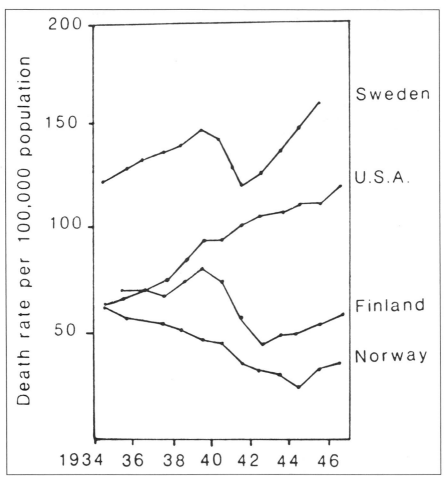

Fig. 1-23. Death rates from heart disease in USA and Scandinavia 1934–1946.

Mortality and Mortality from Heart Disease in 26 Countries from 1950–1978 (International Journal of Epidemiology, 1985; 14:510–520). Instead of sharply diverging trends found by Thom and associates between the sexes for "nonrheumatic heart disease and hypertension"—upward for men, downward for women—Burch found close parallels in the trends for CAD for all 4 age groups in both sexes. These similarities and trends for different age groups of men and women approach those demonstrated earlier for the U.S. white population over the period 1968–1975 (Lancet 1983; 2:743). Reproduced with permission from Thom et al.[79]

References

1. BLACKBURN H: The low risk coronary male. Am J Cardiol 1986 (July 1); 58:161.
2. MULTIPLE RISK FACTOR INTERVENTION TRIAL RESEARCH GROUP: Coronary heart disease death, non-fatal acute myocardial infarction and other clinical outcomes in the Multiple Risk Factor Intervention Trial. Am J Cardiol 1986 (July 1); 58:1–13.
3. CROW RS, RAUTAHARJU PM, PRINEAS RJ, CONNETT JE, FURBERG C, BROSTE S, STAMLER J, MULTIPLE RISK FACTOR INTERVENTION TRIAL RESEARCH GROUP: Am J Cardiol 1986 (May 1); 57:1075–1082.

4. KANNEL WB, NEATON JD, WENTWORTH D, THOMAS HE, STAMLER J, HULLEY SB, KJELSBERG MO: Overall and coronary heart disease mortality rates in relation to major risk factors in 325,348 men screened from the MRFIT. Am Heart J 1986 (Oct); 112:825–836.

5. MARTIN MJ, BROWNER WS, HULLEY SB, KULLER LH, WENTWORTH D: Serum cholesterol, blood pressure, and mortality: implications from a cohort of 361,662 men. Lancet 1986 (Oct 25); 933–936.

6. EUROPEAN COLLABORATIVE GROUP: European collaborative trial of multifactorial prevention of coronary heart disease: Final report on the 6-year results. Lancet 1986 (Apr 19); 869–872.

7. ARONOW WS, STARLING L, ETIENNE F, D'ALBA P, EDWARDS M, LEE NH, PARUNGAO RF: Risk factors for coronary artery disease in persons older than 62 years in a long-term health care facility. Am J Cardiol 1986 (Mar 1); 57:518–520.

8. TREVISAN M, CELENTANO E, MEUCCI C, FARINARO E, JOSSA F, KROGH V, GIUMETTI D, PANICO S, SCOTTONI A, MANCINI M: Short-term effect of natural disasters on coronary heart disease risk factors. Arteriosclerosis 1986 (Sept/Oct); 6:491–494.

9. BLANK DW, HOEG JM, KROLL MH, RUDDEL ME: The method of determination must be considered in interpreting blood cholesterol levels. JAMA 1986 (Nov 28); 256:2767–2770.

10. DELONG DM, DELONG ER, WOOD PD, LIPPEL K, RIFKIND BM: A comparison of methods for the estimation of plasma low- and very low-density lipoprotein cholesterol: The Lipid Research Clinics Prevalence Study. JAMA 1986 (Nov 7); 256:2372–2377.

11. SUPERKO HR, BACHORIK PS, WOOD PD: High-density lipoprotein cholesterol measurements: a help or hindrance in practical clinical medicine? JAMA 1986 (Nov 21); 256:2714–2717.

12. WYNDER EL, FIELD F, HALEY NJ: Population screening for cholesterol determination: a pilot study. JAMA 1986 (Nov 28); 256:2839–2842.

13. WATKINS LO, NEATON JD, KULLER LH: Racial differences in high-density lipoprotein cholesterol and coronary heart disease incidence in the usual-care group of the multiple risk factor intervention trial. Am J Cardiol 1986 (Mar 1); 57:538–545.

14. SRINIVASAN SR, FREEDMAN DS, SUNDARAM GS, WEBBER LS, BERENSON GS: Racial (black-white) comparisons of the relationship of levels of endogenous sex hormones to serum lipoproteins during male adolescence: The Bogalusa Heart Study. Circulation 1986 (Dec); 74: 1226–1234.

15. MAYNARD C, FISHER LD, PASSAMANI ER, PULLUM T: Blacks in the coronary artery surgery study: risk factors and coronary artery disease. Circulation 1986 (July); 74:64–71.

16. WILLIAMS RR, HASSTEDT SJ, WILSON DE, ASH KO, YANOWITZ FF, REIBER GE, KUIDA H: Evidence that men with familial hypercholesterolemia can avoid early coronary death: an analysis of 77 gene carriers in four Utah pedigrees. JAMA 1986 (Jan 10); 255:219–224.

17. DE BACKER G, HULSTAERT F, DE MUNCK K, ROSSENEU M, VAN PARIJS L, DRAMAIX M: Serum lipids and apoproteins in students whose parents suffered prematurely from a myocardial infarction. Am Heart J 1986 (Sept); 112:478–484.

18. FREEDMAN DS, SRINIVASAN SR, SHEAR CL, FRANKLIN FA, WEBBER LS, BERENSON GS: The relation of apolipoproteins A-I and B in children to parental myocardial infarction. N Engl J Med 1986 (Sept 18); 315:721–726.

19. WINOCOUR PH, ISHOLA M, DURRINGTON PN, ANDERSON DC: Lipoprotein abnormalities in insulin-dependent diabetes mellitus. Lancet 1986 (May 24); 1176–1178.

20. LAAKSO M, PYORALA K, SARLUND H, VOUTILAINEN E: Lipid and lipoprotein abnormalities associated with coronary heart disease in patients with insulin-dependent diabetes mellitus. Arteriosclerosis 1986 (Nov/Dec); 6:679–684.

21. NEWMAN WP, FREEDMAN DS, VOORS AW, GARD PD, SRINIVASAN SR, CRESANTA JL, WILLIAMSON GD, WEBBER LS, BERENSON GS: Relation of serum lipoprotein levels and systolic blood pressure to early atherosclerosis: The Bogalusa Heart Study. N Engl J Med 1986 (Jan 16); 314:138–144.

22. GLUECK CJ: Pediatric primary prevention of atherosclerosis. N Engl J Med 1986 (Jan 16); 314:175–177.

23. ROSE G, SHIPLEY M: Plasma cholesterol concentration and death from coronary heart disease: 10 year results of the Whitehall study. Br Med J 1986 (Aug 2); 293:306–307.

24. HAMSTEN A, WALLDIUS G, SZAMOSI A, DAHLEN G, DE FAIRE U: Relationship of angiographically defined coronary artery disease to serum lipoproteins and apolipoproteins in young survivors of myocardial infarction. Circulation 1986 (June); 73:1097–1110.

25. DAHLEN GH, GUYTON JR, ATTAR M, FARMER JA, KAUTZ JA, GOTTO AM: Association of levels of lipoprotein Lp(a), plasma lipids, and other lipoproteins with coronary artery disease documented by angiography. Circulation 1986 (Oct); 74:758–765.

26. STAMLER J, WENTWORTH D, NEATON JD: Is relationship between serum cholesterol and risk of

premature death from coronary heart disease continuous and graded? Findings in 356,222 primary screenees of the Multiple Risk Factor Intervention Trial (MRFIT). JAMA 1986 (Nov 28); 256:2823–2828.

27. POCOCK SJ, SHAPER AG, PHILLIPS AN, WALKER M, WHITEHEAD TP: High density lipoprotein cholesterol is not a major risk factor for ischemic heart disease in British men. Br Med J 1986 (Feb); 292:515–519.

28. CASTELLI WP, GARRISON RJ, WILSON PWF, ABBOTT RD, KALOUSDIAN S, KANNEL WB: Incidence of coronary heart disease and lipoprotein cholesterol levels: The Framingham Study. JAMA 1986 (Nov 28); 256:2835–2838.

29. GORDON DJ, KNOKE J, PROBSTFIELD JL, SUPERKO R, TYROLER HA, FOR THE LIPID RESEARCH CLINICS PROGRAM: High-density lipoprotein cholesterol and coronary heart disease in hypercholesterolemic men: The Lipid Research Clinics Coronary Primary Prevention Trial. Circulation 1986 (Dec); 74:1217–1225.

30. KOTTKE BA, ZINSMEISTER AR, HOLMES DR, KNELLER RW, HALLAWAY BJ, MAO SJT: Apolipoproteins and coronary artery disease. Mayo Clin Proc 1986 (May); 61:313–320.

31. FRANTZ ID: Cardiovascular risk—what should be measured? Mayo Clin Proc 1986 (May); 61:396–397.

32. SEDLIS SP, SCHECHTMAN KB, LUDBROOK PA, SOBEL BE, SCHONFELD G: Plasma apoproteins and the severity of coronary artery disease. Circulation 1986 (May); 73(5):978–986.

33. ARO A, SOIMAKALLIO S, VOUTILAINEN E, EHNHOLM C, WILJASALO M: Serum lipoprotein lipid and apoprotein levels as indicators of the severity of angiographically assessed coronary artery disease. Atherosclerosis 1986; 62:219–225.

34. CUTHBERT JA, EAST CA, BILHEIMER DW, LIPSKY PE: Detection of familial hypercholesterolemia by assaying functional low-density-lipoprotein receptors on lymphocytes. N Engl J Med 1986 (Apr 3); 314:879–883.

35. HOEG JM, GREGG RE, BREWER HB: An approach to the management of hyperlipoproteinemia. JAMA 1986 (Jan 24); 255:512–521.

36. CONNOR SL, ARTAUD-WILD SM, CLASSICK-KOHN CJ, GUSTAFSON JR, FLAVELL DP, HATCHER LF, CONNOR WE: The cholesterol/saturated-fat index: an indication of the hypercholesterolemic and atherogenic potential of food. Lancet (May 31); 1229–1232.

37. GRUNDY SM: Comparison of monounsaturated fatty acids and carbohydrates for lowering plasma cholesterol. N Engl J Med 1986 (Mar 20); 314:745–748.

38. GRUNDY SM, NIX D, WHELAN MF, FRANKON L: Comparison of three cholesterol-lowering diets in normolipidemic men. JAMA 1986 (Nov 7); 256:2351–2355.

39. SACKS FM, HANDYSIDES GH, MARAIS GE, ROSNER B, KASS EH: Effects of a low-fat diet on plasma lipoprotein levels. Arch Intern Med 1986 (Aug); 146:1573–1577.

40. KUUSISTO P, MANNINEN V, VAPAATALO H, HUTTUNEN JK, NEUVONEN PJ: Effect of activated charcoal on hypercholesterolemia. Lancet 1986 (Aug 16); 366–367.

41. HOEG JM, MAHER MB, ZECH LA, BAILEY KR, GREGG RE, LACKNER KJ, FOJO SS, ANCHORS MA, BOJANOVSKI M, SPRECHER DL, BREWER HB: Effectiveness of mevinolin on plasma lipoprotein concentrations in type II hyperlipoproteinemia. Am J Cardiol 1986 (Apr 15); 57:933–939.

42. THE LOVASTATIN STUDY GROUP II: Therapeutic response to lovastatin (Mevinolin) in nonfamilial hypercholesterolemia: a multicenter study. JAMA 1986 (Nov 28); 256:2829–2834.

43. EAST C, GRUNDY SM, BILHEIMER DW: Normal cholesterol levels with lovastatin (mevinolin) therapy in a child with homozygous familial hypercholesterolemia following liver transplantation. JAMA 1986 (Nov 28); 256:2843–2848.

44. MOL MJTM, LEUVEN JAG, ERKELENS DW, SCHOUTEN JA, STALENHOFF AFH: Effects of synvinolin (MK-733) on plasma lipids in familial hypercholesterolemia. Lancet 1986 (Oct 25); 936–939.

45. BROWN WV, DUJOVNE CA, FARQUHAR JW, FELDMAN EB, GRUNDY SM, KNOPP RH, LASSER NL, MELLIES MJ, PALMER RH, SAMUEL P, SCHONFELD G, SUPERKO HR: Effects of fenofibrate on plasma lipids: double-blind, multicenter study in patients with Type IIA or IIB hyperlipidemia. Arteriosclerosis 1986 (Nov/Dec); 6:670–678.

46. A JOINT STATEMENT FOR PHYSICIANS BY THE COMMITTEE ON ATHEROSCLEROSIS AND HYPERTENSION IN CHILDHOOD OF THE COUNCIL OF CARDIOVASCULAR DISEASE IN THE YOUNG AND THE NUTRITION COMMITTEE, AMERICAN HEART ASSOCIATION: Diagnosis and treatment of primary hyperlipidemia in childhood. Arteriosclerosis 1986 (Nov/Dec); 6:685A–692A.

47. GRUNDY SM: Cholesterol and coronary heart disease: a new era. JAMA 1986 (Nov 28); 256:2849–2858.

48. LaRosa JC: Dyslipoproteinemia in North America: introduction. Circulation 1986 (Jan); 73: 1-1–1-3.

49. Williams OD, Stinnett S, Chambless LE, Boyle KE, Bachorik PS, Albers JJ, Lippel K: Populations and methods for assessing dyslipoproteinemia and its correlates. Circulation 1986 (Jan); 73:1-4–1-11.

50. LaRosa JC, Chambless LE, Criqui MH, Frantz ID, Glueck CJ, Heiss G, Morrison JA: Patterns of dyslipoproteinemia in selected North American populations. Circulation 1986 (Jan); 73: 1-12–1-29.

51. Kwiterovitch PO, Stewart P, Probstfield JL, Stinnett S, Chambless LE, Chase GA, Jacobs DR, Morrison JA: Detection of dyslipoproteinemia with the use of plasma total cholesterol and triglyceride as screening tests. Circulation 1986 (Jan); 73:1-30–1-39.

52. Criqui MH, Cowan LD, Heiss G, Haskell WL, Laskarzewski PM, Chambless LE: Frequency and clustering of nonlipid coronary risk factors in dyslipoproteinemia. Circulation 1986 (Jan); 73:1-40–1-50.

53. Glueck CJ, Laskarzewski PM, Suchindran CM, Chambless LD, Barrett-Connor E, Stewart P, Heiss G, Tyroler: Progeny's lipid and lipoprotein levels by parental mortality. Circulation 1986 (Jan); 73:1-51–1-61.

54. Wallace RB, Pomrehn P, Heiss G, Chambless LD, Johnson N, Patten R, Lippel K, Rifkind BM: Alterations in clinical chemistry levels associated with the dyslipoproteinemias. Circulation 1986 (Jan); 73:1-62–1-69.

55. Wallace RB, Hunninghake DB, Chambless LE, Heiss G, Wahl P, Barrett-Connor E: A screening survey of dyslipoproteinemias associated with prescription drug use. Circulation 1986 (Jan); 73:1-70–1-79.

56. Little JA, Graves K, Suchindran CM, Milner J, McGuire V, Beaton G, Feather T, Mattson FH, Christiansen D, Williams OD: Customary diet, anthropometry, and dyslipoproteinemia in selected North American populations. Circulation 1986 (Jan); 73:1-80–1-90.

57. Rubenstein C, Romhilt D, Segal P, Heiss G, Chambless LE, Boyle KE, Ekelund LG, Adolph R, Sheffield LT: Dyslipoproteinemias and manifestations of coronary heart disease. Circulation 1986 (Jan); 73:1-91–1-99.

58. Pomrehn P, Duncan B, Weissfeld L, Wallace RB, Barnes R, Heiss G, Ekelund LG, Criqui MH, Johnson N, Chambless LE: The association of dyslipoproteinemia with symptoms and signs of peripheral arterial disease. Circulation 1986 (Jan); 73:1-100–1-107.

59. Seagal P, Insull W, Chambless LE, Stinnett S, LaRosa JC, Weissfeld L, Halfon S, Kwiterovitch PO, Little JA: The association of dyslipoproteinemia with corneal arcus and xanthelasma. Circulation 1986 (Jan); 73:1-108–1-118.

60. Wilcosky TC, Kwiterovitch PO, Glueck CJ, Suchindran C, Laskarzewski P, Christensen B, Tyroler HA: Dyslipoproteinemia in black participants. Circulation 1986 (Jan); 73:1-119–1-125.

61. LaRosa JC, Levy RI, Hazzard WR: Some clinical implications of the results of the Lipid Research Clinics Program Prevalence Study. Circulation 1986 (Jan); 73:1-126–1-133.

62. Rifkind BM, Lenfant C: Cholesterol lowering and the reduction of coronary heart disease risk. JAMA 1986 (Nov 28); 256:2872–2873.

63. Smoking and Health: A national status report. MMWR 1986 (Nov 21); 35:709–711.

64. Cook DG, Pocock SJ, Shaper AG, Kussick SJ: Giving up smoking and the risk of heart attacks. Lancet 1986 (Dec 13); 1376–1379.

65. Winniford MD, Wheelan KR, Kremers MS, Ugolini V, van den Berg E, Niggemann EH, Jansen DE, Hillis LD: Smoking-induced coronary vasoconstriction in patients with atherosclerotic coronary artery disease: evidence for adrenergically medicated alterations in coronary artery tone. Circulation 1986 (April); 73:662–667.

66. Paffenbarger RS, Hyde RT, Wing AL, Hsieh CC: Physical activity, all-cause mortality, and longevity of college alumni. N Engl J Med 1986 (Mar 6); 314:605–613.

67. Kannel WB, Belanger A, D'Agostino R, Israel I: Physical activity and physical demand on the job and risk of cardiovascular disease and death: The Framingham Study. Am Heart J 1986 (Oct); 112:820–825.

68. Jennings G, Nelson L, Nestel P, Esler M, Korner P, Burton D, Bazelmans J: The effects of changes in physical activity on cardiovascular risk factors, hemodynamics, sympathetic function, and glucose utilization in man: a controlled study of four levels of activity. Circulation 1986 (Jan); 73(1):30–40.

69. Sebrechts CP, Klein JL, Ahnve S, Froelicher VF, Ashburn WL: Myocardial perfusion changes

following 1 year of exercise training assessed by thallium-201 circumferential count profiles. Am Heart J 1986 (Dec); 112:1217–1226.

70. FLETCHER BJ, THIEL J, FLETCHER GF: Phase II intensive monitored cardiac rehabilitation for coronary artery disease and coronary risk factors—A six-session protocol. Am J Cardiol 1986 (Apr 1); 751–756.

71. VAN CAMP SP, PETERSON RA: Cardiovascular complications of outpatient cardiac rehabilitation programs. JAMA 1986 (Sept 5); 256:1160–1163.

72. LERNER DJ, KANNEL WB: Patterns of coronary heart disease morbidity and mortality in the sexes: a 26-year follow-up of the Framingham population. Am Heart J 1986 (Feb); 111:383–390.

73. KHAW KT, BARRETT-CONNOR E: Family history of heart attack: a modifiable risk factor? Circulation 1986 (Feb); 74:239–244.

74. LACROIX AZ, MEAD LA, LIANG KY, THOMAS CB, PEARSON TA: Coffee consumption and the incidence of coronary heart disease. N Engl J Med 1986 (Oct 16); 315:977–982.

75. MEADE TW, BROZOVIC M, CHAKRABARTI RR, HAINES AP, IMESON JD, MELLOWS S, MILLER GJ, NORTH WRS, STIRLING Y, THOMPSON SG: Hemostatic function and ischemic heart disease: principal results of the Northwick Park Heart Study. Lancet 1986 (Sept 6); 533–537.

76. ISNER JM, ESTES NAM, THOMPSON PD, COSTANZO-NORDIN MR, SUBRAMANIAN R, MILLER G, KATSAS G, SWEENEY K, STURNER WQ: Acute cardiac events temporally related to cocaine abuse. N Engl J Med 1986 (Dec 4); 315:1438–1443.

77. CREGLER LL, MARK H: Medical complications of cocaine abuse. N Engl J Med 1986 (Dec 4); 1495–1499.

78. BEAGLEHOLE R: Medical management and the decline in mortality from coronary heart disease. Br Med J 1986 (Jan); 292:33–35.

79. THOM TJ, EPSTEIN FH, FELDMAN JS, LEAVERTON PE: Trends in total mortality and mortality from heart disease in 26 countries from 1950 to 1978. Int J Epidemiol 1986; 14:510–20.

80. SHAPER AG: National trends in mortality from ischaemic heart disease: implications for prevention. Lancet 1986 (Apr 5); 795.

81. BURCH PRJ: National trends in mortality from ischaemic heart disease: implications for prevention. Lancet (May 17); 1155.

Coronary Artery Disease

Cardiac cinefluoroscopy -vs- exercise electrocardiography -vs- thallium scintigraphy

To compare the accuracy of cinefluoroscopy, stress ECG and thallium perfusion imaging in diagnosing CAD, Detrano and associates[1] from Cleveland, Ohio, performed these 3 studies in 297 subjects without prior AMI who were referred for coronary angiography. Of the 137 patients who had >50% angiographic diameter narrowing in at least 1 major coronary artery, 91 (67%) were correctly identified by cinefluoroscopy, 90 (66%) by stress electrocardiography and 100 (73%) by thallium imaging. Of the 164 patients with ≤50% diameter narrowing, the proportion of patients correctly identified as normal were 81%, 72%, and 79%, respectively. Cardiac cinefluoroscopy correctly classified 74% of the 297 subjects as to their disease status (>50% coronary narrowing), compared to 69% for stress electrocardiography and 76% for thallium imaging. There was no significant difference between the sensitivity or specificity of the test combination of stress electrocardiography and cinefluoroscopy and the combination of stress electrocardiography and thallium imaging. Cardiac cinefluoroscopy, a relatively cost-effective diagnostic test, is similar in accuracy to other, more expensive noninvasive diagnostic examinations for CAD.

Calcific deposits in abdominal aortic wall

Witteman and associates[2] from Rotterdam, The Netherlands, studied prospectively 1,359 men and 1,598 women who had ≥2 lateral radiographs of the lumbar spine and examined each of them for the presence of calcific deposits in the wall of abdominal aorta. The radiographs were taken in 1985–1978. In the subsequent 9 years, 50 men and 33 women died from cardiovascular disease. The prevalence of calcific deposits in the abdominal aortic wall was about 10% in middle-aged subjects and rose with age to a maximum of 45% in men and 75% in women. Aortic calcific deposits were associated with a 6-fold increased risk of cardiovascular disease in men aged 45 years, independent of other major cardiovascular risk factors. For each year of age over 45 years, risk associated with the presence of aortic wall calcific deposits declined by 6%. These results suggest that atherosclerosis in arteries other than coronary or cerebral may have predictive relevance for cardiovascular disease death. Its diagnosis should indicate intervention for other cardiovascular disease risk factors.

Duration of QT interval

Extensive narrowing of the major epicardial coronary arteries, impaired LV function, and prolongation of the QT interval are considered risk factors for sudden coronary death. No studies have investigated whether there is a correlation between the QT interval and changes in coronary anatomy or in LV function. Kramer and associates[3] from Heidelberg, Federal Republic of Germany, correlated coronary angiographic data to QT interval in 304 patients who were studied because of suspected CAD. QT intervals, however, were expressed as QTc = QT/ $\sqrt{RR}$ (Bazett's correction for heart rate), LV function was assessed by the EF of the ventricular angiogram, and coronary angiograms were classified according to the Gensini score and into 1-, 2- and 3-vessel CAD (stenoses $\geq$50%): A multidimensional linear regression model was employed to eliminate the effects of varying mean rates still present after application of Bazett's formula. In patients with 1-, 2- and 3-vessel CAD, significant changes of QTc were observed only in patients with impaired LV function (EF <60%). In these patients the QTc interval increased significantly from 1- to 3-vessel CAD. If the critical degree of coronary stenosis was changed from $\geq$50% to $\geq$90%, further prolongations of QTc were noted. In patients with 1-, 2- and 3-vessel CAD the QTc-duration difference was further enhanced if either the proximal part of the LAD or the LM coronary artery were affected (stenoses $\geq$50%). These data reveal that prolongation in the duration of electrical systole correlates with known cardiac risk factors for sudden death, i.e., 3-vessel-CAD, proximal LAD, or LM stenosis and impaired LV function. In the individual patient, however, the prognostic value of a single QTc determination is limited because of a large interindividual variation of the data.

Echocardiography

Sasaki and associates[4] from Los Angeles, California, recorded a 1-D echocardiogram shortly after admission in 46 patients with nondiagnostic chest pain. Eighteen patients were studied during chest pain and 28 were studied after the resolution of chest pain. Of the 18 patients studied during chest pain, 6 who had a regional wall motion abnormality evolved an AMI and the remaining 2 patients had evidence of significant CAD. Only 1 of 10 patients without a regional wall motion abnormality evolved an AMI and none had significant CAD. Of the 28 patients studied after resolution of chest pain, 8 of the 10 patients with a regional wall motion abnormality evolved an AMI and 1 patient had evidence of significant CAD; of 18 patients without a regional wall motion abnormality, none evolved an AMI and 5 had evidence of significant CAD. These data suggest that in patients presenting with nondiagnostic chest pain, an early assessment of regional wall motion by 2-D echocardiography can reliably differentiate patients with myocardial ischemia or early

AMI from patients with nonischemic chest pain when performed during an episode of chest pain; it also can identify patients with early AMI, even when performed after resolution of chest pain, but is not useful for the detection of patients with significant CAD without AMI when performed after resolution of chest pain.

Exercise electrocardiography with or without exercise echocardiography and with or without radionuclide angiography

Gordon and co-investigators[5] from multiple centers examined the results from >3,600 white men aged 30–79 years without a history of AMI who underwent submaximal treadmill exercise tolerance test as part of their baseline evaluation in the Lipid Research Clinics mortality follow-up study. The exercise test was conducted according to a common protocol and coded centrally; depression of the ST segment by >1 mm and/or 10 V-s (ST integral) signified a positive test. Concurrent measurements of age, BP, history of cigarette smoking, and plasma levels of lipids, lipoproteins, and glucose, and other CAD risk factors were obtained. Cumulative mortality from cardiovascular disease was 12% over 8.1 years mean follow-up among men with a positive test -vs- 1% 8.6 years mean follow-up among men with a negative test. Three-fourths of these deaths were due to CAD. The relative risk for cardiovascular mortality associated with a positive exercise test was 9.3 before and 4.6 after age adjustment. Cardiovascular mortality rates were especially elevated among the 82 men whose exercise tests were adjudged strongly positive based on degree and timing of the ischemic electrocardiographic response. A positive exercise test was also moderately associated with noncardiovascular mortality; the relative risk for all-cause mortality was 7.2 before and 3.4 after age adjustment. The positive exercise test was a stronger predictor of cardiovascular death than were high plasma levels of LDL cholesterol, low plasma levels of HDL cholesterol, smoking, hyperglycemia, or systemic hypertension. The impact of the positive exercise test on risk of cardiovascular death was equivalent to that of a 17.4-year increment in age.

Rautaharju et al[6] in Halifax, Nova Scotia, Canada, Minneapolis, Minnesota, Bethesda, Maryland, and Evanston, Illinois, determined the prognostic value of the exercise electrocardiogram in 6,438 men enrolled in the Multiple Risk Factor Intervention Trial as regards the ability of the exercise test to predict fatal and nonfatal CAD events. In this study, an abnormal response to exercise was defined as an ST-depression integral of ≥ 16 μV-s, and it was found in 12.2% of the men tested. There was a nearly 4-fold increase in 7-year coronary mortality among men with an abnormal response to exercise compared with men with a normal ST-segment response to exercise (Table 2-1). The risk ratio for CAD death adjusted for age, diastolic BP, serum cholesterol, and smoking status at baseline was 3.5, and the corresponding adjusted risk ratio for death from all causes was 1.6. There was a similar trend toward excess coronary events for angina. Multivariate analyses of the data obtained indicated that the ST-depression integral was a strong and independent predictor of future coronary death. The data also indicated that men with abnormal electrocardiograms at rest, primarily high-amplitude R waves and with an abnormal ST response to exercise have a 6-fold relative risk for CAD death than men with an abnormal electrocardiogram at rest and a normal ST response to exercise. Thus, these results suggest that exercise testing provides an assessment of future risks that is useful in predicting prognosis for middle-aged men with risk factors for CAD.

TABLE 2-1. *Number and rate of coronary heart disease deaths (per 1,000 person-years of risk), crude relative risk and Cox adjusted relative risk‡ by the presence of exercise electrocardiographic abnormalities for multiple risk factor intervention trial usual care men. Reproduced with permission from Rautaharju et al.*[6]

	EXERCISE ECG					COX ADJUSTED RELATIVE RISK
	NORMAL		ABNORMAL		RELATIVE RISK	
END POINT	NO.	RATE/1,000	NO.	RATE/1,000		
CHD death	73	2.0	38	7.61	3.80†	3.45*
CVD death	90	2.48	40	8.02	3.25†	2.99†
Non-CVD death	101	2.78	5	1.00	0.36*	0.35*
All deaths	191	5.25	45	9.02	1.72†	1.61†
Angina	632	18.34	132	28.26	1.55†	1.58†
Nonfatal MI by serial ECG change	129	3.53	18	3.54	1.04†	0.93
Definite clinical MI	183	5.03	31	6.21	1.25†	1.17
CHD death, serial ECG change or definite clinical MI	356	9.79	85	17.04	1.76†	1.67†

* p <0.05   † p <0.01.

‡ Adjusted for age, diastolic pressure, serum cholesterol and number of cigarettes smoked daily. CHD = coronary heart disease; CVD = cardiovascular disease; ECG = electrocardiogram; MI = myocardial infarction.

Hakki and associates[7] from Philadelphia, Pennsylvania, assessed the determinants of exercise-induced abnormal systolic BP response in 127 patients with documented CAD who underwent exercise thallium-201 scintigraphy. Three types of systolic BP response to exercise were identified: an increase by >20 mmHg (group I, n = 74); an increase by ≤20 mmHg (group II, n = 26); and a decrease of ≥10 mmHg (group III, n = 17). The 3 groups were not significantly different in age, gender or medications. The number of segments with perfusion defects was significantly higher in groups II and III than in group I (group III, 2.9 ± 1.5; group II, 2.9 ± 2.1; and group I, 1.8 ± 1.4). Prior AMI, abnormal LVEF, and multivessel CAD were more common in group III than in groups I and II. Stepwise discriminant analysis of 15 relevant clinical, angiographic and exercise scintigraphic descriptors showed that the number of thallium perfusion defects, abnormal LVEF at rest and multivessel CAD to be important predictors of hypotensive BP response. Multivariate analysis, however, showed that the number of thallium perfusion defects was the only important predictor of the hypotensive response. Thus, it is the functional significance of CAD assessed by the extent of thallium perfusion abnormalities rather than the extent of CAD or LV dysfunction at rest that determines the systolic BP response to exercise.

To evaluate the utility of exercise RNA and electrocardiography in assessing the severity of CAD, 185 patients undergoing coronary angiography were evaluated prospectively in a study carried out by Weintraub and associates[8] from Philadelphia, Pennsylvania. To avoid work-up bias and to provide an appropriate control group, all patients were simultaneously scheduled for exercise RNA and electrocardiography and for coronary arteriography. All test results were interpreted blinded to other data. Of multiple exercise variables analyzed by stepwise linear discriminant analysis, the independent predictors of CAD severity were exercise EF, ST-segment change, and maximum heart rate. These 3 variables were used to create a set of 4 equations that determine probabilities of 0, 1-, 2- or 3-vessel CAD. The noninvasive estimate of number of diseased arteries in each patient was compared to the angiographic result. Patients without significant CAD were classified correctly 71% of the time, while those with 3-vessel CAD were predicted correctly in 80%. Fully 90% of patients with predicted 3-vessel had 2- or 3-vessel CAD. Conversely, 84% of patients predicted to have 0 vessel CAD had 0 or 1-vessel CAD. Thus, the combined use of exercise RNA and electrocardiographic data permits assessment of the presence and severity of CAD.

Ahnve and associates[9] from Long Beach, California, determined whether exercise-induced myocardial ischemia demonstrated by thallium-201 imaging could be detected by ST-segment shifts in patients with abnormal Q waves at rest. Fifty-four patients with CAD and exercise-induced thallium-201 defects were compared to 22 patients with similar Q-wave patterns but without thallium-201 exercise defects and to 14 normal persons. Exercise data were analyzed visually in the 12-lead electrocardiogram and for spatial ST-vector shifts. Both ST-segment depression observed on the 12-lead electrocardiogram and spatial criteria were reasonably sensitive and specific for ischemia when the resting electrocardiogram showed no Q waves or inferior Q waves (range 69% to 93%). However, when anterior Q waves were present, ST-segment shifts could not distinguish patients with ischemia from those with normal perfusion as determined by thallium imaging.

The ST-segment shift relative to exercise-induced increments in heart rate, the ST/heart rate slope, has been proposed as a more accurate electrocardiographic criterion for diagnosing significant CAD. Finkelhor and associates[10] from Cleveland, Ohio, compared the clinical utility of the ST/heart rate slope using a standard treadmill protocol with quantitative stress thallium and standard treadmill criteria in 64 unselected patients who underwent coronary angiography. The overall diagnostic accuracy of the ST/heart rate slope was an improvement over thallium and conventional ST criteria (81%, 67%, and 69%). For patients failing to reach 85% of their age-predicted maximal heart rate, the diagnostic accuracy of the ST/heart rate slope was comparable with thallium (77% and 74%). The sensitivity of the ST/heart rate slope in patients without prior AMI was equivalent to that of thallium (91% and 95%). The ST/heart rate slope was directly related to the angiographic severity of CAD in patients without prior AMI. The ST/heart rate slope was an improved electrocardiographic criterion for diagnosing CAD and compared favorably with thallium imaging.

Kligfield and associates[11] from New York, New York, analyzed rate-related change in exercise-induced ST-segment depression, the ST/heart rate slope (Fig. 2-1), to significantly improve the accuracy of the exercise electrocardiogram for the identification of CAD patients and for the recognition of patients with stable angina who have anatomically or functionally severe CAD (Fig. 2-2). This method, in effect, normalizes the extent of ST-segment depression for heart rate, which serves as an index of exercise-induced augmentation of myocardial oxygen demand. While preserving the specificity of the exercise electrocardiogram at >90%, an ST/heart rate slope value of 1.1 μV/beats a minute as an upper limit of normal improved exercise test sensitivity from 57–91% in patients with stable angina who were examined using standard Bruce protocols and 3 monitoring leads. In addition, an ST/heart rate slope value of 6.0 μV/beats a minute was found to partition patients with and without 3-vessel CAD with a sensitivity of 78%, specificity of 97%, positive predictive value of 93%, and overall test accuracy of 90%. No other criteria based on standard electrocardiographic interpretation performed as well as the ST/heart rate slope for the recognition of 3-vessel CAD in these

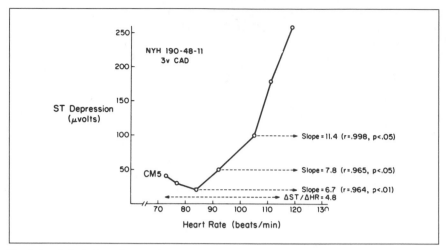

Fig. 2-1. Calculation of ST/HR slope. Cumulative ST segment depression in lead V$_5$ is plotted against exercise-related change in heart rate in patient with three-vessel coronary artery disease. In this case, as heart rate increases, rate of ST segment depression increases progressively. As a result, slope of line relating final three data points by linear regression is higher than slope of lines incorporating earlier data points. When more than one linear correlation is statistically significant, greatest value (in this case 11.4) is accepted as maximum ST/HR slope for lead being examined. Highest ST/HR slope in any lead is taken as test value for patient. Note that value obtained by simply dividing final amount of ST segment depression by change in heart rate does not accurately represent ST/HR slope. Reproduced with permission from Kligfield et al.[11]

patients. Further, patients with high ST/heart rate slopes who did not have 3-vessel CAD could be shown to have functionally severe 2-vessel CAD by RNA. These data suggest that the ST/heart rate slope can improve the evaluation and management of patients with possible CAD. Additional improvement in ST/heart rate slope accuracy and applicability is likely to result from modification of exercise protocols to reduce heart rate increments between stages, an increase in monitoring leads to include CM$_5$, and computer analysis of the ST-segment depression.

Armstrong and associates[12] from Indianapolis, Indiana, performed 2-D echocardiograms during rest and after exercise in 95 patients who subsequently had coronary angiography. Prior AMI was present in 36 patients, 35 of whom had wall motion abnormalities. There was no evidence of prior AMI in 59 patients, 44 of whom had CAD. In these 44 patients, the exercise electrocardiogram showed ischemia in 19, was normal in 13, and was nondiagnostic in 12. Exercise echocardiograms were abnormal in 35 of these 44 patients. In 15 patients without CAD, the treadmill response was nondiagnostic in 6, ischemic in 1, and normal in 8. Exercise echocardiograms were normal in 13 of these 15 patients. The authors concluded that exercise echocardiography is a valuable addition to routine treadmill testing. It may be of special value in patients with an abnormal resting electrocardiogram or a nondiagnostic response to treadmill testing or when a false-negative treadmill test is suspected.

Dipyridamole testing

Stress thallium imaging with intravenous dipyridamole permits assessment of CAD without the need for exercise. Intravenous dipyridamole is available in the USA, however, only on an experimental basis. To study the

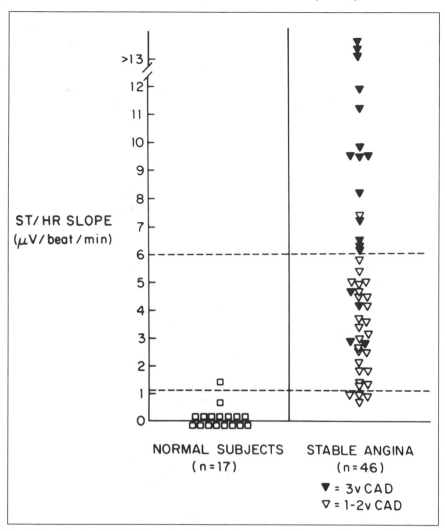

Fig. 2-2.   Calculated ST/HR slopes in 17 clinically normal subjects and in 46 patients with effort-related angina. Exercise was performed on treadmill with use of Bruce protocol, and three monitoring leads were examined. Partition at 1.1 μV/bpm represents upper limit of normal reported by Elamin et al.[18] Reproduced with permission from Kligfield et al.[11]

use of oral dipyridamole as a clinically available alternative to intravenous dipyridamole for this purpose, Homma and associates[13] from Boston, Massachusetts, performed thallium imaging with oral dipyridamole in 100 patients. Each patient received 300 mg of pulverized tablets in a 30-ml suspension. Maximal increase in mean heart rate and decrease in mean BP occurred 30 minutes after ingestion. At 45 minutes, 2 mCi of thallium was given intravenously and serial imaging was begun within 7 minutes. The serum dipyridamole level (mean ± standard deviation) 45 minutes after 300 mg was administered orally (3.7 ± 2.2 μg/ml) was similar to that 5 minutes after 0.56 mg/kg was given intravenously (4.6 ± 1.3 μg/ml). Fifty-five patients had some adverse effects between 15 and 75 minutes after oral ingestion, including nausea, headache, dizziness, chest pain (25 patients) and electrocardiographic changes (14 patients). Intravenous aminophylline was used to resolve these adverse effects in 21 patients. There were no severe arrhythmias, AMIs or deaths. Of the 43 patients with angiographically documented CAD, 39 had an initial perfusion defect that redistributed on the delayed images. When the results in patients who had undergone catheterization were analyzed by individual segment, the presence of thallium redistribution was associated with normal or hypokinetic contrast left ventriculographic wall motion of that segment, whereas the presence of a persistent defect was associated with akinesia or dyskinesia. In conclusion, stress thallium imaging without exercise is feasible with a clinically available form of dipyridamole—the oral suspension. It is safe and may be used for evaluation of CAD to unmask regions of hypoperfused viable myocardium.

Picano and associates[14] from Pisa, Italy, performed a dipyridamole test (infusion of dipyridamole, 0.14 mg/kg/min intravenously for 4 minutes) in 14 consecutive patients with exercise-induced ST-segment elevation in the absence of previous AMI and basal LV asynergy at rest during 12-lead electrocardiography and 2-D echocardiographic monitoring. In 7 of the 14 patients, dipyridamole infusion consistently induced ST-segment elevation in the leads that showed ST elevation on effort; reversible asynergy (occurring in the region corresponding to the electrocardiographic leads with diagnostic changes) could always be documented by echocardiography. In 2 patients, dipyridamole induced reversible asynergy in presence of ST-segment depression. In these 9 patients, angiography invariably revealed a severe organic stenosis in the coronary artery feeding the region that became transiently asynergic after dipyridamole. In the other 5 patients (all of whom had either spontaneous or ergonovine-induced ST-segment elevation), the dipyridamole test yielded no significant echocardiographic or electrocardiographic change; coronary angiography showed absent (2 patients) or significant (3 patients) CAD. The authors concluded that dipyridamole may induce transmural ischemia in humans, as detected by the electrical hallmark of ST elevation; this electrocardiographic pattern, in contrast to ST depression, reliably predicts the presence and site of transient regional asynergy. When dipyridamole induces ST-segment elevation, severe basal stenosis is invariably present in the coronary artery supplying the transiently asynergic myocardial region.

Thallium-201 scintigraphy

The abilities of subjectively determined and quantitative analyses of stress redistribution thallium-201 scintigrams, exercise electrocardiograms, and exercise BP responses were compared for correct identification of extensive CAD, defined as LM or 3-vessel CAD, or both, in 105 consecutive patients with suspected CAD by Maddahi et al[15] in Los Angeles, California. Fifty-six patients had extensive CAD and the remaining patients had less extensive CAD (n = 34) or normal coronary arteriograms (n = 15). For visual interpretation of the thallium-201 images, analog images were displayed on Polaroid® film. For quantitative analyses of the thallium-201 images, 60 radii spaced at 6-degree intervals were constructed from the LV center. Along each radius, the point with maximal thallium-201 activity was chosen and plotted as number of counts -vs- the angle. The combination of all 60 points resulted in a circumferential profile of myocardial thallium-201 activity and these profiles were aligned by the operator so that the 90-degree point in each view corresponded to the scintigraphic apex. The number of counts in each point was then normalized to the maximal count in the stress profile of each view and the stress profile and washout weight circumferential profiles were generated by calculating percent washout for each point from the time of stress to delayed imaging. Exercise BP responses, exercise electrocardiograms and visual thallium-201 analyses were specific (98, 88, and 96%, respectively),

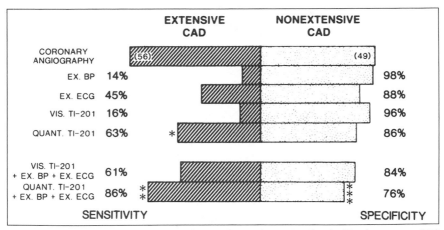

	EXTENSIVE CAD	NONEXTENSIVE CAD
CORONARY ANGIOGRAPHY	(56)	(49)
EX. BP	14%	98%
EX. ECG	45%	88%
VIS. TI-201	16%	96%
QUANT. TI-201	63%	86%
VIS. TI-201 + EX. BP + EX. ECG	61%	84%
QUANT. TI-201 + EX. BP + EX. ECG	86%	76%
	SENSITIVITY	SPECIFICITY

Fig. 2-3. Comparative sensitivity and specificity of exercise (EX.), blood pressure (BP) response, exercise electrocardiography (ECG), stress redistribution thallium-201 (Tl-201) scintigraphy by visual (VIS.) and quantitative (QUANT.) analysis individually and in combination for correct identification of patients with extensive angiographic coronary artery disease. Reproduced with permission from Maddahi et al.[15]

but they were insensitive in identifying patients with extensive CAD (14, 45, and 16%, respectively). However, quantitative thallium-201 analysis significantly improved the sensitivity of thallium-201 analysis in the identification of patients with extensive CAD from 16–63% without an important loss of specificity (96 -vs- 86%) (Fig. 2-3). Eighteen of 28 patients misclassified by visual analysis of the thallium-201 scintigrams were correctly classified as having extensive CAD by the quantitative analysis of regional myocardial thallium-201 washout. When the results of quantitative thallium-201 analyses were combined with those of BP and electrocardiographic responses to exercise, the sensitivity and specificity in the identification of patients with extensive CAD were 86% and 76%, respectively, and the highest overall accuracy of 0.82 was obtained. These data suggest that the quantitative analysis of myocardial thallium-201 stress distribution and washout increases the sensitivity of visual thallium-201 analysis in the correct identification of patients with extensive CAD or LM disease. Furthermore, the sensitivity in identifying these high-risk patients is improved by combining the results of quantitative thallium-201 analyses with those of BP and electrocardiographic responses to exercise.

Ladenheim et al[16] in Los Angeles, California, assessed the utility of determining the presence and extent of exercise-induced myocardial hypoperfusion on thallium scintigraphy in the prediction of coronary events in 1,689 patients with symptoms suggestive of CAD but without prior AMI or CABG. In these studies, the extent of hypoperfusion was measured by exercise and redistribution with thallium myocardial perfusion scintigraphy. Seventy-four patients had a coronary event in the year after testing (12 cardiac deaths, 20 nonfatal AMIs, and 42 referrals for CABG more than 60 days after testing). Logistic regression analysis identified 3 independent predictors: (a) the number of myocardial regions with reversible hypoperfusion; (b) the maximum magnitude of hypoperfusion; and (c) the achieved heart rate. The extent and severity of hypoperfusion were correlated with the event rate, whereas achieved heart rate was linearly correlated with event rate. From these data, a prognostic model was defined employing the extent and severity of thallium-201 determined hypoperfusion during stress. The predicted coronary event rate ranged over 2 orders of magnitude from a low of 0.4% in patients able to exercise adequately without having hypoperfusion to a high of 78% in patients having severe and extensive hypoperfusion at a low heart rate, i.e.,

<85% of their maximal predicted heart rate. Thus, the extent and severity of myocardial hypoperfusion are important independent variables of prognosis in patients with CAD.

Kaul et al[17] in Boston, Massachusetts used exercise thallium images to determine the relative value of different imaging variables in the detection of perfusion defects indicative of physiologically important CAD. Three hundred twenty-five patients were evaluated; 281 patients had cardiac-catheterization-documented CAD and 44 patients had no CAD. Regional initial thallium-201 uptake, redistribution, and clearance between the exercise and rest thallium-201 studies were measured. Normal values were defined in 55 additional clinical normal subjects. Five myocardial segments were analyzed in each view (Fig. 2-4), the sensitivity and specificity for initial thallium uptake were 95 and 50%, respectively; the sensitivity and specificity for thallium-201 redistribution were 60 and 87%, respectively; and the sensitivity and specificity for the thallium-201 clearance were 74 and 66%, respectively. Initial thallium-201 uptake was the most sensitive but least specific, and redistribution of thallium-201 was the least sensitive and most specific. The best correlation with CAD was with the initial thallium-201 uptake. The addition of redistribution to a mathematical model of the probability of CAD did not alter sensitivity, but increased specificity from 50 to 70%. When the 2 basal LV segments were excluded from each view, the specificity increased from 70% to 80% without altering sensitivity. Among the 15 patients (5%) with CAD not detected using this approach, none had LM CAD and 10 (67%) had 1-vessel CAD. Thus, a combination of variables derived from quantification of exercise thallium-201 images provides an enhanced sensitivity and specificity in the detection of CAD compared with the use of a single variable.

Taillefer et al[18] in Montreal, Canada, determined the diagnostic utility of thallium-201 myocardial imaging after dipyridamole infusion compared to the oral administration of dipyridamole. Fifty patients referred for coronary angiography were studied prospectively. During a 2-week period, each patient had cardiac catheterization and thallium-201 myocardial imaging after both oral and intravenous dipyridamole administration. For the oral protocol, patients were randomized to receive either 200 or 400 mg of dipyridamole in tablet form. Coronary artery stenoses ≥70% were considered significant. Twenty-five patients received a 200–mg oral dose of dipyridamole, and the scintigraphic study showed perfusion defects in 65% of patients with significant CAD after the oral dose and 85% of patients after the intravenous dose of dipyridamole. In the 25 patients receiving a 400-mg oral dose, the

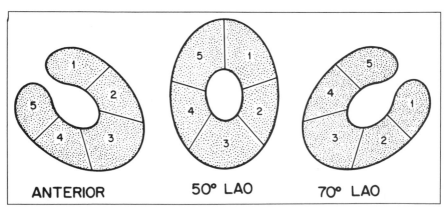

Fig. 2-4. The segmentation of the left ventricle into five segments per view. LAO = left anterior oblique. Reproduced with permission from Kaul et al.[17]

sensitivity of the scintigram was 84% after the oral dose and 79% after the intravenous dose. Side effects were less severe and more frequent with oral than with intravenously administered dipyridamole, and included headaches and nausea. Oral studies required 45–60 minutes of medical supervision and aminophylline was administered empirically after the completion of the first set of thallium-201 images. Thallium-201 myocardial imaging after coronary vasodilatation with a 400-mg oral dose of dipyridamole is a safe and widely available alternative for the evaluation of CAD in patients unable to exercise.

Kaul et al[19] in Boston, Massachusetts, and Charlottesville, Virginia, evaluated the myocardial clearance of Tl-201 in 370 patients attempting to determine whether Tl-201 clearance from LV segments might enhance the diagnostic utility of this scintigraphic approach in detecting CAD. Among the 370 patients, those in group I (n = 45) had less than a 1% probability of having CAD; patients in group II (n = 44) had normal coronary arteries, and patients in group III (n = 281) had significant CAD. Although mean myocardial clearance of Tl-201 in 15 myocardial segments in 3 views in group I subjects was 3.4 ± 0.7 hours, the variability between the slowest and fastest clearing segments in the same subject was as much as 98%. Seventy-eight percent of the slowest clearing segments were basal, whereas 53% of the fastest clearing segments were apical. A comparison of group II and III patients based on group I values demonstrated that the absolute myocardial clearance of Tl-201 had a sensitivity and specificity in detecting CAD of 92 and 16%, respectively. When the myocardial clearance of Tl-201 was considered abnormal in an LV segment (only if the rate was 98% slower than in the fastest clearing LV segment in the same patient) sensitivity and specificity changed to 69 and 86%, respectively. These data suggest that there is significant regional LV variability in the myocardial clearance of Tl-201 even in normal subjects; when myocardial clearance of Tl-201 is considered abnormal after comparison with the fastest clearing segment in the myocardium, its diagnostic utility improved significantly; and using myocardial clearance of Tl-201 to detect CAD enhances its diagnostic utility.

Iskandrian and associates[20] from Philadelphia, Pennsylvania, studied the prognostic value of exercise thallium-201 imaging in 196 men with suspected or known CAD who had nondiagnostic exercise electrocardiograms. The perfusion images in each of 3 projections were divided into 3 segments; each segment was assessed for perfusion defects (fixed or reversible). There were 12 cardiac events at a mean follow-up of 15 months (range, 1–66 months). Of those, 5 patients died of cardiac causes and 7 had nonfatal AMI. Only the number of perfusion defects significantly predicted cardiac events; clinical presentation, history of AMI, presence of Q-wave AMI, exercise duration, and exercise heart rate and double product did not predict cardiac events or add to information provided by the number of defects. Furthermore, actuarial life-table analysis showed that patients with ≥3 perfusion defects had significantly worse prognoses than patients with <3 defects. Exercise thallium-201 imaging helps in risk stratification of men with nondiagnostic exercise electrocardiograms.

Positron emission tomography

Positron emission tomography (PET) can be used with nitrogen-13-ammonia ($^{13}NH_3$) to estimate regional myocardial blood flow, and with fluorine-18-deoxyglucose (^{18}FDG) to measure exogenous glucose uptake by the myocardium. Tillisch and associates[21] from Los Angeles, California, used PET to predict whether preoperative abnormalities in LV wall motion in 17 patients who underwent CABG were reversible. The abnormalities were quantified by radionuclide or contrast angiography, or both, before and after CABG. PET images were obtained preoperatively. Abnormal wall motion in regions in which PET images showed preserved glucose uptake was predicted to be reversible, whereas abnormal motion in regions with depressed glucose uptake was predicted to be irreversible. According to these criteria, abnormal contraction in 35 of 41 segments was correctly predicted to be reversible (85% predictive accuracy), and abnormal contraction in 24 of 26 regions was correctly predicted to be irreversible (92% predictive accuracy). In contrast, electrocardiograms showing pathological Q waves in the region of asynergy predicted irreversibility in only 43% of regions. The authors concluded that PET imaging with $^{13}NH_3$ to assess blood flow and ^{18}FDG to assess the metabolic viability of the myocardium is an accurate method of predicting potential reversibility of wall motion abnormalities after surgical revascularization.

Gould et al[22] in Houston, Texas, determined the clinical feasibility of diagnosing significant CAD by positron imaging of myocardial perfusion without a cyclotron, using generator-produced rubidium-82. Fifty patients underwent positron emission tomography of the heart using a multislice positron camera, and rubidium-82 or nitrogen-13 ammonia were administered intravenously before and after the intravenous administration of dipyridamole combined with handgrip stress. Quantitative coronary arteriography was obtained for the arteriographic correlates of coronary flow reserve and significant CAD was identified when there was an arteriographically determined coronary flow reserve of <3.0 based on a determination of all stenosis dimensions. The sensitivity for identifying patients with physiologically important coronary stenoses was 95% by positron imaging and the specificity was 100%. The single case that was missed was studied with nitrogen-13 ammonia and had a 43% diameter narrowing of a small ramus intermedium from the LM coronary artery with no significant narrowing of other major coronary arteries. Thus, positron emission tomographic evaluation of myocardial perfusion before and after intravenous dipyridamole combined with handgrip stress using rubidium-82 provides a sensitive and apparently specific diagnosis of reduced coronary flow reserve due to significant coronary stenoses.

Coronary angiography

Thompson[23] in Wellington, New Zealand, found that 27 (1.3%) of 2,105 consecutive patients with angiographically defined coronary stenoses had ≥50% stenosis of 1 or both *coronary ostia*. He also found that serious complications occurred during angiography in 3 patients (11%) with 1 death. CABG was performed in 25 patients with 1 early (4%) and 1 late death (mean follow-up, 28 months). Twenty-two patients (group 1) had associated multivessel CAD, of whom 18 (82%) presented with stable angina of variable duration (43 ± 53 months) and 10 (46%) were in New York Heart Association functional class II. The prevalence of risk factors was high, especially among the 8 women, 7 of whom had hyperlipidemia. Five patients (group 2) representing 0.2% of the total had isolated coronary ostial stenosis; each of these patients was a woman with a mean age of 41 ± 6 years. This group presented with a short history (2.0 ± 1.7 months) of severe angina and a low incidence of risk factors. Therefore, isolated coronary ostial stenosis is an uncommon lesion occurring predominantly in young or middle-aged women. Clinical and angiographic profiles suggest a natural history distinctly different from that usually found with atherosclerotic CAD.

Prediction by a data-based multivariable statistical model -vs- prediction by senior cardiologists

To study the accuracy with which long-term prognosis can be predicted in patients with CAD, Lee and associates[24] from Durham, North Carolina, compared prognostic predictions from a data-based multivariable statistical model with predictions from senior clinical cardiologists. Test samples of 100 patients each were selected from a large series of medically treated patients with significant CAD. Using detailed case summaries, 5 senior cardiologists each predicted 1- and 3-year survival and infarct-free survival probabilities for 100 patients. Fifty patients appeared in multiple samples for assessing interphysician variability. Cox regression models (Table 2-2), developed using patients not in the test samples, predicted corresponding outcome probabilities for each test patient. Overall, model predictions correlated better with actual patient outcomes than did the doctors' predictions. For 3-year survival, rank correlations were 0.61 (model) and 0.49 (doctors). For 3-year infarct-free survival predictions, correlations with outcome were 0.48 (model) and 0.29 (doctors). Comparisons by individual doctor revealed Cox model 3-year survival predictions were better than those of 4 or 5 doctors (model predictions added significant prognostic information to the doctor's predictions, whereas the converse was not true). For infarct-free survival, the Cox model was superior to all 5 doctors. Where predictions were made by multiple doctors, the interphysician variability was substantial. In CAD, statistical models developed from carefully collected data can provide prognostic predictions that are more accurate than predictions of experienced clinicians made from detailed case summaries.

TABLE 2-2. *Prognostic patient descriptor used in Cox models for survival and event-free survival. Reproduced with permission from Lee et al.[24]*

Age
Sex
Characterization of angina (progressive versus stable, frequency, nocturnal, preinfarction)
History of Prinzmetal's angina*
Noninvasive indicators of myocardial damage (congestive heart failure, cardiomegaly, previous myocardial infarction by history or electrocardiography, ST-T wave abnormality on electrocardiography, premature ventricular contractions on electrocardiography, ventricular gallop)
Vascular disease (peripheral, cerebral)
Ejection fraction
Maximum luminal diameter narrowing of each coronary artery (left main, left anterior descending, left circumflex, and right coronary artery)
Left ventricular end-diastolic pressure
Arteriovenous oxygen difference†
Mitral insufficiency*
Left ventricular contraction (normal versus abnormal, diffusely abnormal, anterior asynergy, inferior asynergy)†

* Used only in the model for event-free survival.
† Used only in the model for survival.

Of severe narrowing of the left anterior descending coronary artery

To determine the prognostic importance of significant narrowings involving the proximal LAD coronary artery, Klein and associates[25] from Philadelphia, Pennsylvania, followed after cardiac catheterization for a mean of 17 months (range 1–46) 866 medically treated patients with significant CAD. Coronary narrowings in all patients were evaluated based on site relative to large branches and on angiographic severity. Prognosis was best predicted by the presence of ≥70% diameter reduction in the LAD before the first 2 large branches. At 3 years, there was a 94% cumulative survival rate in patients with <70% stenoses at this location, but an 82% survival rate in patients with ≥70% stenoses. In addition, although the presence of proximal LAD narrowings was the best predictor of prognosis in patients with a low global EF, this was not so in patients with a normal EF, as this subgroup had an excellent overall prognosis. Thus, the presence and severity of significant stenoses in the proximal LAD are stronger predictors of prognosis than stenoses elsewhere in the major coronary arteries. The presence of an angiographically significant narrowing in this anatomic location is highly correlated with an increased 1- to 3-year mortality rate.

For survival ≥20 years

Hamby and associates[26] from Roslyn, and Valhalla, New York, and Albuquerque, New Mexico, reviewed clinical, angiographic, and therapeutic aspects of CAD of long duration (≥20 years) in 50 patients (study group) and compared them to a control group of 100 consecutive patients with CAD of shorter duration. All were referred because of symptomatic CAD. The study group had a greater prevalence of clinically evident extracardiac vascular disease (28% -vs- 4%). Transmural AMI was more frequent in the study group (64% -vs- 45%). Triple-vessel and LM CAD were observed, respectively, in 90% and 28% compared to 36% and 7% in the control group. Twenty-nine percent of collaterals were jeopardized in the study group compared to 13% of collaterals in controls. Abnormal LVEF was found in 50% of the study group compared to 28% of controls. Medical therapy was recommended for 36% of the study group with 11 of 18% (61%) considered inoperable, whereas in 39% of the control group medical therapy was continued, with 9 of 39 (23%) considered inoperable. CABG or PTCA was recommended in 64% of the study group and in 61% of the control group. No patient in the study group was considered a candidate for PTCA, whereas in 20% (12 of 61) of the control group PTCA was recommended. Patients with CAD for ≥20 years have severe CAD, with 1 in 4 having LM CAD.

Of patients with angiographically normal and insignificantly narrowed coronary arteries

Papanicolaou and associates[27] from Durham, North Carolina, examined the clinical presentation and prognosis of 1,977 consecutive patients with angiographically normal coronary arteries or "insignificant" CAD (no major epicardial artery with ≥75% luminal diameter narrowing). Compared with patients with significant CAD, these patients had a lower frequency of traditional cardiac risk factors and abnormalities on the rest and exercise electrocardiogram. Cardiac survival was 99% at 5 years of follow-up and 98% at 10 years for patients with normal or insignificantly narrowed coronary arteries (Fig. 2-5). Patients with normal coronary arteries differed from those with

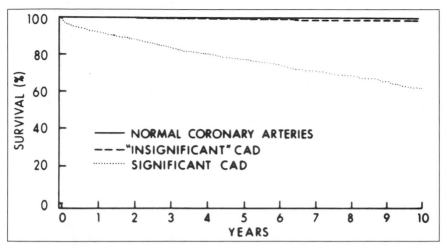

Fig. 2-5. Survival curves for patients with normal, insignificantly diseased and significantly diseased coronary arteries. Cardiac deaths only. Noncardiac deaths are censored at the time of death. CAD = coronary artery disease.

insignificant CAD in their AMI-free survival rate: 99% at 5 years and 98% at 10 years for patients with normal coronary arteries, and 97% at 5 years and 90% at 10 years for patients with insignificant CAD (Fig. 2-6). A strong relation occurred between the amount of insignificant CAD and follow-up cardiac events. Cardiac risk factors were statistically related to the risk of follow-up cardiovascular events when considered alone, but this relation lost significance after adjusting for the effect of coronary anatomy. Patients in both groups continued to have cardiac symptoms that resulted in frequent hospitalizations, medication use and job disability (Fig. 2-7). Almost 50% in any given year of follow-up could not perform activities of high metabolic equivalent requirement and 70% had continuing symptoms of chest discom-

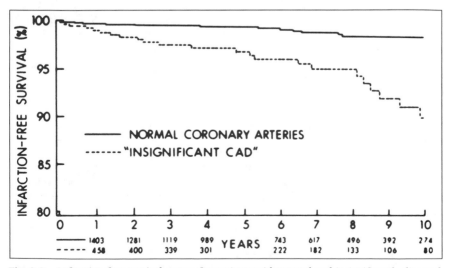

Fig. 2-6. Infarction free survival curves for patients with normal and insignificantly diseased coronary arteries. Numbers at bottom represent numbers of patients followed at each interval. CAD = coronary artery disease.

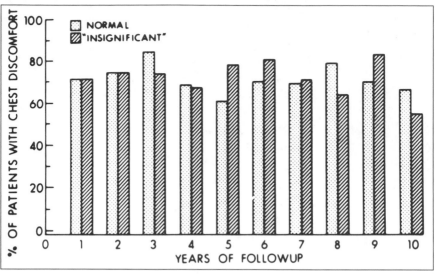

Fig. 2-7. Percentage of patients with continuing chest discomfort over 10 years of follow-up (cross-sectional data).

fort. Although these patients are at low risk of death, many remain functionally impared for years.

ANGIOGRAPHIC PROGRESSION OF CORONARY ARTERIAL NARROWING

Although specific *risk factors* correlate with the development of clinical coronary events, little is known about their importance in patients with established CAD. Raichlen and associates[28] from Baltimore, Maryland, used a numerical scoring system to assess serial coronary angiograms in subjects who had detailed risk factor determinations. Strong linear correlations were demonstrated between the extent of progression of CAD and diastolic BP, systolic BP, the number of cigarette pack-years smoked among current smokers, fasting blood glucose level, and low levels of physical activity at leisure. This analysis of sequential coronary angiograms identified BP, cigarette smoking, diabetes mellitus, and physical activity as important risk factors in the progression of CAD.

Visser and colleagues[29] from Eindhoven, Nijmegen, Nieuwegein, and Leyden, the Netherlands, studied the impact of the evolution of obstructive CAD on LV function in 300 nonoperated patients who had had 2 angiographic studies. The interval between studies ranged from 6–120 months (mean 30). Quantitative analysis of LV contraction in right anterior oblique projections was performed with the use of a computer program for calculation of EF and regional wall motion. No progression of CAD was found in 131 patients. Progression of CAD was found in 169 patients. In the patients without progression and in 75 patients who had progression to less than total obstruction, no changes in EF and regional wall motion were found. In the 67 patients in whom progression from <90% narrowing to occlusion had occurred, a significant decrease in EF and regional wall motion was found. In the 27 patients with progression from subtotal narrowing to occlusion, however, no change in LV function was found. A myocardial protective value of angiographically visible preexistent collaterals could not be demonstrated. It was concluded that absence of progression of CAD implies that LV function does not deteriorate and that slow progression to occlusion, via a stage of subtotal narrowing, generally does not influence LV function.

Shea et al[30] in New York, New York, measured progression of coronary artery stenosis using a quantitative, computer-assisted cinevideodensitometric method in 144 arterial segments in 44 subjects undergoing coronary arteriography on 2 separate occasions ≥6 months apart. Projected coronary arteriograms were digitized into 512 × 512 pixel mode, and percent stenosis was calculated by comparing background-corrected videodensitometric values over stenotic and normal segments. Subjects had repeat coronary arteriograms because of worsening symptoms of angina or CHF. The mean interval between coronary arteriography was 29 months. Overall progression of CAD was found in 40 of the 44 subjects with a mean progression at 24 months of 39%. At 33–36 months, the mean progression was 45% and 48%, respectively. The degree of progression of CAD was related primarily to the length of time between arteriograms and to serum cholesterol values (Fig. 2-8). These data indicate that the risk of progressive CAD in patients is related to serum cholesterol values and time. The data also indi-

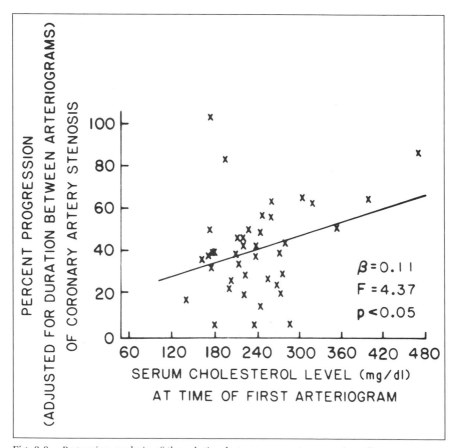

Fig. 2-8. Regression analysis of the relation between percent progression of coronary artery disease and serum cholesterol level at the time of the first arteriogram. Progression of disease has been adjusted for duration of the interval between arteriograms to account for the relation between duration and progression. Reproduced with permission from Shea et al.[30]

cate that an accurate, quantitative method of measuring coronary arteriograms quantitatively may be used to measure progression of CHD.

To evaluate the best method of quantitating the progression of CAD, Ellis and co-investigators[31] in Stanford, California, studied 4 measurements in 114 coronary segments from 35 medically treated patients from whom angiograms were obtained 5 years apart. Only stenoses of <70% that were visualized in nearly identical projections on both angiograms were evaluated. Vessel edges were measured by use of catheter calibration and an automated computer algorithm yielding 2 "absolute dimensions" (mean and minimum diameters) and 2 measurements (percent stenosis and atheroma area) that required a "normal reference" diameter. The coefficient of variation for repeated segment measurements was less for mean and minimum diameter than for percent stenosis and area of atheroma. The best measure of progression of CAD as determined by t-test comparison of different methods was the change in mean diameter over time, whether calculated on a per coronary segment or per patient basis. Based on this measurement and its standard deviation of progression of CAD in this patient subset with relatively benign disease, it was estimated that 470 patients per group would be required for an interventional study to demonstrate a 33% reduction in disease progression (207 patients for 50% reduction) at a 95% confidence level and 90% power.

SILENT MYOCARDIAL ISCHEMIA

Recent studies with ST-segment monitoring in patients with angina, positive exercise tests, and CAD have revealed that most patients had frequent and usually asymptomatic episodes of ST-segment depression. To understand the relation between transient myocardial ischemia observed during an exercise test and ischemic activity out of hospital, Campbell and co-investigators[32] in Boston, Massachusetts, followed 39 patients with well documented CAD and positive treadmill exercise test results for 24–28 hours with continuous ambulatory monitoring during daily activities. A total of 245 episodes of transient ischemia were recorded in 21 of 32 patients with positive exercise electrocardiograms (group 1), whereas 7 patients with negative test results (group II) had no episodes of transient ischemia during monitoring out of hospital. Certain measures in the exercise test were related to the severity of ischemia out of hospital: there were more episodes and a greater total duration of transient ischemia per 24 hours of ambulatory monitoring in patients in whom ischemic electrocardiographic changes developed before 6 minutes of exercise or at a heart rate of <150 beats/minute and in those in whom ST-segment changes persisted for >5 minutes after exercise. In contrast, there was no relation between transient ischemia out of hospital and the commonly quoted exercise variables: chest pain, total exercise duration, and the maximum levels of heart rate, systolic BP, and double product. Thus, patients with CAD and negative exercise electrocardiograms are most unlikely to have active ischemia during normal daily life. Certain features of the positive exercise test, namely the exercise duration at onset of significant ST depression, the heart rate at this threshold point, and the persistence after exercise of these ischemic changes are all related to the level of this disease activity during daily life. These findings may help to assess risk and explain why the early positive exercise test is an adverse sign for coronary events.

Campbell and associates[33] from Boston, Massachusetts, performed ambulatory Holter monitoring of ST segments out of the hospital in 7 asympto-

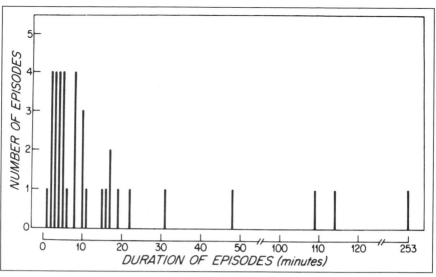

Fig. 2-9. Distribution and frequency of duration of episodes of ST depression during ambulatory monitoring. Episodes ranged from 1 to 253 minutes in duration.

matic subjects with CAD during normal daily activities. Their condition was detected because they all had a silent positive exercise test and angiographically proved CAD. During a total of 384 hours of monitoring, 37 asymptomatic episodes of ST depression (≥ 1 mm and lasting ≥ 30 seconds) were recorded in 5 of the patients. Most episodes (68%) were ≤ 10 minutes in duration but ranged from 1–253 minutes (Fig. 2-9), and most (70%) had a maximal ST depression of 1–2 mm. A small increase in heart rate, ranging from 1 to 34 beats/minute, preceded 65% of the episodes, but 35% were associated with no change or even a decline before the onset of ischemia (Fig. 2-10). Fifty-four percent of the episodes occurred during rest or usual light physical activity, 8% during sleep and only 38% during exercise, including 1 prolonged bout while jogging. During 78% of the episodes, the subjects rated their mental activity as usual and only 14% occurred during mental stress. In addition, a distinct diurnal variation was noted with 57% of the ischemia occurring between 0600 and 1200 hours (Fig. 2-11). Therefore, most asymptomatic subjects had active transient ischemia during daily life, with many of the characteristics already described in symptomatic subjects with CAD.

Cohn and associates[34] from Stoneybrook, New York, studied the effect of beta-adrenergic blockade on regional LV wall motion abnormalities in 11 patients with CAD and silent myocardial ischemia during exercise testing. Four patients were asymptomatic; 7 were asymptomatic after an AMI. LV wall motion abnormalities were characterized by reduced regional EF during exercise as determined by gated left anterior oblique images of the cardiac blood pool. In the 11 patients, 10 anteroseptal and 8 inferoposterior regions were subserved by stenotic coronary arteries. Before beta blockade, regional EF decreased in 15 of 18 regions. After beta blockade, this occurred in only 6 of 18 regions; the other 12 regions showed no change or an actual increase in regional EF. Thus, beta-adrenergic blockade effectively improved the reduction in exercise regional EF usually seen in patients with CAD with silent myocardial ischemia. One probable mechanism of action is a reduction in myocardial oxygen requirement at peak exercise.

Picano and associates[35] from Pisa, Italy, performed a dipyridamole-echocardiography test in 83 patients with angina on effort and either nega-

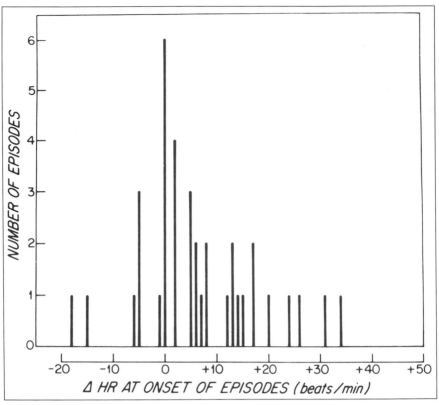

Fig. 2-10.   Distribution of change in heart rate (HR) at onset of ST depression from the minute preceding the episode.

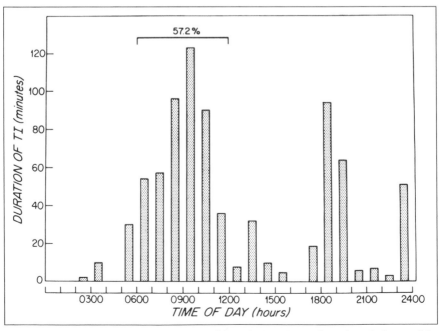

Fig. 2-11.   Duration of ischemic ST-segment depression in minutes throughout 24 hours of the day in 5 of the 7 patients with silent positive exercise tests. Most episodes of ischemia (57.2%) occur between 0600 and 1200 noon. TI = transient ischemia.

tive or nondiagnostic exercise stress test results to determine the usefulness of this test for detection of CAD. The dipyridamole-echo test (2-D echocardiographic monitoring combined with intravenous dipyridamole infusion at a maximal dosage of 0.84 mg/kg over 10 minutes) and coronary angiography were performed in all patients. Positivity of dipyridamole-echocardiography test was based on the detection of regional transient asynergy of contraction. At coronary arteriography, 50 of the 83 patients had significant (>70% diameter reduction) CAD: 27 had 1-vessel, 17 had 2-vessel, and 6 and 3-vessel CAD. Interpretable echocardiograms were recorded in all the patients studied. The dipyridamole-echocardiography test results were positive in 27 of the 50 patients (54%) with CAD. No patient without CAD had a positive test result. In conclusion, the dipyridamole-echocardiography test frequently unmasks electrocardiographically silent effort myocardial ischemia by providing objective mechanical evidence of the ischemic event.

Kaski and associates[36] from London, UK, performed continuous 48-hour electrocardiographic monitoring during unrestricted daily life in 19 patients with syndrome X (typical exertional angina, positive exercise test response [at least 0.1 mV of ST-segment depression]), and no evidence of coronary spasm in angiographically normal coronary arteries. Fifty-eight ischemic episodes of ≥0.1 mV of ST-segment depression were observed in the same electrocardiographic leads that showed ST depression during stress testing: 28 (48%) were accompanied by anginal pain and 30 (52%) were asymptomatic. No significant differences were found between painful and silent ST-segment depression with regard to the number of episodes, their temporal distribution, magnitude, duration or heart rate at onset of ST-segment depression. In the minute preceding ischemic ST shifts, heart rate did not change in 33% of episodes or increased by <10 beats/minute in 28%. Heart rate at onset of ST depression was significantly lower during ambulatory electrographic monitoring than during exercise testing (98 ± 18 -vs- 117 ± 17 beats/minute. During ambulatory monitoring, 85 episodes of sinus tachycardia (exceeding by 10 to 80 beats/minute the heart rate that triggered ischemia during exercise testing) occurred in the absence of angina or ST-segment shifts. The results of this study suggest that in patients with syndrome X, myocardial ischemia frequently develops during daily life, silent ischemia is an important component of this syndrome, and increased oxygen demand in the presence of impaired coronary vasodilatory capacity is not the only cause of AMI. Active mechanisms that transiently reduce coronary flow may act and explain occurrence of angina at rest and with minimal exertion.

Deanfield and associates[37] from London, UK, compared the effect of *smoking a single cigarette on regional myocardial profusion* in 13 chronic smokers with stable angina pectoris using positron emission tomography with rubidium-82 (^{82}Rb). After exercise, 8 patients (61%) had angina, ST depression, and abnormal regional myocardial perfusion (Fig. 2-12). Uptake of ^{82}Rb increased from 49 ± 8–60 ± 7 in remote myocardium, but decreased from 46 ± 3–37 ± 5 in an ischemic area. The remaining 5 patients (39%) had homogeneous increases in ^{82}Rb uptake without angina or ST depression. After smoking, 6 of the 8 patients with positive exercise test responses had a decrease in ^{82}Rb uptake, from 47 ± 3–35 ± 6 in the same segment of myocardium affected during exercise. However, in contrast to exercise, the events during smoking were largely silent. The absolute decreases in regional ^{82}Rb uptake after smoking occurred at significantly lower levels of myocardial oxygen demand than after exercise. This suggests that an impairment of coronary blood supply is responsible. Thus, in smokers with CAD, each cigarette can cause profound silent disturbances of regional myocardial perfusion that are likely to occur frequently during daily life. Such repeated insults

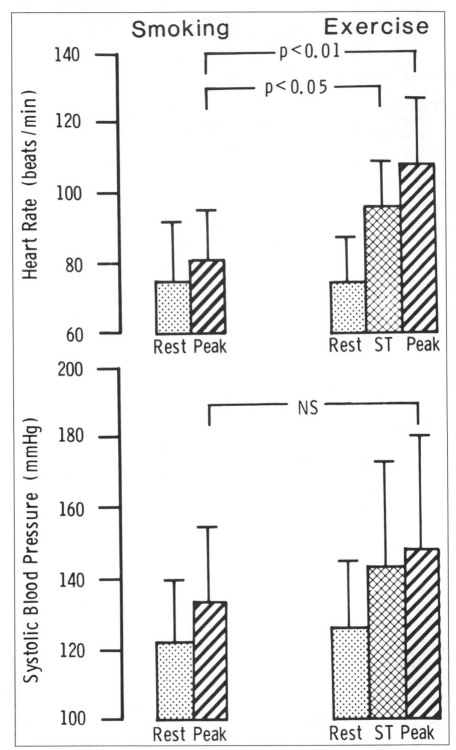

Fig. 2-12. Histogram showing hemodynamic responses in patients to smoking and exercise. The peak heart rate after smoking was significantly lower than both the peak heart rate after exercise and the heart rate at the onset of ST-segment depression (ST) during exercise. The peak systolic blood pressure was also lower after smoking but this did not reach statistical significance.

may represent an important mechanism linking smoking with coronary events.

Gottlieb and associates[38] from Baltimore, Maryland, examined the prevalence and prognostic importance of silent myocardial ischemia detected by continuous electrocardiographic monitoring in 70 patients with unstable angina pectoris. All the patients received intensive medical treatment with nitrates, beta blockers, and calcium channel blockers. Continuous electrocardiographic recordings were made during the first 2 days in the coronary care unit to quantify the frequency and duration of asymptomatic ischemic episodes, defined as a transient ST-segment shift of 1 mm or more. Thirty-seven patients (group 1) had at least 1 episode of silent ischemia, and the other 33 patients had no silent ischemia (group 2). Over the subsequent month, AMI occurred in 6 patients in group 1 and in only 1 in group 2; bypass surgery or angioplasty was required for recurrent symptomatic angina in 10 patients in group 1 and only 3 in group 2 (Fig. 2-13). Survival-curve analysis demonstrated that silent ischemia was associated with these outcomes, and multivariate analysis showed that silent ischemia was the best predictor of these outcomes among the 15 variables tested. Patients in group 1 with ≥60 minutes of silent ischemia per 24 hours had a worse prognosis than those with <60 minutes per 24 hours (Fig. 2-14). Silent ischemia occurred in >50% of the patients with unstable angina, despite intensive medical therapy, and it identified a subset who were at high risk for early unfavorable outcomes.

Previous studies have shown that the severity and duration of myocardial ischemia are necessary but not sufficient factors to explain the occurrence of anginal pain. Glazier and associates[39] from London, UK, studied the responses to a battery of painful stimuli in 12 patients with predominantly painless (group A) and in 15 patients with predominantly painful (group B) ischemic episodes. The severity of myocardial ischemia as assessed by the measurement of ST-segment depression during exercise stress testing and during ambulatory electrocardiographic monitoring was comparable in the 2 groups. Patients in group A had a significantly higher threshold and tolerance for forearm ischemia (+32%, +120%), cold (+100%, +180%) and

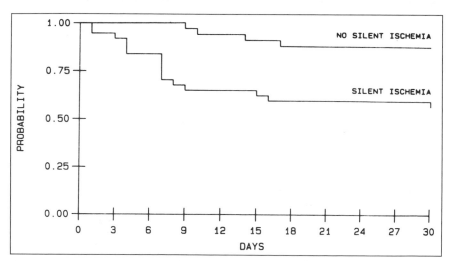

Fig. 2-13. Kaplan–Meier curves comparing the cumulative probabilities of not experiencing myocardial infarction or revascularization for recurrent angina during a period of 30 days for the 37 patients with silent ischemia (group 1) and the 33 patients without it (group 2), as detected by continuous electrocardiographic monitoring (p <0.002). Reproduced with permission from Gottlieb et al.[38]

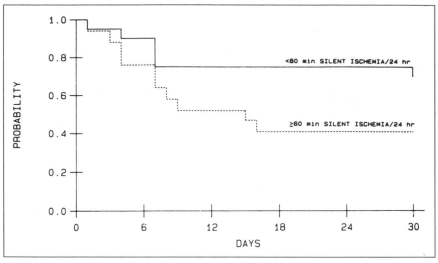

Fig. 2-14. Kaplan–Meier curves showing the cumulative probabilities of not experiencing myocardial infarction or revascularization for recurrent angina during a period of 30 days in the patients with silent ischemia, comparing the patients with less than 60 minutes of silent ischemia per 24 hours and those with more yhan 60 minutes per 24 hours during the two days of electrocardiographic monitoring (p = 0.04). Reproduced with permission from Gottlieb et al.[38]

electrical skin stimulation (+145%, +109%), but the overlap between the 2 groups was often appreciable. In the 6 patients with the longest tolerance times for forearm ischemia pain (all in group A) and in the 5 having the shortest tolerance times (all in group B), plasma levels of B endorphin, metenkephalin, noradrenaline, and adrenaline were similar during both the basal state and the induction of forearm ischemic pain. Thus, a generalized defective perception of painful stimuli plays an important role in many patients with predominantly painless myocardial ischemia. Other mechanisms, however, also may be important, particularly in patients whose threshold and tolerance values overlap with those of patients who have predominantly painful myocardial ischemia.

ANGINA PECTORIS

Survival in mild angina and in healed myocardial infarction with and without angina

Proudfit and associates[40] from Cleveland, Ohio, analyzed 408 catheterized patients who had mild angina pectoris or AMI without angina. The selective criteria were in accord with the criteria used for entry into the Coronary Artery Surgery Study which had been previously reported. Medical treatment had been chosen initially by the cardiologist, referring physician, or the patient, although 27% had late operation. Five-year survival rates were 91% and 72% for mild angina with a high or low EF and 85% for those who had AMI without subsequent angina. Survival rates were 95%, 88%, and 80% for 1, 2, and 3-artery CAD, respectively (Fig. 2-15). For patients who had an EF ≥0.50, 5-year survivals were 95%, 89%, and 83% for 1, 2, and 3-artery involvement, respectively (Fig. 2-16). Good LV function (Fig. 2-17), single artery CAD, and a short history were favorable prognostic variables in multivariate analysis of patients who had angina pectoris. Statistical methods of dealing with patients who had late operation influenced calculated survival, especially for patients at relatively high risk. The lower survival rates for the whole group and most subsets compared with survival rates in the randomized trial may be of clinical importance.

Daly and associates[41] from Dublin, Ireland, examined the course of postcoronary angina pectoris in 555 men who had survived a first AMI or unstable angina. Patients were aged >60 years and were followed yearly for up to 17 years. Only 25 (4.5%) had CABG. Most patients with angina were treated by nitrates alone. One year after AMI 24% of survivors (124/515) reported angina pectoris, and the proportions at 5, 10, and 15 years were 30%, 30%, and 44% respectively. Seventeen years after the initial event, 35% of the survivors had never reported postcoronary angina. The patients who

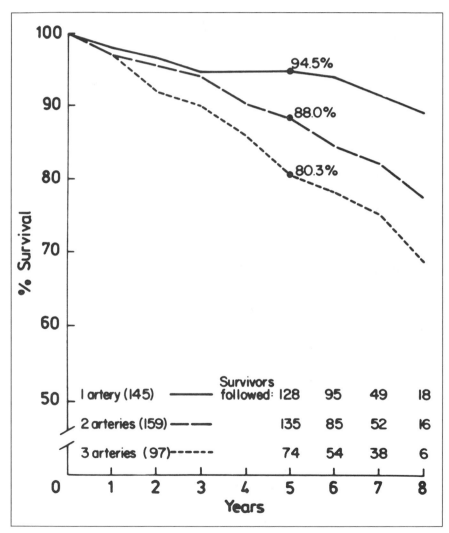

Fig. 2-15. Survival by number of arteries affected. The numerals in parentheses indicate the numbers of patients at zero time; the other numerals refer to the numbers of survivors followed at five, six, seven, and eight years. Bypass surgery was done in 14%, 17%, and 32% of patients with one, two, and three artery disease respectively at five years, and 23%, 27%, and 32% at eight years (p = 0 · 004). Reproduced with permission from Proudfit et al.[40]

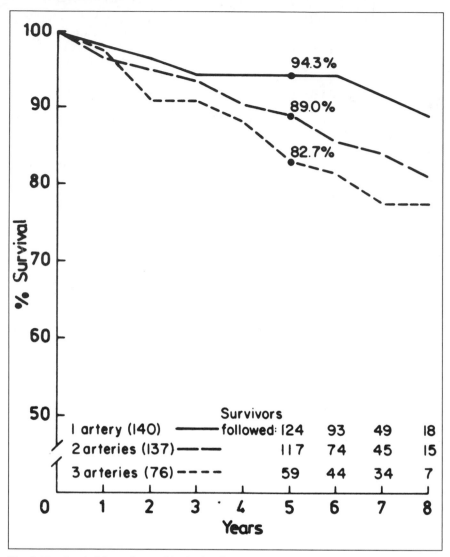

Fig. 2-16. Survival in patients with ejection fraction $\geq 0 \cdot 50$ by number of arteries affected. Reproduced with permission from Proudfit et al.[40]

had angina in the year after their coronary attack had a poorer long-term survival than the group who were symptom free over the first year. These patients also had longer subsequent periods with angina, though in 42% angina resolved before death after a median of 2.9 years. Throughout follow-up, mortality during periods in which patients had angina was higher than in the symptom-free periods. This long-term follow-up study of patients after a coronary event confirms that the presence or absence of angina may vary considerably in patients treated medically and that the presence of angina is associated with a poorer prognosis.

Repeated exercise testing

In patients with stable angina, the variability of results during repeated exercise tests is higher in some than in others. Crea and colleagues[42] from London, England, assessed whether this difference can be explained by a different susceptibility of the coronary arteries to vasoconstrictor stimuli. Ten patients (group A) with stable angina, in whom myocardial ischemia (angina and ST-segment depression >0.1 mV) developed after ergonovine-induced coronary constriction, and 10 other patients (group B) with stable angina but a negative ergonovine test result, were subjected to 2 treadmill exercise tests. The variability of heart rate and heart rate–BP product at 0.1 mV ST-segment depression was significantly higher in group A than in group B (12 ± 4 -vs- 4 ± 4 beats/minute, $p < 0.001$ and $3,366 \pm 1,900$ -vs- 930 ± 960 beat/minute $\times$ mmHg, $p < 0.005$), as was the variability of heart rate–BP product at the onset of angina ($3,887 \pm 2,400$ -vs- $1,428 \pm 1,800$ beats/minute $\times$ mmHg, $p < 0.04$). The remaining exercise parameters were always more variable in group A than in group B, but these differences did not achieve statistical significance. Thus, patients with stable angina in whom

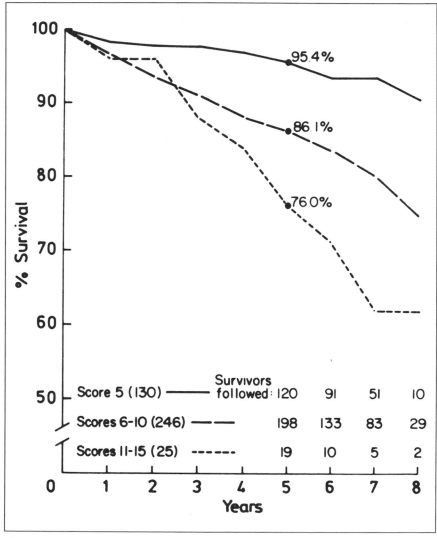

Fig. 2-17.   Ventricular score (Coronary Artery Surgery Study method).[3] Score 5 means normal ventricle, scores 6–10 indicate mild impairment, and scores 11–15 represent moderate impairment. Reproduced with permission from Proudfit et al.[40]

myocardial ischemia develops in response to ergonovine have a larger variability of results during repeat exercise testing.

Significance of ST-segment elevation during unstable period

de Servi and colleagues[43] from Pavia, Italy, delineated the clinical, electrocardiographic and angiographic features of a large series of consecutive patients with angina at rest. Transient ST-segment elevation during pain was observed in 219 patients (group I), whereas 220 patients had ST-segment depression during pain (group II). Group II patients had a higher frequency of systemic hypertension before AMI, exertional angina, and a progressive aggravation of symptoms before hospitalization; group I patients had a prevalence of recent onset angina and more frequently had severe ventricular arrhythmias during pain. Furthermore, a larger number of patients showing ST-segment depression during chest pain had multivessel CAD, LM CAD, and lower values of LVEF than patients with ST-segment elevation during pain. Survival curves of medically treated patients had a significantly better long-term prognosis in patients in group I (Fig. 2-18). The direction of the ST-segment shift during anginal attacks at rest may therefore allow a classification of patients included into the broad spectrum of unstable angina. This distinction should be taken into consideration in studies aimed at evaluating long-term prognosis or the results of medical and surgical therapy.

Sclarovsky and associates[44] from Petah Tikvah and Tel Aviv, Israel, evaluated 46 patients with unstable angina, who had no significant changes in heart rate, BP, and double product (as evidence of increased oxygen demand) during episodes of chest pain. Coronary angiography was performed in all patients during the same hospitalization. Of 26 patients with unstable angina and ST depression (group A), 10 had LM CAD and 8 had LM-equivalent CAD. Of 20 patients with unstable angina and ST elevation (group B), only 1 had LM CAD and 1 had LM-equivalent CAD. All patients in group A had ST

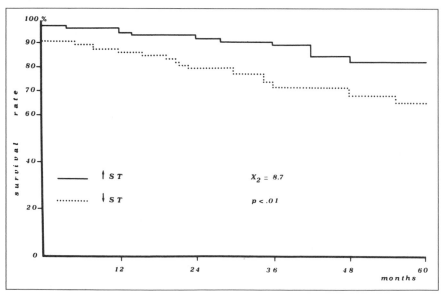

Fig. 2-18. Survival curves in medically treated patients with angina at rest. A significantly worse prognosis is noted in patients showing ST segment depression during pain. Reproduced with permission from de Servi et al.[43]

depression in leads V_4 and V_5, and all patients in group B had ST elevation in leads V_2 and V_3. The presence of ST depression in leads V_4 and V_5 in unstable angina patients without evidence of increased oxygen demand suggests significant LM or LM-equivalent CAD; therefore, coronary angiography is recommended during the same hospitalization.

Exercise testing after stabilization of unstable angina

Butman and associates[45] from Long Beach and Irvine, California, evaluated the safety and diagnostic use of exercise testing in patients with unstable angina: 78 patients underwent submaximal exercise testing and diagnostic cardiac catheterization early after stabilization of their pain. Thirty-six patients (46%) had a positive exercise test manifested as angina or ST-segment depression of ≥ 0.1 mV during or immediately after exercise. Of 36 patients (92%) with a positive exercise test, 33 had multivessel CAD compared to 18 of 42 patients (43%) with a negative exercise study (Fig. 2-19). Of 36 patients (61%) with a positive exercise test, 22 had 3-vessel CAD compared to 12 of 42 patients (29%) with a negative test (Fig. 2-19). The sensitivity of exercise testing in detecting multivessel CAD was 65%, specificity 89%, predictive value of a positive test 92%, predictive value of a negative test 57%, and overall accuracy 73%. When the 42 patients taking beta blockers were examined, these values were essentially unchanged. Ventricular arrhythmias during exercise testing were associated with a lower EF, $61 \pm 13\%$, compared to $68 \pm 11\%$ in patients without ventricular arrhythmias. Submaximal exercise testing after stabilization of patients with unstable angina is safe and useful in evaluating patients for the presence of multivessel CAD.

Dipyridamole echocardiography

Picano et al[46] in Pisa, Italy, studied the dipyridamole echocardiographic test in 93 patients with effort chest pain and in 10 control subjects. Dipyridamole was given intravenously and 2-D echocardiographic monitoring was utilized thereafter. The test was considered positive when regional asynergy appeared after dipyridamole administration. When negative at the low dose of dipyridamole, the test was repeated on a different day with a higher dose (0.56 mg/kg body weight in 4 minutes of dipyridamole at the low dose and 0.84 mg/kg in 10 minutes at the high dose). All 93 patients had coronary arteriography; 72 had significant CAD. Of the 93 patients, 38 had a positive low-dose dipyridamole echocardiographic test; 15 other patients with a negative low dose had a positive high-dose test. All 53 patients with a positive test had significant CAD; 12 had a negative exercise stress test. The dipyridamole echocardiographic test had an overall specificity higher than that of the exercise stress test (100% -vs- 71%) and a similar overall sensitivity (74% -vs- 69%). These data suggest that dipyridamole echocardiography adds to the noninvasive ability to detect significant CAD in patients.

Quantitation of coronary anatomy

Wilson and co-workers[47] in Iowa City, Iowa, postulated that coronary lesions associated with recent AMI or unstable angina would have an angiographic morphology suggesting disruption of an atherosclerotic plaque and would appear morphologically different from lesions associated with chronic stable angina. To test this hypothesis, these investigators performed quanti-

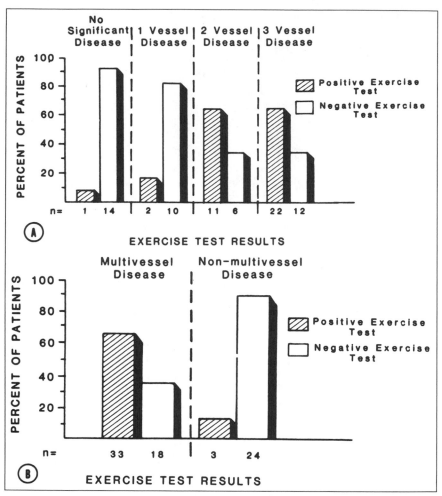

Fig. 2-19. Results of exercise testing in relation to coronary anatomy. *A*, Results of exercise testing in relation to specific anatomic subgroups. *B*, Results of exercise testing in patients with and without multivessel disease. A positive exercise test is defined as angina and/or 0.1 mV ST segment depression. The three patients with left main disease are included in the group with three-vessel disease. Reproduced with permission from Butman et al.[45]

tative coronary angiography with the Brown-Dodge method in 15 patients 4–30 days after AMI in 10 patients with the abrupt onset of unstable angina and 1-vessel CAD, and in 15 patients with chronic stable angina without prior AMI. Serial arterial diameters (20 to 40) within each lesion were determined and the degree of luminal irregularity was quantitated by calculation of an "ulceration" index. The ulceration index was defined as the diameter of the least severe narrowing within the lesion (downward lip of the ulcer) divided by the maximal intralesional diameter (presumably the maximal diameter of the ulcerated portion of the vessel (Fig. 2-20). Most lesions analyzed resulted in severe luminal stenoses (mean 78% area stenosis, all groups). Despite small differences in mean lesion severity among groups, overlap in the degree of luminal compromise prevented precise classification of lesions associated with AMI or unstable angina based on percent stenosis or minimum luminal cross-sectional area. The mean ulceration index of lesions in patients with unstable angina and in the infarct-related artery in those with AMI was 0.62 and 0.61, respectively. These were significantly different from the mean ulceration indexes of lesions in patients with stable angina (0.96) or from indexes of lesions in the noninfarct-related vessel in patients with AMI (0.90). None of 10 lesions associated with unstable angina and 14 to 15 infarct-related lesions had an ulceration index <0.78. All lesions associated with stable angina and each lesion in the noninfarct-related vessel in patients with AMI had an ulceration index of >0.83. The ulceration index did not vary significantly with the degree of luminal stenosis or prior treatment with thrombolytic agents. These data provide quantitative evidence that lesions associated with AMI or the abrupt onset of unstable angina are of a similar characteristic angiographic morphology that is suggestive of plaque disruption and not commonly seen in lesions associated with chronic stable angina.

Ambrose et al[48] in New York, New York, studied the evolution of lesions responsible for unstable angina evaluating coronary anatomy and morphology on angiography in patients with stable angina progressive to unstable angina. Group I comprised 25 patients with a history of stable angina restudied after an acute episode of unstable angina and group II included 21 patients with little or no change in symptoms between cardiac catheterizations. Progression of CAD occurred in 19 (76%) of 25 patients in group I compared with 7 (33%) of 21 patients in group II. Of the 25 lesions with progression in group I, 17 progressed <100% and 8–100% occlusion. Eighteen of the 25 lesions in group I were previously insignificant (<50% narrowing on the first catheterization). In contrast, of the 8 lesions with progression of the stenoses in group II, only 2 were previously insignificant, whereas 6 showed at least 50% stenoses on the initial study. Eccentric stenoses were seen in 71% of all lesions with progression to <100% occlusion in patients in group I, but they were not found in any group II arteries with progression. Progression of stenoses was common with acute presentations of unstable angina and most lesions progressed from previously insignificant stenoses. An eccentric lesion with a narrow neck due to one or more previously insignificant stenoses. An eccentric lesion with a narrow neck due to one or more overhanging edges, irregular, scalloped borders, or both, was the most common anatomic con-

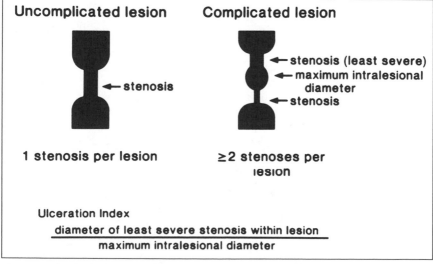

Fig. 2-20. Method for classification of stenoses and calculation of the ulceration index. Reproduced with permission from Wilson et al.[47]

figuration of the coronary lesions in patients having unstable angina subsequently.

Single-vessel disease

Yasue and colleagues[49] from Kumamoto City and Shizuoka City, Japan, examined the pathogenesis of angina pectoris in 101 patients with 1-vessel CAD except those with 99–100% occlusion. The attacks could not be induced or could not be reproducibly induced by maximal treadmill exercise at the same hour of different days within a week period in 54 (54%) of the patients (group A). In the 47 patients whose attacks were reproducibly induced by exercise (group B), propranolol, 80 mg orally, did not suppress the attacks in 87% of these patients. Diltiazem, 90 mg, and nifedipine, 20 mg given orally, suppressed the attacks completely in 83% of group A patients and in 81% of the group B patients. Coronary arteriography showed that dynamic obstruction of the artery supplying the area of myocardium represented by ST-segment deviation appeared during the attacks and disappeared with subsidence of the attacks in all the patients in whom coronary arteriography was done during the attack. It was concluded that angina is usually caused not by increased myocardial oxygen demand but by dynamic coronary obstruction or by a combination of both in most patients with 1-vessel CAD.

With angiographically normal coronary arteries

Schofield and associates[50] from Manchester, UK, assessed LV function in 201 patients who presented with angina pectoris and who were subsequently found to have completely normal coronary arteries by angiography. LV angiograms from 187 patients were suitable for analysis of systolic regional wall motion; 121 had normal and 66 had a total of 115 hypokinetic segments. Patients with hypokinesia had a significantly higher LV end-systolic volume and a significantly lower LVEF and exercise capacity than those in whom regional wall motion was normal: 31% of patients with normal wall motion and 30% of those with hypokinesia had a rest LV end-diastolic pressure >15 mm Hg. There were significantly more smokers in the group with hypokinetic segments. Thus, of patients with angina and normal coronary angiograms, 25% had evidence of LV systolic dysfunction, 20% had evidence of diastolic dysfunction, and 11% had evidence of both systolic and diastolic dysfunction. The results suggest that smoking may be associated with LV regional wall motion abnormalities.

Mosseri and co-workers[51] in Jerusalem, Israel, studied 6 patients who had angina pectoris but angiographically patent major coronary arteries. Two patients also had CHF. Three patients had supraventricular tachyarrhythmias. Three patients had conduction disturbances. During coronary angiography, the patients had significantly reduced flow velocity of angiographic contrast medium compared with that in a control group. Echocardiography and Doppler flow studies showed a tendency for symmetrical thickening of the LV wall, enlargement of the RV cavity, and reduced compliance of both ventricles. RV endomyocardial biopsy revealed abnormal small coronary arteries with fibromuscular hyperplasia, hypertrophy of the media, myointimal proliferation, and endothelial degeneration. Capillaries had swollen endothelial cells encroaching on the lumen. Myocardial hypertrophy, lipofuscin deposition, and patchy fibrosis also were observed. These cases show that small-vessel CAD can cause classic angina pectoris.

Coronary angioscopy

To visualize intracoronary lesions in patients with different clinical expressions of CAD, Sherman and associates[52] from Los Angeles, California, performed coronary angioscopy during CABG in 10 patients with unstable angina and in 10 patients with stable CAD. They examined a total of 32 arteries using flexible fiberoptic angioscopes: 22 arteries had no acute intimal lesions; 3 had complex plaques; 6 had thrombi, and 1 had both. Coronary angiography correctly identified the absence of complex plaque and thrombus in 22 arteries, but it detected only 1 of 4 complex plaques and 1 of 7 thrombi. On angioscopy, none of the 17 arteries in the patients with stable CAD had either a complex plaque or thrombus. In the "offending" arteries of the patients with unstable angina, all 3 patients with accelerated angina had complex plaques and all 7 with angina at rest had thrombi. The authors concluded that angioscopy frequently reveals complex plaques or thrombi not detected by coronary angiography. These observations suggest that angina refractory to medical treatment can be caused by unstable processes in the intima. Ulceration of plaques may increase the frequency and severity of effort angina, and the subsequent development of partially occlusive thrombi may cause unstable rest angina.

Platelet activation

Morphologic and clinical studies have suggested that platelets have a roll in the pathogenesis of unstable angina and AMI. The relation of platelet activation to episodic myocardial ischemia in these patients, however, is unknown. Fitzgerald and associates[53] from Nashville, Tennessee, and Quebec, Canada, assessed the biosynthesis of thromboxane and prostacyclin as indexes of platelet activation in 36 patients admitted to the coronary care unit with chest pain: 16 had unstable angina pectoris; 14 had AMI, and 6 patients with noncardiac chest pain served as controls. Prostacyclin biosynthesis was markedly elevated in patients with AMI and correlated with plasma creatine kinase. The largest increase in thromboxane synthesis was observed in patients with unstable angina, in whom 84% of the episodes of chest pain were associated with phasic increases in the excretion of thromboxane and prostacyclin metabolites. However, 50% of such increases were not associated with chest pain, possibly reflecting silent myocardial ischemia. These data indicate that platelet activation occurs during spontaneous ischemia in patients with unstable angina. The increment in prostacyclin biosynthesis during such episodes may be a compensatory response of vascular endothelium that limits the degree or effects of platelet activation. If so, biochemically selective inhibition of the synthesis or action of thromboxane A_2 would be desirable in the treatment of unstable angina. In contrast, thromboxane inhibitors or antagonists would not be expected to be effective in patients with chronic stable angina, in whom there was no increase in the formation of thromboxane A_2.

This article was followed by an editorial entitled "Mechanisms of Unstable Angina" by Fuster and Chesebro[54] from New York, New York, and Rochester, Minnesota. These 2 editorialists concluded that successful antithrombotic therapy in patients with unstable angina and the efficacy of thrombolytic therapy in opening occluded coronary arteries in AMI represent testimony to the importance of thrombus in the acute and subacute coronary syndromes.

Davies and co-investigators[55] in London, UK, made a specific search for intramyocardial platelet aggregates in 90 patients who died suddenly of

CAD. Platelet aggregates in small intramyocardial vessels were found in 27 (30%). There was a significant difference in the incidence of platelet aggregates in patients with chest pain of recent origin (unstable angina) before death (16/36, 44%) and in those without it (11/54, 20%). Multifocal microscopic necrosis with involvement of the full thickness of the ventricular wall, including the subpericardial zone, was significantly more common in the patients with platelet emboli (56 -vs- 13%). With 1 exception, aggregates were confined to the segment of the myocardium immediately downstream of a major epicardial coronary artery containing an atheromatous plaque that had undergone fissuring and on which mural thrombus had developed. The results support the view that platelet aggregates in the myocardium represent an embolic phenomenon and are a potential cause of unstable angina.

Evolution to acute myocardial infarction

Sclarovsky and colleagues[56] from Petah Tikvah, and Tel Aviv, Israel, retrospectively evaluated 32 patients with unstable angina and no evidence of increased oxygen demand during episodes of chest pain (no significant changes in heart rate and BP), in whom AMI developed during the same hospitalization. Based on the type of ST changes during anginal pain, 2 groups were defined: group A included 19 patients who had ST elevation during AMI; 15 of these 19 patients (79%) were in Killip class I, 2 were in class II, and there was 1 patient each in classes III and IV, respectively. Only 1 of the 19 patients died. Group B included 13 patients who had ST depression during AMI; 9 of these 13 patients were in Killip class IV and the remaining 4 patients died before they could be evaluated. Ten of the 13 patients died (77%), 7 in electromechanical dissociation and 3 in cardiogenic shock. Necropsy, performed in 4 patients, revealed total LM obstruction. It was concluded that patients with unstable angina who, during attacks of chest pain, have ST depression and no evidence of increased oxygen demand, may have a poor prognosis when an AMI develops. This selected group of high-risk patients appears to need immediate intensive medical care and most probably early surgical treatment.

Prognostic significance of previous coronary bypass in unstable angina

Waters and associates[57] from Montreal, Canada, analyzed the effect of previous CABG, a mean of 55 months earlier (range 1–168), among patients hospitalized for unstable angina pectoris in 1982 and 1983. This group was compared with a group of 54 randomly selected patients with unstable angina without previous CABG (control patients). The 2 groups did not differ with respect to clinical characteristics at admission or hospital course. Coronary arteriograms, recorded in all but 4 CABG patients, revealed multivessel narrowing ≥70% luminal diameter in 40 CABG and 32 control patients, but when patent grafts were considered, the groups were comparable. Overall, 48 of 112 grafts were totally occluded and 14 had stenoses ≥70% in diameter. Complete or almost complete revascularization was feasible in 39 of 52 control and only 9 of 42 CABG patients. By 1 year, 46 control patients and 20 CABG patients had undergone CABG or PTCA; 42 of 53 control patients and only 22 of 50 CABG patients were in functional class 0 or 1. Cumulative adverse events (5 deaths, 10 AMI and 15 cases of recurrent unstable angina) were more frequent in the CABG group (20 -vs- 10). Thus, although their clinical features and hospital course are similar, patients with unstable angina who have undergone previous CABG do not do as well as other patients with unstable angina because they are less amenable to revascularization.

TREATMENT

Placebo

Khurmi and associates[58] from Middlesex, UK, studied the effects of placebo in 150 patients aged 42–75 years with stable exertional angina pectoris, using multistage graded exercise testing. Treadmill exercise, using on-line computer analysis of the electrocardiogram, was performed after the basal period, during which time the patients had no treatment for 2 weeks, and after 2 weeks of placebo therapy. Mean exercise time during no treatment was 6.0 ± 0.2 minutes and during placebo was 6.1 ± 0.2 minutes. Similarly, time to development of 1 mm of ST-segment depression of 4.0 ± 0.2 minutes without treatment was 4.1 ± 0.2 minutes after 2 weeks of placebo therapy. Placebo failed to show any effect on rest or maximal heart rate or on maximal ST-segment depression. It also failed to increase exercise tolerance or to improve other objective indexes of effort-induced myocardial ischemia in both single- and double-blind protocols in patients with stable exertional angina pectoris. Therefore, placebo control of antianginal drug trials that use exercise testing for evaluation of effect is unnecessary and can be omitted.

Transdermal nitroglycerin

Thadani and associates[59] from Oklahoma City, Oklahoma, studied the duration of effect of transdermal nitroglycerin patches in 14 patients with angina pectoris. By titrating the dose to achieve specific circulatory effects, they chose a patch size that produced a consistent decrease in systolic BP of ≥ 10 mmHg for each patient (10 cm^2 in 7 patients, 20 cm^2 in 5, and 40 cm^2 in 2; releasing 5, 10, and 20 mg of nitroglycerin per 24 hours, respectively). The effects of these individualized patches were compared with those of placebo patches. Compared with placebo, nitroglycerin patches increased exercise duration to the onset of angina (257 ± 72 compared with 383 ± 130 seconds) and total exercise time (338 ± 89 compared with 456 ± 119 seconds) and decreased ST-segment depression (1.0 ± 0.5 compared with 0.6 ± 0.4 mm) at 4 hours but not at 24 and 48 hours. The authors concluded that nitroglycerin patches do not show objective evidence of antianginal or anti-ischemic effects for 24 hours. Tolerances to the circulatory and antianginal effects probably develops within 24 hours of patch application.

Nitroglycerin ointment has been shown to be effective in the treatment of angina pectoris and CHF. Its duration of action is usually 4 to 6 hours. Klein and associates[60] from Tel-Aviv, Israel, presented data that show that a new slow release nitroglycerin ointment produces hemodynamic improvement over at least 24 hours. Twenty patients with CAD were tested with serial gated equilibrium radionuclide ventriculography before and at various stages of continuous, once-a-day use of slow-release nitroglycerin ointment and 4 days after cessation of therapy. Nitroglycerin ointment significantly decreased LV end-diastolic and end-systolic volumes both at rest (23 and 33%) and during handgrip exercise (22 and 32%) when examined after continuous usage ≥ 24 hours. EF increased 21% at rest (from $0.42 \pm 0.15 - 0.51 \pm -0.18$). The ratio of peak systolic pressure to end-systolic volume increased

85% at rest and 54% during exercise. All values had returned to baseline 4 days after cessation of treatment. Thus, slow-release nitroglycerin ointment may be useful in the treatment of angina pectoris and CHF on a once-a-day basis.

Nitroglycerin lingual spray

Parker and Associates[61] from Kingston, Canada, studied 20 patients with chronic stable, exercise-induced angina pectoris after each received lingual sprays that equalled 0.2, 0.4, and 0.8 mg of nitroglycerin. The hemodynamic effects and changes in exercise time to the onset of angina and to the development of moderate angina were compared with those of placebo spray and 0.4 mg of sublingual nitroglycerin. A dose-response relation was apparent with the 3 doses of active spray for heart rate at rest but not for standing systolic BP. Sublingual nitroglycerin produced effects similar to those with 0.4 and 0.8 mg of nitroglycerin spray, but exceeded the response to 0.2 mg of nitroglycerin spray. Treadmill walking time to the onset of angina and to the development of moderate angina was prolonged with each dose of nitroglycerin spray and showed a dose-response relation with significantly greater effects with increasing doses of nitroglycerin spray. This study indicates that nitroglycerin lingual spray is effective in the prophylaxis of angina and should be effective in the therapy of exercise-induced or spontaneous episodes of angina pectoris. The dose of 0.4 or 0.8 mg would appear to be most effective and similar to 0.4 mg of sublingual nitroglycerin.

Betaxolol

To assess the effect of beta blockade on LV performance in patients with LV dysfunction and stable angina pectoris, Alpert and associates[62] from Columbia, Missouri, studied 18 subjects taking a placebo followed by incremental doses of the cardioselective beta-adrenergic blocking agent betaxolol (5, 10, 20, and 40 mg/day). The study ended with the achievement of optimal clinical beta blockade (heart rate at rest 50–60 beats/minute, a 20% or smaller increase in heart rate during stage I of symptom-limited treadmill exercise using the modified Bruce protocol). Optimal clinical beta blockade produced a decrease in mean frequency of angina, from 6.8 ± 1.7–0.7 ± 0.8 episodes per week and an increase in mean treadmill exercise capacity, from 3.1 ± 1.7–7.7 ± 2.8 minutes. LV systolic function was assessed at rest and during symptom-limited exercise with radionuclide left ventriculography. Mean LVEF during therapy with placebo was 39 ± 7% at rest and 40 ± 8% at peak exercise. Mean LVEF during optimal clinical beta blockade was 43 ± 11% at rest and 45 ± 10% at peak exercise. No patient had clinical or radiographic signs of CHF. The results suggest that optimal clinical beta blockade with betaxolol, in doses sufficient to significantly reduce the frequency of angina and improve exercise capacity in patients with stable angina pectoris and mild-to-moderate LV systolic dysfunction, does not cause significant deterioration of LV systolic function or produce LV failure.

Diltiazem

Weiner and associates[63] from Boston, Massachusetts, assessed the safety and efficacy of a sustained-release preparation of diltiazem (diltiazem-SR), with dose levels of 240 and 360 mg/day in 18 patients with stable angina pectoris of effort. A double-blind, placebo-controlled, randomized, crossover protocol was used. Diltiazem-SR, when given twice daily, reduced the frequency of weekly anginal attacks, from 0.3 ± 10.4 with placebo to 3.7 ± 4.7 with 240 mg/day and to 3.1 ± 4.7 with 360 mg/day. Treadmill time was increased from 410 ± 180 seconds during the placebo phase to 519 ± 177 seconds during the 240-mg/day dose and to 506 ± 182 seconds during the 360-mg/day dose of diltiazem-SR. The time to the onset of angina and ischemic ST-segment depression were similarly prolonged by both doses of diltiazem-SR. The beneficial effects of diltiazem-SR appeared partly due to a reduction in the heart rate during submaximal exercise. Diltiazem-SR is effective at submaximal exercise. Diltiazem-SR is effective and safe for the treatment of angina of effort when given twice daily.

Joyal and associates[64] from Gainesville, Florida, investigated the mechanism of relief of angina pectoris by diltiazem in 14 patients with effort angina. They used a protocol to control heart rate. Coronary, systemic, and LV hemodynamic function was assessed at rest and during tachycardia stress (atrial pacing)–induced angina before and during diltiazem infusion. Angina occurred in all patients during tachycardia stress before diltiazem administration. During tachycardia stress at the heart rate that produced angina after diltiazem infusion, pressure-rate product, coronary sinus flow and resistance, and ST-segment depression were all similar to findings before diltiazem. Although at the onset of angina, systolic BP was usually slightly lower after diltiazem infusion (138 ± 11 -vs- 128 ± 11 mmHg), the pacing rate at onset of angina was higher in only 3 patients and the BP–heart rate product was higher in only 1 patient. After diltiazem, LV end-diastolic pressure increased less frequently after interruption of pacing. The results suggest that diltiazem favorably alters the relation between myocardial oxygen demand and supply at rest, but during tachycardia, anginal threshold and coronary reserve do not change. Diltiazem's potent antianginal action, shown in previous investigations using exercise-induced angina, is not prominent when heart rate is controlled. The major benefit of diltiazem in patients with stress-induced angina is related to reduction of myocardial oxygen demand rather than improved myocardial oxygen delivery.

Joyal and associates[65] from Gainesville, Florida, determined diltiazem serum concentration and the magnitude and time course of systemic and coronary hemodynamic and electrocardiographic responses to intravenous diltiazem (250 μg/kg intravenous bolus plus 1.4 μg/kg/min infusion) in 14 patients with chronic stable angina pectoris. After 3, 8, and 15 minutes this dosing schedule produced serum concentrations of 570 ± 259, 199 ± 62, and 136 ± 30 ng/ml, respectively. These drug levels were associated with a small transient increase in heart rate (6 beats/minute, mean) at 3 minutes, which occurred during the nadir of the BP response. At 8 and 15 minutes, heart rate was unchanged compared to control rates, although BP remained decreased (19% at 15 minutes). BP–heart rate product was significantly reduced as LV end-diastolic pressure and dP/dT remained unchanged. Systemic resistance decreased 17% and stroke index increased 10%. Coronary flow was maintained as coronary resistance declined (14%). PR interval prolongation (14%) occurred at 15 minutes. Correlations between changes in systolic, diastolic, and mean BP and drug concentration were significant. The intercept for each regression line was approximately 96 ng/ml diltiazem concentration, suggesting that this represents the minimum effective diltiazem serum concentration. These results indicate that intravenous diltiazem is well tolerated and promptly reduces BP and both systemic and coronary resistances without oxygen-wasting effects of an increase in heart rate.

Nifedipine

In 1981 a large double-blind, randomized, multicenter trial was started in The Netherlands to evaluate the therapeutic effects of nifedipine or metoprolol in patients with unstable angina pectoris. This study, called The Holland Interuniversity Nifedipine Trial (HINT), included several hundred patients to establish potential therapeutic effects. Van Der Wall and associates[66] from Utrecht, The Netherlands, studied the effects of nifedipine on LV performance in a subgroup of 37 HINT patients using radionuclide techniques. All patients (18 treated with nifedipine, 19 with placebo) underwent radionuclide angiography and 33 underwent thallium-201 scintigraphy just before and 48 hours after the start of treatment with the medication. Radionuclide angiographic studies also were performed 1 hour (29 patients) and 4 hours (31 patients) after the start of treatment. The thallium-201 images showed defects in 24 (73%) of the baseline images and in 21 (64%) of the 48-hour images. No significant differences were seen between patients receiving nifedipine or placebo in the incidence of new defects or in the disappearance of defects at 48 hours. Changes in thallium-201 images were not related to recurrence of myocardial ischemia or the development of AMI. Nineteen of the 37 patients (51%) with baseline blood pool images had a reduced LVEF ($38 \pm 10\%$) and 18 patients (49%) had a normal LVEF of $56 \pm 5\%$. LVEF improved after 48 hours in 8 patients receiving nifedipine and in only 1 patient receiving placebo. This effect was not present at 1 and 4 hours after treatment. Similar to findings with thallium-201, changes in LVEF did not reflect clinical outcome. Thus, nifedipine does not affect myocardial perfusion, but improves LV function in patients with unstable angina after 48 hours. These findings from HINT suggest a predominant afterload-reducing effect of nifedipine in patients with unstable angina 48 hours after starting treatment.

Nicardipine

Nicardipine, a new calcium channel blocking drug of the dihydropyridine family, was administered by Scheidt and associates[67] from New York, New York, to 63 patients at a dose of 30 or 40 mg 3 times daily in a multicenter, randomized, double-blind, placebo-controlled, crossover trial. Nicardipine mildly increased heart rate at rest and mildly decreased BP at rest. When generally similar responses to the 30- and 40-mg doses were averaged, nicardipine produced a 7% increase in peak exercise heart rate, which was balanced by a 6% decrease in peak exercise BP. Thus, no change occurred in the exercise heart rate–BP product. With nicardipine, treadmill exercise duration increased 9%, time to angina increased 15%, time to 1-mm ST-segment depression increased 16%, and oxygen consumption at peak exercise increased 13%. Mean anginal frequency declined, as did mean weekly sublingual nitroglycerin consumption, but not significantly. There were more cardiovascular side effects with nicardipine than with placebo, with at least 3 patients having increased angina judged by investigators as probably related to the drug. Vasodilatory side effects were also more frequent with nicardipine, but were generally mild and well tolerated; the drug had to be discontinued in only 1 patient because of vasodilatory effects. Nicardipine is effective and generally well tolerated in patients with chronic stable angina.

PY 108-068 (a new calcium antagonist)

Buitleir and associates[68] from London, UK, compared the efficacy of PY 108-068 (75 and 150 mg/day), a new dihydropyridine calcium-blocking agent, with placebo for treatment of chronic stable angina. Twelve patients were studied in a placebo-controlled, double-blind, randomized, crossover trial of 2 weeks each. Antianginal efficacy was assessed by the number of episodes of angina and nitroglycerin tablets consumed during each 2-week period, and by the number of episodes of ischemia during 48-hour ambulatory monitoring, and the area and severity of ST-segment depression during 16-point precordial exercise mapping. Nitroglycerin decreased from 6.1 ± 2.9 with placebo to 1.8 ± 1.5 with 75 mg/day of PY 108-068 and to 3.6 ± 2.3 with 150 mg/day of PY 108-068, whereas episodes of angina were reduced significantly only by the high dose (11.1 ± 3.9 with placebo, 6.3 ± 2.4 with 75 mg/day of PY 108-068 and 8.1 ± 3.4 with 150 mg/day of PY 108-068). The low dose alone significantly reduced ST-segment depression during exercise testing (29.6 ± 3.6 with placebo, 23.1 ± 5.6 with 75 mg/day of PY 108-068 and 24.4 ± 5.0 with 150 mg/day of PY 108-068), whereas neither dose significantly altered the number of episodes of ischemia during ambulatory monitoring. Supine and erect BP was significantly decreased in the absence of reflex tachycardia and the PR interval was not prolonged. Adverse effects did not necessitate discontinuation of treatment in any patient. These findings suggest that PY 108-068 has a role and potential advantages in the treatment of angina.

Nitroglycerin -vs- diltiazem

Hossack and associates[69] from Denver, Colorado, performed hemodynamic monitoring and measurement of cardiac output during a controlled treadmill exercise test in 15 patients with exertional angina. Then the patients were randomized to receive sustained release nitroglycerin, 13 mg (group I) or placebo (group II). Repeat exercise testing revealed that in group I, both maximal oxygen consumption and cardiac output increased significantly. In group II neither maximal oxygen consumption nor cardiac output increased significantly. All patients then received diltiazem, 60 mg, and repeat testing was carried out 1 hour later. In group I maximal oxygen consumption and cardiac output were higher than control, but were no higher than after nitroglycerin. In group II, maximal oxygen consumption increased significantly, but the increase in cardiac output was not significant. Thus, sustained-release nitroglycerin, 13 mg, or diltiazem, 60 mg, both improve exercise performance, but the combination does not improve exercise performance to an extent greater than either drug alone.

Propranolol -vs- diltiazem

Humen et al[70] in London, Canada, evaluated 24 patients with symptomatic stable effort angina despite beta blockade to determine whether combined diltiazem and beta blockers were more effective than beta blockers and diltiazem alone in relieving effort-related angina. Diltiazem given as 240 mg/day in divided doses and a combination of propranolol and diltiazem, 240 or 360 mg, were administered to the patients. Treadmill testing was utilized to assess exercise tolerance and radionuclide ventriculography to estimate LV functional responses. Treadmill exercise times were similar when beta blockers and diltiazem were used alone. However, with combined propranolol and diltiazem, 360 mg/day, there was a significant increase in treadmill time. Five patients whose treadmill exercise was limited by angina taking all therapies had a significant improvement in the time to onset of chest pain with both low- and high-dose combinations of propranolol and diltiazem. Thirteen of 24 patients blindly selected a higher dose diltiazem combination with beta blockers as their optimal therapy. Using RNA, LV dilation was observed with exercise with each of the types of therapy. However, cardiac index was higher at rest and during exercise with diltiazem therapy. These data suggest that combination therapy with propranolol and diltiazem, especially with a higher diltiazem dose of 360 mg/day, results in important improvement in exercise capacity and reduction in symptoms without a major increase in adverse effects or deterioration in LV function in patients continuing to have symptoms of angina on diltiazem or propranolol alone.

Propranolol -vs- nifedipine

Higginbotham and associates[71] from Durham, North Carolina, compared the effects of nifedipine (60–90 mg/day) and propranolol (240 mg/day) on symptoms, angina threshold and cardiac function in a placebo-controlled, double-blind, crossover study. Five-week treatment periods with nifedipine and propranolol were compared with 2 weeks of placebo treatment in 21 men with chronic stable angina pectoris, 13 of whom had symptoms both at rest and on exertion. Compared with placebo, New York Heart Association functional class improved in patients equally with nifedipine and propranolol. Frequency of chest pain decreased with nifedipine and propranolol, and nitroglycerin consumption similarly decreased with both treatments. Nifedipine significantly delayed the onset of chest pain and 1 mm of ST-segment depression during bicycle exercise. A preferential clinical response to nifedipine (9 patients) or propranolol (6 patients) was unrelated to the presence or absence of pain at rest or to any baseline hemodynamic finding. Nifedipine and propranolol were equally effective in relieving exertional ischemia as shown by improvements in EF at identical workloads, from 0.48 ± 0.11 to 0.58 ± 0.12 and 0.56 ± 0.14, respectively. Exercise wall motion, assessed by a semiquantitative wall motion score, also improved with both drugs. Propranolol treatment decreased exercise cardiac output by 14% through its effect on heart rate. In contrast, nifedipine treatment had no effect on cardiac output. Thus, nifedipine is as effective as propranolol when administered as single drug therapy in stable angina and has the potential advantage of preserving cardiac output during exercise.

Although the efficacy of beta blockers in the treatment of patients with stable angina had been demonstrated, their use in patients with rest angina has been controversial. Gottlieb and co-investigators[72] in Baltimore, Maryland, conducted a double-blind, randomized, placebo-controlled, 4-week trial of propranolol in 81 patients with unstable angina, 39 of whom were assigned to placebo and 42 of whom received propranolol in a dose of at least 160 mg/day. All patients were also treated with coronary vasodilators, including 80 mg/day of nifedipine and long-acting nitrates. The incidences of cardiac death, AMI, and requirement for CABG or PTCA did not differ between the 2 groups (propranolol = 16; placebo = 18). The propranolol group had a lower cumulative probability of having recurrent rest angina than the placebo, and over the first 4 days of the trial the mean number of clinical episodes of angina, duration of angina, and nitroglycerin requirement also were fewer. Continuous electrocardiographic recording for ischemic ST-segment changes revealed fewer daily ischemic episodes in the propranolol group (2.0) than in the placebo group (3.8), and a shorter duration of ischemia (propranolol 43 minutes, placebo 104 minutes). Thus, propranolol, in patients with unstable angina, in the presence of nitrates and nifedipine, is not detrimental and reduces the frequency and duration of symptomatic and silent ischemic episodes.

Propranolol -vs- nicardipine

In a double-blind, randomized, crossover clinical trial, nicardipine (90 mg/day in 3 divided doses) was compared with propranolol (120 mg/day in 3 divided doses) in 25 patients with chronic stable angina by McGill 'and associates[73] from Sydney, Australia. The mean weekly frequency of angina episodes decreased from 7.8 ± 1.2 (± standard error of the mean) with placebo to 3.8 ± 1.2 with nicardipine treatment and 3.5 ± 1 with propranolol treatment. With exercise testing, 5 patients receiving nicardipine and 3 receiving propranolol had no angina or ST-segment changes. When paired samples of both drugs were compared with placebo, significant improvement occurred in exercise duration (nicardipine, 1.3 ± 0.3 minutes; propranolol, 1.0 ± 0.4 minutes), time to onset of angina (nicardipine, 1.5 ± 0.4 minutes; propranolol, 1.5 ± 0.5 minutes), maximal ST-segment changes (nicardipine, 0.7 ± 0.1 mm; propranolol, 0.06 ± 0.1 mm) and time to 1 mm of ST depression (nicardipine, 2.5 ± 0.4 minutes; propranolol, 2.0 ± 0.3 minutes). Mild side effects occurred in 10 patients receiving propranolol and 5 receiving nicardipine. Nicardipine proved to be safe and effective for patients with chronic stable angina; it had fewer side effects than propranolol in the doses used.

Rousseau and co-investigators[74] in Brussels, Belgium, studied the long-term effects of antianginal therapy on coronary blood flow and myocardial metabolism in 35 patients with chronic stable angina. Arterial and coronary sinus blood samples and coronary blood flow measurements were obtained before and after 1 month of oral administration of propranolol or nicardipine. The data obtained at a fixed heart rate (10–15% above the pretreatment sinus rhythm) were compared, no significant differences were evidenced between the propranolol and the nicardipine groups. Coronary blood flow and myocardial oxygen uptake were unchanged with both drugs. Myocardial lactate uptake increased in 11 patients in the propranolol group and in 11 patients in the nicardipine group. In these 22 patients, increase in lactate uptake was accompanied by reductions in uptake of free fatty acids and by a decrease in the coronary sinus concentration of thromboxane B_2, whereas the transcardiac release of prostacyclin increased. Myocardial lactate uptake decreased more in the patients receiving propranolol than in those receiving nicardipine. Thus, long-term antianginal therapy with propranolol or nicardipine improved several markers of myocardial ischemia in approximately two-thirds of the patients. Although the changes observed at low heart rates were similar with the 2 drugs, the data also suggest that better metabolic protection is provided by the calcium antagonist during pacing-induced tachycardia.

Propranolol -vs- verapamil

Parodi and associates[75] from Pisa, Italy, and London, England, compared the effects of oral verapamil, 400 mg/day, oral propranolol, 300 mg/day, and placebo in 10 patients admitted to the coronary care unit because of frequent attacks of angina at rest. Testing was done according to a randomized, double-blind, multiple-crossover, placebo-controlled trial, consisting of 8 consecutive 48-hour treatment periods with verapamil, propranolol or placebo. Three patients had variant angina, 5 had episodes of both ST-segment elevation and depression and 2 had only ST-segment depression. One patient had no critical coronary stenoses, 1 had 1-vessel CAD, 7 had 2-vessel CAD and 1 had 3-vessel CAD. Electrocardiographic monitoring and tape recording were continued during the 16 days of the trial. A total of 1,602 episodes of transient diagnostic ST shift were recorded during the trial (1,309 episodes of ST-segment elevation, 293 of ST-segment depression); 43% were painless. Mean blood levels of verapamil and propranolol at the end of the active phases were 161 ± 89 and 120 ± 45 ng/ml, respectively. In the group as a whole, the average number of diagnostic ischemic ST-segment shifts per 24 hours was significantly reduced relative to corresponding placebo periods during verapamil (2.6 ± 2.4 vs 11.9 ± 8.6) but not during propranolol treatment (11.9 ± 8.6 vs 12.0 ± 7.3). Similar statistically significant reductions were observed in the number of anginal attacks and nitroglycerin tablets consumed. Considering individual patients, verapamil reduced ischemic episodes during both active phases in all patients, whereas propranolol was effective only in 1. Propranolol was not effective in 3 patients with severe limitation of exercise tolerance, but did not increase consistently the number or duration of episodes in the 3 patients with variant angina.

Propranolol -vs- bepridil

Parker and Farrell[76] from Kingston, Canada, studied 18 patients with chronic stable angina pectoris in a double-blind, placebo controlled 3-way crossover study in which they received 4 weeks of treatment with a once-daily dose of bepridil, 300 mg, a once-daily dose of long-acting propranolol, 160 mg, and placebo. Heart rate at rest during bepridil treatment was less than that during placebo, whereas propranolol reduced heart rate compared with placebo and bepridil. Systolic BP at rest did not change during the 3 treatment phases. Exercise time to onset of angina and to development of moderate angina were reproducible over the 24-hour period during each treatment phase. Treadmill walking time to onset of angina and to development of moderate angina was significantly prolonged during bepridil and during propranolol treatment. Heart rate at peak exercise was similar during bepridil and during placebo, but was markedly reduced with propranolol treatment. Systolic BP during exercise was similar during placebo and bepridil, but was substantially lower during propranolol treatment.

Metoprolol -vs- nifedipine

The Holland Interuniversity Nifedipine/Metoprolol Trial (HINT) Research Group[77] in a multicenter, double-blind, placebo-controlled randomized trial of nifedipine, metoprolol, and nifedipine and metoprolol combined was conducted in 338 patients with unstable angina not pretreated with a beta blocker and of nifedipine in 177 patients pretreated with a beta blocker. The main outcome event was recurrent ischemia or AMI within 48 hours. Trial medication effects were expressed as ratios of event rates relative to placebo. In patients not pretreated with a beta blocker the event rate ratios (with associated 95% confidence intervals) were 1.15 (0.83, 1.64) for nifedipine, 0.76 (0.49, 1.16) for metoprolol, and 0.80 (0.53, 1.19) for nifedipine and metoprolol combined. In patients already taking a beta blocker the addition of nifedipine was beneficial (rate ratio 0.68 (0.47, 0.97)). In equal numbers of patients AMI and reversible ischemia developed. Most AMIs occurred within 6 hours of randomization. In patients not already taking a beta blocker, the nifedipine rate ratio for AMI only was 1.51 (9.87, 2.74). These results suggest that in patients not previously taking beta blockade, metoprolol has a beneficial short-term effect on unstable angina, that fixed combination with nifedipine provides no further gain, and that nifedipine may be detrimental. The addition of nifedipine to existing beta blockade when the patient's condition becomes unstable seems beneficial.

This article was accompanied by an editorial by Fox and Krikler[78] entitled "Early Treatment of Unstable Angina." These authors concluded that clinicians are not really concerned with whether nifedipine is more effective than a beta blocker or vice versa because almost all patients with unstable angina are vigorously treated with intravenous nitrates, oral beta blockers, oral calcium antagonists, and aspirin in combination. In patients who do not respond rapidly to this approach PTCA or CABG are the treatments of choice.

Uusitalo and associates[79] from Tampere and Turku, and Joensuu, Finland, and Volda and Halden, Norway, compared treatment with metoprolol (100 mg twice daily), nifedipine (10 mg 3 times daily), and both drugs combined for effect on clinical variables, bicycle ergometer exercise tolerance, and adverse effects in a randomized double-blind crossover study in 62 patients with stable angina. Nitroglycerin consumption and anginal attack rate as recorded in patient diaries indicated a higher antianginal efficacy with metoprolol and combination therapy than with nifedipine monotherapy. All exercise test variables showed a significantly higher antianginal efficacy with combination therapy than with nifedipine monotherapy (15% -vs- 26%). The combination therapy also was better than metoprolol in all exercise variables (9% -vs- 14%), except for onset and duration of chest pain. Furthermore, metoprolol showed a higher efficacy than nifedipine in all exercise variables (7% -vs- 23%) except total exercise time. More adverse symptoms of peripheral vasodilation were reported for nifedipine than for metoprolol (tachycardia, flushing, headache). It was concluded that combined treatment with metoprolol and nifedipine increased antianginal efficacy compared with the monotherapies without increasing adverse effects. In effort angina, metoprolol in these doses was more effective and better tolerated than nifedipine.

VARIANT ANGINA PECTORIS

Late follow-up

From 37 patients with coronary artery spasm and <70% diameter narrowing treated initially with verapamil and nitrates, Freedman and associates[80] from Sydney, Australia, followed 33 for 41–102 months (mean 62). One patient died from carcinoma of the lung, 3 had AMI, and 10 had either VT and VF or AV block. During follow-up there were no cardiac deaths and no AMIs. Asymptomatic periods of >3 months occurred in 23 patients during follow-up: 18 with asymptomatic periods of >1 year were pain free at the time of study and 5 with asymptomatic periods of 3 to 6 months had infrequent pain. Ten patients had no asymptomatic periods. Symptomatic status at last review was related to initial response to therapy: 13 of 18 patients (72%) currently asymptomatic became asymptomatic with initial therapy compared with 5 of 15 patients (33%) currently having pain. Twenty-six patients were currently receiving therapy; 12 patients were not receiving therapy or were receiving low-dose therapy, including 8 with asymptomatic periods of >1 year. Patients with coronary spasm and <70% diameter narrowing treated medically have low mortality and morbidity rates over a 5-year follow-up. Many have long asymptomatic periods and some may be able to stop therapy indefinitely.

Provocation of spasm by dopamine or acetylcholine

The effects of dopamine on arteries are different depending on the dose, route of administration, and receptor population. Dopamine administration can cause vasodilatation by stimulation of dopaminergic receptors, vasoconstriction by stimulation of alpha-adrenergic and serotonergic receptors, and even spasm of cerebral arteries when given intracisternally in dogs. Crea and co-workers[81] in London, UK, assessed the ability of dopamine to provoke coronary spasm in 18 patients with active vasospastic angina in whom this amine was infused at rates of 5, 10, and 15 μg/kg/min for periods of 5 minutes each. The 12-lead electrocardiogram and (cuff) BP were monitored throughout the whole test. In 9 patients dopamine caused angina and ischemic electrocardiographic changes suggestive of coronary spasm: ST-segment elevation in 6 patients with ST-segment depression in the absence of important coronary stenosis in the remaining 3. Infusion of dopamine was repeated in coronary angiography in 3 patients with positive test results; this provoked occlusive coronary spasm with ST-segment elevation in 2 patients and nonocclusive spasm with ST-segment depression in the remainder. In conclusion, infusion of dopamine provokes coronary spasm in a sizeable proportion of patients with active vasospastic angina. Dopamine administration may be detrimental in patients susceptible to coronary spasm, such as those with AMI.

Since coronary spasm most often occurs when patients are at rest and since the activity of the parasympathetic nervous system is enhanced at rest and suppressed by physical activity, Yasue and co-investigators[82] in Kumamoto City, Japan, postulated that the activity of the parasympathetic nervous system might be related to the pathogenesis of variant angina or coronary spasm. The investigators injected acetylcholine, the neurotransmitter of the parasympathetic nervous system, into the coronary arteries of 28 patients with variant angina. Injection of acetylcholine into the coronary artery responsible for the attack induced spasm together with chest pain and ST-segment elevation or depression on the electrocardiogram in 30 of the 32 arteries of 25 of the 27 patients. The injection of acetylcholine into the coronary artery not responsible for the attack in 18 patients resulted in various degrees of constriction in most of them, but no spasm. After intravenous injection of 1.0–1.5 mg atropine sulfate, the injection of acetylcholine into the coronary artery responsible for the attack did not induce spasm or attack in any of the 9 coronary arteries injected in 8 patients. The investigators concluded that the intracoronary injection of acetylcholine induces coronary spasm and attack in patients with variant angina and that the activity of the parasympathetic nervous system may play a role in the pathogenesis of coronary spasm. They also concluded that the intracoronary injection of acetylcholine is a useful test for provocation of coronary spasm.

Risk factors

To determine the importance of usual risk factors of CAD in patients with coronary artery spasm, Scholl and associates[83] from Paris, France, compared

40 patients with vasospastic angina, normal or nearly normal coronary arteries, and without previous AMI with 2 control groups of 40 patients each, matched for age and sex: 1 group with CAD and 1 without heart disease. Ninety percent of patients with vasospastic angina were cigarette smokers and 70% were heavy smokers (>20 cigarettes daily), compared with 53% and 33% in patients with CAD and 30% and 15% in those without heart disease. Except for cigarette smoking, the risk-factor profile of patients with vasospastic angina appeared more like the profile of patients without heart disease than that of patients with CAD. The results suggest that cigarette smoking may play a role in CAD independent of atherosclerosis and possibly favoring coronary artery spasm.

With esophageal spasm

Rasmussen and associates[84] from Aarhus, Denmark, performed esophageal manometry in 20 patients with chest pain, of whom 10 had coronary artery spasm (group 1) and 10 did not (group 2). In the basal state, esophageal spasms were recorded in 6 patients from group 1 but in none from group 2. In group 1 the duration of esophageal contractions was 4.50 ± 0.65 second compared with 2.86 ± 0.36 second in group 2. Prolonged hyperventilation was performed during manometry by 7 patients from each group. In group 1, this caused chest pain in all 7, with electrocardiographic changes in 6; at the same time esophageal spasms were intensified in 5 patients and began anew in 1. In group II no electrocardiographic changes were seen with hyperventilation, and 1 patient showed esophageal spasm. These observations suggest a relation between spasm of the coronary arteries and spasm of the esophagus. This article was followed by an unsigned editorial entitled "Angina and Esophageal Disease."[85]

With fixed coronary narrowing

Araki and associates[86] from Fukuoka, Japan, performed 12-lead electrocardiography during treadmill exercise in 57 patients with variant angina in whom coronary angiography had been performed. Thirty-six patients performed exercise tests with or without calcium antagonists, and 21 performed them only with calcium antagonists. In 55 patients, calcium antagonists prevented spontaneous attacks of variant angina for >2 days before the test. The other 2 patients were given a single dose of diltiazem (90 mg) 2 hours before the test. Exercise testing without calcium antagonists induced ST-segment elevation with chest pain in 9 patients, ST-segment depression in 10 (9 with chest pain), and no important shift of the ST-segment in 17. Five patients had severe coronary stenosis ($\geq 75\%$) and all of them had a positive response. Thirty-one patients had no important coronary stenosis and 14 of them had a positive response. The sensitivity of the exercise test in detecting a coronary stenosis $\geq 75\%$ was 100% without calcium antagonists but the specificity was low (55%). When the exercise test was done in patients taking calcium antagonists, only 2 (specificity 96%) of 48 patients without severe coronary stenosis had a positive response (elevation of ST segment in 1, depression of ST segment in 6, and elevation in 3 (sensitivity 100%). The authors concluded that exercise testing with calcium antagonists may be a useful method for detecting severe coronary stenosis in patients with variant angina.

PERCUTANEOUS TRANSLUMINAL
CORONARY ANGIOPLASTY

Safety and results by low-frequency operators

Jacob and associates[87] from Washington, D.C., analyzed results of PTCA at their hospital from July 1983 through April 1985. Sixteen physicians performed PTCA in 131 patients from July 1983 through June 1984 (1983/84) (mean 0.7 PTCAs per physician per month) and 279 from July 1984 through April 1985 (1984/85) (mean 1.7 PTCAs per physician per month). Success rates increased from 76% in 1982/84 to 84% in 1984/85. The incidence of emergency CABG decreased from 11% in 1983/84 to 5% in 1984/85. Results for 1984/85 were separated into 2 groups according to the mean number of PTCAs per month performed by each physician. Success rates for group I (≤2 PTCAs per month) and group II (>2 PTCAs per month) were 83% and 84% for all PTCAs attempted and 89% and 88% for PTCAs attempted and 89% and 88% for PTCAs excluding those attempted during AMI or on totally occluded arteries. The similar results of both groups may reflect the performance of the catheterization laboratory PTCA team and the assistance of more experienced physicians, in addition to the performance of each physician. These findings must be applied with caution to laboratories with different organization and with less frequent PTCA experience.

To determine the safety and success rate of a beginning PTCA program using the steerable guidewire system, Harston and associates[88] from Nashville, Tennessee, analyzed results of the initial 100 attempted dilatations. In accordance with recommended guidelines, the operators had extensive experience in cardiac catheterization and attended demonstration courses in PTCA to learn the technique, but had no in-laboratory training or assistance from experienced PTCA operators. Using the same criteria for success and complications, the results with the steerable guidewire system were compared with those of the National Heart, Lung, and Blood Institute Registry of programs beginning PTCA with the nonsteerable, fixed guidewire system. Success rates were 95 and 59%, emergency CABG 1 and 6%, acute coronary occlusion 1 and 5%, and AMI 3 and 5%. The success and complication rates were similar for each decile in the 100 procedures, in contrast to the Registry in which results significantly improved as operator experience increased. The average stenosis was reduced from 86–28% and the average gradient was reduced from 51–14 mmHg. These results indicate that cardiologists experienced in cardiac catheterization can start a PTCA program using the steerable guidewire system and have an improved learning curve compared with previously reported experience in which the nonsteerable, fixed guidewire system was used. With careful case selection, results comparable to those of experienced PTCA operators can be achieved. These findings may provide a more accurate prediction of the results than can be expected in a beginning PTCA program using current techniques and equipment.

These 2 articles above were followed by 2 editorials, 1 by Hartzler[89] from Kansas City, Missouri, and 1 by Roubin and associates[90] from Atlanta, Georgia. Hartzler's summary comments were as follows: "I believe the most effective approach for developing institutional and regional excellence in coronary angioplasty will require limitation and restriction of PTCA privileges. Ideally, selected institutions with higher-volume cardiac catheterization laboratories and with support personnel including an established cardiovascular surgical program would identify a small group of cardiologists to perform the first few to several hundred angioplasty procedures within the institution. These operators should have distinguished themselves by expertly performing at least 1,000 unsupervised coronary angiographic procedures after completion of their formal cardiovascular fellowship. Peer recognition for technical and laboratory excellence should be required. After an initial introduction to coronary angioplasty acquired through attendance at formal courses and by visiting established programs, these individuals ideally would commence their basic training in coronary angioplasty with the assistance of a skilled operator for at least the first 20–25 procedures. Case selection for the first few hundred procedures should be deliberate and rigid to exclude patients with higher anatomic and clinical risk situations. Within the first 200 cases, this group of physicians should be able to achieve at least a 90% primary success rate for well selected cases while experiencing less than a 5% combined incidence of procedure-related infarction and need for urgent bypass surgery and a procedure-related mortality of less than 1%. In this fashion, 2 to 3 skilled invasive cardiologists within an institution should be able to acquire mature judgment, expertise and a technical proficiency allowing cautious entry into the performance of more complex PTCA procedures. Once reaching this level of experience, these persons should be committed, obligated and dedicated to sharing their experience through the teaching of local and regional colleagues in a similar supervised fashion."

The major points made by Roubin and associates[90] might also be summarized in their own words: "As the practice of PTCA increases in complexity and its potential application to a large proportion of patients with obstructive coronary artery disease increases, more formal training of PTCA operators is required. In this era of DRGs and decreasing hospital census, there is an economic incentive on the part of institutions to allow many cardiologists to perform PTCA. This should not be allowed to compromise optimal patient care. Just as it is totally unacceptable for general surgeons to perform coronary artery bypass graft procedures, so it must become unacceptable for untrained cardiologists to attempt instrumentation of the coronary arteries.

Finally, both (above) groups reporting their experience should be commended on recording and auditing their results. The greatest problem confronting the practice of PTCA in this country is the total lack of control over which patients undergo PTCA and who performs the procedure."

Predicting long-term outcome

Berger and associates[91] from Providence, Rhode Island, determined whether the immediate efficacy of PTCA is sustained by obtaining follow-up data in 183 patients who had undergone PTCA at least 1 year earlier. The duration of follow-up ranged from 1 to 5 years. Subjective clinical information was obtained in each patient and objective functional information, determined by exercise stress testing, was obtained in 91. PTCA was initially successful in 141 patients (79%). Of the 42 patients in whom PTCA was unsuccessful, 26 underwent CABG, and 16 were maintained on medical therapy. When compared to the medical therapy patients at time of follow-up, successful PTCA patients had less angina (13% -vs- 47%), used less nitroglycerin (25% -vs- 73%), were hospitalized less often for chest pain (8% -vs- 31%), and subjectively believed their condition had improved (96% -vs- 20%). Furthermore, during exercise testing, the prevalence of angina was reduced (9% -vs- 43%), and exercise duration was greater (8.2 -vs- 5.8 minutes) among PTCA patients. There were no significant differences in the incidence of subsequent AMI, mortality, or need for CABG. For these variables, no differences were seen between the CABG and PTCA groups. Thus, successful PTCA results in long-term relief of subjective and objective manifestations of myocardial ischemia, superior to that of medical therapy and comparable to CABG.

The *final translesional pressure gradient* measured during PTCA <25 mmHg correlates with immediate angiographic and clinical results. Whether this pressure gradient is of value in predicting late clinical outcome has not been determined. Hodgson and colleagues[92] in Providence, Rhode Island, obtained complete follow-up information from 159 patients with 1-vessel CAD who underwent successful PTCA. Mean follow-up time was 15 ± 10 months. The occurrence of repeat PTCA, CABG, recurrent anginal chest pain, or a positive post–PTCA stress test result were considered clinical events indicative of late failure. Of the variables, age, gender, initial and final translesional pressure gradient, extent of initial and final arterial narrowing, site of dilatation, type of balloon catheter used, number of inflations, and maximal inflation pressure, only the final translesional pressure gradient was predictive of late failure when analyzed by multivariate techniques.

Effectiveness in patients >65 years of age

Raizner and associates[93] from Houston, Texas, performed PTCA in 119 patients ≥65 years of age (mean 70). On angiography, elderly patients differed only in the more frequent occurrence of visible calcific coronary arterial deposits (26% -vs- 8% in younger patients). Primary success was achieved in 81% -vs- 80% in patients <65 years. Major complication rates were comparable to those of younger patients: emergency CABG, 4.1% -vs- 4.7%; AMI, 2.5% -vs- 2.9%; and death, 0.8% -vs- 0. Late clinical follow-up ranging from 5 to 50 months (mean 18) showed that symptomatic improvement was achieved in 91% of patients in whom PTCA was successful, with 55% being asymptomatic. Seventy percent of patients were as active or more active (30%) than before PTCA and 47% were taking fewer medications. Four late deaths occurred, none from cardiac causes. These data support the safety and clinical effectiveness of PTCA in elderly patients.

For post–acute myocardial infarction, unstable angina

De Feyter and co-workers[94] in Rotterdam, The Netherlands, performed PTCA in 53 patients in whom unstable angina had reoccurred after 48 hours and within 30 days after sustained AMI. Single-vessel CAD was present in 64% of the patients and multivessel CAD in 36%. The preceding AMI had been small to moderate in size in most patients. The LVEF was >50% in 80% of patients. Forty-five patients were refractory to pharmacologic treatment; 8 were initially stabilized but once again became symptomatic with light exertion. PTCA was performed in 35 patients at 2–14 days and in 18 patients 15–30 days after AMI. The initial success rate was 89% (47/53). The success rate of the patients treated at 2–14 days was lower (29/35, 83%) than that of patients treated at 14–30 days (18/18, 100%). There were no deaths related to the procedure. In 4 of the 6 failures, emergency CABG was performed and 2 patients sustained AMI. AMI complicated the PTCA procedure in 2 other patients; thus the overall procedure-related AMI rate was 8% (4/53). At 6 months follow-up, 26% (14/53) of all the patients who underwent PTCA had recurrence of angina, which was successfully treated with repeat PTCA, CABG, or medical therapy. There were no late deaths. Late AMI occurred in 2 patients. Thus, the total AMI rate after PTCA at 6 months was 11%. In 42 of the 47 (89%) patients with successful PTCA, angiography was repeated a mean 3.3 months after PTCA. The angiographic restenosis rate was 33%. The investigators concluded that in selected patients, PTCA for unstable angina occurring 48 hours to 30 days after AMI is an effective treatment with an acceptable risk, a high initial success rate, and a sustained beneficial effect.

For total coronary occlusion

DiSciascio and associates[95] from Richmond, Virginia, performed PTCA for nonacute total coronary occlusion in 46 patients, with a 63% primary success rate (29 of 46 procedures). None had AMI and none died. There was no difference in success rate according to artery dilated, prior AMI, or lesion morphology. The success rate with occlusions less than 2-weeks' duration was 14 of 19 (74%) -vs- 15 of 27 (55%) with occlusions more than 2-weeks' duration. There was clinical recurrence in 14 of 29 patients (48%). Factors predictive of recurrence included a greater residual post–PTCA stenosis of $47 \pm 6\%$ in recurrences -vs- $31 \pm 3\%$ in nonrecurrences, whereas estimated duration of initial occlusion was 1.1 ± 0.4 months for recurrences -vs- 3.1 ± 1 month for nonrecurrences (Fig. 2-21). PTCA for total occlusion has a lower success rate and higher recurrence rate than PTCA for nontotal stenoses. Recurrence appears to be related to a higher degree of post–PTCA residual narrowing and to a shorter duration of initial occlusion.

For dynamic stenosis

Bertrand et al[96] in Lille, France, evaluated results of PTCA in 132 patients (group A) with fixed coronary stenosis and without spontaneous or ergonovine-provoked spasm and in 97 patients (group B) with dynamic coronary stenosis (spasm superimposed on the stenosis). In these patients, the rate of restenosis defined as a loss of 50% of the initial gain was significantly higher in patients in group B with a dynamic coronary stenosis (35% -vs- 22%). Coronary artery spasm persisted in 44% of the patients in group B despite treatment with a calcium antagonist and was detected for the first time in 15% of the patients in group A. Therefore, in patients with dynamic coronary

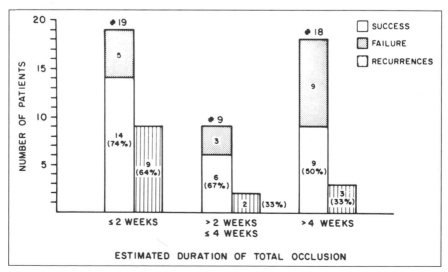

Fig. 2-21. Effect of pre-PTCA estimated duration of total occlusion on initial success and recurrence rates. Reproduced with permission from DiSciascio et al.[95]

stenoses, the results of PTCA are less satisfactory than in patients with fixed coronary stenoses.

For stenoses of aorto-coronary grafts

Reeder and associates[97] from Rochester, Minnesota, reviewed findings in 19 patients who underwent balloon angioplasty for partial or complete stenosis of aortocoronary bypass saphenous vein bypass grafts during a 5-year period. The procedures were performed a mean of 38 months after CABG to relieve recurrent angina of at least class 2 (Canadian Cardiovascular Association). Graft angioplasty was successful in 16 of the 19 patients, and the location of the narrowing (in the origin, body, or distal insertion of the graft) was not an important factor in achieving a successful result (Fig. 2-22). At a mean follow-up interval of 20 months (range, 1–40 months), 14 patients had symptomatic improvement. Two patients required late repeat operation and 4 had repeat PTCA because of restenosis. This experience supports the use of balloon angioplasty in selected patients with bypass graft stenosis.

Significance of "reciprocal" electrocardiographic changes during occlusion

Quyyumi and associates[98] from London, England, investigated ST-segment depression remote from the region of AMI in 3 groups of patients undergoing LAD–PTCA. Ten patients had 1-vessel CAD, 9 concomitant stenoses in ≥1 other major coronary artery, and 2 AMI after occlusion during PTCA. Continuous surface electrocardiograms were recorded from leads I, II, III, V_2, and V_5, before, during, and after PTCA, and ST-segment changes were measured to 0.1 mm. All 10 patients with 1-vessel CAD had ST-segment elevation in lead V_2 and 9 also had changes in lead III. All 9 patients with multivessel CAD had ST-segment changes in lead V_2; 8 of them had concomitant changes in lead III. Both patients with AMI had elevation in lead V_2 and depression in lead III. ST-segment changes began simultaneously in all leads where they occurred. Most (70%) patients with 1-vessel CAD who had inferior ST-segment depression had a right dominant coronary circulation. Therefore, the presence of inferior ST-segment depression during LAD coro-

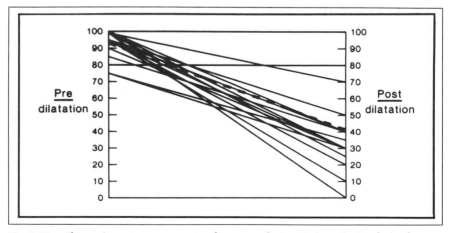

Fig. 2-22.   Change in aortocoronary artery bypass graft stenosis in patients who underwent coronary angioplasty. (Mean change is shown by dotted line.) In two patients who had 100% stenosis and one who had 80% stenosis before dilation, the vessel lumen remained unchanged. Reproduced with permission from Reeder et al.[97]

nary artery occlusion does not indicate the presence or absence of multivessel CAD. Furthermore, it is unlikely that this change always represents ischemia remote from the site of AMI; it is merely an electrical phenomenon.

To assess the relation between the direction of ST-segment response to transient coronary occlusion and collateral function, MacDonald and colleagues[99] in Gainesville, Florida, studied 25 patients with diagnostic ST-segment changes during transient occlusion of the proximal LAD. ECG leads I, II, V_2 and V_5; LV filling, aortic, and distal coronary pressures; and great cardiac vein flow were measured during PTCA of the LAD. During a 1-minute LAD balloon occlusion, 16 patients had reversible ST elevation (group I) and 9 patients had ST depression (group II). The ST responses in individual patients were consistent during repeated occlusions, and ST depression never preceded ST elevation. Angiography before PTCA showed less severe LAD stenosis in group I than in group II and collateral filling of the LAD in no group I patient but in 6 of 9 patients in group II. During LAD occlusion, determinants of myocardial oxygen demand (LV filling pressure, aortic pressure, heart rate, and double product) were similar in both groups. Group I patients, however, had lower distal coronary pressure and residual great cardiac vein flow and higher coronary collateral resistance than group II patients. In patients with ST elevation during LAD occlusion, stenosis before PTCA was less severe, visible collaterals were not present, and hemodynamic variables during LAD occlusion reflected poorer collateral function. Thus, collateral function is an important determinant of the direction of ST-segment response to ischemia during acute coronary occlusion.

Effects of and prevention of myocardial ischemia during balloon dilatation

Catheter balloon inflation performed during PTCA results in temporary interruption of coronary blood flow and subsequent myocardial ischemia. This produces transient but profound regional LV dysfunction. In an effort to mitigate this inflation-related dysfunction, Cleman and colleagues[100] in New Haven, Connecticut, infused oxygenated Fluosol DA 20%, a perfluorochemical oxygen transport fluid, distal to the balloon through the central lumen of the dilating catheter during balloon inflation. Regional wall motion during PTCA was assessed by simultaneous continuous 2-D echocardiography and was quantified by computer analysis. During control inflations accompanied by no intracoronary infusion or by transcatheter infusion of Ringer's lactate solution or nonoxygenated Fluosol DA 20%, there was profound regional LV dysfunction with a >90% decrease in regional contraction. In contrast, regional contraction during transcatheter infusion of oxygenated Fluosol DA 20% remained at normal levels throughout balloon inflation. Distal infusion of Fluosol DA 20% during balloon inflation is a useful adjunct to PTCA, allowing longer inflation times and perhaps permitting PTCA to be performed safely in patients with significant myocardium at ischemic risk or with limited LV reserve for whom the procedure is currently believed to be too hazardous.

Wijns et al[101] in Rotterdam, The Netherlands, and Zurich, Switzerland, evaluated the effects of repeated (3–10 seconds) and transient (15–75 seconds) abrupt coronary occlusions on the global and regional LV stiffness in 9 patients undergoing PTCA of a single proximal narrowed LAD coronary artery. With transient ischemia, there was an upward shift of the pressure-volume relation. The nonlinear simple elastic constant of chamber stiffness increased from 0.0273 ± 0.017 before PTCA to 0.0621 ± 0.026 after 20 seconds of coronary occlusion and 0.0605 ± 0.015 after 50 seconds of occlusion.

Post-PTCA values remained higher than the control values, but at the group level the mean value was not significantly different. Regional stiffness determined from the changes in the length of 6 segmental radii during diastole was unaffected in the nonischemic zones. In the adjacent and ischemic zones, regional stiffness was increased during occlusion. The regional abnormalities in diastolic function persisted at the time of post-PTCA measurements, 12 minutes after the end of the procedure. Thus, recovery of normal diastolic function after repeated ischemic injuries is delayed after restoration of normal blood flow and systolic function.

Wohlgelernter et al[102] in New Haven, Connecticut, evaluated the influence of transient and repetitive balloon inflation during PTCA on regional myocardial responses in patients with CAD. Twenty patients with normal LV function undergoing PTCA for isolated stenosis of a proximal LAD coronary artery were evaluated. Group A patients (14 patients) had 1 inflation-deflation sequence performed; group B (6 patients) had multiple (>5) inflations. The first and last sequences were analyzed. Assessments included continuous 2-D echocardiography with computerized quantitative analysis of regional LV wall motion and continuous 12-lead electrocardiographic recordings. The mean duration of balloon inflation in group A patients was 62 ± 6 seconds. Regional LV dysfunction occurred within 12 ± 5 seconds after balloon inflation and profound LV segmental dysfunction was noted in all patients. With balloon deflation, there was prompt recovery of regional LV function, with full recovery at 43 ± 17 seconds (Fig. 1). In patients in group B, a comparison of regional wall motion alterations from the first and last inflations revealed no significant differences in the time-to-onset of LV dysfunction, magnitude of LV segmental dysfunction, or the time to complete recovery of segmental function. Electrocardiographic changes occurred after the onset of LV regional wall motion abnormalities and only 64% of patients showed evidence of ischemia on 12-lead electrocardiograms at 20 seconds of balloon inflation. However, after 1 minute of balloon inflation, 86% of patients had electrocardiographic alterations consistent with myocardial ischemia. Therefore, balloon inflation during PTCA causes reversible regional LV dysfunction. Repeated occlusions of the coronary artery during PTCA do not appear to have a cumulative ischemic effect. However, it is difficult to apply these findings to patients with underlying severe LV dysfunction in whom the reversibility of dysfunction and lack of cumulative ischemic effect are not certain.

To study myocardial and clinical events during transient coronary occlusion in humans, 2-D echocardiography was continuously performed by Visser and colleagues[103] from Amsterdam and Utrecht, The Netherlands, in 15 patients undergoing 49 balloon inflations during PTCA. Transient segmental asynergy developed in all patients 8 ± 3 seconds after balloon inflation and returned to baseline 19 ± 8 seconds after balloon deflation. Segmental dyskinesia was seen in only 8 of 11 patients undergoing PTCA of the LAD. A wall motion score, based on degree of asynergy of 13 segments of the left ventricle, was significantly higher during LAD than during right coronary artery inflation (7.9 ± 1.3 -vs- 4.0 ± 1.4). LV size index increased significantly during balloon inflation, from 179 ± 9–196 ± 10 mm. Four patients had transient ST-segment changes in the extremity leads of the electrocardiogram and 5 patients had angina pectoris. The first sign of ischemia in 3 patients, who had all of these symptoms together, was consistently asynergy, followed by electrocardiographic changes, and last, angina pectoris. Thus, during PTCA, transient asynergy and LV dilatation develop, which are often clinically silent.

Zalewski and co-investigators[104] in Philadelphia, Pennsylvania, studied patients undergoing PTCA to verify whether myocardial protection could be achieved via the intracoronary administration of propranolol. Accordingly, 21 patients undergoing PTCA were randomly assigned to receive either intracoronary placebo (group A, n = 10) or intracoronary propranolol (group B, n = 11). Three balloon inflations producing coronary artery occlusion were performed in each patient. Inflations I and II (maximum duration 60 seconds) served as control occlusions. Inflation III (maximum duration 120 seconds) was performed either after intracoronary administration of saline solution or propranolol. The following electrocardiographic indexes of myocardial ischemic injury were measured: time to develop ST-segment elevation equal to 0.1 mV and magnitude of ST-segment elevation after 60 seconds of coronary artery occlusion. Both indexes did not differ significantly between the groups during inflations I and II. In group A the time to development of ST-segment elevation of 0.1 mV remained unchanged between the second and third occlusions. In group B subselective injection of propranolol into the affected coronary artery significantly prolonged the time to ST-segment elevation of 0.1 mV from 19–53 seconds. Administration of placebo did not change the magnitude of ST-segment elevation 60 seconds after coronary artery occlusion between the second and third occlusion in group A. In group B, after intracoronary administration of propranolol, ST-segment elevation 60 seconds after occlusion decreased significantly from 0.23–0.12 mV. There were no significant differences in heart rate and mean aortic pressure between groups A and B during inflation I, II, and III. In conclusion, these results suggest that repetitive episodes of transient coronary artery occlusion are associated with similar degrees of myocardial ischemic injury, intracoronary propranolol significantly reduces the electrocardiographic indexes of myocardial ischemic injury, and the myocardial protection afforded by intracoronary propranolol is most likely mediated by a regional effect of the drug.

Significance of coronary collaterals during balloon dilatation

Cohen and Rentrop[105] in New York, New York, have shown improvement in collateral filling immediately after sudden controlled coronary occlusion in human subjects undergoing elective PTCA. Although it has been suggested that collateral circulation can limit myocardial ischemia, clinical proof has been lacking. These investigators prospectively studied 23 patients with isolated LAD (14 patients) or right coronary (9 patients) disease and normal left ventriculograms during elective PTCA. A second arterial catheter was used for injection of the contralateral artery to assess collateral filling before balloon placement and during coronary occlusion by balloon inflation. LV angiography was performed during another inflation. Grading of collateral filling was as follows: 0 = none, 1 = filling of side branches only, 2-partial filling of the epicardial segment, and 3 = complete filling of the epicardial segment. Indexes of myocardial ischemia included percent of the LV perimeter having new hypocontractility and the sum of ST-segment elevation measured on a simultaneous 12-lead electrocardiogram recorded during each inflation. Collateral filling during balloon occlusion and indexes of ischemia were assessed at 30–40 seconds into inflation. Aortic pressure and heart rate did not correlate with the percent hypocontractile perimeter nor the sum of ST-segment elevation. There was a significant correlation between the sum of collateral filling and inflation and both percent hypocontractile perimeter and the sum of ST-segment elevation. Anginal pain occurred in all patients with grade 0 or 1 collateral filling but only 36% of patients with grade 2 or 3 collaterals. These investigators concluded that collateral circulation limits myocardial

ischemia as assessed by the extent of new LV asynergy and electrocardiographic changes during coronary occlusion.

Late coronary arterial luminal changes

Although immediate and late changes in coronary stenoses after PTCA
have been reported, most investigators have utilized qualitative or semiquantitative techniques to analyze the coronary arteriograms. Such data are less
then optimal because of considerable interobserver variability and the use of
relative instead of absolute changes in lesion geometry. Analysis is further
compounded by the indistinct edges that characterize coronary narrowings
immediately after PTCA. To quantify the changes in minimal cross-sectional
area (CSA) of the coronary lumen that occur during and after PTCA, Johnson
and co-investigators[106] in Iowa City, Iowa, analyzed angiograms in 23 patients before and immediately after PTCA, and at 7.2 months follow-up
using 2 computer-assisted methods of angiographic analysis—quantitative
coronary angiography and videodensitometry. Quantitative coronary angiography provides an absolute measure of the area of the lumen; videodensitometry is a nongeometric method that is not dependent on exact border recognition. Based on these quantitative methods, the investigators found that
successful PTCA is associated with about a 3-fold increase in the minimal
CSA of the lesion (from 1.0–3.2 mm). This area is, however, well below
normal and is less than half of the average minimal CSA of the inflated
dilating balloon. Analysis of follow-up angiograms demonstrated that 8 of 23
patients had a substantial late increase in the minimal CSA (from 2.7–4.1
mm^2) after PTCA. Clinical, hemodynamic, and angiographic characteristics
immediately after PTCA were not predictive of minimal CSA of the lumen at
follow-up. Because substantial late increases in minimal CSA of the lumen
occur in about one-third of patients, angiographic and noninvasive analyses
performed immediately after PTCA will not define the ultimate adequacy of
coronary dilation in many patients undergoing PTCA.

Complications—dissection and total occlusion

Coronary dissection and total coronary occlusion leading to emergency
CABG are the most frequent complications of PTCA and their occurrence
usually is unpredictable. To identify angiographic characteristics of coronary
stenoses that may affect the frequency of these complications, Ischinger and
co-workers[107] in Atlanta, Georgia, reviewed diagnostic pre–PTCA coronary
angiograms of 38 consecutive patients (group I) undergoing emergency
CABG for dissection or occlusion and compared them to the angiograms of a
random sample of 38 patients (stratified for LAD and right coronary arteries)
from a group of 1,151 who did not need emergency CABG (group II). Stenosis
morphology before PTCA was considered "complicated" if at least 1 of the
following criteria was present: irregular borders, intraluminal lucency, and
localization of stenosis in a curve or at a bifurcation. Baseline characteristics,
maximum inflation pressure, types of balloon catheters used, and routinely
registered angiographic stenosis properties (severity, length, eccentricity, and
calcium) were similar in both groups. Irregular borders before PTCA were
present in 22 of 38 patients in group I -vs- 10 of 38 in group II, intraluminal
lucency in 22 of 38 -vs- 9 of 38, localization in curve in 27 of 38 patients -vs-
16 of 38, and localization at bifurcation in 11 of 38 -vs- 15 of 38. Complicated
angiographic morphology of coronary stenosis may represent a risk factor for
dissection or occlusion. Although the predictive value of these findings is low,

detailed evaluation of angiographic morphology of coronary stenoses may improve patient selection and reduce complication rates of PTCA.

Complications—restenosis

Sugrue and associates[108] from Rochester, Minnesota, reviewed their experience with acute coronary occlusion during PTCA in patients with coronary artery thrombosis. In their early PTCA experience from October 1979 to March 1983, acute occlusion occurred in 11 of 15 patients with preexisting thrombus compared to 18 of 223 patients without coronary artery thrombus. The effect of improved technology (steerable guiding systems and altered dilatation strategy, full intravenous heparinization for 24 hours after the procedure, and more intensive use of antiplatelet medications) was studied by review of angiograms from 297 consecutive patients without evidence of AMI who underwent PTCA from April 1983 to March 1985 inclusive. Coronary artery thrombus was present in 34 (11%) patients, 8 (24%) of whom had complete occlusion during or immediately after PTCA compared with 34 (13%) of 263 patients without thrombus. Patients with preexisting coronary artery thrombus continue to be at greater risk of complete occlusion than patients without thrombus, but this risk has declined significantly since the modification of the PTCA procedure.

To assess angiographic patterns of restenosis after PTCA of multiple coronary arteries, DiSciascio and associates[109] from Richmond, Virginia, reviewed angiograms in 40 patients with clinical recurrence of stenosis after PTCA of multiple arteries. Clinical recurrence was defined as return of symptoms after successful PTCA of >1 major artery or branch and angiographic evidence of restenosis of ≥1 lesion. In these 40 patients, 83 arteries (2.1 arteries per patient) and 103 narrowings (2.6 narrowings per patient) were successfully dilated. Restenosis developed in 57 of 83 arteries at risk (69%): 23 patients (58%) had restenosis in only 1 artery and 17 (42%) in 2 arteries. Restenosis occurred in 63 of 103 lesions at risk (61%): 20 patients (50%) had restenosis of 2 narrowings and 3 (7%) had recurrence of 3 narrowings. Only 13 patients (33%) had restenosis of all narrowings dilated. Predictors of restenosis of individual narrowings were: higher pre–PTCA percent stenosis (87 ± 10% in narrowings with restenosis -vs- 82 ± 10% in narrowings without), and higher degree of residual stenosis after PTCA (46 ± 13% in narrowings with restenosis -vs- 36 ± 12% in narrowings without). Balloon size or inflation pressure did not predict recurrence of narrowings. Repeat PTCA was successful in 97% of cases attempted (33 of 34), 3 patients underwent elective CABG and 3 were managed with medical therapy. Most patients with clinical recurrence after PTCA of multiple arteries do not have restenosis of multiple arteries or narrowings, and only one-third will have recurrence of all narrowings. A higher degree of pre– and post–PTCA stenosis was associated with recurrence of individual narrowings.

Whitworth et al[110] in Atlanta, Georgia, evaluated the effect of *nifedipine* on restenosis after PTCA. Two hundred forty-one patients with 271 coronary dilatations were randomized at the time of hospital discharge to receive nifedipine (123 patients) or placebo (118 patients) as 10 mg 4 times daily for 6 months. The mean duration of therapy was 4.4 ± 2 months for nifedipine and 4.3 ± 2 months for placebo. A restudy coronary angiogram was available in 100 patients (81%) in the nifedipine-treated group and 98 patients (83%) in the placebo-treated group. A recurrent coronary stenosis, defined as the loss of ≥50% of the gain in luminal diameter accomplished at initial dilation, was found in 28% of patients in the nifedipine group and in 30% of those in the placebo group. The mean diameter stenosis was 36 ± 23% for those in the nifedipine-treated group and 37 ± 23% for those in the placebo-treated group. Thus, these data do not demonstrate a significant beneficial effect of nifedipine on the incidence of recurrent stenosis after successful PTCA in patients.

To determine risk factors for restenosis, Leimgruber and co-workers[111] in Atlanta, Georgia, studied 998 patients who underwent elective PTCA to native coronary arteries between July 1980 and July 1984. Restenosis, defined as a luminal narrowing of >50% at follow-up, was present in 302 patients (30%). Univariate analysis of 29 factors revealed 7 factors related to restenosis: coronary artery dilated (LC 18%, right 27%, LAD 34%); final gradient of ≤ 15 mmHg compared with >15 mmHg; duration of angina >2 months compared with angina of shorter duration; post–PTCA stenosis of ≤30% compared with 31–50%; stable -vs- unstable angina; presence -vs- absence of intimal dissection; and female gender -vs- male gender. Multivariate analysis revealed 5 factors independently related to increased risk of restenosis in the following order of importance: PTCA in the LAD coronary artery, absence of intimal dissection immediately after PTCA, final gradient >15 mmHg, a large residual stenosis after PTCA, and unstable angina. Thus, restenosis after PTCA is a multifactorial problem. The hemodynamic and angiographic result at the time of PTCA significantly influences long-term outcome, but additional measures aimed at reducing the rate of recurrence of atherosclerotic plaque are required.

Cost of surgical standby

Wilson and associates[112] from Cincinnati, Ohio, discussed the cost of surgical standby for PTCA; 699 patients had undergone PTCA at their institutions in 5 years. Simultaneous surgical standby was available in all cases: 124 patients (18%) underwent immediate myocardial revascularization; 45 were operated on because the narrowing could not be dilated; and 79 patients underwent immediate operation for an acute complication of PTCA (coronary occlusion in 45, dissection in 29, coronary perforation in 3, and atrial perforation in 1). Fourteen patients required cardiopulmonary resuscitation on route to the operating room and 10 patients had insertion of an intraaortic balloon pump in the catheterization laboratory. The average time from recognition of a complication to reperfusion was 87 minutes (range 40–165). Of the 79 patients undergoing operation for an acute complication, 1 died, 31 (39%) had an AMI according to enzyme criteria, and 17 patients (22%) had a new Q wave. These excellent results are related to minimizing the time from complication to reperfusion. No patient in whom reperfusion was begun in <75 minutes had a Q-wave AMI or a creatine kinase >40 IU. The authors suggest that surgical standby is the only method allowing immediate access to surgical facilities. However, a standby team of 8 persons and equipment for an average of 3.6 hours range from 1.3–5.4 hours per PTCA attempt, resulting in patient charges of $632 per PTCA attempt or $442,278.00 for the entire series. The actual cost of the standby was >$1,700.00 per attempt, totalling $1,188,843.00. Actual costs were difficult to estimate. At one institution there was no charge for cardiac surgical standby but the standby costs were absorbed in a large surcharge on all cardiac surgical procedures. At another institution, there was a minimal charge for cardiac surgical standby, the actual cost being reflected in an increased cardiac catheterization laboratory fee. Surgeon-man hours equaled 3.6 hours per attempt, only a small portion of this being productively used on other procedures. This multi-institutional study indicates that excellent results can be obtained even when

PTCA is complicated. However, the costs of simultaneous surgical standby must be factored in to the comparative analysis of primary PTCA -vs- primary surgical approaches.

Coronary angioplasty -vs- coronary surgeon (a debate)

A symposium was published in the December 1986 *Chest* discussing PTCA. It was advanced by Hartzler[113] from Kansas City, Missouri, and criticized to some extent by Kirklin[114] from Birmingham, Alabama. This symposium which reviews previously published data is well worth the reading. The most interesting feature is that Hartzler and Kirklin usually were in agreement. They both seemed to say that PTCA and CABG were not competitive therapies but should be viewed as complimentary therapies. Indeed, Hartzler advocated PTCA as an extension of medical therapy to further defer the need for CABG. This symposium provides both enjoyable and informative reading, and it is introduced by King[115] from Atlanta, Georgia.

CORONARY ARTERY BYPASS GRAFTING

Late results

FitzGibbon and associates[116] from Ottawa, Canada, studied 1,179 vein grafts angiographically in unselected survivors of 786 CABG operations. Studies were done at 1 month, 1 year, and 5 years. Ten percent, 17%, and 26% of grafts were occluded early at 1 and at 5 years, respectively. Irregularities in patent grafts increased from 9% at 1 year to 42% at 5 years. All severely narrowed grafts at the 1-year study had been normal in outline early. At the 5-year study, 79% had been disease-free at 1 year. All newly occluded grafts at the 1-year study had been normal in outline, and 82% had had a good patency early. Of newly occluded grafts at the 5-year study, 78% had been disease-free at 1 year, and 77% had had good patency. Thus, normal appearance of the intima in grafts studied at 1 year had no prognostic value for 5-year findings. However, 62% of grafts with the appearance of intimal disease at 1 year had deterioration by 5 years and 28% were occluded. Thus, the appearance of intimal irregularities compatible with atherosclerosis in saphenous vein grafts at 1 year after operation carried a poor prognosis; normally-appearing intima at 1 year had no predictive value for the 5-year study.

Rutherford and associates[117] from Auckland, New Zealand, analyzed the results of 492 consecutive CABG operations performed for angina in the 2-year period from 1976 to 1977 and evaluated them 77 months after CABG. Follow-up was complete in 99%. In 80% of patients angina severity was New York Heart Association functional classes III or IV. An EF of <50% and LV end-diastolic pressure of <15 mmHg were each present in one-third of patients. Thirteen patients (2.6%) died in the hospital and 70 (14%) died later during the follow-up period. Twenty-six reoperations were performed for recurrent angina (5.3%). Angina was initially relieved by operation in 97% of patients, but only 57% were alive and free of angina 6 years after their operation. Despite this, 91% of patients at last follow-up were in functional class I or II and 94% thought their symptoms were better than preoperatively. The mean postoperative time of onset of angina, estimated independently by family physicians and patients, was 33 months. The significant preoperative predictors of late death were a low LVEF, previous AMI, prior cardiac surgery, increased cardiothoracic ratio and the number of coronary arteries with significant narrowing.

Adler and associates[118] from Boston, Massachusetts, analyzed findings in 2,004 patients who underwent their first CABG between January 1970 and December 1980 without concomitant cardiac valve replacement or LV aneurysmectomy. Life-table survival was 89% at 5 years and 80% at 8 years after CABG. In a multivariate Cox model analysis, the independent correlates of long-term survival were emergent operation with cardiogenic shock, use of a postoperative intraaortic balloon pump, EF <50%, preoperative history of CHF, cardiopulmonary bypass time, uncorrected MR, LM coronary artery narrowing and diabetes mellitus. After controlling for these factors, age, sex, and the percentage of narrowings that were bypassed were not independent correlates of long-term survival.

Vigilante and associates[119] from Philadelphia, Pennsylvania, studied the survival of 1,657 patients with angiographically proved CAD for up to 4 years (mean 2 ± 1) during the 1980s to examine the prognostic importance of multiple clinical variables. One hundred of the 1,049 medically treated patients (9.5%) and 31 of the 608 surgically treated patients (5.1%) died. Multivariate analyses revealed that the strongest prognostic variables for survival in the medical group were indexes of LV function, severity of coronary stenoses, and age. However, only age was a significant prognostic variable in the surgically treated group. This study emphasizes the lack of prognostic significance of LV function indexes and severity of coronary stenoses in surgically treated patients with CAD.

Rahimtoola and co-workers[120] in Los Angeles, California, assessed the long-term results of CABG for angina from 1974–1983 in 1,304 patients aged ≥65 years (group 1). Using actuarial techniques, the investigators determined that the 5- and 10-year survival rates for patients ≥65 years were 81% and 65%, respectively. The patients aged 65 years and older were further subdivided into those aged 65–74 (group 1a) and 75–84 years (group 1b) and were compared with 1,700 patients aged 55–64 years (group 2). The operative mortality in the 3 subgroups was 3%, 3%, and 2%, respectively. For CABG, the duration of hospital stay was significantly longer by a mean of 1 to 2 days for group 1 patients and the cost of hospitalization was higher by a mean of $700. The cost of hospitalization was significantly higher only for group 1b patients. The 5-year survival rates for the 3 subgroups were 83%, 73%, and 91%, respectively. The 10-year survival rates were 66%, 65%, and 77%, respectively. The lower survival rates for subgroups 1a and 1b were significant; however, this lower survival was only seen in men. The mortality in the general population is expected to be higher for men than for women and for patients older than 65 years. For men, the mortality observed in these patients was lower than the expected mortality by a similar margin for all 3 subgroups. This suggests that the observed higher mortality of men in subgroups 1a and 1b is at least partly related to their older age. The reoperation rates and angina status at 1–5 years and 6–10 years were not significantly different among the 3 subgroups. The investigators concluded that the immediate and long-term results of CABG in patients aged 65–84 years are similar to those seen in a younger patient group. Therefore, CABG should be offered to the older members of our society for the usual indications.

Results with positive exercise tests

Weiner et al[121] from multiple centers using data from the Coronary Artery Surgery Study (CASS) determined whether exercise testing may identify

patients whose survival might be prolonged by CABG. In 5,303 nonrandomized patients from the CASS study who underwent exercise testing, the results of CABG were compared with those of medical therapy alone. The
patients in the 2 treatment groups differed substantially with regard to important baseline variables and an analysis of 32 variables of Cox's regression
model for survival revealed an independent beneficial effect of CABG on
survival (Table 2-3). Patients were stratified into subsets according to the
results of exercise testing. Surgical benefit was greatest in the 789 patients
who had ≥1 mm of ST-segment depression and who could exercise only into
stage 1 or less. Among the 398 patients with significant 3-vessel CAD with
these characteristics, the 7-year survival was 58% for the medical group and
81% for the surgical group (Fig. 2-23). There were no differences in survival
between the surgically- and medically-treated groups among the 1,545 patients without ST depression during exercise who were able to exercise into
stage 3 or greater. These data indicate that in patients who demonstrate
ST-segment depression on exercise testing and whose exercise capacity is
limited, CABG improves survival compared with medical therapy alone.

Influence of diabetes mellitus on results

To determine the long-term influence of the severity of preoperative diabetes mellitus on the results of CABG, Lawrie and associates[122] from Houston, Texas, reviewed 212 diabetic patients operated on between 1968 and
1973, of whom 87 (41%) were receiving no drugs, 108 (51%) were receiving
oral hypoglycemic agents, and 17 (8%) were receiving insulin. They were
compared with 1,222 nondiabetic patients operated on over the same period.
Perioperative mortality was similar in the diabetics and nondiabetics: 7.1%

TABLE 2-3. *Baseline characteristics of the medical and surgical cohort. Reproduced
with permission from Weiner et al.*[121]

VARIABLE	MEDICAL (N = 3,660)	SURGICAL (N = 1,643)	p VALUE
Clinical			
Age <60 yr	3,126 (85%)	1,284 (78%)	<0.0001
Male gender	2,708 (74%)	1,451 (87%)	<0.0001
Congestive heart failure score ≥3	114 (3%)	37 (2%)	0.259
Angina class III or IV	600 (16%)	635 (39%)	<0.0001
Prior myocardial infarction	1,612 (44%)	862 (53%)	<0.0001
One or more associated illnesses	2,707 (74%)	1,232 (75%)	0.115
Drug therapy			
Digitalis	375 (10%)	163 (10%)	0.721
β-adrenergic blocking agents	1,325 (26%)	812 (49%)	<0.0001
Arteriographic			
One vessel disease	913 (25%)	295 (18%)	
Two vessel disease	639 (18%)	555 (34%)	
Three vessel disease	479 (13%)	779 (47%)	<0.0001
Hemodynamic			
Left ventricular score ≥10	588 (16%)	304 (19%)	<0.001
Left ventricular end-diastolic pressure ≥18	465 (13%)	282 (17%)	<0.001
Exercise test			
ST depression ≥1 mm	1,295 (35%)	1,020 (62%)	<0.0001
Final exercise stage ≤1	762 (21%)	673 (41%)	<0.0001
Angina	963 (26%)	1,019 (62%)	<0.0001

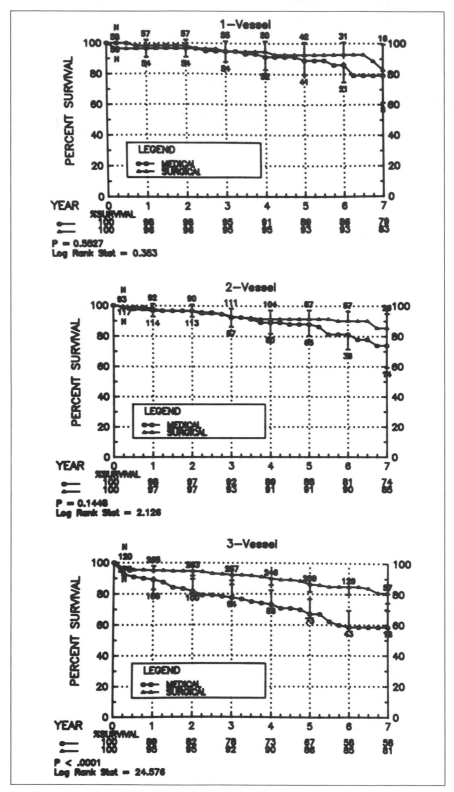

Fig. 2-23. Cumulative survival rates for medical and surgical patients with the higher risk exercise classification and single, double or triple vessel coronary disease. Reproduced with permission from Weiner et al.[121]

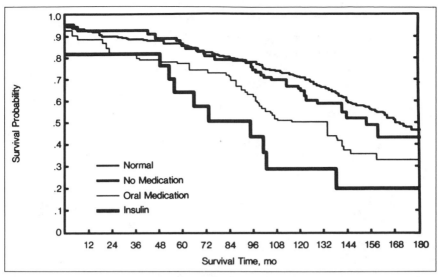

Fig. 2-24. Comparison of 15-year survival probabilities of 1222 nondiabetics, 87 patients not receiving drug treatment, 108 patients receiving oral hypoglycemic agents, and 17 patients treated with insulin. Reproduced with permission from Lawrie et al.[122]

-vs- 4.5%. Improvement in anginal symptoms were similar in all patient groups: 85.9–92.7%. Overall 15-year survival probability was 0.53 for the nondiabetic group, 0.43 for the diabetic patients not receiving drugs, 0.33 for those receiving oral agents, and 0.19 for the insulin-treated patients (Fig. 2-24). Late graft patency ranged from 78–90% and was comparable in all groups. The preoperative blood glucose level was an important predictor of late mortality in all diabetic patients (Fig. 2-25). Thus, CABG was effective in all groups of diabetic patients in long-term relief of anginal symptoms. Intermediate-term survival rates were good in all groups, but the initial severity of the diabetes was an important determinant of long-term survival rates.

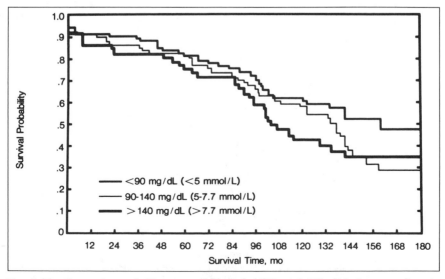

Fig. 2-25. Comparison of 15-year survival probabilities of 212 diabetics according to preoperative blood glucose levels. Reproduced with permission from Lawrie et al.[122]

Benefit of internal mammary artery graft

Loop and associates[123] from Cleveland, Ohio, compared patients who received an internal mammary artery (IMA) graft to the LAD coronary artery alone or combined with ≥1 saphenous vein (SV) grafts (n = 2,306) with patients who had only SV bypass grafts (n = 3625). The 10-year actuarial survival rate among the group receiving IMA graft compared with the group who received SV grafts (exclusive of hospital deaths) was 93.4% -vs- 88.0% for those with 1-vessel CAD (Fig. 2-26); 90% -vs- 79.5% for those with 2-vessel CAD (Fig. 2-27), and 82.6% -vs- 71.0% for those with 3-vessel CAD. After an adjustment for demographic and clinical differences by Cox multivariate analysis, the authors found that patients who had only vein grafts had a 1.61 times greater risk of death throughout the 10 years, compared with those who received an IMA graft. In addition, patients who received only vein grafts had 1.41 times the risk of late AMI, 1.25 times the risk of hospitalization for cardiac events, 2.00 times the risk of cardiac reoperation, and 1.27 times the risk of all late cardiac events, compared with patients who received IMA grafts. IMA grafting for lesions of the LAD coronary artery is preferable whenever indicated and technically feasible (Fig. 2-28). This article was followed by an editorial by Frank Spencer.[124]

Early patency and late patency have consistently been better with single internal mammary artery (IMA) grafts than with saphenous vein (SV) grafts.

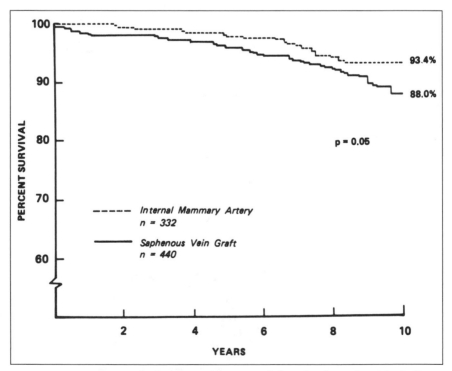

Fig. 2-26. Ten-year survival of patients with one-vessel (anterior descending artery) disease who had either an isolated internal-mammary-artery graft or a vein graft. The survival difference was statistically significant by univariate analysis; however, when preoperative multivariate characteristics were entered, significance was lost. Reproduced with permission from Loop et al.[123]

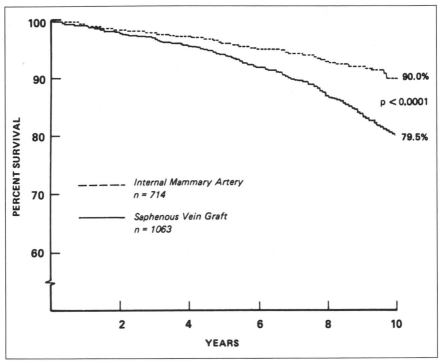

Fig. 2-27.   Ten-year survival of patients with two-vessel disease, including those with lesions of the proximal anterior descending artery. The difference in survival between the patients who received internal-mammary-artery grafts and those who received saphenous-vein grafts was significant by both univariate and multivariate analysis. Reproduced with permission from Loop et al.[123]

To determine the efficacy of these 2 types of grafts in sequential anastomoses, Orszulak and associates[125] from Rochester, Minnesota, performed sequential anastomoses of the left IMA to the LAD and diagonal coronary arteries in 40 patients and compared the results with those in 58 patients who received sequential SV grafts. Treatment with dipyridamole (starting 48 hours before CABG) and aspirin (added 7 hours after operation) was given to the 40 patients with IMA grafts and to 32 of the 58 patients with SV grafts. After CABG, mean blood flows were as follows: 68 ml/minute in patients with IMA grafts, 73 ml/minute in patients with SV grafts and a placebo, and 99 ml/minute in those who received SV grafts, aspirin, and dipyridamole. Early patency of sequential IMA grafts to the diagonal and LAD coronary arteries was comparable to that of sequential SV grafts. Because of a substantial late reduction in patency in sequential SV grafts, sequential IMA grafts appear to be the preferred conduit for CABG.

This article was followed by an editorial by Tector[126] who also concluded that the IMA artery will assume the role as the preferred graft in comparison to the SV graft.

Side-to-side -vs- end-to-side anastomoses

Kieser and associates[127] from Ottawa, Canada, continued their ongoing study of patency in SV CABG. To better define differences between patency in side-to-side -vs- end-to-side SV coronary artery anastomoses, they studied 212 sequential SV grafts early after operation. Ninety percent of these were evaluated again at 1 year and 44% at 5 years after operation. A total of 424 control

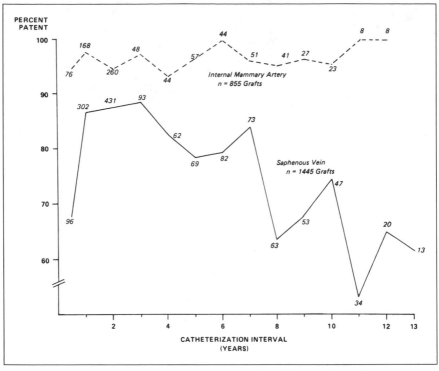

Fig. 2-28. Patency of internal-mammary-artery and saphenous-vein grafts at one-year intervals. The number of patients restudied at each interval is noted. Reproduced with permission from Loop et al.[123]

single grafts were studied similarly. Patency rates of side-to-side anastomoses were much better than those of end-to-side anastomoses whether of sequential or control single grafts (Tables 2-4 and 2-5). When specifically diagonal coronary artery–LAD coronary artery sequential grafts are considered, the combined patency of all sequential anastomoses theoretically exceeded that of a comparable number of single grafts at all times of the study, but the differences were small. However, there is a slightly better patency at a 5-year interval of end-to-side anastomoses of control single grafts than end-to-side anastomoses of sequential grafts. Although data included in their analysis appear to favor the sequential grafts, the authors suggest that, when looking at 3 or 4 sequential grafts, there is better patency of single than sequential grafts. Consequently, they concluded that single SV grafts be placed to each coronary artery unless there is a shortage of venous conduit or local aortic conditions dictate otherwise.

TABLE 2-4. Patency of SSAs and ESAs of 212 sequential grafts. Reproduced with permission from Kieser et al.[127]

TIME	SSA	%	ESA	%	p VALUE
Early	202/212	95	181/212	85	<0.0005
1 yr	168/188	89	146/188	78	<0.001
5 yr	77/91	85	60/91	66	<0.005

Legend: SSA, Side-to-side anastomosis. ESA, End-to-side anastomosis.

TABLE 2-5. *Patency of 212 SSAs and 424 control single grafts. Reproduced with permission from Kieser et al.*[127]

TIME	SSA	%	CONTROL	%	p VALUE
Early	202/212	95	375/424	88	<0.005
1 yr	168/188	89	305/379	80	<0.005
5 yr	77/91	85	162/214	76	<0.005

Legend: SSA, Side-to-side anastomosis.

With coronary endartectomy

Over a 14-year period (1970–1984), 30,464 patients underwent surgical revascularization for CAD at the Texas Heart Institute. Livesay and associates[128] examined the effect of coronary endarterectomy as an adjunct to CABG. CABG alone was done in 27,095 patients and was combined with coronary endarterectomy in 3,369 patients (12.4%). In those patients having endarterectomy, there was an increased incidence of male sex, diabetes mellitus, low EF, and multiple vessel CAD. Early results after CABG indicated a small increase in surgical risk and surgical mortality after endarterectomy: bypass alone 2.6% -vs- 4.4% for coronary endarterectomy. Multivariate analysis identified EF <30%, reoperation, age, absence of hyperlipidemia, endarterectomy, and female sex as indicative of increased operative risk. Early mortality was significantly increased by endarterectomy of the LAD coronary artery (8.5% mortality) compared to endarterectomy in arteries other than the LAD (4.2%). The frequency of perioperative AMI was 2.6% in patients undergoing CABG alone -vs- 5.4% for patients undergoing endarterectomy. Both fatal and nonfatal cardiac arrests were increased by endarterectomy, 3.5% -vs- 1.7%. This finding suggests the failure mode of unsuccessful endarterectomy. Actuarial analysis at 5 years and longer has shown little difference in the long-term survival rate (CABG alone 90%, endarterectomy 86%), freedom from angina (CABG alone 58%, endarterectomy 52%), and freedom from reoperation (CABG alone 97%, coronary endarterectomy 98%). Despite the small increase in surgical risk, the early and late results support the selective application of coronary endarterectomy. Coronary endarterectomy probably allows complete revascularization in patients with multiple vessel CAD who would otherwise be less well revascularized.

With the patient's lungs as oxygenator

Glenville and Ross[129] from London, UK, assessed the use of the patient's own lungs as oxygenator during CABG in 20 patients. This technique maintained the circulation and provided excellent oxygenation, and the lungs did not intrude on the operative field. Blood damage as assessed by platelet function and lung sequestration was less than that reported with other forms of bypass. No microbubbles were produced, since there was no artificial blood/air interface. Complement activation, as assessed by amount of white-cell sequestration in the lungs, was also lower than that reported in other forms of bypass. There were no major complications attributable to the technique. Apart from being substantially cheaper than conventional cardiopulmonary bypass, the use of the patient's lungs as oxygenator offers the potential advantage of reduced trauma to the blood and merits further consideration.

Supraventricular tachyarrhythmias postoperatively

SVT is a common complication of CABG. Dixon and associates[130] from New Orleans, Louisiana, and Kessler Air Force Base, Mississippi, retrospectively reviewed 424 cases of CABG and found that 64 patients (15%) had had clinically significant SVT. Sixty randomly selected arrhythmia-free patients served as controls. The arrhythmia group differed from the control group in age (62 ± 8 years -vs- 57 ± 8 years), radiographic cardiomegaly (19 of 64 patients with arrhythmia -vs- 6 of 60 control subjects), and echocardiographic LA enlargement (16 of 38 -vs- 6 of 37 control subjects). No significant differences existed regarding sex of the patient, prior AMI, reduced EF, history of CHF, occurrence of perioperative AMI or pericarditis, or pump time. The relative risk of SVT developing in patients ≥60 years was 1.91; in patients ≥60 years with LA enlargement, 3.29; and in patients ≥60 years with cardiomegaly and LA enlargement, 3.47. Thus, it may be possible to select patients at relatively higher risk of having SVT who could especially benefit from preventive measures.

SVT is common after CABG and it may have deleterious hemodynamic consequences. To determine if *acebutolol*, a cardioselective beta-blocking drug, prevents SVT after CABG, Daudon and associates[131] from Paris, France, entered 100 consecutive patients aged 30–77 years (mean 53) into a randomized, controlled study. From 36 hours after CABG until discharge (usually on the seventh day), 50 patients were given 200 mg of acebutolol (or 400 mg if weight was >80 kg) orally twice a day (dosage then modified to maintain a heart rate at rest between 60 and 90 beats/minute). The 50 patients in the control group did not receive beta-blocking drugs after CABG. The 2 groups were comparable in angina functional class, EF, number of diseased arteries, antianginal therapy before CABG, number of bypassed arteries, and duration of cardiopulmonary bypass. All patients were clinically evaluated twice daily and had continuous electrocardiographic monitoring and daily electrocardiograms. A 24-hour continuous electrocardiogram was recorded in the last 20 patients. Atrial tachyarrhythmias developed in 20 patients (40%) in the control group (17 patients had AF and 3 patients atrial flutter), but in none in the acebutolol group. This study reveals the efficacy of acebutolol in prevention of supraventricular tachyarrhythmias after CABG.

Conduction defects postoperatively

Wexelman and associates[132] from Brooklyn, New York, studied 200 consecutive patients undergoing only CABG. Forty-five patients (group A) had new fascicular conduction blocks and 155 patients (group B) did not. The 45 patients in group A had the following fascicular conduction blocks: right BBB 47%, right BBB and left anterior hemiblock 8%, right BBB and first-degree AV block 2%, left anterior hemiblock 11%, left BBB 18%, right BBB–left anterior hemiblock and first-degree AV block 5%. There were no significant differences in sex, prevalence of diabetes mellitus, number of grafts performed, EF (<55%) and perioperative AMI. Group A patients were older. Systemic hypertension was found frequently in group A (27 -vs- 45 patients) and was present for a mean of 12 years in group A and 5 years in group B. Preoperative use of digitalis was found in 14 (31%) patients in group A and in 18 (12%) patients in group B. Twenty-one (47%) patients in group A had significant disease (>70%) of the LM coronary artery compared to 17 (11%) in group B. There was no difference in the recurrence of angina or the survival rate at 14 months. In conclusion, the frequency of new fascicular conduction block after CABG is 23%. Long-standing hypertension, LM coronary disease, and the preoperative use of digitalis appear to be predisposing factors. New fascicular conduction block does not affect prognosis.

Usefulness of antithrombotic drugs

Many units have used the aspirin/dipyridamole regimen promulgated by the Mayo Clinic to improve patency in CABG. Jan Pirk and colleagues[133] from Prague, Czechoslovakia, presented their experience with a similar aspirin/ dipyridamole regimen. There were 1,017 bypasses performed in 442 patients. About 10% of the grafts had a flow rate of ≤40 ml/minute, and it is in these patients that the effect of aspirin and dipyridamole was evaluated. Coronary arteriography was performed at 1 month and then at 1 year after CABG. At 1 month postoperatively, 34 of 41 aortocoronary bypasses in the aspirin/dipy- ridamole group were patent compared to 17 of 37 patent in the untreated group. One year after operation, 34 of 37 aortocoronary bypasses in the treated group were patent, whereas in the control group, only 8 of 38 aorto- coronary bypasses were patent. The study indicates that in patients with low flow in grafts, antiplatelet drugs have a beneficial effect on short-term and long-term patency.

Reoperation

Reoperation may be necessary in 20% of patients 7–10 years after saphe- nous vein (SV) CABG. The proper management of SV grafts showing minimal angiographic evidence of atherosclerosis at reoperation for progressive ather- osclerosis in the native coronary arteries or for severe atherosclerosis in other SV grafts is uncertain. Marshall and colleagues[134] from St. Louis, Missouri, reported their policy of elective replacement of all SV grafts, irrespective of angiographic findings, when reoperation was necessary ≥5 years after the initial CABG. Sixteen patients had repeat CABG 6–13 years after initial CABG. In each, the operation included replacement of at least 1 SV graft showing no severe obstruction by angiography. At pathologic examination, 3 of the grafts had minimal, 5 had moderate, and 8 had severe atherosclerotic changes present. These changes were generally more diffuse than those observed by angiography. Because angiography underestimates the severity of the athero- sclerotic degeneration in SV grafts and because of the propensity of athero- sclerotic disease to progress at an unpredictable rate, the authors recom- mend routine replacement of all SV grafts at the time of reoperation if done ≥5 years after the initial procedure.

Lamas et al[135] in Boston, Massachusetts, evaluated 112 patients to deter- mine the efficacy and risks of repeat CABG between 1971 and 1981. Com- pared with patients who did poorly after a first CABG but who did not have repeat CABG, patients undergoing repeat CABG were younger, had a higher smoking rate, and had fewer prior AMIs. They also had fewer narrowed coronary arteries and fewer distal coronary artery narrowings. At least 1 graft was occluded in 83% of patients undergoing reoperation, and a mean of 1.7 grafts were placed at reoperation. Operative mortality rate was 4%, with a follow-up mortality rate of 6% at a mean of 3.8 years. After reoperation, patients initially showed improvement. The main correlate of a better long- term symptomatic response after the second CABG compared to that in the period before the first operation was a lower serum cholesterol level. These data should help identify patients who may benefit from a second CABG operation when angina recurs after the initial procedure. The data also em- phasize the importance of controlling and reducing serum cholesterol values after CABG.

Late morphologic studies

Neitzel and associates[136] from Milwaukee, Wisconsin, obtained segments of aortocoronary saphenous vein (SV) grafts from 42 patients who underwent a second CABG or came to autopsy 6–12 years after the initial CABG. Complex atheromas often associated with an acute thrombus were present in 71% of the grafts. In 14% of the cases, aneurysms of the atherosclerotic type were noted. The medical records of 40 of these patients were reviewed. Special attention was paid to risk factors associated with CAD. A control population of 535 patients who had undergone CABG and had not had recurrence of symptoms requiring reoperation ≥5 years later was drawn from the Milwaukee Cardiovascular Data Registry. Significantly higher triglyceride and cholesterol levels and lower HDL levels were noted in the patients undergoing 2 bypass procedures. In addition, more diabetic patients, cigarette smokers, and patients with abnormal lipoprotein phenotypes were noted in the study group. Systemic hypertension did not appear to be a significant risk factor. Atherosclerosis appears to be an important factor in late graft failure. Vein grafts that develop atherosclerosis appear to be susceptible to aneurysm formation. Risk factors associated with atherosclerosis in coronary arteries also appear to play a role in the development of atherosclerosis in aortocoronary bypass grafts.

KAWASAKI DISEASE

Capannari and associates[137] from Cincinnati, Ohio, evaluated 77 patients with Kawasaki disease using selective coronary angiography and compared results with a systematic 2-D echocardiogram. Aneurysms were demonstrated in 9/70 (13%) and the sensitivity of 2-D echocardiography was 100% for aneurysm detection. Echocardiography did not miss aneurysms when they were present in the proximal region of either coronary artery. Sensitivity was lower in the distal portion of the coronary system, but there were no patients with isolated distal aneurysms. The specificity was 96% for the entire coronary system, 99% for the right, and 95% for the left. The rare false positives occurred because of the difficulty of distinguishing arteries that were large but normal from those that contain a small fusiform aneurysm. This excellent study indicates that the predictive accuracy of a 2-D echocardiogram for coronary aneurysm is about 98%. In addition, the negative predictive value was also quite high, being 95–100%, depending on which coronary artery or region was in question. Thus, with a negative 2-D echo there is a low probability that the patient will have a coronary aneurysm regardless of the region imaged. This study is quite helpful in providing guidelines which indicate that coronary arteriography is probably not useful patients with Kawasaki disease who do not have signs or symptoms suggestive of myocardial ischemia.

Nakano and associates[138] from Shizuoka, Japan, reported 11 patients with AMI after Kawasaki disease. There were 7 male and 4 female patients, aged 3 months to 6 years. The AMI developed from 19–180 days of illness in all but 3 patients. Significant clinical symptoms were recognized in only 5 of 11. The diagnosis of AMI was confirmed by typical electrocardiography in 10 of 11, abnormality of LV wall motion by echo in 9 of 10, elevated cardiac enzymes in 6 of 6, thallium perfusion defect in 6 of 8, and coronary artery occlusion or ventricular aneurysm by angiogram in 9 of 9. All patients had markedly dilated and multiple coronary aneurysms during the course of the illness. These authors presented further valuable data on the rare occurrence of AMI after Kawasaki disease. These patients accounted for 2.3% of the 485 cases of Kawasaki disease seen at their hospital during the study. The time interval between onset of Kawasaki disease and recognition of AMI was 19 days to 14 months with 8 patients having AMI within 6 months after onset of disease. Asymptomatic AMI occurred in 6 of 11. These data provide further guidelines for followup of patients with Kawasaki disease. Of particular importance are patients with giant coronary aneurysms who obviously need close followup and antiplatelet therapy. In addition to the early onset of AMI, Kawasaki disease may set the stage for late sequelae with AMI many years after the initial episode (Am J Cardiol 1983; 52: 427–428, Arch Pathol Lab Med 1985; 109: 874–876, J Pediatr 1986; 108: 256–259).

Newburger and associates[139] from multiple USA medical centers compared the efficacy of intravenous gamma globulin plus aspirin with that of aspirin alone in reducing the frequency of coronary artery abnormalities in children with acute Kawasaki disease. Children randomly assigned to the gamma globulin group received intravenous gamma globulin, 400 mg/kg body weight per day for 4 consecutive days; both treatment groups received aspirin, 100 mg/kg/day, through the fourteenth day of illness, then 3–5 mg/kg/day. Two-D echocardiograms were interpreted blindly and independently by ≥2 readers. Two weeks after enrollment, coronary artery abnormalities were present in 18 of 78 children (23%) in the aspirin group compared with 6 of 75 (8%) in the gamma globulin group. Seven weeks after enrollment, abnormalities were present in 14 of 79 children (18%) in the aspirin group and in 3 of 79 (4%) in the gamma globulin group. No child had serious adverse effects from receiving gamma globulin. The authors concluded that high-dose intravenous gamma globulin is safe and effective in reducing the prevalence of coronary artery abnormalities when administered early in the course of Kawasaki disease. This article was followed by an editorial by Feigin and Barron[140].

MISCELLANEOUS TOPICS

Hlatky and associates[141] from Durham, North Carolina, identified medical, psychologic and social factors that independently affected employment in patients with CAD. At coronary angiography, extensive clinical, psychological, and social profiles were collected on 814 men >60 years of age with documented CAD. Clinical factors studied included measures of symptom severity, prior AMI, coronary anatomy and LV function. Psychosocial factors studied included the Minnesota Multiphasic Personality Inventory (MMPI), Zung Depression and Anxiety Scales, a type A structured interview, Jenkins Activity Survey and measures of education and social support. Multiple logistic regression analyses were used to assess the relative strength of the relation between these different factors and the patients' employment status. Many single factors differed between the 204 men (25%) who were disabled and the 610 (75%) who were not. Disabled men were less educated but no different in age, marital status or number of dependents. Disabled men had lower EF and higher indexes of angina, previous AMI and coexisting vascular disease. Disabled men also were more depressed and anxious and had lower ego strength and higher hypochondriasis scores on the MMPI, but were no different in type A behavior. By multivariable analysis, the most significant independent predictors of work disability were, in decreasing order of importance, low education level, history of AMI, high levels of depression and high levels of hypochondriasis. It was concluded that psychological and social factors are strongly related to work status in patients with CAD, and may be more important than medical factors.

Synchronized coronary sinus (CS) retroperfusion with arterial blood has been extensively tested in animals, and this intervention can offer temporary support to areas of ischemic myocardium while a method of definitive revascularization is being sought. The feasibility and safety of this procedure for patients with unstable angina was tested by Gore and co-workers[142] in Worcester, Massachusetts. A No. 7Fr, autoinflatable retroperfusion balloon catheter (USCI) was inserted percutaneously into the CS of the study patients. Arterial blood was obtained through a No. 8Fr catheter placed in the femoral artery. Arterial blood was infused in a retrograde fashion into the coronary venous system during cardiac diastole by means of a piston-driven pump that was electrocardiographically synchronized with the drainage of the venous system during systole. This procedure was performed in 5 patients with unstable angina refractory to maximum medical therapy. CS retroperfusion significantly decreased the frequency of anginal episodes and the requirement for antianginal medications. CS retroperfusion also provided time for patient stabilization before diagnostic cardiac catheterization of therapeutic intervention. This preliminary experience suggests that synchronized CS retroperfusion is a feasible and safe procedure. It can be performed at the bedside with no apparent adverse effects to the patient. Retroperfusion also appears to be effective in relieving ischemic symptoms.

The Council on Scientific Affairs[143] Panel on Lasers in Medicine and Surgery of the American Medical Association, summarized clinical applications for lasers in a number of medical and surgical specialties. New applications in current areas of use and extension of laser technology to other medical and surgical specialties will continue to occur as investigational uses are pursued. Lasers produce medical and surgical effects in target tissues by heating them to the point of coagulation or vaporization, by ionizing molecular tissue, and by inducing photochemical effects through a mediating photosensitizer. Increased ability to transmit certain laser beams via fiber optics further extends areas of clinical application. Laser safety programs are essential to safeguard physician operators, ancillary personnel, and patients. Federal regulation, under 2 laws, deals with the laser radiation safety of devices and controls to ensure that devices reaching the market are reasonably safe and effective for their intended use. This report emphasized that laser procedures as far as the cardiovascular system is concerned is, of course, still experimental.

Since the early demonstrations that laser radiation can effectively vaporize coronary atherosclerotic obstruction, attempts have been made to minimize its hazards by mounting a metal cap at the distal end of the flexible fiberoptic delivery system. The laser-heated metal cap has been shown to vaporize atherosclerotic plaque on contact. The present report by Lee and associates[144] from San Francisco, California, and Washington, D.C., demonstrated the successful clinical application of this device in LC segmental obstruction during CABG. One week and 5 months after the laser procedure, the LC recanalized site continued to be patent. This initial clinical report demonstrates that the flexible laser fiber with metal cap at its distal end can be effective in both acutely and chronically removing coronary atherosclerotic obstruction.

It has been suggested that CABG is efficacious in patients with severe CAD before they undergo a major noncardiac operation. Foster and associates[145] from Albany, New York, analyzed the CASS registry population to identify variables affecting operative mortality and cardiovascular morbidity for noncardiac procedures, and to assess the influence of prior CABG on the surgical risks. Major noncardiac operations were performed on 1,600 registry patients between June 30, 1978, and June 30, 1981. Operative mortality for patients without significant CAD was 0.5% (2/399 patients), and for patients with CAD having CABG before noncardiac procedure, 0.9% (7/743 patients). Patients with significant CAD undergoing noncardiac operation without prior CABG had an increased operative mortaltiy, 2.4% (11/458 patients). CABG patients had more severe angina symptoms and more extensive CAD on entering CASS than medically treated patients. Postoperative chest pain occurred in 8.7% of the medically treated patients -vs- 4.5% of the nonsignificant CAD patients, and 5.1% of the CABG patients. There were no differences noted for the frequency of perioperative AMI or arrhythmias.

Discriminant analysis revealed that a high LV score, preoperative nitrate use, male sex, diabetes, dyspnea on exertion, and LV hypertrophy noted on the electrocardiogram correlated independently with operative mortality, morbidity, or both. The authors concluded that the study supported the use of CABG in patients with important CAD before their undergoing a major noncardiac operation. Certainly, the patients with CABG had a lower mortality than patients with CAD who did not have CABG before the noncardiac surgical intervention. Dr. Gerald M. Lawrie of Houston, Texas, in discussing this article, emphasized that this, however, was not a study of the value of *prophylactic* CABG but of the outcome of *incidental* surgery performed on survivors of CABG. The distinction is that the CASS mortality of 2.4% for patients in this study must be included in the mortality data if one were going to suggest that a prophylactic operation produced a better result. Additionally, it is claimed that present techniques of anesthesia and perioperative care supersede the state of the art which applied at the time of the CASS study.

References

1. DETRANO R, SALCEDO EE, HOBBS RE, YIANNIKAS J: Cardiac cinefluoroscopy as an inexpensive aid in the diagnosis of coronary artery disease. Am J Cardiol 1986 (May 1); 57:1041–1046.

2. WITTEMAN JCM, KOK FJ, SAASE JLCM, VALKENBURG HA: Aortic calcification as a predictor of cardiovascular mortality. Lancet 1986 (Nov 15); 1120–1122.

3. KRAMER B, BRILL M, BRUHN A, KUBLER W: Relationship between the degree of coronary artery disease and of left ventricular function and the duration of the QT-interval in ECG. European Heart Journal 1986 (Jan); 7:14–24.

4. SASAKI H, CHARUZI Y, BEEDER C, SUGIKI Y, LEW AS: Utility of echocardiography for the early assessment of patients with nondiagnostic chest pain. Am Heart J 1986 (Sept); 112:494–497.

5. GORDON DJ, EKELUND LG, KARON JM, PROBSTFIELD JL, RUBENSTEIN C, SHEFFIELD T, WEISSFELD L: Predictive value of the exercise tolerance test for mortality in North American men: the lipid research clinics mortality follow-up study. Circulation 1986 (Feb); 74:252–261.

6. RAUTAHARJU PM, PRINEAS RJ, EIFLER WJ, FURBERG CD, NEATON JD, CROW RS, STAMLER J, CUTLER JA: Prognostic value of exercise electrocardiogram in men at high risk of future coronary heart disease: multiple risk factor intervention trial experience. J Am Coll Cardiol 1986 (July); 8:1–10.

7. HAKKI A, MUNLEY BM, HADJIMILTIADES S, MEISSNER MD, ISKANDRIAN AS: Determinants of abnormal blood pressure response to exercise in coronary artery disease. Am J Cardiol 1986 (Jan 1); 57:71–75.

120 • CARDIOLOGY 1987

8. Weintraub WS, Schneider RM, Seelaus PA, Wiener DH, Agarwal JB, Helfant RH: Prospective evaluation of the severity of coronary artery disease with exercise radionuclide angiography and electrocardiography. Am Heart J 1986 (Mar); 111:537–542.

9. Ahnve S, Savvides M, Abouantoun S, Atwood JE, Froelicher V: Can myocardial ischemia be recognized by the exercise electrocardiogram in coronary disease patients with abnormal resting Q waves? Am Heart J 1986 (May); 111:909–916.

10. Finkelhor RS, Newhouse KE, Vrobel TR, Miron SD, Bahler RC: The ST segment/heart rate slope as a predictor of coronary artery disease: comparison with quantitative thallium imaging and conventional ST segment criteria. Am Heart J 1986 (Aug); 112:296–304.

11. Kligfield P, Okin PM, Ameisen O, Borer JS: Evaluation of coronary artery disease by an improved method of exercise electrocardiography: the ST segment/heart rate slope. Am Heart J 1986 (Sept); 112:589–598.

12. Armstrong WF, O'Donnell J, Dillon JC, McHenry PL, Morris SN, Feigenbaum H: Complementary value of two-dimensional exercise echocardiography to routine treadmill exercise testing. Ann Intern Med 1986 (Dec); 105:829–835.

13. Homma S, Callahan RJ, Ameer B, McKusick KA, Strauss HW, Okada RD, Boucher CA: Usefulness of oral dipyridamole suspension for stress thallium imaging without exercise in the detection of coronary artery disease. Am J Cardiol 1986 (Mar 1); 57:503–508.

14. Picano E, Masini M, Distante A, Simonetti I, Lattanzi F, Marzilli M, L'Abbate A: Dipyridamole-echocardiography test in patients with exercise-induced ST-segment elevation. Am J Cardiol 1986 (Apr 1); 765–768.

15. Maddahi J, Abdulla A, Garcia EV, Swan HJC, Berman DS: Noninvasive identification of left main and triple vessel coronary artery disease: improved accuracy using quantitative analysis of regional myocardial stress distribution and washout of thallium-201. J Am Coll Cardiol 1986 (Jan); 7:53–60.

16. Ladenheim ML, Pollock BH, Rozanski A, Berman DS, Staniloff HM, Forrester JS, Diamond GA: Extent and severity of myocardial hypoperfusion as predictors of prognosis in patients with suspected coronary artery disease. J Am Coll Cardiol 1986 (Mar); 7:464–471.

17. Kaul S, Boucher CA, Newell JB, Chesler DA, Greenberg JM, Okada RD, Strauss HW, Dinsmore RE, Pohost GM: Determination of the quantitative thallium imaging variables that optimize detection of coronary artery disease. J Am Coll Cardiol 1986 (Mar); 7:527–537.

18. Taillefer R, Lette J, Phaneuf D-C, Léveille J, Lemire F, Essiambre R: Thallium-201 myocardial imaging during pharmacologic coronary vasodilation: comparison of oral and intravenous administration of dipyridamole. J Am Coll Cardiol 1986 (July); 8:76–83.

19. Kaul S, Chesler DA, Newell JB, Pohost GM, Okada RD, Boucher CA: Regional variability in the myocardial clearance of thallium-201 and its importance in determining presence or absence of coronary artery disease. J Am Coll Cardiol 1986 (July); 8:95–100.

20. Iskandrian AS, Hakki AH, Kane-Marsch S: Exercise thallium-201 scintigraphy in men with nondiagnostic exercise electrocardiograms: Prognostic implications. Arch Intern Med 1986 (Nov); 146:2189–2193.

21. Tillisch J, Brunken R, Marshall R, Schwaiger M, Mandelkern M, Phelps M, Schelbert H: Reversibility of cardiac wall-motion abnormalities predicted by positron tomography. N Engl J Med 1986 (Apr 3); 314:884–888.

22. Gould KL, Goldstein RA, Mullani NA, Kirkeeide RL, Wong W, Tewson TJ, Berridge MS, Bolomey LA, Hartz RK, Smalling RW, Fuentes F, Nishikawa A: Noninvasive assessment of coronary stenoses by myocardial perfusion imaging during pharmacologic coronary vasodilation. VII. Clinical feasibility of positron cardiac imaging without a cyclotron using generator-produced rubidium-82. J Am Coll Cardiol 1986 (Apr); 7:775–789.

23. Thompson R: Isolated coronary ostial stenosis in women. J Am Coll Cardiol 1986 (May); 7:997–1003.

24. Lee KL, Pryor DB, Harrell FE, Califf RM, Behar VS, Floyd WL, Morris JJ, Waugh RA, Whalen RE, Rosati RA: Predicting outcome in coronary disease: statistical models versus expert clinicians. Am J Med 1986 (Apr); 80:553–660.

25. Klein LW, Weintraub WS, Agarwal JB, Schneider RM, Seelaus PA, Katz RI, Helfant RH: Prognostic significance of severe narrowing of the proximal portion of the left anterior descending coronary artery. Am J Cardiol 1986 (July 1); 58:42–46.

26. Hamby RI, Hamby B, Hoffman I: Symptomatic coronary disease for 20 or more years: Clinical aspects, angiographic findings, and therapeutic implications. Am Heart J 1986 (July); 112:65–70.

27. Papanicolaou MN, Califf RM, Hlatky MA, McKinnis RA, Harrell FE, Mark DB, McCants B,

ROSATI RA, LEE KL, PRYOR DB: Prognostic implications of angiographically normal and insignificantly narrowed coronary arteries. Am J Cardiol 1986 (Dec 1); 58:1181–1187.

28. RAICHLEN JS, HEALY B, ACHUFF SC, PEARSON TA: Importance of risk factors in the angiographic progression of coronary artery disease. Am J Cardiol 1986 (Jan 1); 57:66–70.

29. VISSER RF, VAN DER WERF T, ASCOOP CAPL, BRUSCHKE AVG: The influence of anatomic evolution of coronary artery disease on left ventricular contraction: an angiographic follow-up study of 300 nonoperated patients. Am Heart J 1986 (Nov); 112:963–972.

30. SHEA S, SCIACCA RR, ESSER P, HAN J, NICHOLS AB: Progression of coronary atherosclerotic disease assessed by cinevideodensitometry: relation to clinical risk factors. J Am Coll Cardiol 1986 (Dec); 8:1325–1331.

31. ELLIS S, SANDERS W, GOULET C, MILLER R, CAIN KC, LESPERANCE J, BOURASSA MG, ALDERMAN EL: Optimal detection of the progression of coronary artery disease: comparison of methods suitable for risk factor intervention trials. Circulation 1986 (Dec); 74:1235–1242.

32. CAMPBELL S, BARRY J, ROCCO MB, NABEL EG, MEAD-WALTERS K, REBECCA GS, SELWYN AP: Features of the exercise test that reflect the activity of ischemic heart disease out of hospital. Circulation 1986 (Jan); 74:72–80.

33. CAMPBELL S, BARRY J, REBECCA GS, ROCCO MB, NABEL EG, WAYNE RR, SELWYN AP: Active transient myocardial ischemia during daily life in asymptomatic patients with positive exercise tests and coronary artery disease. Am J Cardiol 1986 (May 1); 57:1010–1016.

34. COHN PF, BROWN EJ, SWINFORD R, ATKINS HL: Effect of beta blockade on silent regional left ventricular wall motion abnormalities. Am J Cardiol 1986 (Mar 1); 57:521–526.

35. PICANO E, MASINI M, LATTANZI F, DISTANTE A, L'ABBATE A: Role of dipyridamole-echocardiography test in electrocardiographically silent effort myocardial ischemia. Am J Cardiol 1986 (Aug 1); 58:235–237.

36. KASKI JC, CREA F, NIHOYANNOPOULOS P, HACKETT D, MASERI A, WATSON J, O'SULLIVAN C: Transient myocardial ischemia during daily life in patients with syndrome X. Am J Cardiol 1986 (Dec 1); 58:1242–1247.

37. DEANFIELD JE, SHEA MJ, WILSON RA, HORLOCK P, DE LANDSHEERE CM, SELWYN AP: Direct effects of smoking on the heart: silent ischemic disturbances of coronary flow. Am J Cardiol 1986 (May 1); 57:1005–1009.

38. GOTTLIEB SO, WEISFELDT ML, OUYANG P, MELLITS ED, GERSTENBLITH G: Silent ischemia as a marker for early unfavorable outcomes in patients with unstable angina. N Engl J Med 1986 (May 8); 314:1214–1219.

39. GLAZIER JJ, CHIERCHIA S, BROWN MJ, MASERI A: Importance of generalized defective perception of painful stimuli as a cause of silent myocardial ischemia in chronic stable angina pectoris. Am J Cardiol 1986 (Oct 1); 58:667–672.

40. PROUDFIT WL, KRAMER JR, BOTT-SILVERMAN C, GOORMASTIC M: Survival of non-surgical patients with mild angina or myocardial infarction without angina. Br Heart J 1986 (Sept); 56:213–21.

41. DALY LE, NICKEY N, MULCAHY R: Course of angina pectoris after an acute coronary event. British Med J 1986 (Sept 13); 293:653–656.

42. CREA F, MARGONATO A, KASKI JC, RODRIGUEZ-PLAZA L, MERAN DO, DAVIES G, CHIERCHIA S, MASERI A: Variability of results during repeat exercise stress testing in patients with stable angina pectoris: Role of dynamic coronary flow reserve. Am Heart J 1986 (Aug); 112:249–254.

43. DE SERVI S, GHIO S, FERRARIO M, ARDISSINO D, ANGOLI L, MUSSINI A, BRAMUCCI E, SALERNO J, VIGANO M, MONTEMARTINI C, SPECCHIA G: Clinical and angiographic findings in angina at rest. Am Heart J 1986 (Jan); 111:6–11.

44. SCLAROVSKY S, DAVIDSON E, STRASBERG B, LEWIS RF, ARDITTI A, WURTZEL M, AGMON J: Unstable angina: The significance of ST segment elevation or depression in patients without evidence of increased myocardial oxygen demand. Am Heart J 1986 (Sept); 112:463–467.

45. BUTMAN SM, OLSON HG, BUTMAN LK: Early exercise testing after stabilization of unstable angina: Correlation with coronary angiographic findings and subsequent cardiac events. Am Heart J 1986 (Jan); 111:11–18.

46. PICANO E, LATTANZI F, MASINI M, DISTANTE A, L'ABBATE A: High dose dipyridamole echocardiography test in effort angina pectoris. J Am Coll Cardiol 1986 (Oct); 8:848–854.

47. WILSON RF, HOLIDA MD, WHITE CW: Quantitative angiographic morphology of coronary stenoses leading to myocardial infarction or unstable angina. Circulation 1986 (Feb); 73(2):286–293.

48. AMBROSE JA, WINTERS SL, ARORA RR, ENG A, RICCIO A, GORLIN R, FUSTER V: Angiographic evolu-

tion of coronary artery morphology in unstable angina. J Am Coll Cardiol 1986 (Mar); 7:472–478.

49. YASUE H, TAKIZAWA A, NAGAO M, NISHIDA S, HORIE M, KUBOTA J, FUJII H: Pathogenesis of angina pectoris in patients with one-vessel disease: possible role of dynamic coronary obstruction. Am Heart J 1986 (Aug); 112:263–272.

50. SCHOFIELD PM, BROOKS NH, BENNETT DH: Left ventricular dysfunction in patients with angina pectoris and normal coronary angiograms. Br Heart J 1986 (Oct); 56:327–333.

51. MOSSERI M, YAROM R, GOTSMAN M, AND HASIN Y: Histologic evidence for small-vessel coronary artery disease in patients with angina pectoris and patent large coronary arteries. Circulation 1986 (Nov); 74:964–972.

52. SHERMAN CT, LITVACK F, GRUNDFEST W, LEE M, HICKEY A, CHAUX A, KASS R, BLANCHE C, MATLORR J, MORGENSTERN L, GANZ W, SWAN HJC, FORRESTER J: Coronary angioscopy in patients with unstable angina pectoris. N Engl J Med 1986 (Oct 9); 315:913–919.

53. FITZGERALD DJ, ROY MBL, CATELLA F, FITZGERALD GA: Platelet activation in unstable coronary disease. N Engl J Med 1986 (Oct 16); 315:983–989.

54. FUSTER V, CHESEBRO JH: Mechanisms of unstable angina. N Engl J Med 1986 (Oct 16); 315:1023–1025.

55. DAVIES MJ, THOMAS AC, KNAPMAN PA, HANGARTNER JR: Intramyocardial platelet aggregation in patients with unstable angina suffering sudden ischemic cardiac death. Circulation 1986 (Mar); 73(3):418–427.

56. SCLAROVSKY S, DAVIDSON E, LEWIN RF, STRASBERG B, ARDITTI A, AGMON J: Unstable angina pectoris evolving to acute myocardial infarction: significance of ECG changes during chest pain. Am Heart J 1986 (Sept); 112:459–462.

57. WATERS DD, WALLING A, ROY D, THEROUX P: Previous coronary artery bypass grafting as an adverse prognostic factor in unstable angina pectoris. Am J Cardiol 1986 (Sept 1); 58:465–469.

58. KHURMI NS, BOWLES MJ, KOHLI RS, RAFTERY EB: Does placebo improve indexes of effort-induced myocardial ischemia? an objective study in 150 patients with chronic stable angina pectoris. Am J Cardiol 1986 (Apr 15); 57:907–911.

59. THADANI U, HAMILTON SF, OLSON E, ANDERSON J, VOYLES W, PRASAD R, TEAGUE SM: Transdermal nitroglycerin patches in angina pectoris: dose titration, duration of effect, and rapid tolerance. Ann Intern Med 1986 (Oct); 105:485–492.

60. KLEIN HO, NINIO R, BLANK I, SEGNI ED, BEKER B, OREN V, KAPLINSKY E: Prolonged hemodynamic effect of a slow-release nitroglycerin ointment. Am J Cardiol 1986 (Sept 1); 58:436–442.

61. PARKER JO, VANKOUGHNETT KA, FARRELL B: Nitroglycerin lingual spray: clinical efficacy and dose-response relation. Am J Cardiol 1986 (Jan 1); 57:1–5.

62. ALPERT MA, SINGH A, HOLMES RA, SANFELIPPO JF, FLAKER GC, VILLARREAL D, MUKERJI V, MORGAN RJ: Effect of beta blockade with betaxolol on left ventricular systolic function in chronic stable angina pectoris and left ventricular dysfunction. Am J Cardiol 1986 (Apr 1); 57:721–724.

63. WEINER DA, CUTLER SS, KLEIN MD: Efficacy and safety of sustained-release diltiazem in stable angina pectoris. Am J Cardiol 1986 (Jan 1); 57:6–9.

64. JOYAL M, CREMER K, PIEPER J, FELDMAN RL, PEPINE CJ: Effects of diltiazem during tachycardia-induced angina pectoris. Am J Cardiol 1986 (Jan 1); 57:10–14.

65. JOYAL M, PIEPER J, CREMER K, FELDMAN RL, PEPINE CJ: Pharmacodynamic aspects of intravenous diltiazem administration. Am Heart J 1986 (Jan); 111:54–61.

66. VAN DER WALL EE, KERKKAMP J, SIMOONS ML, VAN RIJK PP, REIBER JHC, BOM N, LUBSEN JC, LIE KI: Effects of nifedipine on left ventricular performance in unstable angina pectoris during a follow-up of 48 hours. Am J Cardiol 1986 (May 1); 57:1029–1033.

67. SCHEIDT S, LEWINTER MM, HERMANOVICH J, VENKATARAMAN K, FREEDMAN D: Efficacy and safety of nicardipine for chronic, stable angina pectoris: a multicenter randomized trial. Am J Cardiol 1986 (Oct 1); 58:715–721.

68. BUITLEIR M, KRIKLER S, KRIKLER DM: Usefulness of PY 108-608, a new calcium channel blocker, for angina pectoris. Am J Cardiol 1986 (Jan 1); 57:15–29.

69. HOSSACK KF, ELDRIDGE JE, BUCKNER K: Comparison of acute hemodynamic effects of nitroglycerin versus diltiazem and combined acute effects of both drugs in angina pectoris. Am J Cardiol 1986 (Oct 1); 58:722–726.

70. HUMEN DP, O'BRIEN P, PURVES P, JOHNSON D, KOSTUK WJ: Effort angina with adequate beta-receptor blockade: comparison with diltiazem and in combination. J Am Coll Cardiol

1986 (Feb); 7:329–335.

71. Higginbotham MB, Morris KG, Coleman RE, Cobb FR: Comparison of nifedipine alone with propranolol alone for stable angina pectoris including hemodynamics at rest and during exercise. Am J Cardiol 1986 (May 1); 57:1022–1028.

72. Gottlieb SO, Weisfeldt ML, Ouyang P, Achuff SC, Baughman KL, Traill TA, Brinker JA, Shapiro EP, Chandra NC, Mellits ED, Townsend SN, Gerstenblith G: Effect of the addition of propranolol to therapy with nifedipine for unstable angina pectoris: a randomized, double-blind, placebo-controlled trial. Circulation 1986 (Feb); 73(2):331–337.

73. McGill D, McKenzie W, McCredie M: Comparison of nicardipine and propranolol for chronic stable angina pectoris. Am J Cardiol 1986 (Jan 1); 57:39–43.

74. Rousseau MF, Hanet C, Pardonge-Lavenne E, Van Den Berghe G, Van Hoof F, Pouleur H: Changes in myocardial metabolism during therapy in patients with chronic stable angina: a comparison of long-term dosing with propranolol and nicardipine. Circulation 1986 (June); 73(6):1270–1280.

75. Parodi O, Simonetti I, Michelassi C, Carpeggiani C, Biagini A, L'Abbate A, Maseri A: Comparison of verapamil and propranolol therapy for angina pectoris at rest: a randomized, multiple-crossover, controlled trial in the coronary care unit. Am J Cardiol 1986 (Apr 15); 57:899–906.

76. Parker JO, Farrell B: Comparative anti-anginal effects of bepridil and propranolol in angina pectoris. Am J Cardiol 1986 (Sept 1); 58:449–452.

77. Holland Interunivesity Nifedipine/Metoprolol Trial (HINT) Research Group: Early treatment of unstable angina in the coronary care unit: a randomised, double blind, placebo controlled comparison of recurrent ischemia in patients treated with nifedipine or metoprolol or both. Br Heart J 1986 (Nov); 56:400–413.

78. Fox KM, Krikler DM: Early treatment of unstable angina. Br Heart J 1986 (Nov); 56:398–399.

79. Uusitalo A, Arstila M, Bae EA, Harkonen R, Keyrilainen O, Rytkonen U, Schjelderup-Mathiesen PM, Wendelin H: Metoprolol, nifedipine, and the combination in stable effort angina pectoris. Am J Cardiol 1986 (Apr 1); 57:733–737.

80. Freedman SB, Richmond DR, Alwyn M, Kelly DT: Late follow-up (41 to 102 months) of medically treated patients with coronary artery spasm and minor atherosclerotic coronary obstructions. Am J Cardiol 1985 (June 1); 57:1261–1263.

81. Crea F, Shierchia S, Kaski JC, Davies GH, Margonato A, Miran DO, Maseri A: Provocation of coronary spasm by dopamine in patients with active variant angina pectoris. Circulation 1986 (Feb); 74:262–269.

82. Yasue H, Horio Y, Nakamura N, Fuji Imoto N, Sonoda R, Kugiyama K, Obata K, Morikami Y, Tadashi K: Induction of coronary artery spasm by acetylcholine in patients with variant agina: possible role of the parasympathetic nervous system in the pathogenesis of coronary artery spasm. Circulation 1986 (Nov); 74:955–963.

83. Scholl JM, Benacerraf A, Ducimetiere P, Chabas D, Brau J, Chapelle J, Thery JL: Comparison of risk factors in vasospastic angina without significant fixed coronary narrowing to significant fixed coronary narrowing and no vasospastic angina. Am J Cardiol 1986 (Feb 1); 57:199–202.

84. Rasmussen K, Funch-Jensen P, Ravnsbaek J, Bagger JP: Esophageal spasm in patients with coronary artery spasm. Lancet 1986 (Jan 25); 174–176.

85. Unsigned: Angina and esophageal disease. Lancet 1986 (Jan 25); 191–192.

86. Araki H, Hayata N, Matsuguchi T, Takeshita A, Nakamura M: Diagnosis of important fixed coronary stenosis in patients with variant angina by exercise tests after treatment with calcium antagonists. Br Heart J 1986 (Aug); 56:138–145.

87. Jacob AS, Pichard AD, Ohnmact SD, Lindsay J: Results of percutaneous transluminal coronary angioplasty by multiple relatively low frequency operators. Am J Cardiol 1986 (Apr 1); 57:713–716.

88. Harston WE, Tilley S, Rodeheffer R, Forman MB, Perry JM: Safety and success of the beginning percutaneous transluminal coronary angioplasty program using the steerable guidewire system. Am J Cardiol 1986 (Apr 1); 57:171–720.

89. Hartzler GO: Percutaneous transluminal coronary angioplasty: view of a single relatively high frequency operator. Am J Cardiol 1986 (Apr 1); 57:869–872.

90. Roubin GS, Douglas JS, King SB: Percutaneous coronary angioplasty: influence of operator experience on results. Am J Cardiol 1986 (Apr 1); 57:873–874.

91. Berger E, Williams DO, Reinert S, Most AS: Sustained efficacy of percutaneous transluminal

coronary angioplasty. Am Heart J 1986 (Feb); 111:233–236.

92. Hodgson JM, Reinert S, Most AS, Williams DO: Prediction of long-term clinical outcome with final translesional pressure gradient during coronary angioplasty. Circulation 1986 (Mar); 74:563–566.

93. Raizner AE, Hust RG, Lewis JM, Winters WL, Batty JW, Roberts R: Transluminal coronary angioplasty in the elderly. Am J Cardiol 1986 (Jan 1); 57:29–32.

94. de Feyter PJ, Serruys PW, Soward A, van den Brand M, Bos E, Hugenholtz PG: Coronary angioplasty for early postinfarction unstable angina. Circulation 1986 (Dec); 74:1365–1370.

95. DiSciascio G, Vetrovec GW, Cowley MJ, Wolfgang TC: Early and late outcome of percutaneous transluminal coronary angioplasty for subacute and chronic total coronary occlusion. Am Heart J 1986 (May); 111:833–839.

96. Bertrand ME, LaBlanche JM, Thieuleux FA, Fourrier JL, Traisnel G, Asseman P: Comparative results of percutaneous transluminal coronary angioplasty in patients with dynamic versus fixed coronary stenosis. J Am Coll Cardiol 1986 (Sept); 8:504–508.

97. Reeder GS, Bresnahan JF, Holmes DR, Mock MB, Orszulak TA, Smith HC, Vlietstra RE: Angioplasty for aortocoronary bypass graft stenosis. Mayo Clin Proc 1986 (Jan); 61:14–19.

98. Quyyumi AA, Rubens MB, Rickards AF, Crake T, Levy RD, Fox KM: Importance of "reciprocal" electrocardiographic changes during occlusion of left anterior descending coronary artery: studies during percutaneous transluminal coronary angioplasty. Lancet 1986 (Feb 15); 347–350.

99. MacDonald RG, Hill JA, Feldman RL: ST segment response to acute coronary occlusion: coronary hemodynamic and angiographic determinants of direction of ST segment shift. Circulation 1986 (Nov); 74:973–979.

100. Cleman M, Jaffee CC, Wohlgelernter D: Prevention of ischemia during percutaneous transluminal coronary angioplasty by transcatheter infusion of oxygenated fluosol DA 20%. Circulation 1986 (Mar); 74:555–562.

101. Wijns W, Serruys PW, Slager CJ, Grimm J, Krayenbuehl HP, Hugenholtz PG, Hess OM: Effect of coronary occlusion during percutaneous transluminal angioplasty in humans on left ventricular chamber stiffness and regional diastolic pressure-radius relations. J Am Coll Cardiol 1986 (Mar); 7:455–463.

102. Wohlgelernter D, Cleman M, Highman HA, Fetterman RC, Duncan JS, Zaret BL, Jaffe CC: Regional myocardial dysfunction during coronary angioplasty: evaluation by two-dimensional echocardiography and 12 lead electrocardiography. J Am Coll Cardiol 1986 (June); 7:1245–1254.

103. Visser CA, David GK, Kan G, Romijn KH, Meltzer RS, Koolen JJ, Dunning AJ: Two-dimensional echocardiography during percutaneous transluminal coronary angioplasty. Am Heart J 1986 (June); 111:1035–1041.

104. Zalewski A, Goldberg S, Dervan JP, Slysh S, Maroko PR: Myocardial protection during transient coronary artery occlusion in man: beneficial effects of regional β-adrenergic blockade. Circulation 1986 (April); 73(4):734–739.

105. Cohen M, Rentrop KP: Limitation of myocardial ischemia by collateral circulation during sudden controlled coronary artery occlusion in human subjects: a prospective study. Circulation 1986 (Mar); 74:469–476.

106. Johnson MR, Brayden GP, Ericksen EE, Collins SM, Skorton DJ, Harrison DG, Marcus ML, White CW: Changes in cross-sectional area of the coronary lumen in the six months after angioplasty: a quantitative analysis of the variable response to percutaneous transluminal angioplasty. Circulation 1986 (Mar); 73(3):467–475.

107. Ischinger T, Gruentzig AR, Meier B, Galan K: Coronary dissection and total coronary occlusion associated with percutaneous transluminal coronary angioplasty: significance of initial angiographic morphology of coronary stenoses. Circulation 1986 (Dec); 74:1371–1378.

108. Sugrue DD, Holmes DR, Smith HC, Reeder GS, Lane GE, Vlietstra RE, Bresnahan JF, Hammes LN, Piehler JM: Coronary artery thrombus as a risk factor for acute vessel occlusion during percutaneous transluminal coronary angioplasty: improving results. Br Heart J 1986 (July); 56:62–66.

109. Disciascio G, Cowley MJ, Vetrovec GW: Angiographic patterns of restenosis after angioplasty of multiple coronary arteries. Am J Cardiol 1986 (Nov 1); 58:922–925.

110. Whitworth HB, Roubin GS, Hollman J, Meier B, Leimgruber PP, Douglas JS Jr., King SB III, Gruentzig AR: Effect of nifedipine on recurrent stenosis after percutaneous transluminal

coronary angioplasty. J Am Coll Cardiol 1986 (Dec); 8:1271–1276.

111. Leimgruber PP, Roubin GS, Hollman J, Cotsonis GA, Meier B, Douglas JS, King SB, Gruentzig, AR: Restenosis after successful coronary angioplasty in patients with single-vessel disease. Circulation 1986 (April); 73(4):710–717.

112. Wilson JM, Dunn EJ, Wright CB, Bailey WW, Callard GM, Melvin DB, Mitts DL, Will RJ, Flege JB: The cost of simultaneous surgical standby for percutaneous transluminal coronary angioplasty. J Thorac Cardiovasc Surg 1986 (Mar); 91:362–370.

113. Hartzler GO: Coronary angioplasty is the treatment of choice for multivessel coronary artery disease. Chest 1986 (Dec); 877–882.

114. Kirklin JW: Percutaneous transluminal coronary angioplasty: a response. Chest 1986 (Dec); 883–888.

115. King S: Introduction. Chest 1986 (Dec); 876–877.

116. FitzGibbon GM, Leach AJ, Keon WJ, Burton JR, Kafka HP: Coronary bypass graft fate. Angiographic study of 1,179 vein grafts early, one year, and five years after operation. J Thorac Cardiovasc Surg 1986 (May); 91:773–778.

117. Rutherford JD, Whitlock RML, McDonald BW, Barratt-Boyes BG, Kerr AR: Multivariate analysis of the long-term results of coronary artery bypass grafting performed during 1976 and 1977. Am J Cardiol 1986 (June 1); 57:1264–1267.

118. Adler DS, Goldman L, O'Neil A, Cook EF, Mudge GH, Shemin RJ, Disesa V, Cohn LH, Collins JJ: Long-term survival of more than 2,000 patients after coronary artery bypass grafting. Am J Cardiol 1986 (Aug 1); 58:195–202.

119. Vigilante GJ, Weintraub WS, Klein LW, Schneider RM, Seelaus PA, Parr GVS, Agarwal JB, Helfant RH: Medical and surgical survival in coronary artery disease in the 1980s. Am J Cardiol 1986 (Nov 1); 58:926–931.

120. Rahimtoola SH, Grunkemeier GL, Starr A: Ten year survival after coronary artery bypass surgery for angina in patients aged 65 years and older. Circulation 1986 (Mar); 74:509–517.

121. Weiner DA, Ryan TJ, McCabe CH, Chaitman BR, Sheffield T, Fisher LD, Tristani F: The role of exercise testing in identifying patients with improved survival after coronary artery bypass surgery. J Am Coll Cardiol 1986 (Oct); 8:741–748.

122. Lawrie GM, Morris GC, Glaeser DH: Influence of diabetes mellitus on the results of coronary bypass surgery: follow-up of 212 diabetic patients ten to 15 years after surgery. JAMA 1986 (Dec 5); 256:2967–2971.

123. Loop FD, Lytle BW, Cosgrove DM, Stewart RW, Goormastic M, Williams GW, Golding LAR, Gill CC, Taylor PC, Sheldon WC, Proudfit WL: Influence of the internal-mammary-artery graft on 10-year survival and other cardiac events. N Engl J Med 1986 (Jan 2); 314:1–6.

124. Spencer FC: The internal mammary artery: the ideal coronary bypass graft? N Engl J Med 1986 (Jan 2); 314:50–51.

125. Orszulak TA, Schaff HV, Chesebro JH, Holmes DR: Initial experience with sequential internal mammary artery bypass grafts to the left anterior descending and left anterior descending diagonal coronary arteries. Mayo Clin Proc 1986 (Jan); 61:3–8.

126. Tector AJ: Internal mammary artery—its changing role in coronary artery bypass grafting procedures. Mayo Clin Proc 1986 (Jan); 61:72–74.

127. Kieser TM, FitzGibbon GM, Keon WJ: Sequential coronary bypass grafts. Long-term follow-up. J Thorac Cardiovasc Surg 1986 (May); 91:767–772.

128. Livesay JJ, Cooley DA, Hallman GL, Reul GJ, Ott DA, Duncan JM, Frazier OH: Early and late results of coronary endarterectomy: analysis of 3,369 patients. J Thorac Cardiovasc Surg 1986 (Oct); 92:649–660.

129. Glenville B, Ross D: Coronary artery surgery with patient's lungs as oxygenator. Lancet 1986 (Nov 1); 1005–1006.

130. Dixon FE, Genton E, Vacek JL, Moore CB, Landry J: Factors predisposing to supraventricular tachyarrhythmias after coronary artery bypass grafting. Am J Cardiol 1986 (Sept 1); 476–478.

131. Daudon P, Corcos T, Gandjbakhch I, Levasseur JP, Cabrol A, Cabrol C: Prevention of atrial fibrillation or flutter by acebutolol after coronary bypass grafting. Am J Cardiol 1986 (Nov 1); 58:933–936.

132. Wexelman W, Lichstein E, Cunningham JN, Hollander G, Greengart A, Shani J: Etiology and clinical significance of new fascicular conduction defects following coronary bypass surgery. Am Heart J 1986 (May); 111:923–927.

133. Pirk J, Vojacek J, Kovac J, Fabian J, Firt P: Improved patency of the aortocoronary bypass by antithrombotic drugs. Ann Thorac Surg 1986 (Sept); 42:312–314.

134. Marshall WG, Saffitz J, and Kouchoukos NT: Management during reoperation of aortocoronary saphenous vein grafts with minimal atherosclerosis by angiography. Ann Thorac Surg 1986 (Aug); 42:163–167.

135. Lamas GA, Mudge GH Jr, Collins JJ Jr, Koster K, Cohn LH, Flatley M, Shemin R, Cook F, Goldman L: Clinical response to coronary artery reoperations. J Am Coll Cardiol 1986 (Aug); 8:274–279.

136. Neitzel GF, Barboriak JJ, Pintar K, Qureshi I: Atherosclerosis in aortocoronary bypass grafts: Morphologic study and risk factor analysis 6 to 12 years after surgery. Arteriosclerosis 1986 (Nov/Dec); 6:594–600.

137. Capannari TE, Daniels SR, Meyer RA, Schwartz DC, Kaplan S: Sensitivity, specificity and predictive value of two-dimensional echocardiography in detecting coronary artery aneurysms in patients with Kawasaki disease. J Am Coll Cardiol 1986 (Feb); 7:355–360.

138. Nakano H, Saito A, Ueda K, Nojima K: Clinical characteristics of myocardial infarction following Kawasaki disease: report of 11 cases. J Pediatr 1986 (Feb); 108:198–203.

139. Newburger JW, Takahashi M, Burns JC, Beiser AS, Chung KJ, Duffy CE, Glode MP, Mason WH, Reddy V, Sanders SP, Shulman ST, Wiggins JW, Hicks RV, Fulton DR, Lewis AB, Leung DYM, Colton T, Rosen FS, Melish ME: The treatment of Kawasaki syndrome with intravenous gamma globulin. N Engl J Med 1986 (Aug 7); 315:341–347.

140. Feigin RD, Barron KS: Treatment of Kawasaki syndrome. N Engl J Med 1986 (Aug 7); 315:388–390.

141. Hlatky MA, Haney T, Barefoot JC, Califf RM, Mark DB, Pryor DB, Williams RB: Medical, psychological and social correlates of work disability among men with coronary artery disease. Am J Cardiol 1986 (Nov 1); 58:911–915.

142. Gore JM, Weiner BH, Benotti JR, Sloan KM, Okike ON, Cuenoud HF, Gaca JMJ, Alpert JS, Dalen JE: Preliminary experience with synchronized coronary sinus retroperfusion in humans. Circulation 1986 (Feb); 74:381–388.

143. Council on Scientific Affairs: Lasers in medicine and surgery. JAMA 1986 (Aug 15); 256:900–907.

144. Lee G, Garcia JM, Chan MC, Corso PJ, Bacos J, Lee MH, Pichard A, Reis RL, Mason DT: Clinically successful long-term laser coronary recanalization. Am Heart J 1986 (Dec); 112:1323–1325.

145. Foster ED, Davis KB, Carpenter JA, Abele S and Fray D: Risk of noncardiac operation in patients with defined coronary disease: the coronary artery surgery study (CASS) registry experience. Ann Thorac Surg 1986 (Jan); 41:42–50.

3

Acute Myocardial Infarction and Its Consequences

GENERAL TOPICS

Morphologic studies

Saffitz and associates[1] from Bethesda, Maryland, studied 78 necropsy patients with transmural AMI to correlate the mode of death, the interval between onset of AMI and death, and the presence or absence of coronary thrombus with the extent of the infarct. Infarct size was assessed quantitatively as a percentage of total LV mass. Death was caused by cardiogenic shock in 16 patients (21%), arrhythmia in 31 patients (40%), and cardiac rupture in 24 patients (31%). The mean interval between the onset of AMI and death was 12 ± 13 days. Infarct size averaged 23 ± 14% of LV mass (Fig. 3-1). Patients who died in cardiogenic shock had the largest infarcts (37 ± 11%) and those who died of cardiac rupture had the smallest infarcts (15 ± 9%) and the shortest interval between onset of AMI and death (7 ± 8 days). Coronary thrombi were present in 58 patients (74%). When present, thrombus was observed in the coronary artery that had supplied the infarct area and was superimposed on advanced atherosclerotic plaque, but no relation was found between extent of luminal obstruction by thrombus and AMI size. The absence of coronary thrombus at necropsy was associated with either small infarcts or prolonged survival after AMI.

Changes in attack and survival rates

Goldberg and associates[2] from Worcester, Massachusetts, conducted a community-wide study in all 16 acute general hospitals in Worcester, Massa-

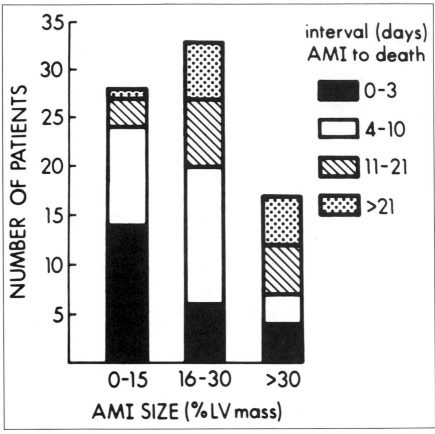

Fig. 3-1. Relation of acute myocardial infarct (AMI) size and the interval between the onset of infarction and death.

chusetts, area during 1975, 1978, and 1981 to examine time trends in the attack and case-fatality rates of patients hospitalized with validated AMI and the occurrence of out-of-hospital CAD deaths. Between 1975 and 1981, there was an increase in the age-adjusted attack rates of initial events of AMI (1975, 254/100,000; 1981, 280/100,000) and recurrent events (1975, 133/100,000; 1981, 156/100,000). These overall increases were due to an increase among those ≥65 years of age, with no significant changes observed in those <65 years old. The age-adjusted in-hospital case-fatality rates declined from 22% in 1975 to 20% in 1978 and 17% in 1981. The age-adjusted mortality rates of out-of-hospital CAD deaths significantly declined between 1975 (229/100,000) and 1981 (147/100,000). The results of this population-based survey suggest that recently observed declines in the mortality rates of CAD may reflect decreases in out-of-hospital coronary deaths and improving trends in the in-hospital survival of patients with AMI.

Circadian variation in onset

Muller et al[3] in the Multicenter Evaluation of the Limitation of Infarct Size (MILIS Study) studied the timing of AMI and determined whether the onset of AMI occurs randomly through the day or in a circadian variation. The time of onset of chest pain in 2,999 patients admitted with AMI was analyzed. A circadian rhythm in the frequency of onset was detected, with a peak frequency of AMI onset between 6 AM and noon (Fig. 3-2). In 703 of the patients, the time of the first elevation in the plasma creatine kinase (CK) MB level could be used to time the onset of AMI objectively; CK-MB–estimated timing of AMI confirmed the presence of a circadian rhythm, with a 3-fold increase in the frequency of onset of AMI at 9 AM compared with lowest frequency of AMI at 11 PM. The data indicated that the circadian rhythm was not present in patients receiving beta blockers before AMI, but it was present in those not receiving such therapy. Therefore, alterations in beta-adrenergic tone perhaps, influencing platelet aggregation at sites of coronary stenosis and endothelial injury, may play a role in the circadian timing of AMI and in leading to vascular thrombosis. Further studies will be necessary to test these hypotheses, but if the mechanisms responsible for the rhythmic processes driving the circadian rhythm of AMI onset can be identified, it may be possible to delay or prevent the occurrence of AMI.

Coronary angiographic findings in non-Q-wave infarction

Complete occlusion of the AMI-related coronary artery is a frequent finding soon after Q-wave AMI. DeWood and associates[4] from Spokane, Washington, performed coronary arteriography to study the frequency of total coronary occlusion and of angiographically visible collateral vessels in 341 patients within 1 week of non-Q-wave AMI. In this cross-sectional study, 192, 94, and 55 patients underwent coronary arteriography within 24 hours of peak symptoms, between 24 and 72 hours after peak symptoms, and between 72 hours and 7 days after peak symptoms, respectively. In the 3 groups, total occlusion of the infarct-related artery was found in 26% (49 of 192), 37% (35 of 94), and 42% (23 of 55) of the patients, respectively. The presence of visible collateral vessels increased in parallel: 27% (52 of 192),

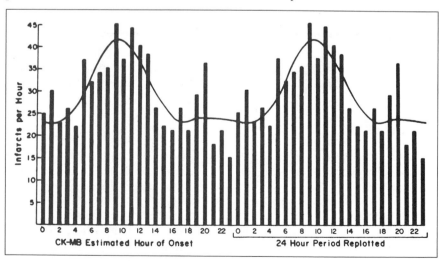

Fig. 3-2. The hourly frequency of onset of myocardial infarction as determined by the CK-MB method in 703 patients. The number of infarctions beginning during each of the 24 hours of the day is plotted on the left side of the figure. On the right, the identical data are plotted again to permit appreciation of the relation between the end and the beginning of the day. A two-harmonic-regression equation for the frequency of onset of myocardial infarction has been fitted to the data (curved line). A prominent circadian rhythm is present, with a primary peak incidence of infarction at 9 a.m. and a secondary peak at 8 p.m. Reproduced with permission from Muller et al.[3]

34% (32 of 94), and 42% (23 of 55), respectively. The frequency of subtotal occlusion (i.e., ≥90% stenosis) decreased inversely: 34% (65 of 192), 25.5% (24 of 94), and 18% (10 of 55), respectively. Thus, in contrast to Q-wave AMI, total coronary occlusion of the infarct-related artery is infrequently observed in the early hours of non-Q-wave AMI, but it increases moderately in frequency over the next several days. These cross-sectional data suggest that non-Q-wave AMI may be related to a preserved but marginal blood supply, which sufficiently disrupts the relation between the supply of and the demand for myocardial oxygen to cause tissue necrosis.

In patients <45 years of age

Since there is a relative paucity of information on the clinical features, natural history, and prognosis in young patients with AMI, Hoit and co-workers[5] in San Diego, California, examined in age subsets, 2,543 patients with AMI. Clinical features and 1-year morbidity and mortality were compared in 203 young patients (<45 years), 1,671 patients 46 to 70 years old, and 769 elderly patients (>70 years). Ninety-two percent of young patients were men, and a family history of premature CAD was more common in young patients (41% compared with 28% of middle-aged and 12% of elderly patients). More young patients were currently smoking cigarettes (82% compared with 56% of middle-aged and 24% of elderly patients), and only 8% of young patients had never smoked. Previous AMI and history of angina pectoris or CHF were less common in the young patients than in middle-aged and elderly patients. In-hospital mortality was 2.5% for young patients, 9% in middle-aged, and 21% in elderly patients. Postdischarge 1-year mortality was low in young patients, at 3% compared with 10% in middle-aged and 24% in elderly patients. The frequency of reinfarction during the 1 year of follow-up was similar in all subsets. The statistical significance of 65 variables as predictors of 1-year mortality and reinfarction was tested and the following found to be significant: hospital discharge on antiarrhythmic drugs, digoxin, or diuretic therapy; history of previous AMI or CHF; chest radiographic findings of CHF; low EF; and AF. Thus, these young patients entering the hospital had an excellent 1-year prognosis, but those with prior AMI in whom there were selected abnormal findings at hospital discharge comprised a subgroup that may benefit from early aggressive management (Fig. 3-3).

In blacks

Over a 12-month period, Cooper and associates[6] from Chicago, Illinois, studied a consecutive series of 111 black patients admitted to a municipal hospital in Chicago. The 2-week mortality rate for the entire group was 19%, and the rate was twice as high for women as for men. A history of systemic hypertension was encountered in 75% of patients, and diabetes mellitus was present in 33%. The delay time from onset of symptoms to arrival at the hospital was markedly prolonged compared with studies of predominantly white populations—twice as long at the median and 3 times as long at the mean. Preventive campaigns aimed at this population should include educating patients on the symptoms of CAD and encouraging them to seek prompt medical care. Attention must also be given to eliminating obstacles to access to care in this group.

Black and associates[7] from New Haven, Connecticut, measured total creatine kinase (CK) in serum samples obtained from 307 asymptomatic healthy subjects, 112 men and 195 women, during screening visits to their

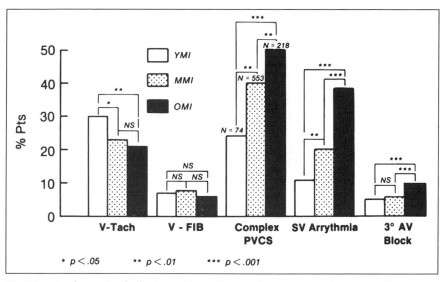

Fig. 3-3.   Incidence of arrhythmias and heart block in the age subsets. Percentage of patients in each subset is shown on the ordinate. V-tach = ventricular tachycardia; V-fib = ventricular fibrillation; SV = supraventricular; YMI = young patients with myocardial infarction; MMI = middle-aged patients with myocardial infarction; OMI = older patients with myocardial infarction. Reproduced with permission from Hoit et al.[5]

Systemic Hypertension Clinic or during prehospital employment physical examination. The group consisted of 147 blacks, 132 whites, and 28 hispanics. BP was measured in all patients and weight and height and serum potassium and creatinine levels were determined in most. Any subject who had engaged in any vigorous exercise in the 12 hours before the visit was excluded. The mean total CK level for black men was 147 ± 137 U/liter (median 108), the mean level for white men was 61 ± 26 U/liter (median 51), and the mean level for Hispanic men was 85 ± 71 U/liter (median 57). The mean level for black women was 66 ± 50 U/liter (median 53), the mean level for white women was 37 ± 18 U/liter (median 32), and the mean level for Hispanic women was 42 ± 36 U/liter for women. Thirty-seven black men (65%) and 49 black women (54%) had abnormal values for total CK. Although sex, race, diastolic BP, serum creatinine level, and presence of hypertension correlated significantly with total CK levels in the entire population, only sex did so in blacks. Multivariate analysis using linear regression techniques clearly demonstrated that sex and race were the only variables that independently predicted the total CK level. These findings show that healthy asymptomatic blacks have higher total CK levels than whites or Hispanics, with most having values in the abnormal range. Thus, different normal values should be used for blacks, just as they are for men and women, and elevated total CK levels should be interpreted with considerable caution.

Elevated MB percentages with or without elevation of creatine kinase levels

To test the hypothesis that patients with normal serum levels of creatine kinase (CK) but elevated percentages of MB isoenzyme fractions in suspected AMI may have sustained clinically significant events, Hong and associates[8] from Boston, Massachusetts, studied the hospital courses of 347 consecutive patients admitted with suspected AMI: 223 patients had normal CK levels

(182 ± 44 IU) and normal MB percentages (normal group); 68 had elevated levels of both CK (1,395 ± 178 IU) and MB percentage (11 ± 1) (macroinfarction group), and 40 had normal CK levels (96 ± 7 IU) but elevated MB percentages (10 ± 1) with typical enzyme curves (microinfarction group). Compared with the normal group, microinfarction patients were older, had more CHF, required more intensive monitoring and therapy during longer stays, and sustained a higher in-hospital mortality rate. Thus, these microinfarction patients are at increased risk and therefore warrant aggressive treatment and further evaluation.

Clinical differences between Q-wave and non-Q-wave Infarction

Ogawa and colleagues[9] from Osaka, Japan, investigated the clinical spectrum and outcome of 119 patients with non-Q-wave AMI in comparison with those of 354 patients with Q-wave AMI. The patients with non-Q-wave AMI had a significantly higher frequency of preinfarction angina (73% -vs- 63%), previous AMI (43% -vs- 22%), multivessel CAD (73% -vs- 51%), postinfarction angina (55% -vs- 21%), and recurrent AMI during follow-up an average of 25 months (17% -vs- 8%). Non-Q-wave AMI patients also had a lower rate of complication of CHF and smaller infarct size estimated by peak creatine kinase levels (1,361 ± 1,243 -vs- 2,711 ± 1,684 IU/liter) than those with Q-wave AMI. There was no difference in in-hospital mortality between the 2 groups (17% -vs- 17%). However, death from cardiac rupture occurred exclusively in the Q-wave AMI group. This study suggests that non-Q-wave AMI is more unstable than Q-wave AMI.

Estimating infarct size by Selvester QRS score and by creatine kinase

Hindman and associates[10] from Durham, North Carolina, and Downey, California, studied the extent of initial AMI and subsequent patient prognosis using 2 independent indicators of AMI size. Two inexpensive, readily available techniques, the complete Selvester QRS score from the standard 12-lead electrocardiogram and the peak value of the isoenzyme MB of creatine kinase (CK), were evaluated in 125 patients with initial AMI. The overall correlation between peak CK-MB and QRS score was fair (0.57), with marked difference according to anterior (0.72) or inferior (0.35) location. The prognostic capabilities of each measurement varied. Peak CK-MB provided significant information concerning hospital morbidity or early mortality (within 30 days) for both anterior and inferior AMI locations; however, the QRS score was significant only for anterior AMI. For total 24-month mortality, the QRS score alone provided the most information, which was not improved with the addition of CK-MB. This study shows a good relation between these 2 independent estimates of AMI size for patients with anterior AMI location. Both QRS and CK-MB results are significantly related to early morbidity and mortality; however, only QRS score is related to total 24-month prognosis.

Transient negative T waves

Granborg and associates[11] from Copenhagen, Denmark, studied diagnostic and prognostic implications of transient isolated negative T waves in 127 patients in whom AMI was suspected. Eighty-four patients with no AMI and no electrocardiographic changes served as the control group. The 2 groups were well matched. Twenty-nine patients (23%) with isolated negative T wave had a significant increase in serum creatine kinase (CK)-MB levels and fulfilled diagnostic criteria for AMI. The increase in serum CK-MB levels did not predict a higher risk of hospital mortality, but during follow-up (median 31 months) a serum CK-MB level >30 U/liter identified patients with a significantly increased risk of dying. Both the number of affected electrocardiographic leads and the sum of negative T-wave amplitudes were significantly related to the follow-up mortality rate. The comparison between control subjects and patients with negative T waves during follow-up showed more events among the patients: AMI (17% -vs- 8%); death (24% -vs- 12%); and AMI or death (31% -vs- 19%). Thus, only 25% of patients with aggravated chest pain and isolated negative T waves had AMI. The long-term prognosis for the entire group of patients with isolated negative T waves was poor.

Reciprocal ST-segment changes

Reciprocal ST-segment changes are frequent during inferior wall AMI, yet their significance remains controversial. To investigate the implications of these changes, Gibelin and associates[12] from Nice, France, obtained electrocardiograms on admission in 83 patients with inferior wall AMI and compared their courses and results of angiographic studies performed an average of 3 weeks after onset of symptoms. Group 1 consisted of 59 patients with ≥ 1 mm of horizontal downsloping ST-segment depression in ≥ 1 of leads V_1 to V_4. Group 2 consisted of 24 patients without precordial ST depression in this area. Group 1 patients were generally older than group 2 patients (59 ± 6 -vs- 54 ± 5 years), had higher total creatine kinase levels and MB fractions (1,835 ± 940 -vs- 875 ± 305, 269 ± 102 -vs- 95 ± 35 for MB fraction) and more complications during the hospital course (80% -vs- 38%) and greater LV dysfunction (EF 52 ± 6% for group 1 -vs- 59 ± 7% for group 2; cardiac index 2 ± 0 1 $min^{-1}m^{-2}$ for group 1 -vs- 3 ± 0 1 $min^{-1}m^{-2}$ for group 2. No difference was observed on biplane angiography in LV wall kinesia. By contrast, coronary arteriography revealed more frequent left CAD in group 1 (84%) than in group 2 patients (37%), the LAD and LC arteries being equally often affected. The persistence of ST-segment depression for >48 hours was associated with a more severe depression of the EF than transient depression (<48 hours). In summary, the presence of ST-segment depression in the precordial leads during inferior AMI was associated with greater myocardial necrosis and more frequent left CAD, thus identifying a subset of high-risk patients.

Lembo and co-workers,[13] in San Antonio, Texas, evaluated prospectively 43 consecutive patients with inferior transmural AMI who had no history or electrocardiographic evidence of prior AMI. To assess the clinical and prognostic importance of persistent precordial (V_1-V_4) ST-segment depression, patients were evaluated within 24 hours of admission by history, physical examination, cardiac enzyme levels, right-sided cardiac catheterization, and RNA; all patients were followed for 1 year. Ten of the 43 patients (group I) had persistent anterior precordial ST-segment depression, defined as ≥ 1 mm in precordial leads 24 hours after admission to the coronary care unit, and 33 patients (group II) did not. Clinical variables that differed between groups I and II, respectively, included age, incidence of Killip class, and average peak creatine kinase concentration. Hemodynamic differences between groups I and II included a higher PA wedge pressure (19 -vs- 11 mmHg) and a lower cardiac index (2.0 -vs- 2.6 liters/min/m²). An evaluation of LVEF and wall motion index by RNA showed that group I had a lower EF and higher wall motion index than group II. Prognostically, group I had a higher frequency of recurrent AMI (30% -vs- 0%) and a higher 1-year mortality (60% -vs- 0). Univariate analysis revealed that several clinical, electrocardiographic, hemodynamic, and RNA variables were predictive of 1-year mortality, with persistent precordial ST-segment depression being the most powerful. Of the variables that had independent value for predicting death within 1 year, the most important was persistent precordial ST-segment depression followed by heart rate.

Ruddy and associates[14] from Boston, Massachusetts, studied the clinical significance of anterior precordial ST-segment depression during AMI in 67 consecutive patients early after onset of symptoms with gated RNA, thallium-201 perfusion images, and 12-lead electrocardiograms. Patients with anterior ST depression (n = 33) had depressed mean values for LVEF (54 ± 2% -vs- 59 ± 2%), cardiac index (3.1 ± 0.2 -vs- 3.6 ± 0.2 liters/m²), and ratio of systolic BP to end-systolic volume (2.0 ± 0.1 -vs- 2.5 ± 0.3 mmHg/ml) compared to patients with no anterior ST depression (n = 34). Patients with anterior ST depression had 1) lower mean LV wall motion values for the inferior, apical, and inferior-lateral segments, and 2) greater reductions in thallium-201 uptake in the inferior and posterolateral regions. However, anterior and septal 1) wall motion and 2) thallium-201 uptake were similar in patients with and without ST depression. Thus, anterior precordial ST-segment depression in patients with inferior wall AMI represents more than a reciprocal electrical phenomenon. It identifies patients with more severe wall motion impairment and greater hypoperfusion of the inferior and adjacent segments. The poorer global LV function in these patients is a result of more extensive inferior AMI and not of remote septal or anterior injury.

Relation of ST-segment elevation and infarct artery patency

Hackworthy and associates[15] from Camperdown, Australia, studied 41 patients with AMI and ST-segment elevation to determine the relation between early changes in ST-segment elevation, time to peak serum creatine kinase (CK), peak serum CK, LV function, and patency of the infarct-related artery. ST-segment elevation decreased by >40% within 8 hours after peak ST sum (sum of ST segments in all leads within 8 hours of symptom onset) in all patients with inferior AMI and in 10 of the 13 patients with anterior AMI and subtotal occlusion, but in none of the patients with anterior AMI and total occlusion. The time to peak serum CK was related to the rate of decrease of ST-segment elevation in patients with anterior and inferior AMI. In patients with anterior AMI, peak serum CK tended to be lower and LVEF higher in those with rapid resolution of ST-segment elevation than in those with persistent ST elevation (1,721 ± 1,422 U/liter -vs- 3,285 ± 1,148 U/liter) for peak CK; and 50 ± 19% -vs- 41 ± 13% for LVEF), but there was no difference in the patients with inferior AMI. Early resolution of ST-segment elevation is an index of early spontaneous anterograde or collateral reperfusion in patients with AMI.

ST segment/heart rate slope

Ameisen et al[16] in New York, New York, evaluated the ability of the exercise electrocardiographic ST segment/heart rate slope to identify accurately 3-vessel CAD in patients with stable angina pectoris after recent (<3 weeks) and remote (>8 weeks) Q-wave AMI. One hundred and thirteen patients were studied, including 58 with stable angina pectoris in whom 17 had remote Q-wave AMI and 55 recent AMI. In patients with stable angina and no prior Q-wave AMI, an ST segment/heart rate slope >6.0 had a sensitivity of 92%, a specificity of 97%, and a positive predictive value of 92% in the identification of 3-vessel CAD by coronary arteriography. In patients with stable angina and remote Q-wave AMI, the sensitivity was 83%, specificity 91%, and positive predictive value 83%. In contrast, after recent AMI, the test specificity for 3-vessel CAD was 95%, but test sensitivity was poor identifying only 3 of 8 patients. Among the combined group of patients with recent AMI, test sensitivity for 3-vessel CAD was 29% (4 of 14); this was significantly lower than in patients with stable angina. Thus, these data indicate a markedly reduced sensitivity and positive predictive value in the utility of exercise electrocardiographic ST segment/heart rate slope in identifying 3-vessel CAD in patients with recent AMI. Nevertheless, the method seems to be considerably more accurate in the identification of 3-vessel CAD in patients with stable angina pectoris.

Ratio of ST depression in V_2 to ST elevation in aVF

Lew and associates[17] from Los Angeles, California, evaluated the potential value of the ratio of precordial ST-segment depression to inferior ST-segment elevation as a sign of concomitant RV ischemia in 68 patients admitted within 3 hours of the onset of inferior wall AMI in whom there was no evidence of prior AMI. In 27 of the 34 patients in whom inferior AMI was the result of right coronary artery occlusion proximal to the RV branch, the magnitude of ST-segment depression in lead V_2 was ≤50% of the magnitude of ST-segment elevation in lead aVF, whereas in only 3 of the 34 patients in whom the site of occlusion was either distal to the RV branch or in the LC artery was this ratio 50%; in no patient was it <50%. All 34 patients with occlusion of the right coronary artery proximal to the RV branch also had regional or global ischemic RV dysfunction by radionuclide ventriculography, with a mean RVEF of 30 ± 10% compared with 42 ± 6% in patients with occlusion distal to the RV branch or in the LC artery. In conclusion, in patients with evolving inferior AMI, ST-segment depression in lead V_2 of ≤50% of the magnitude of ST-segment elevation in lead aVF may be a useful sign (sensitivity 79%, specificity 91%, positive predictive value 90%, and negative predictive value 82%) for identifying patients with concomitant RV ischemia.

Q waves in leads I, aVL, V_5 and V_6

To determine the diagnostic significance for CAD of abnormally large Q waves in leads I, aVL, V_5 and V_6—the "lateral" electrocardiographic leads—Warner and associates[18] from Syracuse, New York, studied the electrocardiograms of 240 patients who had undergone cardiac catheterization. The electrocardiograms of 99 subjects proved normal by cardiac catheterization (group 1) were studied to determine the values of the durations of Q waves in leads I, aVL, V_5, and V_6 that should be exceeded to be considered abnormal. These values were 30, 30, 20, and 25 ms, respectively. Then, 67 patients were identified who had abnormal Q waves in ≥1 of these leads (group 2) and 74 patients with ≥1 angiographic abnormality but without abnormal Q waves in any of these leads (group 3). Group 2 had generally more extensive LV disease and a higher prevalence of anterior, inferior, and apical healed myocardial infarction than group 3. However, compared with group 3, group 2 had lower prevalences of significant narrowing of the coronary arteries that supply the LV lateral wall. Within group 2, abnormal Q waves in leads I and aVL (traditionally designated high lateral myocardial infarction) were associated with inferior and apical myocardial infarction. Thus, abnormal Q waves in leads I, aVL, V_5, and V_6 tend to reflect apical rather than lateral myocardial infarction and the term anterolateral myocardial infarction is especially misleading.

QT interval

Juul-Moller[19] from Malmo, Sweden, investigated with exercise electrocardiography and rest LVEF within 1 month of AMI and at 6 and 12 months, 101 unselected patients <66 years of age who had had an AMI. QTC was measured at rest (QTc^{rest}) and at maximal exercise (QTc^{work}). In patients with $QTc^{work} > QTc^{rest}$, LVEF was lower (mean 0.42) and QTc^{rest} longer (mean 0.467 second) than in patients with $QTc^{work} > QTc^{rest}$. In this latter group LVEF was 0.50 (mean value) and QTc^{rest} 0.426 second (mean value). A negative correlation was found between LVEF and QTc^{rest}. A negative correlation was also found between QTc^{work}-QTc^{rest} (i.e., the change in QTc during maximal exercise) and QTc^{rest}. In patients with $QTc^{rest} > 0.480$ second at the first investigation, the 1-year mortality was 50%, compared with 9% in patients with $QTc^{rest} < 0.480$ second. It is concluded that in post-AMI patients, QTc^{rest} reflects the condition of the LV myocardium, a prolonged QTc^{rest} being found with impaired myocardial function.

Body surface potential maps

Kornreich and associates[20] from Halifax, Canada, described a practical approach for identifying electrocardiographic leads which allow the earliest and most accurate diagnosis of the presence and electrocardiographic type of AMI. The authors took advantage of the increased information content of body surface potential maps over standard electrocardiographic techniques for facilitating clinical use of body surface potential maps for such a purpose. Multivariate analysis was performed on 120-lead electrocardiographic data, simultaneously recorded in 236 normal subjects, 114 patients with anterior and 144 patients with inferior AMI, using as features instantaneous voltages on time-normalized QRS and ST-T waveforms. Leads and features for optimal separation of normal subjects from, respectively, anterior and inferior AMI patients were selected. Features measured on leads originating from the upper left precordial area, lower midthoracic region, and the back correctly identified 97% of anterior AMI patients, with a specificity of 95%; in patients with inferior AMI, features obtained from leads located in the lower left back, left leg, right subclavicular area, upper dorsal region, and lower right chest correctly classified 94% of the group, with specificity of 95%. Most features were measured in early and mid-QRS, although very potent discriminators were found in the late portion of the T wave. Repeatability of the results was investigated by separating the study population in training and testing sets; no deterioration was observed when the discriminant functions computed on the training sets were run on the testing sets. In comparison, at the same level of specificity and with the same number of features, the standard 12-lead electrocardiogram correctly diagnosed 89% of anterior and 85% of inferior AMI patients. Thus, diagnosis of anterior and inferior AMI can be substantially improved by appropriate selection of electrocardiographic leads and features.

Serum potassium levels, arrhythmias and acebutolol

Nordrehaug and Von Der Lippe[21] from Bergen, Norway, determined serum potassium concentrations in 1,033 consecutive patients with AMI and related these admission K values to frequency of AF and atrial flutter and of VT and VF. In multivariant analysis, with serum K concentrations as a continuous variable, age, the presence of VT and VF, and maximum level of aspartate aminotransferase >4 times the upper limit of normal were significantly associated with the occurrence of AF and atrial flutter, while serum K concentration was not. Serum potassium concentrations and time from onset of the AMI to hospital admission were significantly negatively associated with the occurrence of VT and fibrillation, while age, cardiomegaly, transient hypotension, pathological Q waves in the electrocardiogram, AF and flutter, and VPC were positively related to these arrhythmias. Thus, there is an independent inverse relation between serum K concentrations and ventricular arrhythmias in AMI.

Hypokalemia frequently occurs in AMI and may be caused by elevated serum levels of adrenaline, allegedly by beta 2-adrenergic mediated influx of potassium into cells. Jardine and associates[22] from Johannesburg, South Africa, investigated the effect on serum K of intravenous *acebutolol* in 50 patients with AMI. Serum K was measured before and 1 hour after drug administration. The same measurements were made in a comparable control group of 30 patients who did not receive the drug. Mean serum K increased from 3.58–3.81 mEq/liter in the treated group. No significant change occurred in the control group. The increase in serum K could not be correlated with prior beta-blocker therapy, zone of infarction, prior diuretic therapy, or gender of the patient. The authors concluded that the administration of intravenous acebutolol after AMI raises serum K, despite the fact that this beta-receptor blocking agent is relatively beta 1-selective. Because hypokalemia is associated with an increased risk of VF, it should no longer be assumed from acute intervention trials with beta blockers in AMI that had mortality or arrhythmias as end-points, that beneficial effects were necessarily due to limitation of infarct size or to a direct antiarrhythmic action of the drugs. Future trials should take the effect on serum K levels into consideration.

Serum magnesium levels

Rasmussen et al[23] from Copenhagen, Denmark, studied serum magnesium concentrations and rate of urine magnesium excretion in 24 patients with suspected AMI. Blood and urine samples were taken on admission, at 3-hour intervals for the first 24 hours after admission, and every 8 hours for the next 24 hours. Thirteen patients had AMI, and the 11 who did not served as controls. During the first 32 hours, the AMI group had significantly lower serum magnesium concentrations (Fig. 3-4); the concentrations were unchanged in the control group. Results of urine samples disproved the authors' hypothesis that the drop in serum magnesium concentrations was due to increased renal magnesium loss. These results indicate a magnesium migration associated with AMI, from extracellular to intracellular space.

Atrial pacing early

Figueras and associates[24] from Barcelona, Spain, carried out atrial pacing within 5 days of uncomplicated AMI in 28 patients to detect the existence of a "menaced area." A positive pacing response (≥1.0 mm of ST-segment

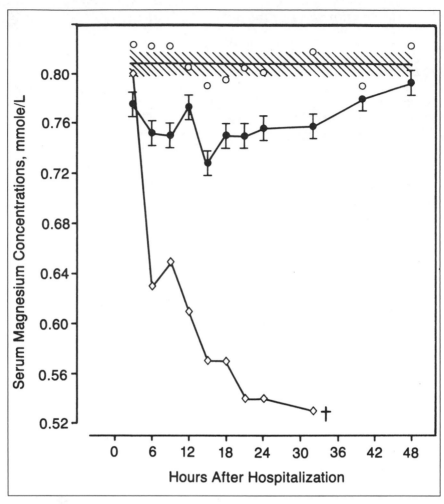

Fig. 3-4.   Mean serum concentrations of magnesium measured 11 times during first 48 hours after hospitalization in 12 patients with acute myocardial infarction (AMI; solid circles), in one patient with AMI who died (dagger) after 35 hours (diamonds), and in 11 patients without AMI (open circles). Hatched area indicates mean ± 3.3 SEs in 11 patients without AMI (3.3 SEs of mean = 1 SE of each mean observed at three hours, six hours, etc); bars, ±1 SE of each corresponding mean value. Reproduced with permission from Rasmussen et al.[23]

shift) was observed in 23 patients (82% in group I), whereas pacing results were negative in 5 (18% in group II). Pacing-induced electrocardiographic changes involved the leads affected by AMI in patients with transmural necrosis. A well-defined thallium-201 redistribution, mostly localized near or within the AMI site, was present in 10 patients from group I (43%), in 1 from group II (20%), and in 1 of 12 comparable patients (8%) in whom pacing was not performed. During pacing, abnormal lactate metabolism was observed in 11 of 17 patients from group I (65%) and in 0 of 5 from group II. A ≥90% stenosis of ≥1 artery was found in 19 of 23 patients from group I (83%) and in 1 of 5 from group II; 2- to 3-vessel disease (>70% diameter stenosis) was present in 14 patients from group I (61%) and 1 from group II (20%). During a 15-month follow-up (range 9–25), effort angina developed in 9 patients from group I (39%) and in none from group II. No deaths or reinfarctions occurred in either group. Thus, early after a first AMI, most patients have a jeopardized periinfarction area that is usually associated with a critical coronary stenosis and that heralds effort angina in a significant proportion of them.

Echocardiography early

Kumar and associates[25] from Los Angeles, California, assessed LV wall motion by 2-D echocardiography in 17 patients admitted with a first trans- mural AMI. The LV myocardium was divided into 17 segments and wall motion was scored from 1 (dyskinesia) to 6 (hyperkinesia) in each segment. Reproducibility of the wall motion scoring system was 90%. Seven patients had anterior and 10 inferior wall AMI on the electrocardiogram. Abnormal wall motion was present in 7.3 ± 2.8 segments (mean ± standard deviation) on the initial 2-D echocardiogram. On follow-up echocardiograms, wall mo- tion was unchanged in 7 patients. In 5, wall motion improved by at least 2 in 2 or more contiguous segments. In 5 other patients wall motion returned to normal in all segments that had shown an abnormality on the initial echocardiogram. These 5 patients (group A), compared with the 12 patients in whom wall motion did not return to normal in all segments (group B), had fewer involved segments (5.4 ± 1.7 -vs- 8 ± 2.8) and a higher total wall motion score (76 ± 4 -vs- 63 ± 7) on the initial echocardiogram. Duration from the time of the AMI to return of normal wall motion in group A varied from 2–8 weeks. Thus, wall motion abnormalities seen on 2-D echocardiog- raphy after transmural AMI often improve and wall motion returns to nor- mal in some patients.

To determine the clinical significance of regional hyperkinesia and re- mote asynergy of noninfarcted areas in patients with a first AMI, Jaarsma and associates[26] from Amsterdam, The Netherlands, performed 2-D echo- cardiography in 113 consecutive patients within 12 hours after admission to a coronary care unit. In 98 patients (87%) all segments of the LV wall were recorded. Infarct-associated asynergy was anterior in 63 and inferior in 35 patients. Regional hyperkinesia was present in 66 patients (67%)—44 of 63 with anterior (69%) and 22 of 35 with inferior (63%) infarcts—and was more frequent in patients with 1- and 2-vessel CAD than in patients with 3-vessel CAD (87% and 72% -vs- 25%). In contrast to enzymatic infarct size, absence of regional hyperkinesia was significantly associated with a higher LV wall motion score. Twenty patients died within 30 days after onset of AMI; in 15 (75%) regional hyperkinesia was absent. Absence of regional hyperkinesia, especially in anterior AMI, was associated with a high mortal- ity rate (13 of 19 patients [68%]). Remote asynergy, i.e., not adjacent to the infarct area and supposed to be related to another vascular region, was pres- ent in 17 of 98 patients (17%)—11 of 63 with anterior (17%) and 6 of 35 with inferior (17%) infarcts. Remote asynergy was present only in patients with multivessel CAD and was significantly related to a higher wall motion score, but not to enzymatic infarct size. Also, the presence of remote asynergy was associated with a high mortality rate (9 of 17 patients [53%]). Thus, regional hyperkinesia and remote asynergy of the noninfarcted areas in patients with a first AMI provide useful information about the extent of CAD and may identify patients at high risk for early (within 30 days) mortality.

To determine the clinical significance of transient remote asynergy after the first AMI, Jaarsma and associates[27] from Amsterdam, The Netherlands, performed 2-D echocardiography at rest and directly after dynamic exercise in 49 consecutive patients within 3 weeks of AMI. In 43 patients (88%), technically adequate 2-D echocardiographic examinations were obtained. Asynergy was found in all patients at rest. Immediately after exercise, new

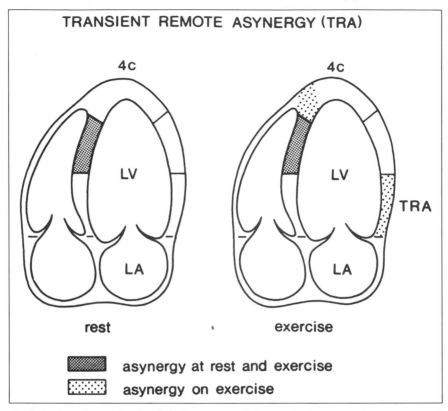

Fig. 3-5. An apical 4-chamber (4c) view at rest and during exercise. At rest three is only septal asynergy. During exercise the basal portion of the opposite, remote wall shows asynergy (transient remote asynergy [TRA]). Note the asynergy during exercise directly adjacent to the distal part of the septum. LA = high atrium; LV = left ventricle.

areas of asynergy, not adjacent to the infarcted area (i.e., transient remote asynergy), were present in 18 patients (Fig. 3-5). Of these patients, 17 had multivessel CAD, compared with 5 of 25 patients without transient remote asynergy. Sensitivity of transient remote asynergy for detecting multivessel CAD was 77% and specificity was 95%. LVEF at rest and after exercise was measured in 39 patients (90%) and could only identify patients with 3-vessel CAD. New ischemic events, defined as reinfarction or recurrent angina pectoris, within a mean of 12 weeks (range 8 to 16) after discharge, occurred in 16 patients. Transient remote asynergy was present in 12 of these patients (75%). It was concluded that exercise-induced transient remote asynergy early after AMI can identify patients with multivessel CAD and a subgroup of patients prone to early new ischemic events. LVEF, however, is not only more laborious but also of lesser value in identifying patients with multivessel CAD.

Radionuclide assessment of left ventricular function early

Ong and associates[28] from New York, New York, examined the prognostic value of early radionuclide imaging in 222 patients in Killip class I and II with Q-wave AMI. Each was studied prospectively within 24 hours of onset of symptoms. The 30-day mortality rate for the entire group was 11% (25 of

222). Univariate analysis indicated that an initial radionuclide LVEF <0.30 was associated with the greatest relative risk, although the percent of abnormally contracting regions and thallium-201 defect index were also significant risk factors. Stepwise logistic regression indicated that addition of EF resulted in the greatest improvement over the best clinical model (Killip class and chest radiographic findings) for the prediction of 30-day mortality. Using the optimal model for prediction of mortality (EF and Killip class), a high-risk group with a 30-day mortality rate of 39% (90-day mortality 47%) and a low-risk group with a 30-day mortality rate of 3% (90-day mortality 4%) was identified. In clinically stable patients with transmural AMI, early assessment of EF in conjunction with clinical evaluation, is a valuable method for early identification of high-risk subsets.

To determine changes in global and regional LV function after AMI, 17 patients underwent RNA at 3 and 10 days post-AMI by Buda and colleagues[29] from Ann Arbor, Michigan, and Ontario, Canada. Five patients had nontransmural AMI and 12 had transmural AMI (6 anterior and 6 inferior). There were no previous infarcts in 16 (94%) patients. Regional EF was calculated by dividing the left ventricle into 4 quadrants using the geometric center of the left ventricle on the end-diastolic frame as a reference point. At 3 days post-AMI, 8 of 17 (47%) patients had an abnormality of global LVEF, whereas 16 of 17 (94%) patients had abnormalities of ≥1 regional EF. Between 3 and 10 days, global LVEF did not change (51% to 49%). There were significant changes in 23 of 68 (34%) regional LVEFs. These changes did not relate to type, electrocardiographic location, creatine kinase, size of AMI, or initial global LVEF. These data suggest that regional LVEF is a sensitive technique for identifying segmental dysfunction associated with AMI. In addition, significant changes occur in regional LV function during AMI despite stable serial global LV performance.

Gjorup and associates[30] from Copenhagen, Denmark, in a controlled, randomized, double-blind study determined whether knowledge of the LVEF could reduce the frequency of left-sided CHF after AMI. The LVEF was determined a few days before hospital discharge in 60 patients. Subsequently, the patients were randomly assigned to 2 groups. The cardiologist responsible for their treatment was aware of the LVEF result in group 1 but not in group 2. A month after hospital discharge there was no significant difference in the LVEF between the groups. Two months after discharge there was no significant differences between the groups in clinical and radiologic signs of LV CHF or the use of drugs. The cardiologist's clinical estimate of the LVEF and the result of the radionuclide determination were significantly correlated. Thus, use of LVEF did not change the clinical outcome.

To determine the spectrum and prognostic implications of LV and RVEF in AMI, Shah and associates[31] from Los Angeles, California, performed radionuclide ventriculography in 114 consecutive patients admitted without (Killip class I, 78 patients) or with (Killip class II, 36 patients) clinical signs of pulmonary congestion within 24 hours of onset of symptoms of transmural AMI. Mean LVEF was significantly lower in patients in Killip class II than in those in class I (0.32 ± 0.11 -vs- 0.46 ± 0.15) and in patients with anterior than inferior AMI (0.34 ± 0.11 -vs- 0.52 ± 0.14). Of the 36 patients with a severely depressed (≤0.30) LVEF, 14 (42%) were in Killip class I. Mean RVEF did not differ significantly between Killip class I and II patients (0.42 ± 0.11 -vs- 0.40 ± 0.12) but was significantly lower in patients with inferior than anterior AMI (0.38 ± 0.09 -vs- 0.44 ± 0.11). In patients with inferior AMI, a depressed RVEF (≤0.38) was associated with a normal LVEF in 30% and a depressed LVEF in 20%, whereas in those with anterior AMI, a depressed RVEF, observed in 25% of patients, occurred only in association with a depressed LVEF. At 1 year of follow-up, the 21 nonsurvivors differed significantly from the 93 survivors with respect to LVEF (0.35 ± 0.11 -vs- 0.45 ± 0.14), RVEF (0.35 ± 0.11 -vs- 0.43 ± 0.10), proportion in Killip class II (57% -vs- 28%) and age (69 ± 13 years -vs- 61 ± 11 years). Mortality rate was 47% in patients with an LVEF of ≤0.30 (group I) compared with 5% in patients with an LVEF >0.30 (group II). In group I patients, the mortality rate was 75% when RVEF was ≤0.38, compared with 25% when RVEF was >0.38). An RVEF < or >0.38 did not influence mortality in group II patients. Multivariate analysis identified LVEF ≤0.30, RVEF ≤0.38 and age as significant independent predictors of mortality. These results show the wide variability in global ventricular function among a subset of patients with AMI with clinical evidence of no or only mild LV failure. They also show independent and additional adverse prognostic implications of a depressed RVEF among a subset of patients with severely depressed LVEF (≤0.30).

Tamaki and associates[32] from Boston, Massachusetts, assessed the incidence of improvement in regional wall motion of segments with severe contractile abnormalities in the first 10 days after a first AMI using serial gated pool scans in 95 patients who received standard medical therapy. Regional wall motion was quantitatively assessed as percent chord shortening in 4 segments in the anterior view and 4 segments in the 45° left anterior oblique view. Among 237 segments with no more than 15% shortening (severely hypokinetic or akinetic [SH/A] segments), 59 (25%) improved at least 15% at 10 days, 166 (70%) did not change and 12 (5%) deteriorated by at least 15%. Among 91 patients who had SH/A segments, 37 (41%) had improvement in at least 1 SH/A segment (group 1) and 54 had no improvement in SH/A segments (group 2). Group 1 had a higher initial EF (50 ± 12%) than group 2 (45 ± 13%). The changes in percent shortening of SH/A segments were compared with coronary anatomy in 37 patients who underwent coronary angiography. The 17 patients with 1-vessel CAD had significantly improved wall motion (8 ± 13%), in contrast to the 20 patients with multivessel CAD (2 ± 12%). Among patients with 1-vessel CAD, the improvement was greater in patients with right coronary or LC artery disease (13 ± 14%). These data indicated that improved wall motion is seen in initially SH/A segments in 41% of AMI patients with akinesia. Patients with a higher initial EF and less severe CAD usually involving the inferoposterior wall are more likely to have improved wall motion in SH/A segments.

Thallium-201 imaging early

Weiss et al,[33] in Los Angeles, California, found "reverse redistribution" on thallium-201 scintigrams on day 10 poststreptokinase rest thallium-201 studies in patients receiving therapy during AMI. The characteristic pattern of thallium-201 scintigrams with myocardial ischemia is a perfusion defect noted on the early postinjection images, either at rest or during stress that normalizes after a time delay of several hours (reversible defect) and it is indicative of myocardial ischemia. A region of AMI usually demonstrates a perfusion defect that remains unchanged with delayed imaging. However, occasionally a thallium-201 perfusion defect first appears or becomes more evident on the delayed rather than on the immediate image; this pattern is referred to as reverse redistribution. To investigate why reverse redistribution patterns are noted frequently on day 10 poststreptokinase therapy, 67 patients were studied before and 10 days after streptokinase therapy. Among the 67 patients, 50 (75%) demonstrated the reverse redistribution pattern on day 10 on the rest thallium-201 studies (group I), 9 (13%) had a nonreversible defect (group II), and the remaining 8 (12%) had a normal study or showed a defect that had become smaller (group III). The reverse redistribution pattern was associated with patency of the infarct-related artery (100%), quantitative improvement in rest thallium-201 defect size from day 1 to 10 (94%), and normal or near-normal wall motion on day 10 as evaluated by RNA. Nonreversible defects were associated with less frequent patency of the infarct-related artery (67%), improvement in defect size (11%), and normal or near normal wall motion (21%). Group III patients were similar to group I with respect to these same variables. The quantitated thallium-201 percent washout was higher in regions with reverse redistribution patterns (49 ± 15%) compared with the contralateral normal zones (24 ± 15%). These data indicate that the reverse redistribution thallium-201 pattern on rest thallium-201 scintigrams is associated with a higher than normal washout rate of thallium-201 and suggest that this pattern is a sign of non-Q-wave AMI with a patent infarct-related coronary artery.

Abraham and associates[34] from Sydney, Australia, performed exercise electrocardiography and thallium scanning a mean of 24 days after uncomplicated AMI in 103 patients, aged 36–60 years, who also underwent coronary angiography. The study determined the ability of the noninvasive tests to predict multivessel CAD and prognosis. Patients were followed up to document medical complications (incidence 12%; 3 deaths, 1 resuscitated cardiac arrest, 4 recurrent AMI, 4 admissions with unstable angina) and combined events (medical events or CABG, incidence 23%). The sensitivity, specificity and predictive accuracy for predicting multivessel CAD were 64%, 77%, and 64% for a positive exercise electrocardiographic response, 64%, 88%, and 80% for a remote thallium defect, and 42%, 96%, and 88% for a combination of the 2 tests. With 2 tests yielding negative findings the probability of multivessel CAD was 13%. No variable (positive exercise electrocardiographic response, remote thallium defect, and presence of multivessel CAD) predicted medical events, although there were nonsignificant trends to more events in patients with any of those findings. The relative risk of combined events was 2.5 for a positive exercise electrocardiographic response; 1.8 for a remote thallium defect; 2.6 for multivessel CAD; and 3.1 for both positive electrocardiographic response and remote defect. A combination of exercise electrocardiography and thallium scanning early after AMI helps to identify subsets of patients with high and low probabilities of multivessel CAD and combined medical or surgical events.

Magnetic resonance imaging early

Johnston and associates[35] from Boston, Massachusetts, obtained electrocardiographic-gated spin-echo magnetic resonance images of the LV short axis in 34 patients a mean of 11 ± 6 days after AMI. This magnetic resonance imaging (MRI) technique allowed division of the LV segments corresponding to the LV segments on angiography. Patients were separated into 2 groups; the first 16 patients (group I) were examined using a variety of imaging techniques. Information derived from this experience resulted in a standard imaging protocol and development of criteria for the presence of AMI. The imaging protocol and interpretation criteria were used in the assessment of a subsequent group of 18 patients (group II). Of the 14 patients in group II with satisfactory image quality, all showed an increase in myocardial signal intensity consistent with an AMI. In addition, the anterior or inferior location of the abnormal magnetic resonance segments corresponded to the electrocardiographic infarct location. Magnetic resonance segments showing increased signal intensity corresponded with severely hypokinetic or akinetic segments on the left ventriculogram in 8 patients having both procedures. In a group of volunteers who underwent imaging and whose images were interpreted in the same manner as those of the patients with AMI, 1 of 9 subjects had regional variation in myocardial signal intensity compatible with an AMI. In summary, AMI is readily detected, located, and characterized by electrocardiographic-gated MRI. These findings suggest that MRI techniques may have a role in the evaluation of AMI in humans.

Filipchuk and associates[36] from Dallas, Texas, evaluated the potential of MRI to detect and localize AMI in 27 patients a mean interval of 15 days after AMI. Eighteen asymptomatic volunteers also were studied to determine the specificity of the observations. The diagnosis of AMI was established by conventional criteria; the infarct was localized by electrocardiography in all patients, technetium pyrophosphate scintigraphy in 19 and necropsy in 1 patient. MRI detected increased myocardial signal intensity in 88%, cavitary signal in 74%, and regional wall thinning in 67% of the patients. At least 1 of these 3 features was seen in the area of the infarct in each patient. The sensitivity of these MRI observations was not influenced by location of the infarct or presence of Q waves. Asymptomatic volunteers also had increased myocardial signal in 83%, cavitary signal in 94%, and wall thinning in 11% of cases. Some patients had these findings in myocardial segments not suspected of being involved by recent or remote AMI. It is concluded that AMI can be detected by MRI performed an average of 15 days after infarction. However, the hearts of normal volunteers and apparently normal myocardial segments of patients with AMI may have the MRI findings previously associated with AMI. Of these findings, wall thinning was the most predictive of and specific for AMI.

Positron emission tomography early

Brunken and co-investigators[37] in Los Angeles, California, used positron emission tomography with ^{13}N-ammonia and ^{18}F-2-deoxyglucose to assess regional perfusion and glucose utilization in 31 chronic electrocardiographic Q-wave regions in 20 patients. With previously published criteria, regions of AMI were identified by a concordant reduction in regional perfusion and glucose utilization, and regions of ischemia were identified by preservation of glucose utilization in regions of diminished perfusion. Only 10 of the 31 regions (32%) exhibited myocardial infarction tomographically. In contrast, positron tomography revealed ischemia in 6 regions (20%) and was normal in 15 regions (48%). Even when Q-wave regions were reassigned and consolidated to enhance the specificity of the electrocardiogram, uptake of ^{18}F-2-deoxyglucose was noted in most (54%) regions. Neither electrocardiographic ST-T changes nor severity of associated wall motion abnormality reliably distinguished tomographically identified regions of ischemia from infarction. Thus, positron tomography reveals evidence of persistent tissue metabolism in a high proportion of chronic electrocardiographic Q-wave regions, and commonly used clinical tests do not reliably distinguish hypoperfused but viable regions from tomographically defined regions of myocardial infarction. This important work should have wide application in selection, as well as assessment of interventions in acute myocardial infarction since metabolically preserved myocardium may be present in a high percentage of patients despite Q waves on the electrocardiogram, ST-T wave changes, or wall motion abnormalities.

Schwaiger et al[38] in Los Angeles, California, used positron emission tomography to evaluate its ability to distinguish between reversibly and irreversibly injured tissue after AMI in 13 patients studied within 72 hours of onset of symptoms. Positron emission tomography was used to evaluate regional blood flow and glucose metabolism with nitrogen-13 ammonia and fluorine-18 deoxyglucose, respectively. Serial noninvasive assessments of regional wall motion were performed to determine the prognostic value of metabolic indexes for functional tissue recovery. Segmental blood flow and glucose utilization were evaluated using a circumferential profile technique and compared with previously established semiquantitative criteria. Myocardial perfusion was decreased in 32 LV segments in these patients. Sixteen segments demonstrated a concordant decrease in flow and glucose metabolism. Among these patients, regional segmental function did not change over time in these segments. However, in 16 additional segments with reduced blood flow, persistent metabolic viability was identified as evidenced by uptake of F-18 deoxyglucose. In these ventricular segments, average wall motion score improved significantly, yet the degree of recovery varied considerably among patients. Coronary anatomy was defined in 9 of 13 patients: patent infarct arteries supplied 8 of 10 segments where F-18 deoxyglucose uptake occurred, whereas 10 of 13 segments in the region of an occluded coronary artery showed concordant decreases in flow and metabolism. Thus, positron emission tomography demonstrates a high incidence of residual tissue viability in ventricular segments with reduced flow and impaired function during the subacute phase of AMI. The absence of regional tissue metabolism is generally associated with irreversible injury, while preservation of metabolic activity identifies ventricular segments with a variable outcome.

Left ventricular angiography early

Dilatation of infarcted segments or infarct expansion may occur during recovery from AMI, but the fate of noninfarcted segments is uncertain. McKay and co-workers[39] in Boston, Massachusetts, assessed LV geometric changes by LV angiography and M-mode echocardiography on admission and 2 weeks later in 30 patients with their first Q-wave AMI. The patients had chest pain, ST-segment elevation with subsequent development of Q waves (15 anterior, 15 inferior), and elevation of cardiac enzymes. Because the patients participated in a study of thrombolysis in AMI, those treated successfully underwent repeat cardiac catheterization. At 2 weeks there was a significant decrease in LV and PA wedge pressures, whereas both LV end-diastolic and end-systolic volume indexes increased. The increase in end-diastolic volume correlated directly with the percentage of the ventriculographic silhouette that was akinetic or dyskinetic at the initial catheterization. Serial endocardial perimeter lengths of both the akinetic-dyskinetic segments (infarction zone) and of the remaineder of the cardiac silhouette (noninfarction zone) were measured in all patients who had a ≥20% increase in their end-diastolic volume at 2 weeks after AMI. There was a mean increase of 13% in the endocardial perimeter length of infarcted segments and a 19% increase in the endocardial perimeter length of the noninfarcted segments. Serial M mode echocardiographic studies revealed no significant change in the wall thickness of noninfarcted myocardial segments. Hemodynamic changes that occurred in this subgroup of patients included significant decreases in LV end-diastolic and PA wedge pressures and significant increases in angiographic cardiac index and end-systolic volume index. The investigators concluded that in patients who manifest cardiac dilatation in the early convalescent period after AMI, there is remodeling of the entire left ventricle including infarct expansion of akinetic-dyskinetic segments and volume-overload hypertrophy of noninfarcted segments. The magnitude of the remodeling process appears directly proportional to infarct size as assessed by the extent of wall motion abnormality present during the acute phase of infarction. The remodeling changes are associated with hemodynamic improvement, including lower LV filling pressures and increased cardiac output, and these hemodynamic improvements appear to occur at the expense of a significant increase in LV chamber volumes.

Early Doppler measurement of aortic flow velocity

Mehta and associates[40] from London, UK, assessed LV function by Doppler ultrasound measurement of ascending aortic blood velocity and maximal acceleration in 165 patients 3 to 4 weeks after AMI; all were undergoing routine 12-lead electrocardiographic exercise stress testing. Patients were grouped according to electrocardiographic stress test response; a positive response was defined as ≥1 mm of ST-segment depression in any lead. The Doppler velocity signal yielded 3 variables of interest: peak velocity, maximal acceleration (an index of inotropic state), and the systolic velocity integral (an index of stroke volume). All 3 Doppler ejection variables were significantly lower at peak exercise in patients with a positive electrocardiographic stress test response than in those with negative response, with maximal acceleration showing the most significance. Coronary angiography was performed in 63 of the 67 patients with positive responses, and patients were separated into 2 groups according to extent of CAD: 1- and 2-vessel or 3-vessel CAD. Peak velocity and maximal acceleration were significantly lower in patients with 3-vessel CAD than in those with 1- and 2-vessel CAD. Discriminant analysis showed maximal acceleration and peak velocity values at peak exercise to be 65% predictive of 3-vessel CAD, onset time to ST-segment depression was 74% predictive, and the combination of Doppler and electrocardiographic variables increased 3-vessel CAD predictive value to 80%. This was considerably higher than the 62% predictive value of the exercise BP response. (No improvement in predictive value was seen when combined with the onset time.) Rapid and accurate measurement of LV functional response to exercise using the Doppler technique may be a useful adjunct to routine exercise stress testing in identifying patients at high risk of dying in the setting of AMI.

COMPLICATIONS

Right-axis deviation

Sclarovsky, et al[41] in Petah Tikva and Tel Aviv, Israel, studied 11 patients, 3 with AMI and 8 with anterior ischemia, who had transient right-axis deviation with a left posterior hemiblock pattern during AMI or ischemia. Correlations were made between clinical variables and angiographic findings. Arteriographic findings were compared with those from a separate group of 24 patients with anterior AMI or ischemia without transient right-axis deviation. In the patients demonstrating transient shifts toward a right-axis pattern, the following electrocardiographic features were noted: 1) an average shift in the mean frontal axis to the right of 42°; 2) increased voltage of R waves in leads II, III, and aVF; 3) decreased voltage of R waves and the development of deep S waves in lead aVL; and 4) inverted T waves and isoelectric ST segments. Coronary arteriography demonstrated that the patients with transient right-axis deviation had a higher incidence of significant right CAD and collateral circulation between the left coronary system and the posterior descending coronary artery. There were no differences between the groups with regard to LAD and LC coronary artery stenoses. Transient right-axis deviation during anterior AMI or ischemia represents different degrees of left posterior hemiblock, most likely a consequence of decreased blood flow to the left posterior fascicle and correlated with the presence of significant right coronary artery stenoses.

Atrioventricular heart block

Lamas and associates[42] as part of the Multicenter Investigation of the Limitation of Infarct Size (MILIS) analyzed data from 698 patients with proved AMI to develop a method to predict the occurrence of complete heart block (CHB). The presence of electrocardiographic abnormalities of AV or intraventricular conduction during hospitalization was determined for each patient. The electrocardiographic risk factors considered were: first-degree AV block, Mobitz type I AV block, Mobitz type II AV block, left anterior hemiblock, left posterior hemiblock, right BBB, and left BBB. A CHB risk score was developed that consisted of the sum of each patient's individual risk factors. CHB risk scores of 0, 1, 2 or ≥3 were associated with incidences of CHB of 1.2, 7.8, 25.0, and 36.4%, respectively. When applied to an independent AMI data base and to the summed results of 6 previously reported series that identified predictors of CHB during AMI, a similar incremental risk of CHB as predicted by the risk score method was demonstrated (Fig. 3-6).

Bassan et al[43] in Rio de Janeiro, Brazil, studied 51 consecutive patients surviving inferior AMI who underwent coronary arteriography to determine the significance of AV block. Eleven patients had some degree of AV block with AMI that disappeared within a few days but was considered by electrocardiographic analysis to be located in the AV node. Patients with AV block during inferior AMI had a significantly greater prevalence of LAD obstructions (91 -vs- 55%) than did patients without AV block, and the obstruction occurred before the first septal perforator branch in 73% of patients with and in 30% of patients without block. The sensitivity, specificity, and predictive

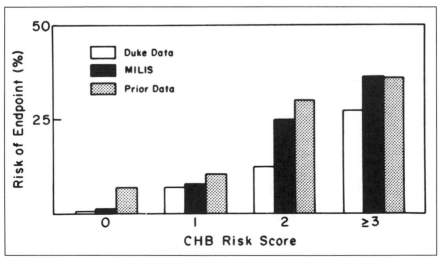

Fig. 3-6. Comparison between the incidence of complete heart block (CHB) predicted by the CHB risk score method (*solid bars*), observed incidence of CHB in the Duke University myocardial infarction data base (*open bars*) and the observed incidence of CHB or CHB and Mobitz II in 6 reported studies (*screened bars*).

values were 31, 95, and 91%, respectively, for the presence of LAD obstruction when AV block occurred during inferior AMI, and 40, 90, and 73%, respectively, for LAD obstruction before the first septal perforator branch. Therefore, patients with inferior AMI and LAD obstruction have a 6-fold greater likelihood of having heart block during AMI than do patients with inferior AMI without similar LAD obstructions. The proximal AV conduction system usually has a dual arterial blood supply from both the right and LAD arteries, thus explaining the transient development of heart block found in some of these patients.

Supraventricular tachyarrhythmias

Berisso and associates[44] from Genova, Italy, evaluated 160 survivors of AMI to assess the significance of SVT occurring at discharge from the hospital after the acute event. All variables considered for the study were estimated before hospital discharge; arrhythmias were quantified with a 24-hour Holter electrocardiographic monitoring system. SVT occurred in 88 patients (55%). Single or repetitive supraventricular premature complexes were found in 65 (41%), paroxysmal atrial or junctional tachycardias in 20 (12%), and bouts of atrial flutter or AF in 3 (2%). Bivariate statistical analysis showed no relation between sex, previous cardiovascular history, type, and location of AMI and SVT occurrence. A close positive relation was found between age, LA dimension, cardiothoracic ratio, and SVT occurrence; an inverse relation was found for LVEF. The presence of SVT appeared significantly related to age >55 years, to LA dimension >40 mm, to LVEF <45%, to serum creatine kinase peak levels >1,400 U 1^{-1} and to cardiothoracic ratio >.49.

Ventricular tachycardia

Bigger and associates[45] of the Multicenter Post Infarction Research Group made 24-hour continuous electrocardiographic recordings 11 ± 3 days after AMI in 820 of the 867 participants in the Multicenter Post Infarction Program. Ninety patients (11%) had unsustained VT and 2 had sustained VT (>15 seconds). In 53 of the 92 patients (58%) with VT, only 1 episode of VT was in the recording. In 26 patients the longest episode of VT was 3 consecutive complexes (28%); in 56 patients (61%) it was 4–10 complexes; and in only 10 patients (11%) were there >10 consecutive complexes per minute (range 75–240). Most episodes of VT started well after the T wave. Occurrence of VT was strongly related to the frequency of VPC in the 24-hour recording; 46% of the patients with ≥100 VPCs/hour had VT. The 92 patients who had VT were compared to the 728 who did not with respect to relevant clinical characteristics. Several variables were significantly more common in the VT group: age >60 years, previous AMI, history of angina pectoris, occurrence of VT or VF in the coronary care unit, LVEF <30%, rales greater than bibasilar in the coronary care unit, and use of antiarrhythmic drugs, digitalis or diuretic drug at the time of discharge from hospital. Based on Kaplan-Meier survival curves, the cumulative probability of surviving 3 years was 0.67 for patients with VT and 0.85 for patients without VT (Fig. 3-7). There were no statistically significant associations between individual VT characteristics and mortality. However, patients with longer runs of VT tended to have a higher mortality rate, and both patients with sustained VT died in the first month after the index infarct. VT had a strong and statistically significant association with all-cause and arrhythmic mortality independent of

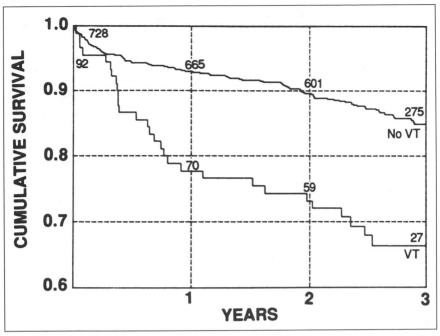

Fig. 3-7. Kaplan-Meier survival curves for patients with and without ventricular tachycardia (VT), using all-cause mortality as the endpoint. The numbers of patients at the start of follow-up and the numbers known to be alive after 1, 2 and 3 years of follow-up are indicated on these curves.

other risk variables that were associated with VT. Adjusted for other risk indicators, VT nearly doubled the risk of dying during an average follow-up of 31 months (Fig. 3-8).

Ventricular fibrillation

Dubois and associates[46] from Liege, Belgium, analyzed 1,265 patients admitted to the coronary care unit with AMI, 96 (8%) of whom had VF within 72 hours of admission. Of these 96 patients, 35 (37%) had VF associated with LV failure; they had an in-hospital mortality of 57%. The remaining 61 patients (64%) had VF occurring in the absence of significant LV failure. Fourteen (23%) of these 61 patients died in hospital, 9 during VF. This mortality percent was significantly higher than the mortality of 10% seen in patients who did not have VF. Compared with the 1,061 patients who left the hospital without VF, the 61 patients with VF unassociated with LV failure were older, had larger infarcts and more frequent complications, such as pericarditis, conduction abnormalities, frequent VPC and signs of RV failure.

Pericardial effusion

To evaluate the frequency and significance of pericardial effusion in patients with AMI, Galve and co-workers[47] in Barcelona, Spain, studied prospectively 138 consecutive patients with AMI. An echocardiogram was obtained in each 1, 3, 10, 90, and 180 days after admission. Fifty-four patients with unstable angina and 57 without heart disease were studied as controls.

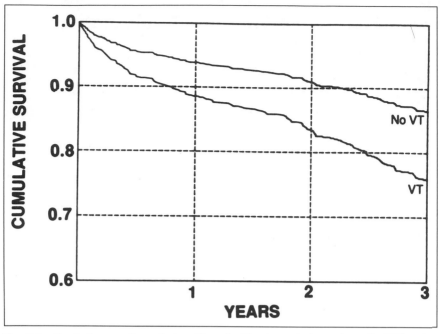

Fig. 3-8. Survival curves for patients with and without ventricular tachycardia (VT), using all-cause mortality as the endpoint. These curves were fitted by Cox's method and adjusted for the following risk factors: radionuclide ejection fraction, rales, age, history of angina, previous infarction and VT/fibrillation in the coronary care unit. The numbers of patients at the beginning of follow-up and those alive and being followed after 1, 2, and 3 years are the same as in Figure 2.

Echocardiographic diagnostic criteria of pericardial effusion were established from 33 additional patients undergoing surgery. Pericardial effusion was found in 28% of patients with AMI. Twenty-five percent of patients with AMI had pericardial effusion on the third day, 8% of patients with unstable angina, and 5% of patients without heart disease. At 1, 3, 10, 90, and 180 days prevalence of pericardial effusion was 17%, 25%, 21%, 11%, and 8%, respectively. There was no case of tamponade. Pericardial effusion was more common in anterior AMI and in patients with CHF, but it was not significantly associated with early pericarditis, peak creatine kinase-MB, the level of anticoagulation, or mortality. Thus, pericardial effusion is a common event in patients with AMI, but does not result in specific complications.

Pierard et al[48] in Liege, Belgium, evaluated the frequency and clinical significance of pericardial effusion after AMI using 2-D echocardiography in 66 consecutive patients. Pericardial effusions were found in 17 (26%). Effusions were small in 13 patients, moderate in 3, and large with signs of cardiac tamponade in 1 patient. In the patient with a large effusion, 2-D echocardiography suggested myocardial rupture. The development of pericardial effusions in these patients was not associated with age, sex, prior AMI, AF, or treatment with heparin. However, it occurred more frequently in patients with anterior than inferior AMI, and patients with pericardial effusions had higher peak serum levels of creatine kinase and lactic dehydrogenase and an apparently larger infarct. More patients with pericardial effusions had CHF or ventricular arrhythmias, had LV aneurysm, and died within 1 year of their AMI.

Left ventricular thrombi

Goldstein and associates[49] from San Francisco, California, compared contrast-enhanced computed tomography (CT) with 2-D echocardiography for evaluation of LV thrombus. Thirteen patients with CAD who had LV thrombus initially documented by 1 of the 2 techniques were then studied with the other technique. The findings of the studies were concordant in 8 of 13 patients, with a similar description of the presence, location, and size of the LV thrombus and associated regional LV wall abnormalities. In 5 of 13 patients, the 2 techniques produced discordant data. Of these, 2 patients had false-negative results on 2-D echocardiography owing to poor visualization of the LV apex; 1 patient had a false-positive result on 2-D echocardiography related to misinterpretation of a prominent papillary muscle; 2 patients had false-negative CT results, 1 related to insufficient contrast infusion. The findings demonstrate that CT is a useful technique for evaluating LV thrombus, and may be particularly helpful when 2-D echocardiography is technically limited or equivocal. A good review of this subject was provided by Meltzer and associates[50] from New York, New York.

Right ventricular infarction

Bellamy and associates[51] from St. Leonards, Australia, evaluated noninvasive tests for the diagnosis of RV infarction—2-D echocardiography, ST elevation V_4R, clinical parameters, and RNA—in 50 patients after inferior AMI: 22 patients had RV wall motion abnormalities on RNA and 20 on 2-D echocardiography. Sensitivity and specificity of 2-D echocardiography was 82% and 93%, ST elevation in V_4R was 50% and 71%, elevation of venous pressure was 77% and 85%, and a positive Kussmaul's sign was found in 59% and 89% for the detection of RV infarction compared with RNA. Patients with RV infarction had higher peak creatine kinase levels and lower LVEF than patients without RV infarction. At 20 weeks of follow-up, two-thirds of the patients had no residual RV wall motion abnormalities, and all but 2 patients had substantial recovery.

Infarct expansion

Pirolo et al[52] in Baltimore, Maryland, studied the hearts of 204 patients with a single AMI to determine reasons for marked variability and "expansion" of myocardial infarcts. There were 58 (28%) of the hearts with marked, 34 (17%) with moderate, and 112 (55%) with no or minimal expansion. Degree of infarct expansion was greater in larger, more transmural infarcts and infarcts with greater expansion had more endocardial thrombus and fibroelastosis. Infarct expansion was more limited in hearts of larger weight and with more severe degrees of LV hypertrophy. A greater degree of infarct expansion was found in 101 hearts (50%) associated with lesions in the distribution of the LAD. Expansion implies that the investigator knows the size of the infarct before expansion begins. Since it is impossible to precisely know the size of an AMI in life, I (WCR) have a major problem with the concept of expansion.

Left ventricular aneurysm

Cohen and Vogel[53] of Ann Arbor, Michigan, determined whether or not LV aneurysm in patients with CAD is a risk factor independent of LV function. Thirty-nine patients with angiographically demonstrated segmental dyskinesia (LV aneurysm group) were retrospectively compared to 28 patients with segmental akinesia and EF <60% (control group). There was no significant difference in age, EF, severity of CAD, cardiac index, or frequency of cardiac surgery between the 2 groups. Compared to control subjects, the LV aneurysm group had a significantly higher LV end-diastolic pressure and greater tendency to have apical involvement. Although, electrocardiography, echocardiography, and RNA were each highly specific, their sensitivities were only 40%–60%. Follow-up data were available for a mean of 33 months after catheterization. No significant benefit from aneurysmectomy could be demonstrated. There was an insignificant trend in the LV aneurysm group toward more severe CHF and less angina. There was no significant difference in the reinfarction rate, frequency of VT, or embolism. Mortality rate was 38% in the LV aneurysm group and 32% in the control group. It was concluded that LV aneurysm is not an independent risk factor for CHF, angina, VT, reinfarction, embolism, or death.

Visser and associates[54] from Amsterdam, The Netherlands, performed serial 2-D echocardiography in 158 consecutive patients with their first AMI to determine the incidence of LV aneurysm formation and the time course required for, and the clinical significance of, onset of LV aneurysm formation. Studies were performed throughout the first 5 days and after 3 months and 1 year. LV aneurysm was defined as an abnormal bulge in the LV contour during both systole and diastole. Eighty-four patients had anterior, 68 posterior, and 6 anteroposterior AMI defined echocardiographically. LV aneurysm was found in 35 of 158 patients (22%): in anterior AMI in 27, in posterior AMI in 6, and in anteroposterior AMI in 2. No new aneurysm developed after 3 months. Early aneurysm formation, during the first 5 days after AMI, was seen in 15 patients with anterior AMI. Twelve of these 15 (80%) died within 1 year (10 within 3 months), in contrast to 5 (25%) of the remaining 20 patients with LV aneurysm. Dyskinesia of the anterior wall in the acute stage usually resulted in aneurysm formation. Thus, LV aneurysm formation was seen in 22% of mostly anterior AMI and occurs within 3 months after AMI. Early aneurysm formation is associated with a high 3-month (67%) and 1-year (80%) mortality rate.

Forman et al[55] in Nashville, Tennessee, determined the factors involved in LV aneurysm formation after transmural AMI in 79 patients with their first AMI who underwent cardiac catheterization within 6 months of AMI. Patients who had received thrombolytic therapy were excluded from these analyses. Patients were classified into 4 groups depending on the status of the LAD and presence or absence of an LV aneurysm. Patients in group I (n = 25) had an LV aneurysm with an occluded LAD; patients in group II (n = 27) did not have an aneurysm but had an occluded LAD; patients in group III (n = 23) had no LV aneurysm and a patent LAD; patients in group IV (n = 4) had an LV aneurysm with patent LAD. Single-vessel CAD was more common in group I than in group II and III patients. Collateral coronary blood flow in the presence of an occluded LAD occurred significantly less frequently in patients in group I than in group II. The extent of CAD and collateral blood flow in patients in groups I and II were directly related. Age, sex, and risk factors for CAD did not correlate with the presence of an LV aneurysm. After a mean follow-up of 48 months, there were no differences in the frequency of recurrent angina, new AMI, embolic events, or sudden death. More patients in group II underwent CABG than in the other groups. Total occlusion of the LAD in association with relatively poor collateral blood flow appears to be a significant determinant of LV aneurysm formation after anterior AMI. Multivessel stenoses with either good collateral circulation or a patent LAD are uncommonly associated with the development of an LV aneurysm.

To evaluate the role of quantitative 2-D echocardiography in the preoperative assessment of patients undergoing LV aneurysmectomy, Ryan and colleagues[56] from Indianapolis, Indiana, identified 37 patients who were studied with 2-D echocardiography 1 to 56 (mean 13) days before surgery. Diastolic and systolic minor axis dimensions at the base were measured and fractional shortening was calculated. Global and basilar half EF were measured from right anterior oblique left ventriculograms. At follow-up (mean 18 months), 27 patients were alive and clinically improved (group A) and 10 patients either died or were symptomatically unimproved (group B). Basilar half EF was significantly greater among patients in group A (0.50 ± 0.09) than in group B (0.37 ± 0.10). Echocardiographic fractional shortening provided the best separation between groups. Mean fractional shortening was 0.25 ± 0.06 in group A and 0.15 ± 0.04 in group B. All 7 patients with fractional shortening <0.17 were in group B, whereas 25 of 27 patients with fractional shortening >0.17 were in group A. Considering all patients, basilar half EF and fractional shortening were highly correlated.

CABG with or without LV aneurysmectomy has been used to treat patients with angiographically defined LV aneurysm. To evaluate whether surgery benefits such patients, Faxon and co-workers[57] in Boston, Massachusetts, analyzed the data from 1,131 patients who were enrolled in the registry of the Coronary Artery Surgery Study. Four hundred sixty-seven patients underwent CABG, of which 238 had LV resection and 30 had resection alone. The overall operative mortality was 8%; the operative mortality was 7% for CABG alone, 9% for CABG plus LV resection. Long-term survival by life-table analysis was similar for both medically and surgically treated patients (69% -vs- 67%). Cox survival analysis identified CHF score, duration of chest pain, extent of CAD, LV end-diastolic pressure, age, and surgical therapy as important predictors of outcome. Patients subsets that showed improved survival with surgical therapy after adjustment of inequities in baseline characteristics were patients with 3-vessel CAD and patients in moderate and high-risk subgroups. Although surgical therapy significantly reduced symptoms of angina and use of cardiac medications, the frequency of recurrent AMI was similar for both therapies.

Mitral regurgitation

The systolic murmur of papillary muscle dysfunction is a well recognized feature of AMI, but no large prospective studies have determined its incidence, associated variables, and prognostic implications. Maisel and associates[58] from San Diego, California, and Vancouver, Canada, studied 1,653 patients with AMI, 283 (17%) of whom had a systolic murmur suggesting MR. At hospital discharge, there was a 5% frequency. There was a higher frequency of systolic murmur in non-Q-wave AMI than in inferior or anterior Q-wave AMI (24% -vs- 13% and 15%). Advanced age, previous AMI, and CHF were all associated with systolic murmur. Persistent pain in the coronary care unit occurred more often in those with systolic murmur (45% -vs- 26%). Systolic murmur was associated with an S_3 and bibasilar rales in the hospital; it was inversely related to peak creatine kinase and unrelated to CHF or EF at discharge. Univariate predictors of mortality associated with systolic murmur included VPC at discharge and a non-Q-wave location. Patients with systolic murmur had higher hospital and 1-year mortality than those without systolic murmurs. When systolic murmur was present during hospitalization, the average time to reinfarction was 2.5 times earlier than when no systolic murmur was present (84 -vs- 214 days). Thus, although systolic murmur of papillary muscle dysfunction in AMI appears transient in most cases, its presence is associated with prior AMI, persistent pain, CHF, and greater mortality despite small infarct size. The presence of systolic murmur may also represent a subset of patients at high risk for early reinfarction.

Loperfido and associates[59] from Rome, Italy, assessed in 72 patients with healed myocardial infarction, the frequency and severity of MR by pulsed-wave Doppler echocardiography and compared it with physical and 2-D echocardiographic findings. MR was found by Doppler in 29 of 42 patients (62%) with anterior AMI, 11 of 30 (37%) with inferior AMI, and in none of 20 normal control subjects. MR was more frequent in patients who underwent Doppler study 3 months after AMI than in those who underwent Doppler at discharge (anterior AMI = 83% -vs- 50%; inferior AMI = 47% -vs- 27%). Of 15 patients who underwent Doppler studies both times, 3 (all with anterior AMI) had MR only on the second study. Of the patients with Doppler MR, 12 of 27 (44%) with a LVEF >30% and 1 of 13 (8%) with an EF of ≤30% had an MR systolic murmur. Mitral prolapse or eversion and papillary muscle fibrosis were infrequent in AMI patients, whether or not Doppler MR was present. The degree of Doppler MR correlated with EF, LV systolic volume, and systolic and diastolic mitral anulus circumference. Doppler MR was present in 24 of 28 patients (86%) with an EF of ≤40% and in 16 of 44 (36%) with EF >40%. The septum and anterobasal free wall were more frequently dyssynergic in patients with than in those without Doppler MR (difference significant for patients with anterior myocardial infarction). Thus, Doppler MR is common in patients with previous AMI; the murmur may be absent in patients with Doppler MR, particularly in those in whom EF is depressed; and in patients with anterior AMI, the degree of Doppler MR is inversely related to LV function.

Connolly and associates[60] from New York, New York, attempted to analyze the surgical results for MR when associated with CAD. Between 1980 and 1984, a total of 1,475 patients underwent CABG. These patients were separated into 3 groups: 1) patients without ischemic MR who had isolated CABG (1,374 patients); 2) patients with ischemic MR who had isolated CABG without valve replacement (85 patients); and 3) patients with ischemic MR who underwent combined MVR and CABG (16 patients). Patients with ischemic MR were older, had more severe CAD, had a higher frequency of CHF, a greater frequency of recent AMI, and a lower mean EF than those without MR. Operative mortality was significantly increased in patients with ischemic MR who underwent CABG alone, and in those who underwent CABG and MVR—11% and 19%, respectively—than in the CABG patients without ischemic MR, 4%. The severity of MR was the most significant predictor of operative mortality. The actuarial survival rate at 5 years for the CABG patients with ischemic MR was 85%, compared to 91% for the CABG patients without ischemic MR (Fig. 3-9). These results indicate that patients with ischemic MR have a high prevalence of cardiac risk factors and are at an increased risk of operative mortality. Although predictive of early survival, the severity of MR had an unexpectedly modest effect on long-term survival after surgical treatment.

In a previous retrospective study of patients with acute MR, investigators from the Mayo Clinic concluded that early emergency operation was the proper course to take. In the present publication, Nishimura and associates[61] from Rochester, Minnesota, described 9 patients subsequently seen at the Mayo Clinic (7 with acute MR and 2 with acute VSD) who underwent emergency operation within 4 days of evaluation. Four patients were operated on within 4 hours after the onset of their complications. All 9 patients survived the perioperative period and 8 are alive and well over a mean follow-up

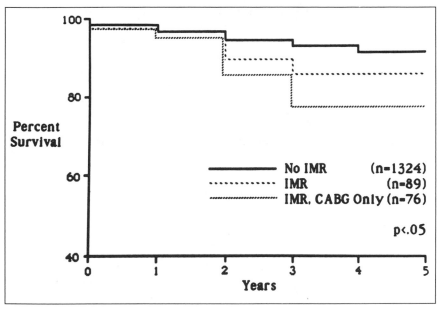

Fig. 3-9. Actuarial survival for coronary bypass *(CABG)* patients with ischemic mitral regurgitation *(IMR)*, which includes those patients with and without mitral valve replacement, compared to CABG patients without ischemic mitral regurgitation *(No IMR)*. CABG patients with ischemic mitral regurgitation, excluding those who required mitral valve replacement, are also represented *(IMR, CABG only)*. Operative mortality was excluded from the actuarial analysis. Survival rates for both groups of patients with ischemic mitral regurgitation *(IMR* and *IMR, CABG only* groups) are significantly less (p <0.05) than that of CABG patients without ischemic mitral regurgitation. All 13 operative surviving CAB/MVR patients were alive at the end of the follow-up period, for a 100% late survival rate. Reproduced with permission from Connolly et al.[60]

period of 10 months. These investigators recommended early operative repair of acute MR or acute VSD during AMI.

Ventricular septal rupture

Over a 5.5-year period, 1,264 consecutive patients with AMI confirmed by enzyme levels were prospectively identified by Moore and colleagues[62] in Charlottesville, Virginia. Of this group, 25 (2%) had ventricular septal rupture an average of 7 days after onset of AMI. Death occurred in 14 patients (56%) and was more common after inferior than anterior wall AMI (11 of 15 [73%] -vs- 3 of 10 [30%]). Among 133 variables analyzed, survivors, and nonsurvivors were similar with respect to all premorbid clinical characteristics, infarct size as assessed by peak creatine kinase values, shunt size, 2-D echocardiographic and hemodynamic indexes of LV function, and extent of CAD. Compared with survivors, the nonsurvivors had greater impairment of RV function as determined by a higher 2-D echocardiographically derived RV wall motion index, greater elevation of RV end-diastolic pressure, and greater mean RA pressure. Two of the 3 patients who presented with anterior AMI and who died had inferiorly extended infarcts and all had abnormal RV wall motion indexes. Cardiogenic shock shortly after onset of ventricular septal rupture was associated with a 91% mortality, but was more common after inferior than anterior AMI (60% -vs- 20%). The mean effective cardiac index was also higher in survivors than in nonsurvivors. Finally, multivariate analysis indicated that all nonsurvivors could be identified based on: 1) an effective cardiac index of <1.75 liters/min/m², 2) the presence of extensive RV and septal dysfunction on the 2-D echocardiogram, 3) a mean RA pressure of >12 mm Hg, and 4) early onset of ventricular septal rupture (Fig. 3-10). Thus, these data demonstrate that mortality is higher when ventricular septal rupture complicates inferior that when it complicates anterior AMI, survivors

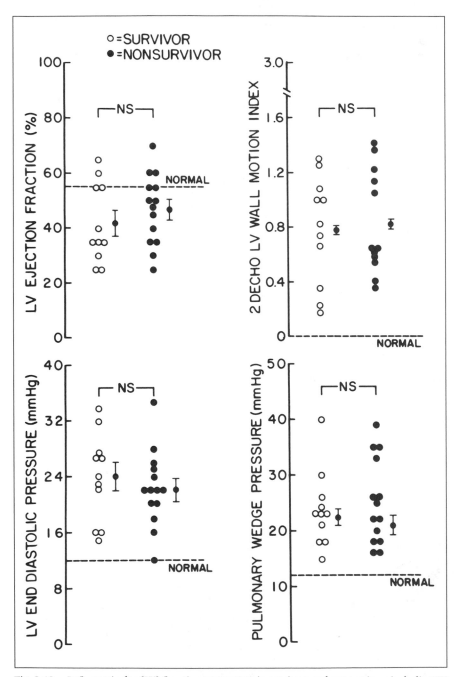

Fig. 3-10.   Left ventricular (LV) function parameters in survivors and nonsurvivors including LV ejection fraction (*upper left*), echocardiographic (2DECHO) LV wall motion index (*upper right*), LV end-diastolic pressure (*lower left*), and pulmonary wedge pressure (*lower right*). Group data are presented as mean ± SEM. Reproduced with permission from Moore et al.[62]

can be distinguished from nonsurvivors and the prediction of outcome is highly accurate, and combined RV and septal dysfunction has a substantial impact on prognosis.

Ischemic cardiomyopathy

Ross and Roberts[63] of Washington, D. C., and Bethesda, Maryland, described necropsy observations in 81 patients aged 29 to 91 years (mean 62) (77 [95%] men) with severe CHF >3 months in duration, LV transmural scar and >75% cross-sectional area narrowing by atherosclerotic plaque of ≥1 of the 4 major epicardial coronary arteries. The duration of symptoms from initial onset of AMI (59 patients) or CHF (18 patients) or angina pectoris (2 patients) to death ranged from 0.5 to 18 years (mean 7.1) (2 unknown) (Fig. 3-11). Angina pectoris occurred at some time, however, in 31 patients (38%). Cause of death was CHF in 48 patients (59%), sudden (arrhythmia) in 16 (20%), AMI in 11 (14%), and emboli in 6 (7%). The heart weight ranged from 410 to 800 g (mean 585). LV or RV thrombi or both occurred in 37 patients (46%), only 4 (10%) of whom had systemic emboli; of the 44 patients without intracardiac thrombi, none had emboli. The severity of coronary narrowing was variable. In 24 patients (30%) only 1 artery was narrowed >75% in cross-sectional area; in 22 patients (27%), 2 arteries were so narrowed; in 32 patients (39%), 3 arteries; and in 3 patients (4%), 4 arteries. The size of the LV scar also varied. Of the 81 patients, 58 (72%) had large scars (involving >40% of the LV wall); 10 (12%) had moderate-sized scars (6 to 40% of the LV wall); and 13 (16%) had small scars (≤5% of the LV wall). Size of the LV scar correlated with a history of habitual alcoholism: of the 16 habitual alcoholics, 6 (38%) had small and 8 (50%) had large LV scars; of the 65 nonalcoholics, 7 (11%) had small and 50 (77%) had large LV scars (Fig. 3-12). Chronic CHF in the 68 patients with either moderate or large-sized LV scars is readily attributed to the LV damage; in the 13 patients with small LV

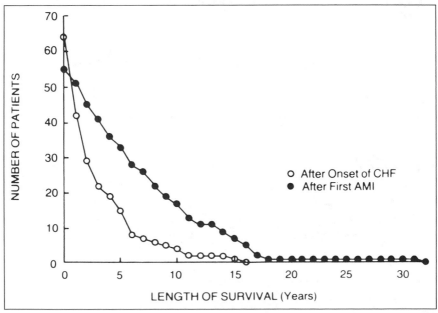

Fig. 3-11. Length of survival after onset of either congestive heart failure (CHF) (65 patients) or acute myocardial infarction (AMI) (55 patients).

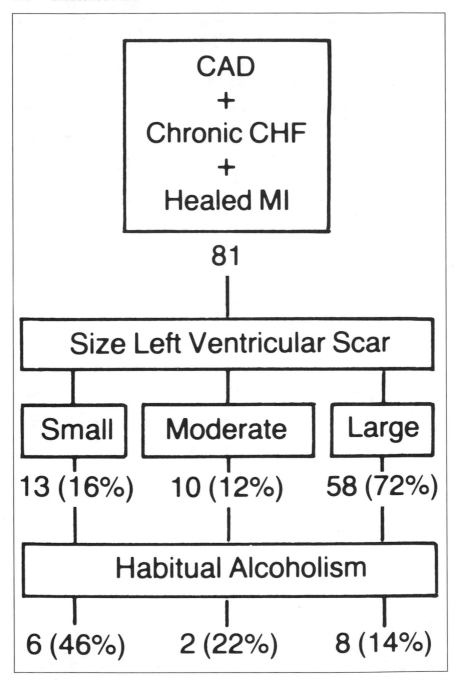

Fig. 3-12. Relation of healed myocardial infarct size to frequency of a history of habitual alcoholism in the 81 patients. Patients with small left ventricular scars had a high frequency of alcoholism and those with large infarcts, a relatively low frequency. CAD = coronary artery disease; CHF = congestive heart failure; MI = myocardial infarction.

scars, however, chronic CHF more reasonably may be attributed to another factor, e.g., alcoholism, despite coronary artery narrowing similar in severity to that in the patients with large LV scars.

PROGNOSTIC INDEXES

Interval from onset of symptom to hospital arrival

Turi and associates[64] from Boston, Massachusetts, St. Louis, Missouri, and Dallas, Texas, studied the time from onset of symptoms to arrival in the hospital emergency room in 778 patients randomized into a study of AMI-size limitation. Patients at relatively high risk of death after AMI (including those with preexisting diabetes mellitus, systemic hypertension, or CHF), women, and older patients arrived significantly later in the emergency room than did patients without these characteristics. A significantly higher mortality rate was observed in patients who arrived late, i.e., those who arrived >2 hours after the onset of chest pain, even though patients with hemodynamic compromise (bradycardia, hypotension) tended to arrive earlier. The difference in long-term mortality between those who arrived early (within 2 hours of onset of chest pain) and those who arrived late was accounted for by the baseline differences between these 2 groups. These baseline differences may influence the effects of early interventions in AMI. In addition, these findings have implications for education of high-risk patients who could benefit the most from aggressive early intervention.

Electrocardiographic site of the infarct

Anterior AMI is associated with more myocardial damage than inferior AMI and the prognosis of patients with anterior AMI is significantly worse than that of patients with inferior AMI. To assess whether the site of AMI is an independent prognostic indicator, Hands and colleagues[65] in Nedlands, Australia, compared the outcome of patients with anterior AMI with that of patients with inferior AMI. A consecutive series of patients who had had their first AMI was analyzed (398 with anterior and 391 with inferior). Patients with anterior AMI had a higher 1-year mortality than those with inferior AMI (18% -vs- 11%). When patients were matched for infarct size determined by peak creatine kinase (CK) level expressed as a multiple of the upper limit of normal, those with anterior AMI tended to have a higher 1-year mortality that those with inferior AMI for all subgroups of peak CK. Early mortality (day 1–28 days) was greater in the anterior than in the inferior AMI group (10% -vs- 6%) (Fig. 3-13); this was most significant when peak CK was >4 times normal (12% -vs- 7%). Late mortality was also higher in the anterior (8% -vs- 4%) than the inferior AMI group and this was most significant when peak CK was <2 times normal or >8 times normal (10% -vs- 4%). Multivariate analysis with proportional-hazards regression confirmed the prognostic significance of location of AMI independent of peak CK levels. Thus, infarct location was found to be a predictor of prognosis that is independent of infarct size based on peak CK levels.

Prolonged QT interval

Wheelan and associates[66] of the Multicenter Investigation of the Limitation of Infarct Size (MILIS) assessed in 533 patients who survived 10 days

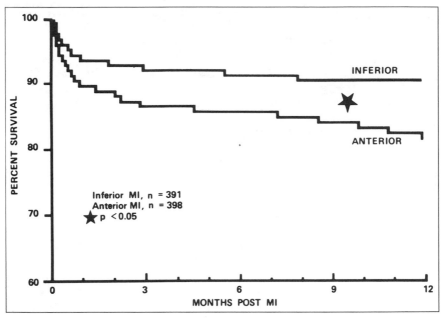

Fig. 3-13. Survival curve for patients who have suffered their first myocardial infarction (MI). n = number of patients. Reproduced with permission from Hands et al.[65]

after onset of AMI and were followed up to 24 months (mean 18) the risk of sudden death. Analysis of clinical and laboratory variables measured before hospital discharge revealed that the QT interval, either corrected (QTc) or uncorrected for heart rate, did not contribute significantly to prediction of subsequent sudden death or total mortality. In this population, frequent VPC >10/hour) on ambulatory electrocardiographic monitoring and LV dysfunction (radionuclide LVEF of ≤0.40) identified patients at high risk of sudden death. In patients with these adverse clinical findings, the QTc was 0.468 ± 0.044 second among those who died suddenly and 0.446 ± 0.032 second in survivors, not statistically significant as an additional predictor of sudden death. Consideration of the use of type I antiarrhythmic agents, digoxin, presence of U waves and correction for intraventricular conduction delay did not alter these findings. Although QT-interval prolongation occurs in some patients after AMI, reduced LVEF and frequent VPC are the most important factors for predicting subsequent sudden death in this patient population.

Transient pulmonary congestion

In a prospective multicenter study of 866 patients after AMI, Dwyer and associates[67] from multiple medical centers analyzed the increased or excessive mortality rate (13%) in the first 6 months after AMI (Fig. 3-14). In the subsequent 18 months of follow-up, the mortality rate (4%) was similar to that in coronary patients in chronic stable conditions. Analysis of patients who died in the first 6 months revealed that 55% had had pulmonary congestion at the time of the index AMI. Neither these patients nor the others who died in the early period were found to have more severe LV dysfunction, more malignant arrhythmias or more severe ischemia than patients who died after 6 months. The reason for the high and early mortality in patients with pulmonary congestion is not clear, particularly because 30% had reasonable LV

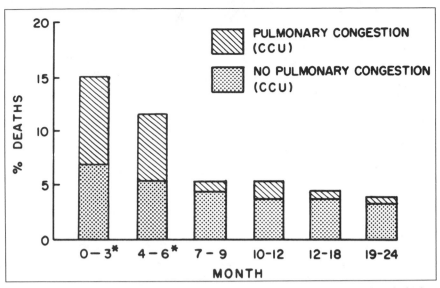

Fig. 3-14. Sequential average 3-month annualized mortality rates. A significantly higher percentage of the deaths occurred among patients with pulmonary congestion in the coronary care unit (CCU) in the first 6 months. After 6 months, there is a significant decline in overall deaths primarily due to the decline in deaths in patients who had pulmonary congestion. These patients account for most of the excessive mortality rate in the early postinfarction period.

function, with an EF >40%. However, given the poor prognosis of these patients, early and aggressive diagnostic efforts should be undertaken to exclude jeopardized regions remote from the initial AMI.

After discharge from a coronary care unit

Smyllie[68] from Doncaster, UK, analyzed 298 patients from 371 consecutive admissions to a coronary care unit who survived to 28 days and divided them on discharge into 2 diagnostic categories: those with and those without AMI. One hundred seventy-five patients had AMI and 123 did not. These patients were surveyed at 3 and 10 years. The patients without AMI were divided into subgroups with and without myocardial ischemia according to whether they had had a history of angina pectoris or AMI preceding the index admission or electrocardiographic features of ischemia during admission. After the adverse prognostic effects of age, smoking, and preceding myocardial ischemia had been allowed for, coronary mortality in the first year was virtually the same in the subgroups of patients without AMI who did and did not have ischemia. Ten-year mortality was also similar, being 29% in those with ischemia and 24% in those without (Fig. 3-15). These findings do not support the theory that patients without AMI who do not have evidence of ischemia have a more favorable prognosis.

Early exercise testing

To determine the relative value of clinical findings, Starling and associates[69] from San Antonio, Texas, studied results of low-level treadmill electrocardiographic exercise testing and LVEF for predicting cardiac events in the year after an AMI in 72 patients who had had an uncomplicated AMI. The

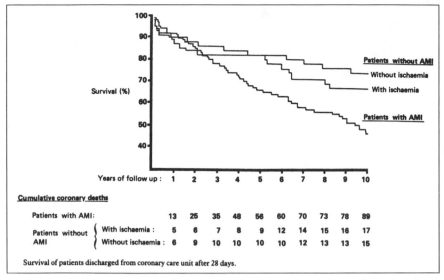

Fig. 3-15. Survival of patients discharged from coronary care unit after 28 days. Reproduced with permission from Smyllie.[68]

patients were studied with either RNA or 2-D echocardiography to assess LVEF and a low-level treadmill exercise test before hospital discharge. All patients were followed for 1 year. Nineteen patients (26%) had ≥1 cardiac event: CABG (11 patients), recurrent AMI (6 patients), or cardiac death (6 patients). Multiple logistic regression analysis revealed that total cardiac events were predicted by exercise electrocardiographic ST-segment depression or angina, prior AMI, ventricular ectopic activity during exercise, and digoxin therapy. CABG was predicted by exercise electrocardiographic ST-segment depression or angina. Recurrent AMI was predicted by exercise electrocardiographic ST-segment depression or angina, prior AMI, and ventricular ectopic activity during exercise. Cardiac death was predicted by an LVEF of ≤40% (Fig. 3-16). The presence of both an LVEF of ≤40% and electrocardiographic ST-segment depression on treadmill exercise testing defined a subgroup of patients with a high incidence of early cardiac death (33%).

Sia and associates[70] from Heidelberg, Australia, assessed the value of an early symptom-limited maximal exercise test in predicting coronary anatomy, LVEF, and hemodynamics in 64 patients after a *non-Q-wave AMI*. Exercise tests and cardiac catheterization were performed at a median of 6 and 7 days, respectively, after non-Q AMI. Forty-one percent of the patients had a negative exercise test response (no angina, <1 mm of ST depression and normal BP responses); 25% had a positive response (1 to 1.9 mm of ST depression or angina); 34% had a "strongly positive" exercise test response (≥2 mm ST depression or abnormal BP responses). A negative response predicted the absence of 3-vessel disease (≥70% stenosis) or critical stenoses (≥90% stenosis) involving major coronary arteries (negative predictive accuracy 92%), whereas a strongly positive response predicted their presence (positive predictive value 77%, specificity 88%). Cardiac index and mean PA wedge pressure did not vary significantly among the 3 exercise groups, whereas LVEF was slightly higher in the exercise test group with a positive response. Thus, in patients who have had a non-Q AMI, early exercise testing can be used to predict the extent and severity of CAD, and the decision to perform coronary angiography should be guided by the exercise test results.

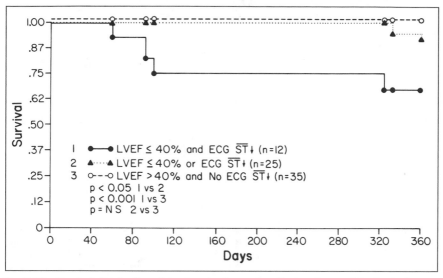

Fig. 3-16. Survival distribution plots given by the product-limit estimate of Kaplan-Meier are shown for 3 patient groups: (1) those with a left ventricular ejection fraction (LVEF) of 40% or less *and* electrocardiographic (ECG) ST-segment depression; (2) those with an LVEF of 40% or less *or* ECG ST-segment depression; and (3) those with an LVEF or more than 40% *and* no ECG ST-segment depression. Significant differences between group 1 and groups 2 and 3 given by the Mantel-Cox statistic are also shown. NS = not significant.

Late exercise testing

Stone et al[71], in Boston, Massachusetts, utilizing data obtained from the Multicenter Investigation of the Limitation of Infarct Size (MILIS) determined whether a maximal exercise test performed 6 months after AMI is useful in predicting prognosis later in the convalescent period. Performance characteristics during the exercise test 6 months after AMI were related to the development of death, recurrent nonfatal AMI, and CABG in the subsequent 6 months in 473 patients. Among these patients, mortality was significantly greater in patients who had any of the following: inability to perform the exercise test because of cardiac limitations; the development of ST-segment elevation of ≥1 mm during the exercise test; and inadequate BP response during exercise; the development of any VPC during exercise or the recovery period; and the inability to exercise beyond stage I of a modified Bruce protocol. Using a combination of 4 high-risk prognostic features from the exercise test, it was possible to stratify patients in terms of risk of mortality from 1% if none of the features was present to 17% if 3 or 4 features were present (Fig. 3-17). Recurrent nonfatal AMI was predicted by an inability to perform the exercise test because of cardiac limitations, but not by any of the variables determined from exercise test performance. CABG in the future was associated with the development of ST-segment depression of ≥1 mm during the exercise test. At rest, the presence of angina and CHF 6 months after AMI were predictive of subsequent mortality among all survivors. Among the low risk patients, the exercise test itself provided unique prognostic information not available from clinical assessment alone. Thus, these data indicate that a maximal exercise test performed 6 months after AMI is a valuable, noninvasive tool to predict future prognosis.

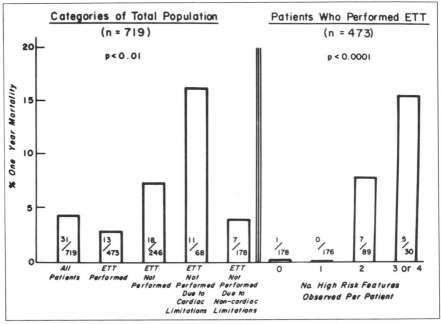

Fig. 3-17. One year death rate after health visit 6 months after myocardial infarction. For patients who performed the treadmill exercise test (ETT), death rate is based on consideration of the number of high risk features observed. The high risk features considered were an inadequate systolic blood pressure response, inability to exercise beyond stage 1 of the modified Bruce protocol, development of any ventricular premature depolarizations or exertional ST segment elevation during the test. The denominator for each *bar* indicates the number of patients manifesting the number of high risk features observed. The numerator indicates the number of patients in the group who died. Of the 473 patients who performed the test, 447 were capable of exhibiting each of the four high risk features, and 26 were capable of exhibiting only three high risk features. Twenty-five patients were excluded from the ST segment analysis because of an uninterpretable ST segment (24 with left or right bundle branch block and 1 with technical failure of the electrocardiograph) and 1 patient could not have his blood pressure determined during exercise or in the recovery period. Reproduced with permission from Stone et al.[71]

Wall motion abnormality early or late

Kan and associates[72] from Amsterdam and Utrecht, The Netherlands, used a score of LV segmental wall motion as a convenient rapid way to assess overall LV function in AMI (Fig. 3-18). Its success in risk stratification at admission was assessed by a blind review of cross-sectional echocardiographic tape recordings from multiple acoustic windows. Sixty-nine (20%) of the 345 patients died during hospital stay or within a 1-year follow up. The mean wall motion score in those who died was significantly higher than in those who survived (16.2 ± (5.9) -vs- 5.7 ± (3.9)). There were no differences between 3 and 12 months after discharge. Among the 31 patients who died in the hospital, however, wall motion score was highest in 15 patients dying of cardiogenic shock (19.2 ± 4.2). In 16 patients with lethal cardiac ruptures, it was 13.5 ± 6.1. The 9 patients with free wall rupture had higher wall motion scores than those with ventricular septal rupture or papillary muscle rupture (15.7 ± 6.9 -vs- 8.5 ± 5.3).

Shiina and associates[73] from Rochester, Minnesota, correlated the results of 2-D echocardiographic and angiographic analysis of LV wall motion abnormalities and their prognostic significance in 50 consecutive patients with

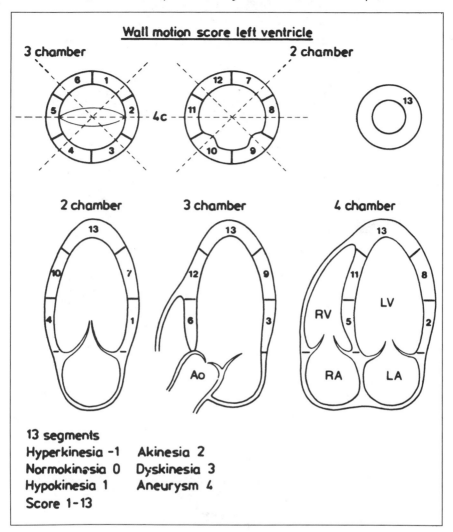

Fig. 3-18. Diagram of the three apical long axis views (lower panel) used for calculation of the left ventricular wall motion score. In each of the three views the left ventricular myocardium was divided into five segments; the apex was considered to be common to all three apical views. If the apical views were not adequate for analysis, the same segments could be evaluated from short axis cross sections (upper panel). The three chamber view was a long axis view or right anterior oblique equivalent. Ao, aorta; LA, left atrium; LV, left ventricle; RA, right atrium; RV, right ventricle. Reproduced with permission from Kan et al.[72]

prior AMI (Fig. 3-19). There was overall good agreement (88%) between the 2 methods. In general, the greater the LV dysfunction, the worse the prognosis. The 3-year survival was significantly reduced for patients with LV wall motion index of ≥2.5 (Fig. 3-20). These findings were similar to the reduced survival rate associated with decreased angiographic EF (<40%) (Fig. 3-21). This study suggests that 2-D echocardiography can provide prognostic information in patients with prior AMI.

Ejection fraction near discharge

Ahnve and associates[74] from San Diego, California, and Vancouver, Canada, determined LVEF close to the time of hospital discharge in 750 patients

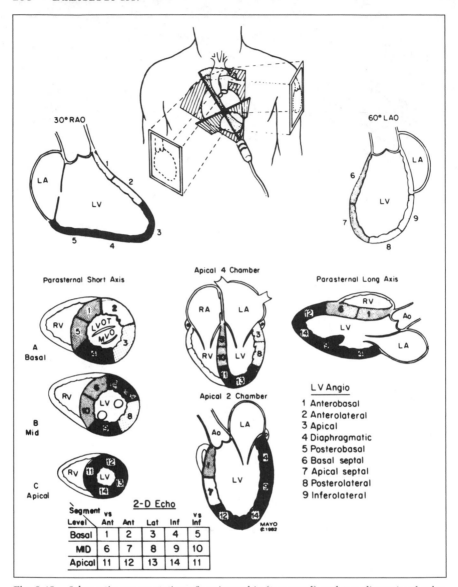

Fig. 3-19. Schematic representation of angiographic (top panel) and two-dimensional echocardiographic (other diagrams) segments of left ventricular wall. *Ant* = anterior; *Ao* = aorta; *Inf* = inferior; *LA* = left atrium; *LAO* = left anterior oblique projection; *Lat* = lateral; *LV* = left ventricle; *LVOT* = left ventricular outflow tract; *MVO* = mitral valve orifice; *RA* = right atrium; *RAO* = right anterior oblique projection. Reproduced with·permission from Shiina et al.[73]

with AMI enrolled in a collaborative study (Fig. 3-22). Used alone, an LVEF <0.45 best defined a high-risk group (39% of the population) yielding 62% sensitivity and 64% specificity for total cardiac mortality by 1 year; it was 77% sensitive for sudden death alone. In a multivariate analysis together with other factors, LVEF was an independent predictor, but other markers of LV dysfunction entered before LVEF with similar sensitivity for total cardiac deaths, but with increased specificity (75%). When an LVEF of <0.45 was used together with the presence of complex arrhythmias to define a high-risk group (19% of the population), sensitivity decreased to 39% and specificity

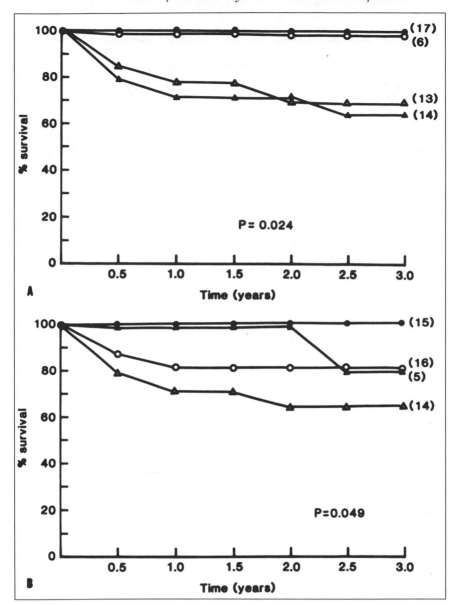

Fig. 3-20.   Correlation between cumulative survival and two-dimensional echocardiographic (A) and angiographic (B) measurements of left ventricular wall motion score index (LVSI). *Closed circles* = LVSI less than 2.0; *open circles* = LVSI 2.0 to 2.4; *open triangles* = LVSI 2.5 to 2.9; *closed triangles* = LVSI 3.0 or greater. Reproduced with permission from Shiina et al.[73]

increased to 84%. Thus, LVEF is a simple and effective alternative to multivariate analysis for risk assessment after AMI. It is more sensitive and produces a high-risk group of more reasonable size than an approach based on LVEF together with complex arrhythmias.

Three-vessel disease

In a study by Castaner and colleagues[75] from Barcelona, Spain, prevalence of 3-vessel CAD was prospectively analyzed in a series of 462 consecutive infarct survivors aged ≤60 years. Eight-seven percent (403) of the pa-

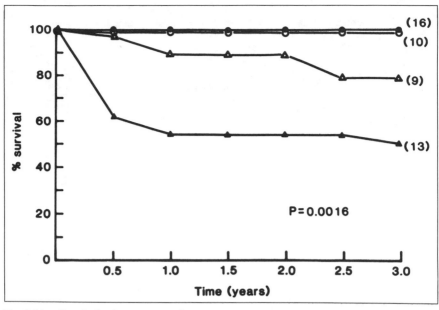

Fig. 3-21.   Correlation between cumulative 3-year survival and angiographic measurement of ejection fraction (EF). *Closed circles* = EF of 50% or greater; *open circles* = EF of 40 to 49%; *open triangles* = EF of 30 to 39%; *closed triangles* = EF of less than 30%. Reproduced with permission from Shiina et al.[73]

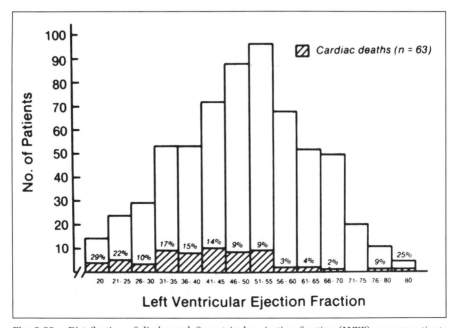

Fig. 3-22.   Distribution of discharge left ventricular ejection fraction (LVEF) among patients followed 1 year (n = 632). The height of the bars represents the number of patients with LVEF in the interval indicated. The *cross-notched portion* indicates numbers of patients within the specific interval who suffered a cardiac death during the 1 year follow-up. The percentage this represents of the total number of patients within the interval is indicated *above* the *cross-notched portion* of the *bar*.

tients underwent catheterization within 1 month of the acute event, and were followed for a mean of 43 months (range 21–69). Three-vessel CAD was present in 96 cases (24%) and these patients formed the study population. The primary goals of this study were to determine the prevalence of 3-vessel CAD and to identify predictors of survival and new coronary events among this subset of infarct survivors. During follow-up, 15 patients died, 17 had recurrent nonfatal AMI, and 54 had angina (4-year probability of each cardiac event being 0.20, 0.22, and 0.59, respectively). Cox's stepwise multivariate analysis identified the EF as the only predictor of survival. No predictors for nonfatal ischemic events were found among the independent variables considered. Patients were stratified in risk categories according to the EF. Four-year probability of survival was 1.0 in participants with EF = >50% (n = 23), 0.77 for those with EF = 21–49% (n = 66), and 0.22 in patients with more severe LV dysfunction, EF = <21% (n = 7). Probability of occurrence of nonfatal reinfarction or angina was similar in the 3 risk categories. Thus, these results indicate that a normal EF is found in 25% of infarct survivors with 3-vessel CAD, and that this subset of patients has a low frequency of early and intermediate range coronary events.

Uptake of thallium-201 by the right ventricular wall

Nestico and associates[76] from Philadelphia, Pennsylvania, examined the correlates of abnormal RV thallium uptake in 116 patients with documented AMI who underwent predischarge thallium-201 scintigraphy at rest, RNA and 24-hour ambulatory electrocardiography. The patients were separated into 2 groups: patients group 1 (n = 31) had increased RV thallium uptake and those in group 2 (n = 85) had no such uptake. The 2 groups were comparable in age, type and site of AMI, peak creatine kinase level, systolic BP, and heart rate. However, compared with group 2, group 1 had a lower mean LVEF (33 ± 15% -vs- 39 ± 14%), higher prevalence of increased lung thallium uptake (45% -vs- 22%), more extensive LV perfusion defects (4.4 ± 2.9 -vs- 3.0 ± 3.0 segments), and more complex ventricular arrhythmias (55% -vs- 35%). At a mean follow-up of 6 months, 17 patients (8 in group 1 and 9 in group 2) died from cardiac causes. Actuarial life-table analysis showed that the survival rate was better in group 2 than in group 1 (Mantel-Cox statistics = 4.62). Thus, patients with AMI and abnormal RV thallium uptake have worse LV function, more complex ventricular arrhythmias and worse prognosis.

Type A behavior

Friedman and associates[77] from San Francisco and Stanford, California, Cambridge, Massachusetts, and New Haven, Connecticut, observed 1,013 post-AMI patients for 4.5 years to determine whether their type A (coronary-prone) behavior could be altered and the effect such alteration might have on the subsequent cardiac morbidity and mortality rates of these persons. Eight hundred and sixty-two of these subjects were randomly assigned either to a control section of 270 participants who received group cardiac counseling or an experimental section of 592 participants who received both group cardiac counseling and type A behavioral counseling. The remaining 151 patients, serving as a comparison group, did not receive group counseling of any kind. Using the intention-to-treat principle, these investigators observed markedly reduced type A behavior at the end of 4.5 years in 35% of participants given cardiac and type A behavior counseling compared with 10% of participants given only cardiac counseling. The cumulative 4.5-year cardiac recurrence rate was 13% in the 592 participants in the experimental group that received type A counseling (Fig. 3-23). This recurrence rate was significantly less than either the recurrence rate (21%) observed in the 270 participants in the control group or the recurrence rate (28%) in those of the comparison group not receiving any special treatment. After the first year, a significant difference in number of cardiac deaths between the experimental and control participants was observed during the remaining 3.5 years of the study. Overall, the results of this study demonstrate for the first time, within a controlled experimental design, that altering type A behavior reduces cardiac morbidity and mortality in postinfarction patients.

ELECTROPHYSIOLOGIC STUDIES DURING ACUTE AND HEALED INFARCTION

To determine if the ability of programmed stimulation to initiate VT varies according to the interval between AMI and electrophysiologic testing, Stevenson and associates[78] from Maastricht, The Netherlands, analyzed clinical and electrophysiologic data of 42 patients with spontaneous sustained VT and 12 patients with VF >3 days after a single AMI. For patients with VT, there were no significant differences in the frequency of initiation of sustained monomorphic VT among those evaluated 1–3 weeks (100%), 3–8 weeks (75%), 2–6 months (100%), 6–18 months (80%) or >18 months (81%) after AMI, and the mean number of extrastimuli required for initiation did not differ among the groups. Patients evaluated >4 weeks after the

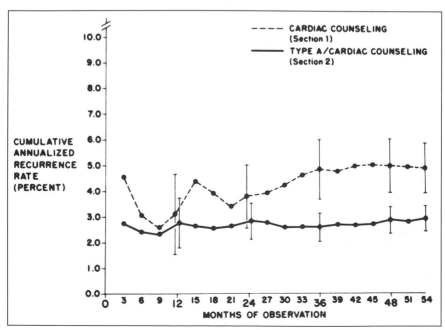

Fig. 3-23. Cumulative annualized recurrence rate in section 1 (cardiac-counseled) and section 2 (type A and cardiac-counseled) participants calculated quarterly for 4.5 years. Note that 95% confidence limits of quarterly calculated cardiac recurrence rates of two sections no longer intersect at end of 36 months. Reproduced with permission from Friedman et al.[77]

initial episode of VT had a lower frequency of inducible VT than those studied earlier (14 of 21 [71%] -vs- 21 of 21 [100%]. The 14 patients evaluated within 8 weeks of AMI had significantly faster VT rates (mean cycle length 269 ± 45 ms) than the 28 patients studied later (320 ± 75 ms). More patients studied within 3 weeks of AMI had anterior AMI (100%), but there were no differences in age or ejection fraction. Among patients with VF, 5 of 7 studied <8 weeks and 3 of 5 patients studied >8 weeks after AMI had inducible VT. Thus, the ability to induce sustained VT in patients with spontaneous episodes of sustained VT or VF after AMI appears to be independent of the interval between AMI and programmed stimulation.

Kienzle and associates[79] from Philadelphia, Pennsylvania, studied by catheter techniques *LV refractoriness* using the strength-interval relation and activation by local electrographic characteristics in 8 patients with and 6 patients without previous AMI. Noninfarcted myocardium in patients with and without healed AMI was similar overall with respect to refractoriness and excitability, whereas local electrographic duration in AMI patients was longer (66 ± 2 -vs- 52 ± 3 ms) and amplitude lower (3.9 ± 2.1 -vs- 6.1 ± 2.0 mV). Comparisons of infarcted and noninfarcted regions in AMI patients revealed an increased threshold of excitability at infarct sites (1.9 ± 1.0 -vs- 0.7 ± 0.4 mA) and prolongation of refractory periods (375 ± 118 -vs- 275 ± 13 ms) at the lowest level of stimulating current. Shortening of refractory period as a result of change in pacing cycle length was not affected by AMI. The local electrographic duration (95 ± 17 ms) was longer in infarcted regions than at noninfarcted sites, but the electrographic amplitude (3.4 ± 3.0 mV) differed only in noninfarct patients. Thus, considerable electrophysiologic disparity exists between infarcted and noninfarcted myocardium. Whether or not arrhythmogenic tissue possesses unique alterations in electrophysiologic characteristics remains to be established.

Vassallo and associates[80] from Philadelphia, Pennsylvania, performed endocardial catheter mapping in 27 patients with anterior wall AMI and in 10 patients with inferior wall AMI. All patients had a history of VT. LV breakthrough occurred at 10 ± 4 ms after the QRS complex in inferior AMI and 11 ± 7 ms after the QRS complex in anterior AMI. Total electrical activity recorded during sinus rhythm was 164 ± 46 ms in inferior and 144 ± 28 ms in anterior AMI. Nine of the 10 patients with anterior AMI had complete activation of the anterior wall within the initial one-half of the QRS complex, compared with only 15 of the 27 patients with anterior AMI. All 10 patients with inferior AMI had activation of the ventricular septum within the initial half of the QRS complex compared with only 13 of 27 with anterior AMI. No patient with inferior AMI had activation of the inferoposterior base within the initial one-half of the QRS complex, compared with 21 of 27 patients with anterior AMI. Complete activation of the anterior wall occurred at 33 ± 15 ms in inferior and 58 ± 30 ms in anterior AMI. Complete activation of the septum occurred at 38 ± 12 ms in inferior and 63 ± 28 ms in anterior AMI. Complete activation of the inferoposterior base occurred at 100 ± 38 ms in inferior and 50 ± 21 ms in anterior AMI. The latest site of endocardial activation was located at the inferoposterior base in 8 of the 10 patients with inferior AMI and was variable in those with anterior AMI.

Roy et al[81] in Montreal, Canada, evaluated long-term reproducibility and significance of inducible ventricular arrhythmias in survivors of AMI. Programmed ventricular stimulation performed a mean of 12 ± 2 days after AMI caused VF in 2 patients, sustained monomorphic VT in 8, and nonsustained VT in 11 patients. Patients were restudied using the same protocol a mean of 8 ± 2 months after AMI. At that time, all patients had programmed ventricular stimulation studies while not receiving antiarrhythmic drug treatment. VT was reinitiated in 16 patients (76%), VF in 2, sustained VT in 5, and nonsustained VT in 9. Among the patients with reinducible tachycardias, 9 of 16 had inferior AMI, whereas none of 5 patients with noninducible tachycardia had inferior AMI. There was no significant difference in clinical variables between patients with and without reinducible arrhythmias in severity of CAD, LV dysfunction, occurrence of VF in the acute phase of AMI, and ventricular arrhythmia as detected by 24-hour electrocardiographic monitoring. In addition, there were no differences between patients with and without inducible arrhythmias late in the study regarding stimulation thresholds, ventricular refractory periods, time interval between initial and repeat testing, and use of beta-blocking agents. One patient with inducible sustained VT at both studies died suddenly during follow-up (mean follow-up of 17 months). All of the remaining patients survived without having a major arrhythmic event. Thus, ventricular arrhythmias induced early after AMI can be reproduced after a mean of 8 months in survivors of AMI, but this persistent "electrical instability" is not a predictor of the risk of sudden death in the first year after AMI.

Kuck et al[82] in Hamburg, West Germany, evaluated the influence of time on the inducibility by programmed electrical stimulation of ventricular arrhythmias after AMI. Eighteen patients were studied on days 5 and 24 after AMI with a stimulation protocol employing a maximum of 3 RV extrastimuli during sinus rhythm and at 3 paced cycle lengths. All patients were without documented sustained ventricular arrhythmias before the investigation. Sustained ventricular arrhythmias were produced in 2 patients on day 5 and in 9 patients on day 24 after AMI. The types of arrhythmias induced on day 24 were sustained VT with a mean cycle length of 207 ms in 6 cases (1 polymorphic) and VF in 3 cases. These 9 patients did not differ in their clinical characteristics from the remaining 9 patients after AMI in maximal serum creatine kinase, infarct site, number of narrowed coronary arteries, LVEF, or results of 24-hour ambulatory electrocardiographic monitoring. However, they did have a significantly shorter RV effective refractory period (223 ± 10 ms -vs- 259 ± 28 ms). During a follow-up period of 24 ± 5 months, no patient died, had syncopal attacks, or had spontaneous episodes of sustained ventricular arrhythmias. These data indicate that the timing of programmed electrical stimulation after AMI with a maximum of 3 RV extrastimuli strongly influences the inducibility of sustained ventricular arrhythmias. The relatively high inducibility on day 24 after AMI of sustained ventricular arrhythmias with a short cycle length does not appear to correlate with a different clinical course in these patients.

Denniss and co-investigators[83] in Westmead, Australia, compared the relative prognostic significance of VT and VF inducible at programmed stimulation within 1 month of AMI in a prospective study of 403 clinically well survivors of transmural AMI who were ≤65 years of age. The prognostic significance of delayed potentials on the signal-averaged electrocardiogram also was examined in a subset of 306 patients without BBB. Among the study patients, 20% had inducible tachycardia, 14% had inducible VT, and 66% had no inducible arrhythmias. The 2-year probability of remaining free from cardiac death or nonfatal VT or VF was 0.73 for those with inducible VT, 0.93 for those with inducible VF, and 0.92 for those with no inducible arrhythmias (Fig. 3-24). The cycle length of inducible VT was ≥230 ms in 70% of the patients with inducible tachycardia who died. Of the patients studied by signal-averaged electrocardiography, 26% had delayed potentials. At 2 years, the probability of remaining free from cardiac death or nonfatal VT or VF was 0.73 for patients with delayed potentials and 0.95 for patients with no

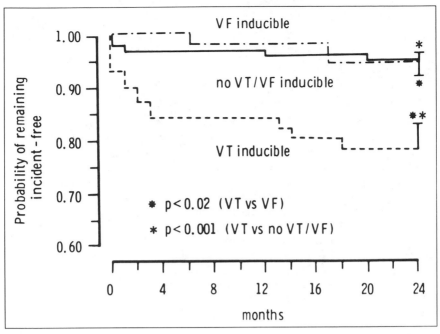

Fig. 3-24. Prediction of instantaneous death and nonfatal ventricular tachycardia or fibrillation (VT or VF) by programmed stimulation. Reproduced with permission from Denniss et al.[83]

delayed potentials. There was a significant correlation between the presence of delayed potentials and the ability to induce VT. Thus, in survivors of recent AMI who have not had spontaneous VT or VF, inducible VT (but not inducible VF) at programmed stimulation predicts a significant risk of death or spontaneous tachycardia or fibrillation. A similar risk was found for patients with delayed potentials on the signal-averaged electrocardiogram.

Brugada et al[84] in Maastricht, The Netherlands, used programmed electrical stimulation of the heart in 160 patients with healed AMI to determine the frequency and characteristics of ventricular arrhythmias that were induced. Thirty-five patients had neither documented nor suspected ventricular arrhythmias (group A); 37 patients had documented nonsustained VT (group B); 31 patients had been resuscitated from VF (group C); and 57 patients had documented sustained monomorphic VT (group D). No electrophysiologic differences were found between patients in groups A and B, but patients in both groups differed significantly from patients in groups C and D. In the last 2 groups, sustained monomorphic VT was more frequently induced, the cycle length of the induced VT was slower, and a lesser number of premature stimuli were required for induction of VT. No differences were found in the incidence or rate or mode of induction of nonsustained VT, but nonsustained VT and VF were more frequently induced in patients in groups A and B. Thus, the substrate for sustained VT is present in ≥40% of patients after AMI. Electrophysiologic characteristics of the substrate for VT appear to be the major determinant of the clinical occurrence of sustained VT. Changes in the electrophysiologic properties of the substrate of VT, either spontaneously with time or induced by ischemia or antiarrhythmic drugs, may contribute to the clinical occurrence of sustained VT in patients with previous AMI.

TREATMENT

Tocainide or lidocaine

Keefe and associates[85] from Bronx, New York, studied 29 patients with AMI in a randomized, double-blind trial of intravenous lidocaine and tocainide, followed by either oral tocainide or placebo without regard to previous therapy, for the prophylaxis of arrhythmias associated with AMI. No patient had symptomatic VT or VF. Tocainide was administered to 16 patients and lidocaine to 13. Seven of the 13 patients receiving lidocaine had VT or accelerated idioventricular rhythm, compared with 2 of 16 receiving tocainide. Adverse effects were noted in 11 of the 13 patients receiving lidocaine and in 6 of the 16 patients receiving tocainide. The infusions used provided therapeutic levels of lidocaine or tocainide and the transition to oral tocainide was accomplished safely with maintenance of therapeutic antiarrhythmic levels. Thus, tocainide appears to be at least as efficacious and may be safer than lidocaine for the prophylaxis of ventricular arrhythmias associated with AMI. The transition to oral tocainide is well tolerated and can be accomplished with minimal difficulty.

Magnesium

Rasmussen and associates[86] from Copenhagen, Denmark, randomized 273 patients with suspected AMI to receive either magnesium intravenously or placebo immediately on admission to hospital. Of 130 patients with proved AMI, 56 received magnesium and 74 received placebo. During the first 4 weeks after treatment, mortality was 7% in the magnesium group and 19% in the placebo group. In the magnesium group, 21% of patients had arrhythmias that needed treatment, compared with 47% in the placebo group. No adverse effects of intravenous magnesium were observed. The findings suggest that the patients with suspected AMI should be treated with intravenous infusion of magnesium immediately after admission to the hospital to counteract postinfarctional hypomagnesemia. The treatment is cheap and easy to administer and appears to be without serious side effects.

Digoxin

Recent studies have led to controversy about whether long-term digoxin therapy after confirmed or suspected AMI increases mortality. Muller and associates[87] from Boston, Massachusetts, analyzed the mortality experience in 903 patients enrolled in the Multicenter Investigation of Limitation of Infarct Size (MILIS). As in previous studies, the decision to treat or not to treat with digoxin was made by the patient's personal physician on the basis of the usual clinical indications. Cumulative mortality was 28% for the 281 digoxin-treated patients compared with 11% for the 622 patients who did not receive digoxin (follow-up interval, 6 days–36 months; mean, 25 months). However, patients treated with digoxin had more baseline characteristics predictive of mortality than did their counterparts. These studies provide no evidence for a significant excess mortality associated with digoxin. Thus, the findings in the MILIS population do not support the assertion that digoxin therapy is excessively hazardous after AMI, but the existence of an undetected harmful effect can only be excluded with a randomized study. Until the results of such a study are available, the authors recommended careful consideration of alternatives to digoxin therapy, and restriction of digoxin use to the subgroup of patients (with severe chronic CHF and a dilated LV) previously shown to have a beneficial clinical response.

Aspirin and/or dipyridamole (or Persantine)

Three thousand, one hundred twenty-eight patients recovering from AMI 1–4 months previously were randomized into 2 groups: dipyridamole (Persantine) and aspirin (n = 1,563) and placebo (n = 1,565) in the Persantine-Aspirin Reinfarction Study, Part II (PARIS II)[88]. The average length of follow-up was 23 months. Primary endpoints were coronary incidence (definite nonfatal AMI and death resulting from recent or acute cardiac event), coronary mortality (death due to recent or acute cardiac event), and total mortality, each at 1 year of patient follow-up and at the end of the study. Patients in the combination treatment group received 1 asantine capsule 3 times a day; each asantine capsule contained 75 mg of dipyridamole and 330 mg of aspirin. The placebo capsules were identical in appearance to asantine capsules, but contained lactose and were given in similar doses. Coronary incidence in the Persantine plus aspirin group was significantly lower than in the placebo group, both at 1 year (30% reduction) and at the end of the study (24% reduction) (Fig. 3-25). The improved prognosis in patients receiving Persantine and aspirin at 1 year and at the end of the study persisted after adjustment for multiple baseline variables and for multiple testing. Coronary mortality was 20% lower in the Persantine plus aspirin group than in the placebo group, and 6% lower overall. The reduced rates of coronary incidence largely reflected lower rates of definite nonfatal AMI in the patients treated with Persantine and aspirin. The beneficial effects of Persantine and aspirin compared with placebo therapy on coronary incidence were greater in the following groups of patients: a) those who had a non-Q-wave infarct; b) those who were not taking digitalis; c) those who were receiving beta-receptor antagonists at baseline; d) those who were in New York Heart Association functional class I; e) those who had only 1 AMI; and f) those who were enrolled in the study early, that is, within 85 days of the qualifying AMI.

Heparin or warfarin

To determine the effect of early anticoagulation on the frequency of LV thrombi complicating anterior wall AMI, Davis and Ireland[89] from Perth, Australia, studied 82 consecutive patients admitted within 12 hours of symptom onset and with electrocardiographic changes consistent with anterior wall AMI, randomly assigning them to 1 or 2 treatment groups. Group I patients received high-dose intravenous heparin to maintain the whole blood clotting time between 15 and 20 minutes, and commenced warfarin therapy within 48 hours. Group 2 patients received low-dose subcutaneous heparin and warfarin therapy if the peak creatine kinase level was >1,000 U/liter. Eighteen group 2 patients received warfarin, but none had a therapeutic prothrombin ratio within 5 days. The presence and morphologic characteristics of thrombus were assessed by serial 2-D echocardiography. Thirty patients were excluded because AMI was not confirmed or because of technically unsatisfactory echocardiograms, death, surgery or, in group 1 patients, inadequate anticoagulation. Thrombi were identified in 29 of 52 patients (56%): in 14 of 25 group 1 patients (56%) and in 15 or 27 group 2 patients (56%). Twenty-three thrombi formed within 3 days. Thrombi were protruding rather than mural only in 3 group 2 patients. The groups did not differ in baseline characteristics or in incidence, time of appearance, or morphologic

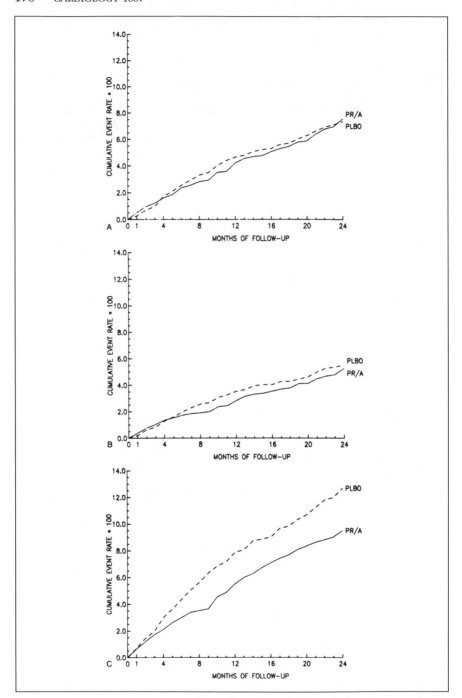

Fig. 3-25. Cumulative events rates, all patients. A, Death, all causes; B, coronary death; C, coronary incidence, PLBO placebo; PR/A Persantine-aspirin group. Reproduced with permission from Klimt et al.[88]

characteristics of thrombus. Systemic embolism occurred only in 1 group 2 patient with mural thrombus. LV thrombus frequently complicates anterior AMI despite early anticoagulation. High-dose heparin may favorably alter thrombus morphologic pattern but prevents its formation no better than low-dose subcutaneous heparin.

Gueret et al [90] in Boulogne Sur Seine, France, evaluated 90 patients admitted within 5.2 ± 4.6 hours after the onset of symptoms suggestive of their first AMI to determine the frequency of LV thrombus after Q-wave AMI using 2-D echocardiography. Patients were randomly assigned either to therapeutic anticoagulation with heparin or to no anticoagulant therapy. Serial 2-D echocardiograms were recorded on the day of admission, the next day, days 4–7, and days 20–50 to detect LV thrombi and to assess LV function. On the first echocardiogram (10 ± 8 hours after the onset of symptoms), no thrombus was visualized. In 44 patients with inferior AMI, including 23 receiving and 21 not receiving heparin, no further LV thrombus developed. In 46 patients with anterior AMI, 21 additional thrombi developed within 4 ± 3 days after AMI. Thrombus developed in 8 of 21 patients receiving heparin compared with 13 of 25 patients not receiving heparin. There was no difference between the subgroups in terms of clinical variables, including estimated infarct size, hemodynamic impairment, and 2-D echocardiographic and cine-angiographic estimates of LV function. Therefore, these data suggest that early anticoagulation with heparin reduced by 27% the frequency of LV thrombus formation in anterior AMI, but this risk reduction was not statistically significant when compared with findings in the untreated group.

Atenolol

Between mid-1981 and January 1, 1985, in the first International Study of Infarct Survival (ISIS-1)[91], 16,027 patients entered 245 coronary care units in 4 European cities (Oxford, Bruxelles, Gent, and Milano) at a mean of 5 hours after the onset of chest pain suggesting AMI. The patients were randomized either to a control group or to a group receiving atenolol (5–10 mg intravenously immediately, followed by 100 mg/day orally for 7 days). Cardiovascular mortality during the treatment period (0–7 days) was significantly lower in the treated group 3.9% -vs- 4.6%, but this 15% difference had wide 95% confidence limits (Fig. 3-26). No subgroups were identified in which the proportional difference in days 0–7 was clearly better or clearly worse than 15%. After the treatment period, there was only a slight further divergence (691 -vs- 703 additional vascular deaths by January 1, 1985). Thus, overall vascular mortality was significantly lower in the atenolol group at 1 year (life-table estimates: 10.7% atenolol -vs- 12.0% control) but not by January 1, 1985 (crude percentages: 12.5% -vs- 13.4%). Atenolol patients were more likely than controls to be discharged on beta blockers, which can account for much of the additional difference in vascular mortality after day 7. Immediate beta blockade increased the extent of inotropic drug use (5.0% -vs- 3.4%), chiefly on days 0–1, but despite this most of the improvement in vascular mortality was seen during days 0–1 (121 -vs- 171 deaths). Treatment did not appear to decrease the number in whom cardiac enzymes increased to above twice the upper limit of normal. Slightly fewer nonfatal cardiac arrests (189 -vs- 198) and reinfarctions (148 -vs- 161) were recorded in the atenolol group. Systematic review of fatal and of nonfatal events in ISIS-1 and in all other randomized trials of intravenous beta blockade reinforces the suggestion that treatment reduces mortality in the first week by about 15%, but

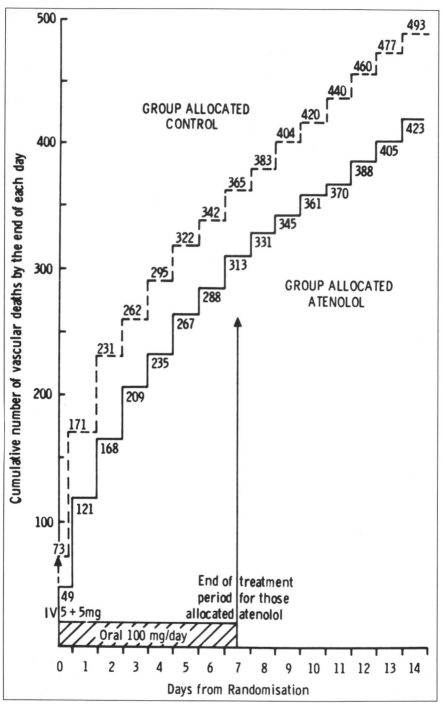

Fig. 3-26. Vascular mortality during scheduled treatment period (days 0-7) and immediately after (to day 14). Reprinted with permission from the First International Study of Infarct Survival Collaborative Group.[91]

with a rather less extreme effect in days 0–1 than was observed in ISIS-1 alone. It also provides highly significant evidence of an effect on the combined endpoint of death, arrest, or reinfarction, suggesting that treatment of about 200 patients would lead to the avoidance of 1 reinfarction, 1 arrest, and 1 death during days 0–7. ISIS-1 suggests these early gains will persist. This article was followed by an editorial entitled Intravenous Beta Blockade During Acute Myocardial Infarction.[92] The anonymous author of this editorial concluded that intravenous administration of a beta blocker to selected patients early during the evolution of AMI is safe and modestly beneficial. The choice of agent—whether cardiac specific or not—is not resolved.

Metoprolol

Murray and associates[93] from Birmingham, UK, studied the effects of metoprolol administered in the early stages of AMI in 126 patients. Patients were treated in a double-blind randomized fashion, with metoprolol (15 mg, intravenously followed by 100 mg twice daily for 15 days, or placebo) with a mean delay of 8 hours from onset of symptoms. All patients underwent 24-hour Holter monitoring on days 1, 5, and 15 after randomization. Although there was no antiarrhythmic effect on day 1, metoprolol reduced the number of hours with warning arrhythmias (>30 VPCs/hour, any R/T ectopics, or VT) on both day 5 (35 ± 16% -vs- 8 ± 11%) and day 15 (13 ± 37% -vs- 4 ± 13%). Metoprolol also reduced the incidence of VF and VT requiring cardioversion (6% -vs- 0). Metoprolol, administered in the early stages of AMI, had an antiarrhythmic effect that was evident only in the later phase of the study.

Olsson and associates[94] from Danderyd, Sweden, compared in a double-blind, randomized study of 154 patients with AMI assigned to metoprolol (100 mg twice daily) and 147 patients assigned to placebo the effects of treatment in relation to health state over 3 years. Health state was evaluated by a new method based on the average number of days spent in each of 7 mutually exclusive categories of health. The scale took into account death, history of serious complications, functional state, and side effects of treatment. Of the maximum attainable 1,095 days alive during the 3 years, patients given metoprolol attained 992 days and those given placebo 964 days. During the period alive the metoprolol-treated group spent an average of 278 days in an optimal functional state compared with 176 days for the placebo-treated group. This included 221 and 156 days, respectively, in a completely asymptomatic state. The time spent with a serious nonfatal complication was shortened by 56 days in the metoprolol group. The overall differences between the groups were statistically significant. Aside from bringing an improved quality of life after AMI, metoprolol may add up to 1 month to life expectancy for 3 years of treatment.

Propranolol

Chadda and co-workers[95] in Hyde Park, New York, studied the frequency of CHF in the Beta Blocker Heart Attack Trial in which post-AMI patients aged 30–69 years with no contraindication to propranolol, were randomly assigned to receive placebo (n = 1,921) or propranolol 180 or 240 mg/day (n = 1,916) 5–21 days after admission to the hospital for the event. Survivors of AMI with compensated or mild CHF, including those on digitalis and diuretics, were included. A history of CHF before randomization characterized 710 (19%) patients; 345 (18%) in the propranolol group and 365 (19%)

in the placebo group. The frequency of definite CHF after randomization and during the study was 7% in both groups. In patients with a history of CHF before randomization, 51 of 345 (15%) in the propranolol group and 46 of 365 (13%) in the placebo group had CHF during an average 25 month follow-up. In the patients with no history of CHF, 5% in both propranolol and placebo groups had CHF. Baseline characteristics predictive of the occurrence of CHF by multivariate analyses included an increased cardiothoracic ratio, diabetes mellitus, increased heart rate, low baseline weight, prior AMI, age, and more than 10 VPCs/hour. Patients with CHF in the propranolol group had a similar decrease in the total mortality (27%) compared with those without CHF (25%), whereas propranolol decreased the occurrence of sudden death by 47% in the patients with prior CHF compared with 13% without CHF (Fig. 3-27).

Croft et al[96] in Dallas, Texas, studied the effect of abrupt beta-blocker withdrawal in patients with AMI. The effects of abrupt withdrawal or continuation of beta-blocker therapy during AMI were evaluated in 326 patients participating in the Multicenter Investigation of the Limitation of Infarct Size (MILIS). Thirty-nine patients previously receiving a beta blocker and randomly selected for withdrawal of beta blockers and placebo treatment during AMI (group 1) were compared with 272 patients previously untreated with beta blockers who were also randomly assigned to placebo therapy

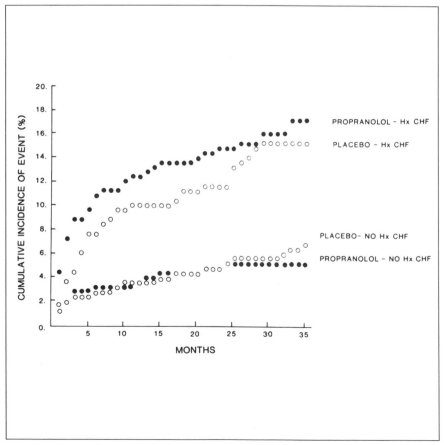

Fig. 3-27. Cumulative incidence of congestive heart failure (CHF) by prior history of congestive heart failure and by treatment group. Reproduced with permission from Chadda et al.[95]

(group 2). There were no significant differences between the 2 groups in creatine kinase-MB estimates of infarct size, radionuclide-determined LVEF within 18 hours of AMI (0.44 ± 0.15 -vs- 0.47 ± 0.16) or 10 days later (0.42 ± 0.14 -vs- 0.47 ± 0.16), creatine kinase-determined incidence of infarct extension (13% -vs- 6%), CHF (43% -vs- 37%), nonfatal VF (5% -vs- 7%), or in-hospital mortality (13% -vs- 9%). The patients in group 1 had more recurrent ischemic chest pain within the first 24 hours after AMI, but not thereafter. The increased frequency of angina post-AMI in patients in whom beta blockers were withdrawn did not appear to be related to a rebound increase in systolic BP, heart rate, or double product. A separate analysis of 20 propranolol-eligible group 1 patients randomly selected for withdrawal of beta blockers (group 3) was performed and these patients were compared with 15 patients randomly selected for continuation of prior beta-blocker therapy (group 4). Careful analyses of clinical variables among these patients demonstrated similar results to those found in the comparisons between group 1 and 2 patients. Thus, these data indicate that beta-blocker withdrawal after AMI may be accomplished safely when necessary without major risk of new AMI, sudden death, or life-threatening arrhythmias.

Timolol

Long-term timolol treatment after AMI is associated with a significant reduction in mortality and nonfatal AMI. To evaluate whether the reduction in mortality and morbidity is exclusively or partly dependent on a reduction in heart rate (HR), Gundersen and associates[97] from Arendal and Oslo, Norway, analyzed cardiac events in the Norwegian Timolol Multicenter Study according to resting HR at baseline and at 1 month of follow-up. Resting HR at baseline was a significant predictor of total death and all events (total death plus nonfatal reinfarction) in both placebo- and timolol-treated patients. In the placebo group and median resting HR was unchanged from baseline to 1 month control (72 beats/minute), but was reduced from 72 beats/minute to 56 beats/minute in the timolol group. Resting HR during follow-up remained a significant predictor of total death. Further, mortality at a given HR during treatment was not markedly different whether the HR was spontaneous or caused by timolol. Timolol treatment was related to a significant reduction in mortality, and this study suggests that the major effect of timolol treatment on mortality after AMI may be attributed to the reduction in HR. Timolol treatment was also associated with an overall reduction in nonfatal reinfarction. However, nonfatal reinfarction was inversely related to resting HR during follow-up, indicating that although coronary artery occlusion in low-risk patients may cause nonfatal reinfarction, the outcome in high-risk patients is more likely to be death. When analyzing mortality and nonfatal reinfarction combined, timolol treatment was related to a reduction in cardiac events at any given HR, suggesting that factors in addition to HR reduction are important in the protective effects of timolol.

Diltiazem

Gibson and associates[98] from multiple medical centers as part of the Diltiazem Reinfarction Study Group performed a multicenter, double-blind, randomized study to evaluate the effect of diltiazem on reinfarction after a *non-Q-wave AMI*. Nine centers enrolled 576 patients: 287 received diltiazem (90 mg every 6 hours) and 289 received placebo. Treatment was initiated 24–72 hours after the onset of AMI and continued for up to 14 days. The primary endpoint, reinfarction, was defined as an abnormal reelevation of

MB-creatine kinase in plasma within 14 days. Reinfarction occurred in 27 patients in the placebo group (9.3%) and in 15 in the diltiazem group (5.2%)—a 51% reduction in cumulative life-table incidence. Diltiazem reduced the frequency of refractory post-AMI angina (a secondary end point) by 50%. Mortality was similar in the 2 groups (3.1 and 3.8%, respectively, in the placebo and diltiazem groups), but adverse drug reactions (most of which were mild) were more common in the diltiazem group. Nevertheless, the drug was well tolerated, despite concurrent treatment with beta blockers in 61% of the patients. The authors concluded that diltiazem was effective in preventing early reinfarction and severe angina after non-Q-wave infarction and that it was also safe and generally well tolerated.

This article was followed by an editorial by Kennedy.[99] Kennedy concluded that diltiazem does appear to be useful in reducing the incidence of reinfarction in patients with initial non-Q-wave AMI, although how it does so has not been defined. Because evidence points to thrombosis as a major event in patients with non-Q-wave AMI, Kennedy recommended anticoagulation followed by early angiography and intracoronary thrombolytic therapy or PTCA as the most attractive therapeutic options for this subset of patients at this time. Supplemental therapy with diltiazem and intravenous nitroglycerin and beta blockers is often indicated, but Kennedy believes that treatment should be directed primarily toward the prevention of progressive coronary artery thrombus and early therapy of severe coronary artery stenosis. He suggested that systemic thrombolytic therapy may be the best initial treatment for patients with non-Q-wave AMI, but because of the hemorrhagic risks associated with the use of thrombolytic agents, Kennedy believed that a control trial of this therapy is needed before the widespread use of systemic thrombolytic therapy for these relatively low-risk patients can be recommended.

Nifedipine

Wilcox and associates[100] from multiple centers in the UK analyzed over a 30-month period, 9,292 consecutive patients admitted to 9 coronary care units with suspected AMI and considered them for admission to a randomized double-blind study comparing the effects on mortality of nifedipine 10 mg 4 times daily with that of placebo. Among the 4,801 patients excluded from the study, the overall 1-month mortality rate was 18%, and the 1-month fatality rate in those with definite AMI 27%. A total of 4,491 patients fulfilled the entry criteria and were randomly allocated to nifedipine or placebo immediately after assessment in the coronary care unit. Roughly 64% of patients in both treatment groups sustained an AMI. The overall 1-month fatality rates were 6.3% in the placebo-treated group and 6.7% in the nifedipine-treated group. Most of the deaths occurred in patients with an in-hospital diagnosis of AMI, and their 1-month fatality rates were 9.3% for the placebo group and 10.2% for the nifedipine group. These differences were not statistically significant. Subgroup analysis also did not suggest any particular group of patients with suspected AMI who might benefit from early nifedipine treatment in the dose studied.

Therapeutic guidelines and exercise

DeBusk and associates[101] from multiple medical centers in the USA developed guidelines for the identification and care of low-risk patients after AMI. The care of patients who are at low risk after AMI is largely concerned with 3 issues: establishing that the prognosis is favorable, i.e., that the probability of subsequent cardiac events is low; quantifying functional capacity as the basis for recommendations regarding physical activity; and reassuring patients about their capacity to resume their customary activities safely, including their occupational work. The same factors that determine prognosis after AMI, namely myocardial ischemia and LV dysfunction, also determine the capacity of patients to resume their customary physical activities with safety and physician's confidence in recommending that their patients do resume such activities. Thus, methods to evaluate prognosis and functional capacity provide a unifying theme for the care of patients who have had an AMI or CABG. The guidelines described by DeBusk and associates represent a consensus on the following related issues: distinguishing high-risk from low-risk patients through the optimal use of diagnostic testing; facilitating the best treatment for the high-risk and low-risk patient subset; and hastening the resumption of customary activities in low-risk patients. The authors also stated that among hospital survivors of AMI, coronary angiography and possible PTCA or CABG are indicated for approximately 30% of patients with rest or exercise-induced severe myocardial ischemia that is manifested by persistent or recurrent ischemic pain at rest $\geq$24 hours after AMI; angina pectoris or ischemic ST-segment depression $\geq$0.2 mV; a reduction of 10 mmHg in systolic BP; a thallium-201 redistribution in multiple myocardial segments; or a decrease in LVEF $\geq$5%, as indicated by RNA or submaximal exercise testing before discharge; and ischemic ST-depression $\geq$0.2 mV at a heart rate <135 beats/minute on symptom-limited treadmill testing at 3 or more weeks after AMI.

To assess functional capacity after AMI, DeBusk and colleagues recommended symptom-limited exercise testing $\geq$3 weeks after an AMI. This test is usually the most strenuous physical effort the patient has undergone since the onset of AMI. Such testing is useful in shaping realistic expectations about the capacity of low-risk patients to resume their customary activities. In general, the well-preserved functional capacity of low-risk patients reflects the absence of severe myocardial ischemia and LV dysfunction. The ability of a patient to carry a high treadmill workload increases the patient's and spouse's confidence in his or her ability to engage in a number of physical activities, including rapid walking, cycling, yard work, and sexual activity. Symptom-limited exercise testing at 21 days or later after AMI is superior to submaximal testing before discharge in determining peak functional capacity and hence the capacity for patients to resume their customary activities. The confidence of patient and spouse will increase even further after a physician has explained the test results and provided specific guidelines for resumption of physical activity, including occupational work.

Previous studies have suggested that exercise training does not improve myocardial blood supply and LV contractile function at the same myocardial oxygen requirement. To determine whether prolonged and intense exercise training can improve LV function in patients with CAD, Ehsani and co-workers[102] from St. Louis, Missouri, studied 25 patients averaging 52 years of age who completed a 12-month program of endurance exercise training and 14 additional patients with comparable maximal exercise capacity and EF who did not exercise. The training program consisted of endurance exercise of progressively increasing intensity, frequency, and duration. During the last 3 months, patients were running an average of 18 miles per week or doing an equivalent amount of exercise on a cycle ergometer. Maximal attainable VO_2 increased 37%. Of the 10 patients with effort angina, 5 became asymptomatic, 3 experienced less angina, and 2 were unchanged after training. EF was determined by equilibrium radionuclide ventriculography. At rest, EF was 53% before and 54% after training. EF did not change during maximal supine exercise before training (52%) but after training it increased to 58%. During maximal exercise, systolic BP and the heart rate–BP product were higher after training. The systolic BP–end-systolic volume relation was shifted upward and to the left, with an increase of maximal systolic BP and a smaller end-systolic volume providing evidence for improvement in contractile state after training. In patients who did not participate in training, neither this relation nor the EF response to exercise was changed after 12 months. These findings that prolonged, intense exercise training can bring about an improvement in LV contractile function independent of cardiac loading conditions in some patients with CAD provide evidence for a reduction in the severity of myocardial ischemia despite an increase in the myocardial O_2 requirement.

Hetherington and associates[103] from Edmonton, Canada, determined in patients who had an AMI 13 ± 0.4 months earlier, using conventional methods, the nature of stroke volume changes during training regimens. Twenty-seven patients (mean age 52 ± 2 years; rest EF 49 ± 2%; New York Heart Association functional class I or II) and 9 normal, age-matched sedentary control subjects (mean age 50 ± 1 years) exercised in the upright position on a bicycle ergometer. Stroke volume was measured by impedance cardiography at rest and after each workload. Ten patients (group A) had a stroke volume response similar to that of the normal sedentary subjects. In 8 patients (group B) the stroke volume increased initially, then decreased (more than 15%) at heart rates >100–105 beats/minute. Nine patients (group C) had a flattened stroke volume response throughout exercise. Training heart rate determined by conventional methods corresponded to a maximal stroke volume in the normal subjects. Training heart rate in group A corresponded to a stroke volume that was maximal or near maximal. Training heart rate in group B corresponded to a maximal or diminishing stroke volume. In group C, the training heart rate corresponded to a stroke volume no different from that at rest. Thus, training heart rate determined by conventional methods based solely on the chronotropic responses to exercise may place patients who have abnormal stroke volume responses to upright exercise in a situation during training sessions in which an inappropriately high heart rate, excessive fatigue, or silent ischemia may develop.

Thrombolysis

Tissue-type plasminogen activator

Jaffe and Sobel[104] from St. Louis, Missouri, reviewed findings pertinent to coronary thrombolysis with conventional activators or tissue-type plasminogen activator (TPA) in the treatment of AMI. These authors concluded that intravenous administration of activator is imminently more practical than is intracoronary administration. It avoids the otherwise required delay associated with preinterventional coronary angiography. Conventionally available activators, including streptokinase and urokinase, entail an unavoidable risk of bleeding as do not clot-selective activators currently undergoing evaluation, such as acyl plasmin and its congeners. Impaired hemostasis accompanying their use may result in unjustified compromise of a patient who may soon require CABG or other invasive procedures. Rarely, it may result in catastrophic bleeding. Activators with relative clot selectivity, such as TPA, are therefore particularly attractive. In therapeutically effective doses, TPA does not include marked depletion of fibrinogen, elevation of fibrinogen degradation products, or persistent hemostatic compromise associated with the systemic lytic state seen with streptokinase or urokinase. Thus, constraints limiting intravenous administration of TPA in patients with suspected, incipient, or early evolving AMI will undoubtedly be less stringent than those applicable to currently available activators. Nevertheless, coronary thrombolysis may not be a panacea. It can benefit the heart only during a brief interval after the onset of coronary occlusion. Recanalization later may gratify the angiographer but confer no benefit on the patient. Early, successful thrombolysis is likely to be only a first step in preserving myocardium subserved by a diseased artery prone to reocclusion or having high-grade residual stenosis with constant persistent or intermittent ischemia. The ultimate capacity of coronary thrombolysis with TPA to prolong life directly or by making possible a series of subsequent steps because of its initial efficacy remains to be defined. These authors concluded in view of these considerations that coronary thrombolysis with conventionally available activators for the fibrinolytic systems has a limited role and that it should not be used routinely for patients with AMI. An attractive strategy may involve implementation of therapy as rapidly as possible with intravenous administration of activator in those patients known to be free from factors compromising hemostasis who are most likely to benefit—namely, those who can be treated within the first 1 or 2 hours after the unequivocal onset of ischemia likely to be caused by an occlusive coronary thrombus in a coronary artery supplying substantial quantities of ventricular myocardium, e.g., patients with anterior wall ischemia. It should be used only in a setting in which prompt delineation of coronary vascular patency can be accomplished after initially successful coronary thrombolysis and in which prompt implementation of PTCA or CABG is feasible, if mandated. Although the rigidity of these constraints may be lessened modestly when TPA becomes available for general use, the principles are unlikely to change. Indiscriminate use of activators of the fibrinolytic system is not likely to be justified presently nor likely to be justifiable in the years to come.

Williams and participants[105] in the NHLBI thrombolysis and myocardial infarction trial investigated the efficacy and safety of a 3-hour, 80-mg intravenous infusion of recombinant TPA in 47 patients with AMI. Coronary angiography, performed before the administration of TPA and for 90 minutes thereafter, demonstrated that 37 patients had total coronary occlusion before therapy. After 90 minutes of TPA (50 mg), reperfusion of the infarct-related artery was observed in 25 patients (68%). Continuous infusions of heparin for anticoagulation were administered for 8–10 days. Of 36 patients who underwent follow-up coronary cineangiography, 21 had initially presented with total occlusion and had had reperfusion at 90 minutes. Sustained perfusion of the infarct-related artery was observed in 14 (67%) of these 21 initially reperfused patients. Late angiography was performed in 9 patients who initially had subtotal occlusion of the infarct-related artery; sustained perfusion was observed in 8. Significant bleeding was observed in 15 patients (32%). A hematoma at the site of the acute catheterization accounted for most instances of significant bleeding (11/15, 73%). Administration of TPA resulted in a significant decline in fibrinogen and plasminogen while amounts of fibrin degradation products increased. In no patient, however, did fibrinogen levels decline to less that 140 mg/dl. If combined with heparin anticoagulation and invasive vascular procedures, significant bleeding is a common complication. Despite anticoagulation with heparin after rt-PA, reocclusion of the reperfused infarct-related artery occurs in one-third of patients.

Gold and associates[106] gave intravenous TPA at a rate of 0.4 to 0.75 mg/kg over 60–120 minutes after angiographic documentation of complete coronary occlusion to 29 patients and reperfusion was accomplished within 1 hour in 24 (83%) and was associated with a decrease of the plasma fibrinogen level by 30%. In a first group of 13 patients, 11 of whom were successfully reperfused, prevention of reocclusion was attempted with heparin anticoagulation. Acute reocclusion within 1 hour after cessation of TPA was demonstrated angiographically in 5 of these patients. Quantitative angiographic analysis indicated that acute reocclusion only occurred in patients with ≥80% residual stenosis. In patients with <80% residual stenosis, heparin anticoagulation was sufficient to maintain patency during the hospital stay in 4 of 5 patients. In a second group of 16 patients, 13 of whom underwent reperfusion with intravenous TPA, 7 had a residual stenosis of ≥80%. These patients were given heparin and, in addition, 10 mg/hour of TPA for 4 hours. In no patient did acute angiographic reocclusion or clinical signs of reocclusion develop during the hospital stay. Repeat angiography at 10–14 days confirmed persistent patency in 6 of the 7 patients. The maintenance infusion resulted in only a moderate additional drop in fibrinogen, while a steady-state plasma TPA level of 750 ng/ml was maintained. In 5 of the 6 patients with <80% residual stenosis maintained on heparin therapy alone, follow-up angiography demonstrated persistent patency. These findings strongly suggest that a maintenance infusion of TPA may prevent or greatly reduce the reocclusion rate in patients with ≥80% residual stenosis after coronary reperfusion with TPA.

Coagulation and fibrinolysis were studied by Collen and co-investigators[107] in Leuven, Belgium, in patients with AMI during intravenous infusion of recombinant human TPA (0.75 mg/kg over 90 minutes) in 101 patients streptokinase (1,500,000 IU over 60 minutes) in 61 patients, or placebo in 40 patients. In the TPA group, the plasma level of TPA antigen was 1.2 μg/ml and the euglobulin fibrinolytic activity (EFA) was 910 IU t-PA/ml. In the streptokinase group, the EFA was equivalent to 430 IU t-PA/ml. At the end of the infusion, the plasma fibrinogen level measured with a coagulation rate assay was decreased to 57% of the preinfusion rate in the TPA group, to 7% in the streptokinase group, and remained unchanged in the placebo group. Fibrinogen-fibrin degradation products increased to 0.75 mg/ml in the streptokinase group but to only 0.10 mg/ml in the TPA group. The plasma levels of a_2-antiplasmin, plasminogen, and factor V decreased to between 30% and 45% in the rt-PA group but significantly more in the streptokinase group (to between 15% and 25%). Thus, TPA induced much less systemic fibrinolytic activation than streptokinase.

Garabedian and associates[108] from Boston, Massachusetts, Leuven, Belgium, and Burlington, Vermont, studied in 45 patients with AMI the pharmacokinetics, thrombolytic profile, and effects on hemostasis of graded intravenous doses of recombinant human TPA. Infusion of TPA at a rate of 4 to 8.3 μg/kg/min resulted in plateau levels of the drug in plasma of 0.52 to 1.4 μg/ml. A linear relation between infusion rate and plasma TPA concentration was observed, although plasma drug levels varied substantially among subjects who received infusions at the same rate. The ratio between plateau levels of TPA in plasma and infusion rate was inversely related to initial distribution volume (7.3 ± 2.9 liters). The initial and terminal half-lives of TPA in the blood were 5 ± 2 and 46 ± 14 minutes, respectively. The efficacy of TPA for coronary thrombolysis was dose-dependent. With 4 μg/kg/min of TPA for 90 minutes, no reperfusion was achieved, whereas infusion rates of ≥5 μg/kg/min for 90 minutes accomplished reperfusion in >80% of the patients. However, the frequency of occurrence of residual intraluminal thrombus was significantly lower with an infusion rate of 7 μg/kg/min for 90 minutes. A dose-related decrease of the plasma fibrinogen level was also observed to a maximum of 53 ± 12% of baseline when measured with a coagulation rate assay and to 76 ± 8% when measured as coagulable protein, at the end of an infusion of 7 μg/kg/min for 90 minutes. At this dose, plasminogen and α_2-antiplasmin levels declined to 57 ± 5% and 20 ± 10% of baseline, respectively. In 9 patients the initial TPA infusion of 5.5 to 7 μg/kg/min for 90 minutes was followed by an intravenous maintenance infusion of 2 μg/kg/min for 4 hours. This treatment resulted in plateau levels of TPA in plasma of 0.43 ± 0.14 μg/ml and was associated with only modest additional fibrinogen breakdown.

Streptokinase

Simoons et al[109] in Rotterdam, The Netherlands, evaluated the influence of thrombolysis in patients with AMI on infarct size, LV function, clinical course, and patient survival in a randomized evaluation comparing thrombolysis with intracoronary streptokinase (269 patients) with conventional therapy (264 patients). These 533 patients were admitted to a coronary care unit within 4 hours after the onset of symptoms suggestive of AMI. Baseline clinical characteristics were similar in patients in both groups. The infarct-related artery was occluded in 169 patients and recanalization was achieved in 133 patients by intracoronary streptokinase. The median time to angiographic documentation of vessel patency was 200 minutes after the onset of symptoms. In the patients admitted within 1 hour after the onset of symptoms, there was a 51% reduction in infarct size with intracoronary streptokinase therapy as evidenced by the measurement of alpha-hydroxybutyric dehydrogenase release over 72 hours. In patients admitted between 1 and 2 hours after the onset of symptoms, the apparent reduction in infarct size was 31%, and in those admitted later than 2 hours, it was only 13%. LV function estimated from RNA before hospital discharge was better after thrombolysis than in control subjects (48 ± 15% -vs- 44 ± 15%). Improvement in LVEF between the treated and control patients was also observed in patients with their first AMIs (50 ± 14% -vs- 46 ± 15%), in patients with anterior infarcts (44 ± 16% -vs- 35 ± 14%), and in those with inferior infarcts (52 ± 12% -vs- 40 ± 12%). Mortality was also reduced by thrombolysis; after 28 days, 16 patients receiving intracoronary streptokinase had died and 31 control patients had died. At 1 year, 91% of patients receiving intracoronary thrombolysis survived, whereas 84% of the control patients survived. However, nonfatal reinfarction occurred more frequently after thrombolysis than in control patients (36 -vs- 16 patients, respectively). These data suggest that early thrombolytic therapy by intracoronary streptokinase may result in a smaller infarct size as estimated by enzyme release, better preservation of LV function, and an improved 1-year survival.

The effects of early intracoronary streptokinase on enzymatic infarct size and rate of enzyme release were studied in a randomized multicenter trial by van der Laarse and associates[110] of the Netherlands Interuniversity Cardiology Institute, Leiden, The Netherlands. A total of 533 patients with AMI were allocated to either the streptokinase treatment group (n = 269) or the conventional (control) treatment group (n = 264). Enzymatic infarct size was represented by the cumulative quantity of alpha-hydroxybutyrate dehydrogenase released by the heart per liter of plasma in the first 72 hours. Rate of enzyme release was represented by the ratio of alpha-hydroxybutyrate dehydrogenase quantities released in 24 and 72 hours. On an intention-to-treat basis, the streptokinase group had a smaller (by 30%) median enzymatic infarct size and a higher (by 35%) median rate of enzyme release than the control group. Limitation of infarct size was less apparent in patients treated with intracoronary streptokinase only (25%) than in patients treated with intravenous plus intracoronary streptokinase (34%). Compared to the control group, the enzyme release rate in patients treated with intracoronary streptokinase only was slightly less (34%) than that in patients treated with intravenous plus intracoronary streptokinase (38%). Patients with a patent infarct-related coronary artery at acute angiography had a median infarct size that was 55% smaller than the median infarct size of the control group, and the median rate of enzyme release was 38% higher than the median release rate of the control group. Patients with successful recanalization during intracoronary streptokinase infusion had a median infarct size that was 31% smaller than the median infarct size of the control group and a median rate of enzyme release that was 42% higher than the median release rate of the control group. Patients with persistent coronary occlusion despite thrombolytic therapy had a median infarct size that was 11% higher than the median infarct size of the control group, although the median rate of enzyme release was still 23% higher than the median release rate of the control group. It was concluded that thrombolysis in the early phase of AMI limits infarct size and that intracoronary streptokinase treatment itself accelerates the process of enzyme release from infarcted myocardium, independent of the angiographic result.

Fine and associates[111] from Jerusalem, Israel, evaluated the importance of timing of intravenous streptokinase administration in 88 patients with AMI. Intravenous streptokinase, 750,000 units, was administered within 4 hours of onset of ischemic chest pain to 72 consecutive patients with their first AMI. Six days later, cardiac catheterization was performed to calculate global EF, and computer-derived infarct-related regional EF and dysfunction index were also determined; electrocardiograms were recorded from which QRS scores could be calculated to estimate infarct size. Of 19 patients who had an anterior AMI, 12 (63%) who received intravenous streptokinase within 2 hours after onset of pain sustained only minimal damage in terms of global EF, infarct-related EF, dysfunction index, and QRS score. All 10 patients who received streptokinase 2–4 hours after pain onset had large infarcts. Of the former group, 11 of 12 patients whose pain was relieved within 1.5 hours of intravenous streptokinase administration (presumably due to successful reperfusion) had a good outcome, whereas all 7 whose pain lasted longer did poorly. Furthermore, among patients with anterior AMI, 11 of 14 (79%) whose pain was relieved within 3.5 hours of onset had small infarcts, compared with none of the 12 patients whose pain lasted longer. In inferior AMI, the critical time between onset of pain and initiation of intravenous SK was 1.5 hours. The timing of initiation of thrombolytic therapy and the total pain duration are critical in determining outcome in AMI, and time intervals vary depending on infarct localization.

Mikell and associates[112] from Springfield, Illinois, determined the frequency of electrocardiographic Q-wave formation and the relation of Q-wave and QRS score to regional and global LV performance in 131 patients with AMI receiving thrombolytic therapy. Thrombolytic therapy was successful in reperfusing the occluded infarct artery in 100 patients and was unsuccessful in 31. The number of patients who had 1 or more Q waves (88% -vs- 87%) and 2 or more Q waves (70% -vs- 74%) was similar. In contrast, normal wall motion was significantly more common in the infarct area in patients in whom reperfusion was successful. Total QRS scores were similar in patients in whom reperfusion was successful and in those in whom it was not (6.0 ± 3.2 -vs- 6.4 ± 4.2). Despite similar QRS scores, successfully treated patients had significantly higher LVEF (53 ± 13% -vs- 46 ± 15%). Thus, Q-wave formation after successful thrombolytic therapy for AMI is common but does not faithfully reflect regional or global LV performance. Electrocardiographic analysis alone is not a reliable method to assess efficacy of reperfusion therapy.

Schofer and colleagues[113] from Hamburg, Germany, performed intracoronary thallium-201/technetium-99m pyrophosphate planar scintigraphy in 60 patients with AMI undergoing intracoronary thrombolysis to predict salvage of myocardium immediately after thrombolysis. In 8 patients, a significant overlap of new thallium uptake and technetium pyrophosphate accumulation was found after thrombolysis. Intravenous planar thallium scintigraphy revealed thallium uptake in the region of overlap in all patients; circumferential profile analysis showed no difference in the thallium scintigrams before and after technetium injections. Both findings indicate that overlap is not the result of scattering of technetium into the thallium window. Emission-computed tomography revealed thallium/technetium pyrophosphate uptake in identical slices and regions. Regional wall motion in the area of overlap remained depressed in all patients, in contrast to patients with similar thallium uptake without overlap. These data suggest that thallium/technetium pyrophosphate overlap reflects the close proximity of viable and necrotic myocardial cells and predicts depressed wall motion after thrombolysis.

"Stunned" myocardium prevents the assessment of myocardial salvage after streptokinase. To unmask "stunning", Satler and associates[114] from Washington, D.C., sought to evaluate LV inotropic contractile reserve of patients after streptokinase. RNA was obtained in 75 consecutive patients 2 weeks after AMI, at rest, and during intravenous isoproterenol infusion. Rest and isoproterenol-stressed EF was compared in the patent and closed-infarct vessel groups. Although there was no difference in rest EF between the patent group (0.48 ± 0.02) and the closed group (0.48 ± 0.02), isoproterenol increased EF in the patent group (increase of 0.14 ± 0.01) significantly more than in the closed group (increase of 0.06 ± 0.01) (Fig. 3-28). Thus, despite identical ventricular function at rest, the greater inotropic contractile reserve in the patent infarct vessel group suggests that restoration of blood flow in AMI salvages myocardium.

Serruys et al[115] in Rotterdam, The Netherlands, evaluated the influence of early myocardial reperfusion within 4 hours after the onset of symptoms on regional LV function in patients with AMI. Thrombolytic therapy consisted of intracoronary streptokinase sometimes preceded by intravenous streptokinase at the time of hospital admission. In addition, patients with severe residual coronary stenoses had immediate PTCA. Five hundred thirty-three patients were randomized either to control conventional therapy or to the reperfusion strategy outlined above. In 332 patients, high-quality angiograms were obtained 2–8 weeks after AMI. Angiographic data were also available after acute reperfusion in patients assigned to thrombolytic therapy. Analyses were based on an "intention to treat" basis and revealed significant preservation of LV function after thrombolytic therapy with LVEF of 53% (mean values) in patients receiving thrombolytic therapy compared with 47% in patients treated conventionally. LV segmental wall motion analysis also showed significant improvement of regional function in the infarct zone in patients with both inferior and anterior AMI. These data suggest that improved regional and global LV function occurs in patients with early reperfusion achieved using a combination of intravenous and intracoronary streptokinase.

Valentine and associates[116] from Indianapolis, Indiana, enrolled 192 consecutive patients with AMI in a prospective trial of coronary thrombolysis in which either intracoronary or intravenous streptokinase was administered. First-pass radionuclide EF was measured early (within 24 hours of admis-

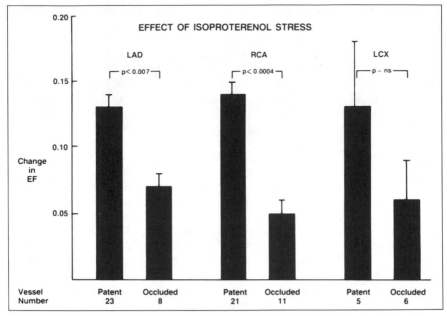

Fig. 3-28. A comparison between the changes in ejection fractions in the patent and occluded infarct vessel groups by infarct vessel. In both the left anterior descending artery and right coronary artery infarct groups, a patent vessel was associated with a greater increase in ejection fraction. The left circumflex artery group did not show this difference, probably due to the small number of patients. *EF* = ejection fraction; *Patent* = patent infarct vessel; *Occluded* = occluded infarct vessel; *LAD* = left anterior descending artery; *RCA* = right coronary artery; *LCX* = left circumflex artery. Reproduced with permission from Satler et al.[114]

sion) and late (10–14 days after admission) to assess changes in LV function. In 68 patients in whom reperfusion was successful, mean EF increased from 39 ± 11% early to 47 ± 13% late. In 36 patients in whom reperfusion was not successful, the mean EF increase was significantly smaller (from 38 ± 10% to 42 ± 11%). Patients in whom reperfusion was successful were then grouped according to extent of LV functional change. The extent of EF change was not significantly influenced by time to lysis at intervals up to 7 hours (EF change = 9.1 ± 10% at 2–3 hours, 8.7 ± 12% at 3–4 hours, 10 ± 10% at 4–5 hours, and 7.0 ± 10% at 5–7 hours; difference not significant), location of the infarct (EF change = 8.9 ± 11% for inferior and 5.7 ± 8.0% for anterior, difference not significant), or presence of Q waves on the initial electrocardiogram (EF change = 8.8 ± 11% in patients with and 7.8 ± 9.9% in patients without Q waves). Only the initial EF was predictive of subsequent EF change. In patients with an initial EF <40%, mean EF increased 13 ± 10%, whereas in patients with an initial ≥EF 40%, mean EF increased 3.8 ± 8.4%.

Res and associates[117] from the Working Group on Thrombolytic Therapy and Acute Myocardial Infarction of the Inner University Cardiology Institute, The Netherlands, studied the effect of reperfusion achieved by early intracoronary streptokinase in AMI on LV function in 533 patients enrolled in a prospective randomized multicenter study. Two hundred and sixty-four patients were allocated to conventional treatment and 269 patients to thrombolysis. At the end of the procedure, patency of the infarct-related artery was achieved in 198 (85%) of 234 patients in whom coronary angiography was performed. The median interval from onset of symptoms until the angiographic documentation of patency was 200 minutes. Data were analyzed according to the original treatment allocation. Global LVEF was determined by RNA in 418 patients within 2 days of admission, in 361 patients after 2 weeks, and in 307 patients after 3 months. Global LV function remained unchanged throughout the observation period in the control group, whereas it improved during the first 2 weeks in patients allocated to thrombolytic treatment. Improved function in these patients persisted up to 3 months after the infarction. Global LVEF was significantly better in the thrombolysis group than in the control group at 2 days, 2 weeks, and at 3 months. In patients with anterior AMI the LVEF was 9% better than in the control group at 2 weeks and at 3 months. In the patients with inferior AMI, differences between the 2 treatment groups were smaller because of photon attenuation within the body. Angiographic evidence suggested that the improvement in function seen after thrombolysis is indeed associated with the patency of the infarct-related artery.

Vermeer and co-workers[118] in Maastricht, The Netherlands, studied the effect of thrombolysis in AMI on enzymatic infarct size, LV function, and early mortality in subsets of patients in a randomized trial. Early thrombolytic therapy with intracoronary streptokinase (152 patients) or with intracoronary streptokinase preceded by intravenous streptokinase (117 patients) was compared with conventional treatment (264 patients). All 533 patients were admitted to the coronary care unit within 4 hours after onset of symptoms indicative of AMI. Four hundred eighty-eight patients were eligible for this detailed analysis, and 245 of these were allocated to thrombolytic therapy and 243 to conventional therapy. Early angiographic examinations were performed in 212 patients allocated to thrombolytic therapy. Patency of the infarct-related artery was achieved in 181 patients (85%). Enzymatic infarct size measured from cumulative alpha-hydroxybutyrate dehydrogenase release was smaller in patients allocated to thrombolytic therapy. LVEF measured by RNA before discharge from the hospital was higher after thrombolytic therapy (50% -vs- 43% in control patients). Three-month mortality was lower in patients allocated to thrombolytic therapy (6% -vs- 14% in the control group). With the use of multivariate regression analysis, infarct size limitation, improvement in LVEF, and 3-month mortality were predicted by sum of the ST-segment elevation, time from onset of symptoms to admission, and Killip class at admission. Thrombolysis was most effective in patients admitted within 2 hours after onset of symptoms and in patients with a sum of ST-segment elevation of ≥ 1.2 mV. No beneficial effects of streptokinase on enzymatic infarct size, LV function, or mortality were observed in the subset of patients with a sum of ST-segment elevation of <1.2 mV who were admitted between 2 and 4 hours after onset of symptoms.

Stadius and colleagues[119] in Seattle, Washington, evaluated the relation between baseline factors defined at 4.6 hours after onset of AMI and 1-year survival in 245 patients entered in the Western Washington Intracoronary Streptokinase Trial. Univariate statistics identified a significant relation between 10 of these factors and survival. Multivariate analysis identified 3 factors as being most closely related to survival: 1) LVEF, 2) treatment with streptokinase, and 3) location of the AMI. Mathematic models based on this analysis and applied to patients in these identified high- and low-risk subgroups for 1-year mortality. Patients receiving standard, not interventional, therapy with anterior AMI and an EF of $\leq 50\%$ and those with inferior AMI and an EF $<40\%$ comprised the high-risk group. For patients receiving standard therapy, 1-year mortality was 41% in the high-risk group and 4% in the low-risk group. Investigators concluded that LVEF determined in the first hours of AMI is the most important of all baseline factors for prediction of

192 • CARDIOLOGY 1987

1-year survival, and mathematic models based on LV function measured as EF are useful for risk stratification in this setting.

In an unblinded trial of intravenous streptokinase in early AMI, the Italian Group for the Study of Streptokinase in Myocardial Infarction (GISSI) chaired by Rovelli[120] enrolled 11,806 patients in 176 coronary care units over 17 months. Patients admitted within 12 hours after onset of symptoms and with no contraindications to streptokinase were randomized to receive streptokinase in addition to usual treatment, and complete data were obtained in 11,712 patients. At 21 days overall hospital mortality was 11% in streptokinase recipients and 13% in controls, an 18% reduction. The extent of the beneficial effect appears to be a function of time from onset of pain to streptokinase infusion (relative risks 0.74, 0.80, 0.87, and 1.19 for the 0–3, 3–6, 6–9, and 9–12 hour subgroups). This article was followed by an unsigned editorial[121]; the author had the following comment: " . . . although the results of the GISSI trial are encouraging it would be inappropriate for streptokinase immediately to become routine treatment for patients with suspected myocardial infarction. The results so far apply only to the initial 21 days after myocardial infarction. A similar benefit shown in the Western Washington Study of intracoronary streptokinase had disappeared when treated and control groups were compared after a year, and, since in the GISSI study there was a higher rate of reinfarction in the streptokinase group, the outlook for treated patients may be less good in the long term. To accept the results of GISSI prematurely would make it both illogical and impracticable to continue with other studies of streptokinase in acute infarction, or with studies of other thrombolytic agents, such as acylated SK-plasminogen complex and tissue plasminogen activator, which have at least theoretical advantages over streptokinase. Although streptokinase is cheaper than the new thrombolytic agents are likely to be, it is still expensive and should not be used wholesale until its effects have been clarified beyond doubt . . . "

The I.S.A.M. Study Group[122] sponsored by the German Federal Ministry for Research and Technology and led by Rolf Schroder and associates, randomly assigned 1,741 patients ≤75 years of age to a 1-hour intravenous infusion of 1.5 million IU of streptokinase or placebo within 6 hours after the onset of symptoms of AMI. At 21 days, mortality was 6.3% in the streptokinase group and 7.1% in the placebo group. Of those treated within 3 hours of the onset of symptoms, 5.2% died in the streptokinase group (n = 477), compared with 6.5% in the placebo group (n = 463). These differences were not significant. The time to peak serum levels of creatine kinase (CK) of myocardial origin after the onset of symptoms was significantly shorter (13.9 -vs- 19.2 hours), and the integrated area under the CK-MB curve (CK-MB infarct size) was significantly smaller, in the streptokinase group. Angiograms obtained in 848 patients 3–4 weeks after AMI revealed that the streptokinase group had higher global EF (57 -vs- 54%) and regional EF (all patients in group; patients with anterior or inferior AMI). The authors concluded that beginning intravenous streptokinase infusion early after the onset of AMI limits the size of the infarct regardless of its location. There was, however, only a trend toward reduced mortality at 21 days. Immediately after randomization, in addition to the 1.5 million IU of streptokinase or placebo, each patient received 5,000 IU of heparin, 0.5 g of acetylsalicylic acid, and 250 mg of methylprednisolone administered intravenously to each patient.

Hartmann and associates[123] from Naperville, Downers Grove, Elmhurst and Maywood, Illinois, studied 58 consecutive patients, ages 37–78 years, who were given intravenous streptokinase early in the course of AMI in 3 community hospitals served by the same mobile intensive care system. Forty-four patients (76%) received intravenous streptokinase within 3 hours and 53 patients (92%) received it within 4 hours of onset of chest pain. Half the patients were brought to the hospital by paramedics. The average time from pain to administration of intravenous streptokinase for paramedic patients was 100 minutes -vs- 198 minutes for those brought by other modes. Fifty of 58 patients (86%) showed clinical evidence of reperfusion. Forty-six of 54 patients (85%) studied with coronary angiography an average of 6 days after infarction had patent vessels subtending the infarcted region of the myocardium. The average angiographic EF was 47% for patients with reperfused vessels -vs- 34% for those with occluded vessels. The in-hospital mortality was 2 of 58 patients (3.4%). There was 1 late death at 8 months (total 5.2%). Twenty-one patients eventually had CABG and 5 patients had PTCA. The remaining 29 patients had conventional therapy including 6 months of warfarin sodium. Fifty-four of 5 surviving patients (98%) are in functional class I or II and none have angina at 2 to 18 months of follow-up. Fifty-one of 55 patients are back at work. It was concluded that 1) intravenous streptokinase is effective in coronary thrombolysis in a high percentage of AMI patients; 2) intravenous streptokinase is safely administered in community hospitals; 3) paramedics act as an early warning system and allow for earlier treatment of patients than do patients presenting without paramedic involvement; and 4) successful coronary reperfusion with intravenous streptokinase results in low mortality rates for AMI patients and minimizes functional disability.

Since there may be considerable observer variability in the conventional estimation of severity of coronary stenosis, Brown and colleagues[124] in Seattle, Washington, believe that the recanalized arterial lumen has structural features that make accurate visual interpretation even more difficult after thrombolytic therapy. These investigators examined thrombolytic recanalization of the obstructed coronary lumen in 32 patients receiving intracoronary streptokinase for 60–90 minutes during AMI. The process was viewed at high arteriographic magnification and was quantified with computer-assisted measurements from repeated single-plane views. The variability of the method for this application was 0.15–1.18 mm on minimum diameter estimates. Structural details were seen that are not commonly appreciated at conventional magnification. The recanalized lumen appears to form along an interface between the thrombus and the vessel wall, progressively enlarging its minimum arteriographic diameter to 1.65 mm at the end of the short-term infusion of streptokinase, reflecting a final percent stenosis of 77%. In 9 infarct lesions found patent 5 weeks later, the recanalized lumen further improved an average of 0.34 mm in minimum diameter and 13% stenosis. A thin film of contrast medium surrounding the obstructing thrombus faintly defined the boundaries of the original atherosclerotic lumen in all but 2 cases. The original stenosis measured 1.25 mm in minimum diameter and 56% stenosis when first visualized; it was unchanged throughout the course of infusion of streptokinase. In 5 patients catheterized 10 weeks after their AMI, the original stenosis averaged 1.15 mm in the preinfarct angiogram, compared with 1.17 mm in its faintly defined form during thrombolytic therapy. In 10 cases, this original lesion was <50% stenosis, and in 21 cases <60%. These measurements permit an objective evaluation of the thrombolytic process; they demonstrate that mild-to-moderate atherosclerotic coronary lesions are subject to acute thrombotic occlusion and that intracoronary streptokinase administered over 60–90 minutes only partially lyses the obstructing thrombus.

Krucoff and associates[125] from Washington, D.C., analyzed continuous ST-segment Holter recordings from 46 patients with AMI receiving intracoronary streptokinase during the first 48 hours of hospitalization. Changes in ST deviation and the time periods of these changes were quantitated and correlated with angiographic evidence of reperfusion. Thirty-six patients had total occlusion of the infarct artery and 10 had subtotal occlusion. Of the 36 arteries that were totally occluded, 19 were reperfused and 17 were not. In patients in whom reperfusion was successful, an ST steady state was achieved 55 ± 32 minutes after streptokinase administration. In patients in whom it was not successful, a steady state was achieved in 219 ± 141 minutes. Achievement of steady state within 100 minutes after streptokinase reperfusion indicated successful reperfusion with 89% sensitivity and 82% specificity. All patients with subtotal occlusion achieved an ST steady state before streptokinase infusion. No patient with total occlusion achieved a steady state before streptokinase. Achievement of ST steady state before streptokinase infusion was 100% sensitive and 100% specific for subtotal occlusion at initial angiography. Continuous, quantitative ST-segment analysis is a sensitive and specific noninvasive technique for following coronary artery patency during AMI.

Buckingham and associates[126] from St. Louis, Missouri, hypothesized that patients having AMI who have reperfusion arrhythmias during intracoronary streptokinase infusion would have different clinical and angiographic characteristics and a larger infarct than those who had achieved reperfusion without reperfusion arrhythmias. Of the 27 patients having successful reperfusion, arrhythmias followed the reperfusion in 8 patients and no arrhythmias occurred in 19 patients. AMI size was calculated using CK-MB isoenzyme time-activity curves using standard methods. The mean CK-MB equivalent for those with reperfusion arrhythmias was 71 ± 25 and for those without reperfusion arrhythmias, 45 ± 24. In patients with reperfusion arrhythmias, EF increased 5 ± 14% before discharge but decreased 10 ± 13% in those with reperfusion arrhythmias. These authors concluded that patients having AMI and reperfusion arrhythmias during intracoronary streptokinase had, for the most part, larger AMI size or a more "stunned myocardium," as indicated by greater CK-MB release and decrease in EF, which is not due to increased time of ischemia.

Accelerated idioventricular rhythm has been used as a marker for coronary reperfusion. Miller and colleagues[127] from Washington, D.C., evaluated the incidence of accelerated idioventricular rhythm (≥3 VPC <100 beats/minute) and VT (≥3 VPC ≥100 beats/minute) in 52 consecutive patients undergoing thrombolysis with intracoronary streptokinase during AMI. Complete 12-hour Holter recordings during and after intracoronary streptokinase were obtained in 39 patients. Reperfusion was documented in 17 patients (44%), no reperfusion in 14 (36%), and subtotal occlusion in 8 (20%). Accelerated idioventricular rhythm occurred in 83%, 57%, and 63% of patients by group, respectively. VT occurred in 100%, 71%, and 100% of patients by group, respectively. These data demonstrate that accelerated idioventricular rhythm is not specific for reperfusion and cannot be used as a marker for this event, and that VT is more common with reperfusion and subtotal occlusion.

AMI, particularly of the inferior wall, is frequently associated with bradycardia and hypotension. Koren and associates[128] from Jerusalem, Israel, reported the occurrence of transient bradycardia hypotension (Bezold-Jarisch reflex) after thrombolytic therapy with intravenous streptokinase. Of the 52 patients, 42 had successful reperfusion, and 12 of the latter had reflex transient bradycardia hypotension. The Bezold-Jarisch reflex occurred in 10 of 24 patients with inferior AMI and in 2 of 28 patients with anterior AMI. The reflex was associated with significantly more with non-Q-wave AMI and also with reduction of LV damage, as evidenced by a lower QRS score (4 ± 3.8 -vs-

8.9 ± 5.6) and a higher EF (61 ± 13% -vs- 49 ± 16%). Patients with inferior AMI were divided into those with transient bradycardia hypotension (10 patients) and those without transient bradycardia hypotension (14 patients). Transient bradycardia hypotension was associated with a significantly higher infarct-related regional EF (60 ± 19% -vs- 35 ± 18%). The results of this study confirm previous findings that reperfusion of the inferoposterior myocardium is capable of stimulating reflex transient bradycardia hypotension. Furthermore, transient bradycardia hypotension is associated with patency of infarct-related coronary arteries and myocardial salvage.

Mentzer and associates[129] from Philadelphia, Pennsylvania, measured the effects in the circulating blood of a 1-hour intravenous infusion of 1.5×10^6 U of streptokinase during the subsequent 24-hour period in 7 patients with AMI. At the end of the infusion, the activator activity, expressed in streptokinase units, averaged 65 U/ml, all of the plasminogen had disappeared, only a small amount of free plasmin was still present and functionally active alpha$_2$ antiplasmin had been reduced to 21% of the preinfusion level. All of the native fibrinogen had been degraded and the thrombin-coagulable protein was composed entirely of fragment X species, but the circulating plasma also contained significant amounts of the more extensively degraded fragments Y, D, and E. The biologic half-life of the streptokinase-induced activator activity was 23 minutes and that of the fibrinogen degradation products was 6.3 hours. The lytic effects persisted for 4 hours before any signs of recovery from the hemostatic defect were evident; considerable recovery was present at 25 hours.

Lew and associates[130] from Los Angeles, California, examined the relation between the level of residual plasma fibrinogen and coronary artery reperfusion after administration of 750,000 IU of intravenous streptokinase in 76 patients with AMI. Both the frequency and rapidity of reperfusion were greater in the 53 patients in whom the residual fibrinogen level was ≤50 mg/dl (low fibrinogen) than in the 23 patients in whom it was >50 mg/dl (high fibrinogen). Reperfusion occurred in all 53 patients in the low-fibrinogen group, compared with only 15 patients in the high-fibrinogen group. The interval from initiation of streptokinase to clinical signs of reperfusion was 50 ± 34 minutes in the low-fibrinogen group and 110 ± 54 minutes in the high-fibrinogen group. A high fibrinogen level occurred in 58% of patients who weighed >85 kg and in 25% of patients who weighed ≤85 kg. No patient who weighed ≤60 kg had a high fibrinogen level. The high-fibrinogen group also had a greater incidence of a high antistreptokinase antibody titer: 8 of 13 patients tested, compared with none of the 8 patients tested in the low-fibrinogen group. The data indicate that a high residual fibrinogen level after administration of intravenous streptokinase identifies patients in whom streptokinase is relatively ineffective, probably because of inadequate dosage or inactivation of the drug. Because 30% of patients in our study had a high residual fibrinogen level after receiving 750,000 IU of streptokinase the data suggest that the dose of intravenous streptokinase in patients (especially obese patients) with AMI should be substantially more than 750,000 IU.

Eisenberg et al[131] from St. Louis, Missouri, evaluated factors responsible for initial success or failure of coronary thrombolysis in the infarct-related artery in 19 patients treated with intravenous streptokinase. The fibrinogen product liberated by thrombin when it is activated, fibrinopeptide A, was measured serially in these 19 patients. Nine patients had recanalization after the administration of streptokinase and decreases in plasma fibrinopeptide A concentration before the administration of heparin. In patients without initially apparent recanalization, fibrinopeptide A increased suggesting ongoing thrombosis, but subsequently decreased promptly after heparin. In patients with initial recanalization followed by reocclusion, fibrinopeptide A increased markedly and remained elevated despite the administration of heparin. These data suggest that inhibition of activation of thrombin is associated with successful recanalization. However, persistent activation of thrombin may be a predisposing factor to initial failure of thrombolytic therapy and leading to early reocclusion of the infarct-related artery.

Sharma and associates[132] from Little Rock, Arkansas, gave intracoronary infusion of prostaglandin E_1 (PGE$_1$) and streptokinase to 14 patients with AMI (duration of chest pain ± 2 hours). Intracoronary PGE$_1$ was followed by intracoronary streptokinase in 10 patients (group A) with successful recanalization in all 10. Of 4 patients in whom recanalization failed with intracoronary streptokinase given first (group B), 2 had successful recanalization after addition of intracoronary PGE$_1$. Immediately after successful recanalization, LVEF increased from 50 ± 9%–62 ± 10%, LV end-diastolic pressure decreased from 20 ± 10–16 ± 10 mmHg and stroke volume index increased from 34 ± 10–44 ± 12 ml/m^2. Infarct-segment shortening improved from 9 ± 5–18 ± 4%. Transient hypotension in 1 patient was the only complication. Follow-up catheterization in recanalized patients at 2–10 days showed maintained improvement in LV global and infarct-segment function. Reocclusion occurred in 1 patient. Thus, intracoronary infusion of PGE$_1$ was effective in establishing reperfusion in all patients when followed by streptokinase and was associated with immediately improved LV global and regional function. PGE$_1$ deserves further evaluation in AMI.

Streptokinase activator complex

Marder and associates[133] from Rochester, New York, assessed the ability of anisoylated plasminogen: streptokinase activator complex (APSAC) to induce coronary artery reperfusion after bolus intravenous injection in 2–4 minutes in 29 patients with transmural AMI and complete coronary artery occlusion. A 5-mg dose resulted in reperfusion in 3 of 14 patients (21%); a 5-mg plus 10-mg regimen was successful in 3 of 7 (43%); and a 30-mg dose induced reperfusion in 9 of 15 (60%). Rethrombosis occurred in only 1 of 15 patients (7%) who received 30 mg, as determined by repeat angiography at 24 hours. The mean interval after injection until reperfusion was 35 minutes with the 30-mg dose, and bleeding occurred at the femoral artery catheterization site in only 3 of 15 patients (20%). Intracoronary streptokinase therapy achieved reperfusion in only 2 of the 6 patients in whom the 30-mg dose failed, indicating that this dose of APSAC was sufficient by itself in 9 of 11 (83%) successfully treated patients. Because therapy can be completed within 2–4 minutes, APSAC appears to be a most suitable fibrinolytic agent for early treatment of the coronary artery thrombosis associated with AMI.

Hyaluronidase

The cooperating institutions of the Multicenter Investigation of the Limitation of Infarct Size (MILIS)[134] conducted a randomized, double-blind, multicenter study of the value of hyaluronidase therapy for AMI. Patients were eligible for enrollment if they were <76 years old, had ≥30 minutes of pain typical of myocardial ischemia and had electrocardiographic changes suggestive of acute ischemia or evolving AMI. A total of 851 patients were randomly assigned to hyaluronidase (500 National Formulary U/kg intravenously every 6 hours for 48 hours) or placebo therapy with a mean of 9.4 ± 0.1 hours after the onset of pain. There were no significant differences between the hyaluronidase- and placebo-treated patients in incidence of AMI

(86 -vs- 88%), creatine kinase-MB infarct size index (14.6 ± 0.8 -vs- 15.1 ± 0.7 CK-MB-gEq/m^2), change in total R wave from time 0 to 72 hours for anterior transmural ischemia or infarction (−34 ± 7 -vs- −35 ± 8 mV), infarct size determined by pyrophosphate scintigrams (27 ± 1 -vs- 27 ± 1 cm^2), change in LVEF from day 0 to day 10 (+2.4 ± 0.7 -vs- +1.2 ± 0.7%) or cumulative proportion surviving 4 years (0.70 ± 0.03 -vs- 0.68 ± 0.03). These findings indicate there is no overall benefit from administration of hyaluronidase >9 hours after the onset of AMI, but do not exclude the possibility that such therapy could be of value if given earlier, or if given to a subgroup of patients with sufficient residual flow to the area of AMI.

PTCA *with or without thrombolysis*

O'Neill and associates[135] from Ann Arbor and Royal Oak, Michigan, randomly assigned 56 patients who presented within 12 hours of their first symptoms of AMI to treatment with either intracoronary streptokinase or PTCA. The mean duration of symptoms (3.0 ± 1.2 hours in the group treated with PTCA -vs- 3.6 ± 1.8 in the group treated with streptokinase) and time to recanalization (4.1 ± 1.4 hours -vs- 4.8 ± 1.7 hours) were similar in both groups. Coronary recanalization was achieved in 83% of those treated with streptokinase. Residual luminal stenosis in the coronary artery was significantly decreased after PTCA, compared with streptokinase therapy (43 ± 31% -vs- 83 ± 17 of patients) (Fig. 3-29). Residual stenosis of ≥70% was present in 4% of the PTCA-treated patients and in 83% of the streptokinase-treated patients. Ventricular function after therapy was assessed by serial contrast ventriculograms. Increases in both global EF (8 ± 7% -vs- 1 ± 6) and regional wall motion (+1.32 ± 1.32 -vs- +0.59 ± 0.79) were greater for the PTCA group (Fig. 3-30). The authors concluded that PTCA and streptokinase produce similar rates of early coronary reperfusion during evolving AMI. However, PTCA is significantly more effective in alleviating the underlying coronary stenoses, and this may result in more effective preservation of ventricular function after therapy.

Prida and associates[136] from Gainesville, Florida, performed PTCA in 29 patients with AMI of the infarct-related coronary artery. Before PTCA, angi-

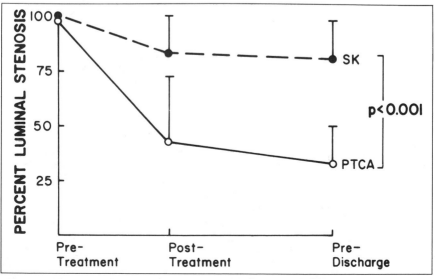

Fig. 3-29. Arteriographic changes in luminal stenosis. Reproduced with permission from O'Neill et al.[135]

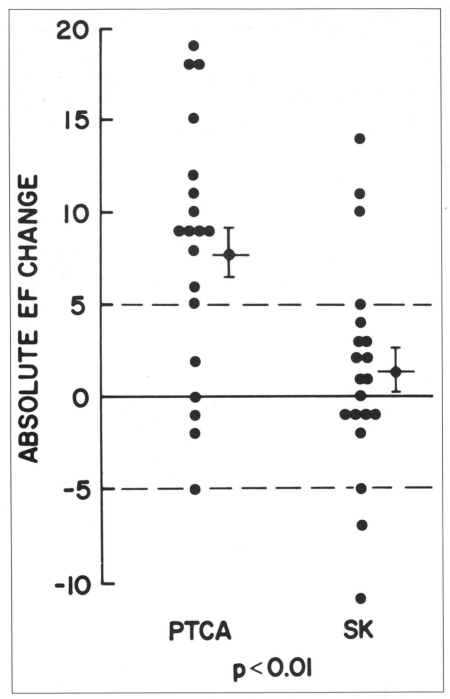

Fig. 3-30. Changes in ejection fraction (EF). Reproduced with permission from O'Neill et al.[135]

ography showed 23 totally occluded and 6 severely stenotic infarct-related coronary arteries. PTCA was initially successful in 15 of 29 patients (86%). Reocclusion occurred in 4 patients within 12 hours after successful PTCA and was associated with new electrocardiographic changes or recurrence of symptoms. In 17 patients the infarct-related coronary artery remained patent at early follow-up; late stenosis occurred in 4 patients. Recurrence of stenosis was accompanied by development of angina. No clinical or angiographic features distinguished those with ultimate vessel patency, occlusion, or recurrence of stenosis. On follow-up, ventricular function appeared better preserved or improved in those with a patent infarct-related coronary artery.

Kitazume and associates[137] from Tokyo, Japan, used combined thrombolytic therapy and PTCA to treat 22 cases of AMI. Initial coronary angiograms showed total obstruction in 13 and severe stenosis in 9. Intracoronary infusion of urokinase reopened 7 of 13 totally occluded lesions but left a residual severe stenosis. PTCA opened all of the remaining totally obstructed lesions and decreased the stenosis in 14 of 16 stenosed lesions. These procedures were performed 0.5–24 hours after the onset of chest pain. Lesions were not successfully dilated in 2 patients. Eighteen of the 20 successfully dilated lesions were patent at repeat angiography performed 1–3 weeks later. One successfully dilated lesion occluded 8 days after the procedure and was redilated by a larger-sized balloon.

Erbel et al[138] in Mainz, West Germany, studied 162 patients with Q-wave AMI in whom continuous intravenous and intracoronary thrombolytic therapy with streptokinase was initiated. In infarct-related arteries that remained occluded, PTCA was performed with a 3Fr recanalization catheter (group I, n = 79) or a 4Fr Grüntzig balloon catheter (group II, n = 83). After reperfusion, intracoronary streptokinase was administered superselectively. After termination of streptokinase infusion, PTCA was performed in 83 patients dilated with a 4Fr Grüntzig balloon. There was no difference between the groups in relation to sex, age, infarct location, serum creatine kinase levels, and time between onset of symptoms and start of treatment. Coronary angiography initially demonstrated an open artery in 27 (34%) of 79 patients in group I and 21 (25%) of 83 patients in group II. The final reperfusion rate was 90% (71 of 79) in group I and 86% (71 of 83) in group II. PTCA was attempted in 69 of the 71 patients in group II with a success rate of 65% and an immediate reocclusion rate of 3%. Coronary reocclusion occurred in 14 (20%) of 71 patients in group I. After thrombolytic therapy, coronary luminal narrowing in group I was 75 ± 17% in patients without and 87 ± 6% in patients with reocclusion. In patients in group II, reocclusion was found in 10 (14%) of 71 patients. After PTCA, the degree of coronary stenosis in group II patients was reduced from 82 ± 12–51 ± 30%. Reocclusion occurred in 3 (7%) of the 45 patients with successful PTCA and in 7 (32%) of the 22 patients with unsuccessful PTCA. Regional LV function improved only in patients in group II with anterior AMI.

Fung and associates[139] from Ann Arbor, Michigan, assessed the effect of sequential high-dose intravenous streptokinase (1.4 million units) followed by emergency PTCA on preserving LV function in 34 patients with AMI. Intravenous streptokinase therapy was initiated 2.6 ± 1.3 hours after the onset of chest pain. Urgent coronary angiography showed persistent total occlusion in 13 patients, significant diameter stenosis (70 to 99%) in 18 patients and a widely patent artery (<50% stenosis) in 3 patients. Emergency PTCA was performed in 29 patients 5.0 ± 2.1 hours after symptom onset. Successful recanalization was achieved in 33 of the 34 patients (97%) treated with sequential therapy. Repeat contrast ventriculograms recorded 7–10 days after intervention in 23 patients showed that the LVEF increased from 53 ± 12%– 59 ± 13% (area-length method). Regional wall motion of the infarcted segments improved from −2.7 ± 1.1 to −1.5 ± 1.7 standard deviation/chord (centerline method). In the subgroup of patients with an occluded artery on initial PTCA (group A), both global LVEF (49 ± 12% -vs- 59 ± 12%) and regional wall motion (−32 ± 1.0 -vs- −1.9 ± 1.7 standard deviation/chord) improved significantly. In contrast, no significant improvement was seen in patients with a patent artery on initial PTCA. Thus, sequential intravenous SK and emergency PTCA is efficacious in achieving coronary reperfusion and in improving both global and regional LV function. When thrombolytic therapy fails, successful recanalization usually can be achieved by emergency PTCA, resulting in significant myocardial salvage.

Fung et al[140] in Ann Arbor, Michigan, compared the efficacy of emergency PTCA and intracoronary streptokinase in preventing exercise-induced peri-infarct ischemia in 28 patients presenting within 12 hours of the onset of symptoms of AMI. Of these, 14 were treated with emergency PTCA and 14 received intracoronary streptokinase. Recatheterization and submaximal exercise thallium-201 single-photon-emission-computed tomography were performed before hospital discharge. Peri-infarct ischemia was defined as a reversible thallium-201 defect adjacent to a fixed defect in the LV. In 86% of patients treated with emergency PTCA, successful reperfusion occurred. Similarly, in 86% of patients treated with intracoronary streptokinase acutely, reperfusion occurred. However, the residual stenosis of the infarct-related coronary artery at predischarge angiography was 44 ± 31% in patients treated with PTCA and 75 ± 16% for the streptokinase-treated group. Among the patients treated with PTCA, 9 had exercise-induced peri-infarct ischemia compared with 60% of the streptokinase-treated group.

CABG

Phillips and associates[141] from Des Moines, Iowa, have had a long experience in the surgical treatment of AMI. They report an analysis of 738 patients who had successful reperfusion in the catheterization laboratory or in the operating room. Factors that predicted wall motion recovery related to the onset of clinical symptoms, time to reperfusion, coronary anatomy, and collateral network. Comparisons were made between patients with stable -vs- those with unstable hemodynamics and between successful or unsuccessful reperfusion. Of the 738 patients, the initial attempt at reperfusion was made in the catheterization laboratory with success in 331. These patients all had primarily 1-vessel CAD. With multiple vessel CAD, 189 patients were immediately treated by surgical reperfusion. This method of surgery was also used for an additional 72 patients in whom reperfusion could not be achieved in the catheterization laboratory. Of the entire group of 738 patients, 146 (20%) could not be reperfused. Overall mortality for the 592 patients reperfused was 5% compared to 17% for those who could not be reperfused. The catheterization reperfusion mortality was 4.2% and the surgical mortality was 5.2% in those reperfused. In 189 patients who were reperfused surgically by first choice, these had a 3.7% (7 patients) mortality. There was a subgroup of 78 patients who were in cardiogenic shock before therapy; 60 of these were successfully reperfused. In 26, reperfusion was achieved with streptokinase and PTCA and there were 6 deaths (23%). Thirty-four patients with multiple-vessel CAD were reperfused surgically with 8 deaths (24%). When reperfusion in the catheterization laboratory failed in 18 of these patients, 9 (50%) died. Time was critical for wall motion recovery if no collaterals were demonstrated on angiography. If collaterals were present, time to reperfusion was not critical. Wall motion recovered in 90% of the patients if the endocardial anatomy of the initial angiogram was smooth. However, if the endocardial anatomy looked mottled and irregular, <10% of patients had recovery of wall motion. Successful reperfusion resulted in significantly lower mortality and morbidity in patients with AMI. In addition, wall motion recovered in most.

From Salt Lake City, Utah, comes a report by Anderson and associates[142] comparing 23 consecutive patients undergoing CABG a median of 5 days, range 1–23, after thrombolytic therapy to a control group of 169 concurrent patients having CABG for standard indications. EF for the control patients was 68 ± 14%, and 61 ± 14% in the streptokinase group. The number of narrowed arteries averaged 2.6 in control and 2.3 in streptokinase patients. Aortic cross-clamp time, cardiopulmonary bypass time were similar, and there were 3.7 ± 1.5 grafts per patient for the controls -vs- 2.8 ± 1.1 for the streptokinase patients. Inotropic support was given postoperatively to 11% of the controls and 13% of the streptokinase patients. Difficult operative hemostasis was noted in 4% of each group. Measured blood loss during the first 48 hours postoperatively was similar (809 ml in the control -vs- 776 ml in the streptokinase group). Blood-product replacement was also comparable (713 ml in the control -vs- 759 ml in the streptokinase group). Postoperative AMI occurred in 2.4% of the controls and in none of the streptokinase patients. There was 1 hospital death among the controls and none among the streptokinase patients. It was concluded that CABG a median of 5 days after administration of streptokinase for AMI may be associated with a similar excellent prognosis as routine bypass procedures. These patients generally had an excellent EF before CABG and, although 57% of the 23 streptokinase patients were said to be emergencies, none were in cardiogenic shock. The report demonstrates that postoperative hemostasis was not a problem.

References

1. SAFFITZ JE, FREDERICKSON RC, ROBERTS WC: Relation of size of transmural acute myocardial infarct to mode of death, interval between infarction and death and frequency of coronary arterial thrombus. Am J Cardiol 1986 (June 1); 57:1249–1254.
2. GOLDBERG RJ, GORE JM, ALPERT JS, DALEN JE: Recent changes in attack and survival rates of acute myocardial infarction (1975 through 1981). JAMA 1986 (May 23); 255:2774–2779.
3. MULLER JE, STONE PH, TURI ZG, RUTHERFORD JD, CZEISLER CA, PARKER C, POOLE WK, PASSAMANI E, ROBERTS R, ROBERTSON T, SOBEL BE, WILLERSON JT, BRAUNWALD E, MILIS STUDY GROUP: Circadian variation in the frequency of onset of acute myocardial infarction. N Engl J Med 1985 (Nov 21); 313:1315–1322.
4. DEWOOD MA, STIFTER WF, SIMPSON CS, SPORES J, EUGSTER GS, JUDGE TP, HINNEN ML: Coronary arteriographic findings soon after non-Q-wave myocardial infarction. N Engl J Med 1986 (Aug 14); 315:417–423.
5. HOIT BD, GILPIN EA, HENNING H, MAISEL AA, DITTRICH H, CARLISLE J, ROSS J: Myocardial infarction in young patients: an analysis by age subsets. Circulation 1986 (Oct); 74:712–721.
6. COOPER RS, SIMMONS B, CASTANER A, PRASAD R, FRANKLIN C, FERLINZ: Survival rates and prehospital delay during myocardial infarction among black persons. Am J Cardiol 1986 (Feb 1); 57:208–211.
7. BLACK HR, QUALLICH H, GARELECK CB: Racial differences in serum creatine kinase levels. Am J Med 1986 (Sept); 81:479–486.
8. HONG RA, LICHT JD, WEI JY, HELLER GV, BLAUSTEIN AS, PASTERNAK RC: Elevated CK-MB with normal total creatine kinase in suspected myocardial infarction: Associated clinical findings and early prognosis. Am Heart J 1986 (June); 111:1041–1047.
9. OGAWA H, HIRAMORI K, HAZE K, SAITO M, SUMIYOSHI T, FUKAMI K, GOTO Y, IKEDA M: Comparison of clinical features of non-Q wave and Q wave myocardial infarction. Am Heart J 1986 (Mar); 111:513–518.
10. HINDMAN N, GRANDE P, HARRELL FE, ANDERSON C, HARRISON D, IDEKER RE, SELVESTER RH, WAGNER GS: Relation between electrocardiographic and enzymatic methods of estimating acute myocardial infarct size. Am J Cardiol 1986 (July 1); 58:31–35.

11. GRANBORG J, GRANDE P, PEDERSEN A: Diagnostic and prognostic implications of transient isolated negative T waves in suspected acute myocardial infarction. Am J Cardiol 1986 (Feb 1); 57:203–207.

12. GIBELIN P, GILLES B, BAUDOUY M, GUARINO L, MORAND P: Reciprocal ST segment changes in acute inferior myocardial infarction: clinical, hemodynamic and angiographic implications. Eur Heart J 1986 (Feb); 7:133–139.

13. LEMBO NJ, STARLING MR, DELLITALIA LJ, CRAWFORD MH, CHAUDHURI TK, O'ROURKE RA: Clinical and prognostic importance of persisten precordial (V_1-V_4) electrocardiographic ST segment depression in patients with inferior transmural myocardial infarction. Circulation 1986 (Jan); 74:56–63.

14. RUDDY TD, YASUDA T, GOLD KH, LEINBACH RC, NEWELL JB, MCKUSICK KA, BOUCHER CA, STRAUSS HW: Anterior ST segment depression in acute inferior myocardial infarction as a marker of greater inferior, apical, and posterolateral damage. Am Heart J 1986 (Dec); 112: 1210–1216.

15. HACKWORTHY RA, VOGEL MB, HARRIS PJ: Relationship between changes in ST segment elevation and patency of the infarct-related coronary artery in acute myocardial infarction. Am Heart J 1986 (Aug); 112:279–284.

16. AMEISEN O, KLIGFIELD P, OKIN PM, MILLER DH, BORER JS: Effects of recent and remote infarction on the predictive accuracy of the ST segment/heart rate slope. J Am Coll Cardiol 1986 (Aug); 8:267–273.

17. LEW AS, LARAMEE P, SHAH PK, MADDAHI J, PETER T, GANZ W: Ratio of ST-segment depression in lead V_2 to ST-segment elevation in lead aVF in evolving inferior acute myocardial infarction: an aid to the early recognition of right ventricular ischemia. Am J Cardiol 1986 (May 1); 57:1047–1051.

18. WARNER RA, HILL NE, MOOKHERJEE S, SMULYAN H: Diagnostic significance for coronary artery disease of abnormal Q waves in the "lateral" electrocardiographic leads. Am J Cardiol 1986 (Sept 1); 58:431–435.

19. JUUL-MOLLER S: Corrected QT-interval during one year follow-up after an acute myocardial infarction. Eur Heart J 1986 (Apr); 7:299–304.

20. KORNREICH F, MONTAGUE TJ, RAUTAHARJU PM, BLOCK P, WARREN JW, HORACEK MB: Identification of best electrocardiographic leads for diagnosing anterior and inferior myocardial infarction by statistical analysis of body surface potential maps. Am J Cardiol 1986 (Nov 1); 58:863–871.

21. NORDREHAUG JE, VON DER LIPPE G: Serum potassium concentrations are inversely related to ventricular, but not to atrial, arrhythmias in acute myocardial infarction. Eur Heart J 1986 (Mar); 7:204–209.

22. JARDINE RM, OBEL IWP, SMITH AM: Intravenous acebutolol raises serum potassium in acute myocardial infarction. Eur Heart J 1986 (Feb); 7:140–145.

23. RASMUSSEN HS, AURUP P, HOJBERG S, JENSEN EK, MCNAIR P: Magnesium and acute myocardial infarction: Transient hypomagnesemia not induced by renal magnesium loss in patients with acute myocardial infarction. Arch Intern Med 1986 (May); 146:872–874.

24. FIGUERAS J, CANDEL J, CINCA J, SEGURA R, ORTEGA D, ANGEL J, RIUS J: Risk of myocardium adjacent to infarcted myocardium: electrocardiographic, metabolic and scintigraphic evidence within the first week of acute myocardial infarction. Am J Cardiol 1986 (May 1); 57:1034–1040.

25. KUMAR A, MINAGOE S, CHANDRARATNA AN: Two-dimensional echocardiographic demonstration of restoration of normal wall motion after acute myocardial infarction. Am J Cardiol 1986 (June 1); 57:1232–1235.

26. JAARSMA W, VISSER CA, EENIGE MJ, RES JCJ, KUPPER AJF, VERHEUGT FWA, ROOS JP: Prognostic implications of regional hyperkinesia and remote asynergy of noninfarcted myocardium. Am J Cardiol 1986 (Sept 1); 58:394–398.

27. JAARSMA W, VISSER CA, KUPPER AJF, RES JCJ, VAN EENIGE MJ, ROOS JP: Usefulness of two-dimensional exercise echocardiography shortly after myocardial infarction. Am J Cardiol 1986 (Jan 1); 57:86–90.

28. ONG L, GREEN S, REISER P, MORRISON J: Early prediction of mortality in patients with acute myocardial infarction: a prospective study of clinical and radionuclide risk factors. Am J Cardiol 1986 (Jan 1); 57:33–38.

29. BUDA AJ, DUBBIN JD, MEINDOK H: Radionuclide assessment of regional left ventricular function in acute myocardial infarction. Am Heart J 1986 (Jan); 111:36–41.

30. GJORUP T, VESTERGAARD B, KELBAEK H, MUNCK O, GODTFREDSEN J: Prospective, randomised,

double-blind study of radionuclide determination of left-ventricular ejection fraction in acute myocardial infarction. Lancet 1986 (Mar 15) I: 583–585.

31. SHAH PK, MADDAHI J, STANILOFF HM, ELLRODT AG, PICHLER M, SWAN HJC, BERMAN DS: Variable spectrum and prognostic implications of left and right ventricular ejection fractions in patients with and without clinical heart failure after acute myocardial infarction. Am J Cardiol 1986 (Sept 1) 58:387–393.

32. TAMAKI N, YASUDA T, LEINBACH RC, GOLD HK, McKUSICK KA, STRAUSS HW: Spontaneous changes in regional wall motion abnormalities in acute myocardial infarction. Am J Cardiol 1986 (Sept 1); 58:406–410.

33. WEISS AT, MADDAHI J, LEW AS, SHAH PK, GANZ W, SWAN HJC, BERMAN DS: Reverse redistribution of thallium-201: A sign of nontransmural myocardial infarction with patency of the infarct-related coronary artery. J Am Coll Cardiol 1986 (Jan); 7:61–67.

34. ABRAHAM RD, FREEDMAN SB, DUNN RF, NEWMAN H, ROUBIN GS, HARRIS PJ, KEELY DT: Prediction of multivessel coronary artery disease and prognosis early after acute myocardial infarction by exercise electrocardiography and thallium-201 myocardial perfusion scanning. Am J Cardiol 1986 (Sept 1); 58:423–427.

35. JOHNSTON DL, THOMPSON RC, LIU P, DINSMORE RE, WISMER GL, SANINI S, KAUL S, ROSEN BR, BRADY TJ, OKADA RD, BEAULIEU PA: Magnetic resonance imaging during acute myocardial infarction. Am J Cardiol 1986 (May 1); 57:1059–1065.

36. FILIPCHUK NG, PESHOCK RM, MALLOY CR, CORBETT JR, REHR RB, BUJA LM, JANSEN DE, REDISH GR, GABLIANI GI, PARKEY RW, WILLERSON JT: Detection and localization of recent myocardial infarction by magnetic resonance imaging. Am J Cardiol 1986 (Aug 1); 58:214–219.

37. BRUNKEN R, TILLISCH J, SCHWAIGER M, CHILD JS, MARSHALL R, MANDELKERN M, PHELPS ME, SCHELBERT HR: Regional perfusion, glucose metabolism, and wall motion in patients with chronic electrocardiographic Q wave infarctions: evidence for persistence of viable tissue in some infarct regions by positron emission tomography. Circulation 1986 (May); 73(5): 951–963.

38. SCHWAIGER M, BRUNKEN R, GROVER-McKAY M, KRIVOKAPICH J, CHILD J, TILLISCH JH, PHELPS ME, SCHELBERT HR: Regional myocardial metabolism in patients with acute myocardial infarction assessed by positron emission tomography. J Am Coll Cardiol 1986 (Oct); 8:800–808.

39. McKAY RG, PFEFFER MA, PASTERNAK RC, MARKIS JE, COME PC, NAKAO S, ALDERMAN JD, FERGUSON JJ, SAFIAN RD, GROSSMAN W: Left ventricular remodeling after myocardial infarction: a corollary to infarct expansion. Circulation 1986 (Oct); 74:693–702.

40. MEHTA N, BENNETT D, MANNERING D, DAWKINS K, WARD DE: Usefulness of noninvasive Doppler measurement of ascending aortic blood velocity and acceleration in detecting impairment of the left ventricular functional response to exercise three weeks after acute myocardial infarction. Am J Cardiol 1986 (Nov 1); 58:879–884.

41. SCLAROVSKY S, SAGIE A, STRASBERG B, LEWIN RF, REHAVIA E, AGMON J: Transient right axis deviation during acute anterior wall infarction or ischemia: electrocardiographic and angiographic correlation. J Am Coll Cardiol 1986 (July); 8:27–31.

42. LAMAS GA, MULLER JE, TURI ZG, STONE PH, RUTHERFORD JD, JAFFE AS, RAABE DS, RUDE RE, MARK DB, CALIFF RM, GOLD HK, ROBERTSON T, PASSAMANI ER, BRAUNWALD E, MILIS STUDY GROUP: A simplified method to predict occurrence of complete heart block during acute myocardial infarction. Am J Cardiol 1986 (June 1); 57:1213–1219.

43. BASSAN R, MAIA IG, BOZZA A, AMINO JGC, SANTOS M: Atrioventricular block in acute inferior wall myocardial infarction: Harbinger of associated obstruction of the left anterior descending coronary artery. J Am Coll Cardiol 1986 (Oct); 8:773–778.

44. BERISSO MZ, FERRONI A, DE CARO E, CARRATINO L, MELA GS, VECCHIO C: Clinical significance of supraventricular tachyarrhythmias after acute myocardial infarction. Eur Heart J 1986 (Sept); 7:743–748.

45. BIGGER JT, FLEISS JL, ROLNITZKY LM, MULTICENTER POST-INFARCTION RESEARCH GROUP: Prevalence, characteristics and significance of ventricular tachycardia detected by 24-hour continuous electrocardiographic recordings in the late hospital phase of acute myocardial infarction. Am J Cardiol 1986 (Dec 1); 58:1151–1160.

46. DUBOIS CH, SMEETS JP, DEMOULIN JC, FOIDART G, HENRARD L, TULIPPE CH, PRESTON L, CARLIER J, KULBERTUS HE: Incidence, clinical significance and prognosis of ventricular fibrillation in the early phase of myocardial infarction. Eur Heart J 1986 (Nov); 7:945–951.

47. GALVE E, GARCIA-DEL-CASTILLO H, EVANGELISTA A, BATLLE J, PERMANYER-MIRALDA G, SOLER-SOLER J: Pericardial effusion in the course of myocardial infarction: incidence, natural history,

and clinical relevance. Circulation 1986 (Feb); 73(2):294–299.

48. PIERARD LA, ALBERT A, HENRARD L, LEMPEREUR P, SPRYNGER M, CARLIER J, KULBERTUS HE. Incidence and significance of pericardial effusion in acute myocardial infarction as determined by two-dimensional echocardiography. J Am Coll Cardiol 1986 (Sept); 8:517–520.

49. GOLDSTEIN JA, SCHILLER NB, LIPTON MJ, PORTS TA, BRUNDAGE BH: Evaluation of left ventricular thrombi by contrast-enhanced computed tomography and two-dimensional echocardiography. Am J Cardiol 1986 (Apr 1); 57:757–760.

50. MELTZER RS, VISSER CA, FUSTER V: Intracardiac thrombi and systemic embolization. Ann Intern Med 1986 (May); 104:689–698.

51. BELLAMY GR, RASMUSSEN HH, NASSER FN, WISEMAN JC, COOPER RA. Value of two-dimensional echocardiography, electrocardiography, and clinical signs in detecting right ventricular infarction. Am Heart J 1986 (Aug); 112:304–309.

52. PIROLO JS, HUTCHINS GM, MOORE W: Infarct expansion: Pathologic analysis of 204 patients with a single myocardial infarct. J Am Coll Cardiol 1986 (Feb); 7:349–354.

53. COHEN DE, VOGEN RA: Left ventricular aneurysm as a coronary risk factor independent of overall left ventricular function. Am Heart J 1986 (Jan); 111:23–30.

54. VISSER CA, KAN G, MELTZER RS, KOOLEN JJ, DUNNING AJ, VAN CORLER M, DE KONING H: Incidence, timing and prognostic value of left ventricular aneurysm formation after myocardial infarction: a prospective, serial echocardiographic study of 158 patients. Am J Cardiol 1986 (Apr 1); 57:729–732.

55. FORMAN MB, COLLINS HW, KOPELMAN HA, VAUGHN WK, PERRY JM, VIRMANI R, FRIESINGER GC: Determinants of left ventricular aneurysm formation after anterior myocardial infarction: a clinical and angiographic study. J Am Coll Cardiol 1986 (Dec); 8:1256–1262.

56. RYAN T, PETROVIC O, ARMSTRONG WF, DILLOW JC, FEIGENBAUM H: Quantitative two-dimensional echocardiographic assessment of patients undergoing left ventricular aneurysmectomy. Am Heart J 1986 (Apr); 111:714–720.

57. FAXON DP, MYERS WO, McCABE CH, DAVIS KB, SCHAFF HV, WILSON JW, RYAN TJ: The influence of surgery on the natural history of angiographically documented left ventricular aneurysm: the Coronary Artery Surgery Study. Circulation 1986 (Jan); 74:110–118.

58. MAISEL AS, GILPIN EA, KLEIN L, LE WINTER M, HENNING H, COLLINS D: The murmur of papillary muscle dysfunction in acute myocardial infarction: clinical features and prognostic implications. Am Heart J 1986 (Oct); 112:705–711.

59. LOPERFIDO F, BIASUCCI LM, PENNESTRI F, LAURENZI F, GIMIGLIANO F, VIGNA C, ROSSI E, FAVUZZI A, SANTARELLI P, MANZOLI U: Pulsed Doppler echocardiographic analysis of mitral regurgitation after myocardial infarction. Am J Cardiol 1986 (Oct 1); 58:692–697.

60. CONNOLLY MW, GELBFISH JS, JACOBOWITZ IJ, ROSE DM, MENDELSOHN A, CAPPABIANCA PM, ACINAPURA AJ, CUNNINGHAM JN: Surgical results for mitral regurgitation from coronary artery disease. J Thorac Cardiovas Surg 1986 (Mar); 91:379–388.

61. NISHIMURA RA, SCHAFF HV, GERSH BJ, HOLMES DR, TAJIK J: Early repair of mechanical complications after acute myocardial infarction. JAMA 1986 (July 4); 256:47–50.

62. MOORE CA, NYGAARD TW, KAISER DL, COOPER AA, GIBSON RS: Postinfarction ventricular spetal rupture: the importance of location of infarction and right ventricular function in determining survival. Circulation 1986 (July); 74:45–55.

63. ROSS EM, ROBERTS WC: Severe atherosclerotic coronary artery disease, healed myocardial infarction and chronic congestive heart failure: analysis of 81 patients studied at necropsy. Am J Cardiol 1986 (Jan 1); 57:44–50.

64. TURI ZG, STONE PH, MULLER JE, PARKER C, RUDE RE, RAABE DE, JAFFE AS, HARTWELL TD, ROBERTSON TL, BRAUNWALD E, MILIS STUDY GROUP: Implications for acute intervention related to time of hospital arrival in acute myocardial infarction. Am J Cardiol 1986 (Aug 1); 58:203–209.

65. HANDS ME, LLOYD BL, ROBINSON JS, DE KLERK N, THOMPSON PL: Prognostic significance of electrocardiographic site of infarction after correction for enzymatic size of infarction. Circulation 1986 (May); 73(5):885–891.

66. WHEELAN K, MUKHARJI J, RUDE RE, POOLE WK, GUSTAFSON N, THOMAS LJ, STRAUSS HW, JAFFE AS, MULLER JE, ROBERTS R, CROFT CH, PASSAMANI ER, WILLERSON JT, MILIS STUDY GROUP: Sudden death and its relation to QT-interval prolongation after acute myocardial infarction: two-year follow-up. Am J Cardiol 1986 (Apr 1); 57:745–750.

67. DWYER EM, GREENBERG H, CASE RB, MULTICENTER POSTINFARCTION RESEARCH GROUP: Association between transient pulmonary congestion during acute myocardial infarction and high

incidence of death in six months. Am J Cardiol 1986 (Nov 1); 58:900–905.

68. SMYLLIE HC: Prognosis of patients discharged from a coronary care unit. Br Med J 1986 (Aug 30); 293:441–542.

69. STARLING MR, CRAWFORD MH, HENRY RL, LEMBO NJ, KENNEDY GT, O'ROURKE RA: Prognostic value of electrocardiographic exercise testing and noninvasive assessment of left ventricular ejection fraction soon after acute myocardial infarction. Am J Cardiol 1986 (Mar 1); 57:532–537.

70. SIA STB, MACDONALD PS, HOROWITZ JD, GOBLE AJ, DOYLE AE: Usefulness of early exercise testing after non-Q-wave myocardial infarction in predicting prognosis. Am J Cardiol 1986 (Apr 1); 57:738–744.

71. STONE PH, TURI ZG, MULLER JE, PARKER C, HARTWELL T, RUTHERFORD JD, JAFFE AS, RAABE DS, PASSAMANI ER, WILLERSON JT, SOBEL BE, ROBERTSON TL, BRAUNWALD E, MILIS STUDY GROUP: Prognostic significance of the treadmill exercise test performance 6 months after myocardial infarction. J Am Coll Cardiol 1986 (Nov); 8:1007–1017.

72. KAN G, VISSER CA, KOOLEN JJ, DUNNING AJ: Short and long term predictive value of admission wall motion score in acute myocardial infarction. A cross sectional echocardiographic study of 345 patients. Br Heart J 1986 (Nov); 556:422–427.

73. SHIINA A, TAJIK AJ, SMITH HC, LENGYEL M, SEWARD JB: Prognostic significance of regional wall motion abnormality in patients with prior myocardial infarction: a prospective correlative study of two-dimensional echocardiography and angiography. Mayo Clin Proc 1986 (Apr); 61:254–262.

74. AHNVE S, GILPIN E, HENNING H, CURTIS G, COLLINS D, ROSS J: Limitations and advantages of the ejection fraction for defining high risk after acute myocardial infarction. Am J Cardiol 1986 (Nov 1); 58:872–878.

75. CASTANER A, BETRIU A, ROIG E, COLL S, DE FLORES T, MAGRINA J, SERRA A, BASSAGANYES J, SANZ G: Clinical course and risk stratification of myocardial infarct survivors with three-vessel disease. Am Heart J 1986 (Dec); 112:1201–1209.

76. NESTICO PF, HAKKI A, FELSHER J, HEO J, ISKANDRIAN AS: Implications of abnormal right ventricular thallium uptake in acute myocardial infarction. Am J Cardiol 1986 (Aug 1) 58: 230–234.

77. FRIEDMAN M, THORESEN CE, GILL JJ, ULMER D, POWELL LH, PRICE VA, BROWN B, THOMPSON L, RABIN DD, BREALL WS, BROUG E, LEVY R, DIXON T: Alteration of type A behavior and its effect on cardiac recurrences in postmyocardial infarction patients: summary results of the recurrent coronary prevention project. Am Heart J 1986 (Oct); 112:653-665.

78. STEVENSON WG, BRUGADA P, KERSSCHOT I, WALDECKER B, ZEHENDER M, GEIBEL A, WELLENS HJJ: Electrophysiologic characteristics of ventricular tachycardia or fibrillation in relation to age of myocardial infarction. Am J Cardiol 1986 (Feb 1); 57:387–391.

79. KIENZLE MG, DOHERTY JU, CASSIDY D, BUXTON AE, MARCHLINSKI FE, WAXMAN HL, JOSEPHSON ME: Electrophysiologic sequelae of chronic myocardial infarction: local refractoriness and electrographic characteristics of the left ventricle. Am J Cardiol 1986 (July 1) 58:63–69.

80. VASSALLO JA, CASSIDY DM, MARCHLINSKY FE, MILLER JM, BUXTON AE, JOSEPHSON ME: Abnormalities of endocardial activation pattern in patients with previous healed myocardial infarction and ventricular tachycardia. Am J Cardiol 1986 (Sept 1); 58:479–484.

81. ROY D, MARCHAND E, THEROUX P, WATERS DD, PELLETIER GB, CARTIER R, BOURASSA MG: Long-term reproducibility and significance of provokable ventricular arrhythmias after myocardial infarction. J Am Coll Cardiol 1986 (July); 8:32–39.

82. KUCK K-H, COSTARD A, SCHLÜTER M, KUNZE K-P: Significance of timing programmed electrical stimulation after acute myocardial infarction. J Am Coll Cardiol 1986 (Dec); 8:1279–1288.

83. DENNISS AR, RICHARDS DA, CODY DV, RUSSELL PA, YOUNG AA, COOPER MJ, ROSS DL, UTHER JB: Prognostic significance of ventricular tachycardia and fibrillation induced at programmed stimulation and delayed potentials detected on the signal-averaged electrocardiograms of survivors of acute myocardial infarction. Circulation 1986 (Oct); 74:731–745.

84. BRUGADA P, WALDECKER B, KERSSCHOT Y, ZEHENDER M, WELLENS HJJ: Ventricular arrhythmias initiated by programmed stimulation in four groups of patients with healed myocardial infarction. J Am Coll Cardiol 1986 (Nov); 8:1035–1040.

85. KEEFE DL, WILLIAMS S, TORRES V, FLOWERS D, SOMBERG JC: Prophylactic tocainide or lidocaine in acute myocardial infarction. Am J Cardiol 1986 (Mar 1); 57:527–531.

86. RASMUSSEN HS, NORREGARD P, LINDENEG O, McNAIR P, BACKER V, BALSLEV S: Intravenous magnesium in acute myocardial infarction. Lancet 1986 (Feb 1); I: 234–235.

87. MULLER JE, TURI ZG, STONE PH, RUDE RE, RAABE DS, JAFFE AS, GOLD HK, GUSTAFSON N, POOLE WK, PASSAMANI E, SMITH TW, BRAUNWALD E, MILIS STUDY GROUP: Digoxin therapy and mortality after myocardial infarction: experience in the MILIS study. N Engl J Med 1986 (Jan 30); 314:265–271.

88. KLIMT CR, KNATTERUD GL, STAMLER J, MEIER P: Persantine-aspirin reinfarction study. Part II. Secondary coronary prevention with Persantine and aspirin. J Am Coll Cardiol 1986 (Feb); 7:251–269.

89. DAVIS MJE, IRELAND MA: Effect of early anticoagulation on the frequency of left ventricular thrombi after anterior wall acute myocardial infarction. Am J Cardiol 1986 (June 1); 57:1244–1247.

90. GUERET P, DUBOURG O, FERRIER A, FARCOT JC, RIGAUD M, BOURDARIAS J-P: Effects of full dose heparin anticoagulation on the development of left ventricular thrombosis in acute transmural myocardial infarction. J Am Coll Cardiol 1986 (Aug); 8:419–426.

91. FIRST INTERNATIONAL STUDY OF INFARCT SURVIVAL COLLABORATIVE GROUP (ISIS-1): Randomized trial of intravenous atenolol among 16,027 cases of suspected acute myocardial infarction: ISIS-1. Lancet 1986 (July 12); II: 57–65.

92. ANONYMOUS: Intravenous B-Blockade during acute myocardial infarction. Lancet 1986 (July 12); II: 79–80.

93. MURRAY DP, MURRAY RG, LITTLER WA: The effects of metoprolol given early in acute myocardial infarction on ventricular arrhythmias. Eur Heart J 1986 (Mar); 7:217–222.

94. OLSSON G, LUBSEN J, VAN ES G, REHNQVIST N: Quality of life after myocardial infarction: effect of long term metoprolol on mortality and morbidity. Br Med J 1986 (June); 292:1491–1493.

95. CHADDA K, GOLDSTEIN S, BYINGTON R, CURB JD: Effect of propranolol after acute myocardial infarction in patients with congestive heart failure. Circulation 1986 (Mar); 73(3):503–510.

96. CROFT CH, RUDE RE, GUSTAFSON N, STONE PH, POOLE WK, ROBERTS R, STRAUSS HW, RAABE DS Jr, THOMAS LJ, JAFFE AS, MULLER J, HOAGLAND P, SOBEL BE, PASSAMANI ER, BRAUNWALD E, WILLERSON JT, MILIS STUDY GROUP: Abrupt withdrawal of beta-blockade therapy in patients with myocardial infarction: effects on infarct size, left ventricular function, and hospital course. Circulation 1986 (June); 73:1281–1290.

97. GUNDERSEN T, GROTTUM P, PEDERSEN T, KJEKSHUS JK: Effect of timolol on mortality and reinfarction after acute myocardial infarction: Prognostic importance of heart rate at rest. Am J Cardiol 1986 (July 1); 58:20–24.

98. GIBSON RS, BODEN WE, THEROUX P, STRAUSS HD, PRATT CM, GHEORGHIADE M, CAPONE RJ, CRAWFORD MH, SCHLANT RC, KLEIGER RE, YOUNG PM, SCHECHTMAN K, PERRYMAN B, ROBERTS R, DILTIAZEM REINFARCTION STUDY GROUP: Diltiazem and reinfarction in patients with non-Q-wave myocardial infarction: results of a double-blind, randomized, multicenter trial. N Engl J Med 1986 (Aug 14); 315:423–429.

99. KENNEDY JW: Non-Q-wave myocardial infarction. N Engl J Med 1986 (Aug 14); 315:451–453.

100. WILCOX RG, HAMPTON JR, BANKS DC, BIRKHEAD JS, BROCKSBY IAB, BURNS-COX CJ, HAYES MJ, JOY MD, MALCOLM AD, MATHER HG, ROWLEY JM: Trial of early nifedipine in acute myocardial infarction: the Trent study. Br Med J 1986 (Nov 8); 293:1204–1208.

101. DEBUSK RF, BLOMQVIST CG, KOUCHOUKOS NT, LUEPKER RV, MILLER HS, MOSS AJ, POLLOCK ML, REEVES TJ, SELVESTER RH, STASON WB, WAGNER GS, WILLMAN VL: Identification and treatment of low-risk patients after acute myocardial infarction and coronary-artery bypass graft surgery. N Engl J Med 1986 (Jan 16); 314:161–166.

102. EHSANI AA, BIELLO DR, SCHULTZ J, SOBEL BE, HOLLOSZY JO: Improvement of left ventricular contractile function by exercise training in patients with coronary artery disease. Circulation 1986 (Feb); 74:350–358.

103. HETHERINGTON M, HAENNEL R, TEO KK, KAPPAGODA T: Importance of considering ventricular function when prescribing exercise after acute myocardial infarction. Am J Cardiol 1986 (Nov 1); 58:891–895.

104. JAFFE AS, SOBEL BE: Thrombolysis with tissue-type plasminogen activator in acute myocardial infarction: potentials and pitfalls. JAMA 1986 (Jan 10); 255:237–239.

105. WILLIAMS DO, BORER J, BRAUNWALD E, CHESEBRO J, COHEN LS, DALEN J, DODGE HT, FRANCIS CK, KNATTERUD G, LUDBROOK P, MARKIS JE, MUELLER H, DESVIGNE-NICKENS P, PASSAMANI ER, POW-

ERS ER, RAO AK, ROBERTS R, ROSS A, RYAN TJ, SOBEL BE, WINNIFORD M, ZARET B: Intravenous recombinant tissue-type plasminogen activator in patients with acute myocardial infarction: a report from the NHLBI thrombolysis in myocardial infarction trial. Circulation 1986 (Feb); 73(2):338–346.

106. GOLD HK, LEINBACK RC, GARABEDIAN HD, YASUDA T, JOHNS JA, GROSSBARD EB, PALACIOS I, COLLEN D: Acute coronary reocclusion after thrombolysis with recombinant human tissue-type plasminogen activator: prevention by a maintenance infusion. Circulation 1986 (Feb); 73(2):347–352.

107. COLLEN D, BOUNAMEAUX H, DE COCK F, LIJNEN HR, VERSTRAETE M: Analysis of coagulation and fibrinolysis during intravenous infusion of recombinant human tissue-type plasminogen activator in patients with acute myocardial infarction. Circulation 1986 (Mar); 73(3): 511–517.

108. GARABEDIAN H, GOLD HK, LEINBACH RC, YASUDA T, JOHNS JA, COLLEN D: Dose-dependent thrombolysis pharmacokinetics and hemostatic effects of recombinant human tissue-type plasminogen activator for coronary thrombosis. Am J Cardiol 1986 (Oct 1); 58:673–679.

109. SIMOONS ML, SERRUYS PW, VAN DEN BRAND M, RES J, VERHEUGT FWA, KRAUSS XH, REMME WJ, BÄR F, DE ZWAAN C, VAN DER LAARSE A, VERMEER F, LUBSEN J: Early thrombolysis in acute myocardial infarction: limitation of infarct size and improved survival. J Am Coll Cardiol 1986 (Apr); 7:717–728.

110. VAN DER LAARSE A, VERMEER F, HERMENS WT, WILLEMS GM, DE NEEF K, SIMOONS ML, SERRUYS PW, RES J, VERHEUGT FWA, KRAUSS XH, BAR F, DE ZWAAN C, LUBSEN J: Effects of early intracoronary streptokinase on infarct size estimated from cumulative enzyme release and on enzyme release rate: a randomized trial of 533 patients with acute myocardial infarction. Am Heart J 1986 (Oct); 112:672–681.

111. FINE DG, WEISS AT, SAPOZNIKOV D, WELBER S, APPLEBAUM D, LOTAN C, HASIN Y, BEN-DAVID Y, KOREN G, GOTSMAN MS: Importance of early initiation of intravenous streptokinase therapy for acute myocardial infarction. Am J Cardiol 1986 (Sept 1) 58:411–417.

112. MIKELL FL, PETROVICH J, SNYDER MC, TAYLOR GJ, MOSES HW, DOVE JT, BATCHELDER JE, SCHNEIDER JA, WELLONS HA: Reliability of Q-wave formation and QRS score in predicting regional and global left ventricular performance in acute myocardial infarction with successful reperfusion. Am J Cardiol 1986 (Apr 15); 57:923–926.

113. SCHOFER J, SPIELMANN RP, BROMEL T, BLEIFELD W, MATHEY DG: Thallium-201/technetium-99m pyrophosphate overlap in patients with acute myocardial infarction after thrombolysis: prediction of depressed wall motion despite thallium uptake. Am Heart J 1986 (Aug) 112:291–295.

114. SATLER LF, KENT KM, FOX LM, GOLDSTEIN HA, GREEN CE, ROGERS WJ, PALLAS RS, DEL NEGRO AA, PEARLE DL, RACKLEY CE: The assessment of contractile reserve after thrombolytic therapy for acute myocardial infarction. Am Heart J 1986 (May); 111:821–825.

115. SERRUYS PW, SIMOONS ML, SURYAPRANATA H, VERMEER F, WIJNS W, VAN DEN BRAND M, BÄR F, ZWAAN C, KRAUSS XH, REMME WJ, RES J, VERHEUGT FWA, VAN DOMBURG R, LUBSEN J, HUGENHOLTZ PG: Preservation of global and regional left ventricular function after early thrombolysis in acute myocardial infarction. J Am Coll Cardiol 1986 (Apr); 7:729–742.

116. VALENTINE RP, PITTS DE, BROOKS-BRUNN JA, WOODS J, NYHUIS A, VAN HOVE E, SCHMIDT PE: Effect of thrombolysis (Streptokinase) on left ventricular function during acute myocardial infarction. Am J Cardiol 1986 (Nov 1); 58:896–899.

117. RES JCJ, SIMOONS ML, VAN DER WALL EE, VAN EENIGE MJ, VERMEER F, VERHEUGT FWA, WIJNS W, BRAAT S, REMME WJ, SERRUYS PW, ROOS JP: Long term improvement in global left ventricular function after early thrombolytic treatment in acute myocardial infarction. Br Heart J 1986 (Nov); 56:414–21.

118. VERMEER F, SIMOONS ML, BAR FW, TIJSSEN JGP, VAN DOMBURG RT, SERRUYS PW, VERHEUGT FWA, RES JCJ, DE ZWAAN C, VAN DER LAARSE A, KRAUSS XH, LUBSEN J, HUGENHOLTZ PG: Which patients benefit most from early thrombolytic therapy with intracoronary streptokinase? Circulation 1986 (Dec); 74:1379–1389.

119. STADIUS ML, DAVIS K, MAYNARD C, RITCHIE JL, KENNEDY JW: Risk stratification for 1 year survival based on characteristics identified in the early hours of acute myocardial infarction: The Western Washington Intracoronary Streptokinase Trial. Circulation 1986 (Oct); 74:703–711.

120. GISSI: Effectiveness of intravenous thrombolytic treatment in acute myocardial infarction. Lancet 1986 (Feb 22); I: 397–401.

121. UNSIGNED: Streptokinase in acute myocardial infarction. Lancet 1986 (Feb 22); 421–422.

122. I.S.A.M. STUDY GROUP: A prospective trial of intravenous streptokinase in acute myocardial infarction (I.S.A.M.): mortality, morbidity, and infarct size at 21 days. N Engl J Med 1986 (June 5); 314:1465–1471.

123. HARTMANN JR, McKEEVER LM, BUFALINO VB, AMIRPARVIZ F, SCANLON PJ: Intravenous streptokinase in acute myocardial infarction: experience of community hospitals served by paramedics. Am Heart J 1986 (June); 111:1030–1034.

124. BROWN BG, GALLERY CA, BADGER RS, KENNEDY JW, MATHEY D, BOLSON EL, DODGE HT: Incomplete lysis of thrombus in the moderate underlying atherosclerotic lesion during intracoronary infusion of streptokinase for acute myocardial infarction: quantitative angiographic observations. Circulation 1986 (Apr); 73(4):653–661.

125. KRUCOFF MW, GREEN CE, SATLER LF, MILLER FC, PALLAS RS, KENT KM, DEL NEGRO AA, PEARLE DL, FLETCHER RD, RACKLEY CE: Noninvasive detection of coronary artery patency using continuous ST-Segment monitoring. Am J Cardiol 1986 (Apr 15); 57:916–922.

126. BUCKINGHAM TA, DEVINE JE, REDD RM, KENNEDY HL: Reperfusion arrhythmias during coronary reperfusion therapy in man: Clinical and angiographic correlations. Chest 1986 (Sept); 90:346–352.

127. MILLER FC, KRUCOFF MW, SATLER LF, GREEN CE, FLETCHER RD, DEL NEGRO AA, PEARLE DL, KENT KM, RACKLEY CE: Ventricular arrhythmias during reperfusion. Am Heart J 1986 (Nov); 112:928–932.

128. KOREN G, WEISS AT, BEN-DAVID Y, HASIN Y, LURIA MH, GOTSMAN MS: Bradycardia and hypotension following reperfusion with streptokinase (Bezold-Jarisch reflex): a sign of coronary thrombolysis and myocardial salvage. Am Heart J 1986 (Sept); 112:468–471.

129. MENTZER RL, BUDZYNSKI AZ, SHERRY S: High-dose, brief-duration intravenous infusion of streptokinase in acute myocardial infarction: description of effects in the circulation. Am J Cardiol 1986 (June 1); 57:1220–1226.

130. LEW AS, CERCEK B, HOD H, SHAH PK, GANZ W: Usefulness of residual plasma fibrinogen after intravenous streptokinase for predicting delay or failure of reperfusion in acute myocardial infarction. Am J Cardiol 1986 (Oct 1); 58:680–685.

131. EISENBERG PR, SHERMAN L, RICH M, SCHWARTZ D, SCHECHTMAN K, GELTMAN EM, SOBEL BE, JAFFE AS: Importance of continued activation of thrombin reflected by fibrinopeptide A to the efficacy of thrombolysis. J Am Coll Cardiol 1986 (June); 7:1255–1262.

132. SHARMA B, WYETH RP, GIMENEZ HJ, FRANCIOSA JA: Intracoronary prostaglandin E$_1$ plus streptokinase in acute myocardial infarction. Am J Cardiol 1986 (Dec 1); 58:1161–1166.

133. MARDER VJ, ROTHBARD RL, FITZPATRICK PG, FRANCIS CW: Rapid lysis of coronary artery thrombi with anisoylated plasminogen: streptokinase activator complex: treatment by Bolus intravenous injection. Ann Intern Med 1986 (Mar); 104:304–310.

134. MILIS STUDY GROUP: Hyaluronidase therapy for acute myocardial infarction: results of a randomized, blinded, multicenter trial. Am J Cardiol 1986 (June 1); 57:1236–1243.

135. O'NEILL W, TIMMIS GC, BOURDILLON PD, LAI P, GANGHADHARHAN V, WALTON J, RAMOS R, LAUFER N, GORDON S, SCHORK A, PITT B: A prospective randomized clinical trial of intracoronary streptokinase versus coronary angioplasty for acute myocardial infarction. N Engl J Med 1986 (Mar 27); 314:312–318.

136. PRIDA XE, HOLLAND JP, FELDMAN RL, HILL JA, MacDONALD RG, CONTI R, PEPINE CJ: Percutaneous transluminal coronary angioplasty in evolving acute myocardial infarction. Am J Cardiol 1986 (May 1); 57:1069–1074.

137. KITAZUME H, IWAMA T, SUZUKI A: Combined thrombolytic therapy and coronary angioplasty for acute myocardial infarction. Am Heart J 1986 (May); 111:826–832.

138. ERBEL R, POP T, HENRICHS K-J, VON OLSHAUSEN K, SCHUSTER CJ, RUPPRECHT H-J, STEUERNAGEL C, MEYER J: Percutaneous transluminal coronary angioplasty after thrombolytic therapy: a prospective controlled randomized trial. J Am Coll Cardiol 1986 (Sept); 8:485–495.

139. FUNG AY, LAI P, TOPOL EJ, BATES ER, BOURDILLON PDV, WALTON JA, MANCINI GBJ, KRYSKI T, PITT B, O'NEILL WW: Value of percutaneous transluminal coronary angioplasty after unsuccessful intravenous streptokinase therapy in acute myocardial infarction. Am J Cardiol 1986 (Oct 1); 58:686–691.

140. FUNG AY, LAI P, JUNI JE, BOURDILLON PDV, WALTON JA JR, LAUFER N, BUDA AJ, PITT B, O'NEILL WW: Prevention of subsequent exercise-induced periinfarct ischemia by emergency coro-

nary angioplasty in acute myocardial infarction: comparison with intracoronary strepto-kinase. J Am Coll Cardiol 1986 (Sept); 8:496–503.

141. Phillips SJ, ZEFF RH, SKINNER JR, TOON RS, GRIGNON A, KONGTAHWORN C: Reperfusion protocol and results in 738 patients with evolving myocardial infarction. Ann Thorac Surg 1986 (Feb); 41:119–125.

142. ANDERSON JL, BATTISTESSA SA, CLAYTON PD, CANNON CY, ASKINS JC, NELSON RM: Coronary by-pass surgery early after thrombolytic therapy for acute myocardial infarction. Ann Thorac Surg 1986 (Feb); 41:176–183.

Arrhythmias, Conduction Disturbances, and Cardiac Arrest

Intracardiac electrophysiologic testing: technique, indications, therapeutic uses—a review

A superb review article discussing the methods of electrophysiologic testing, its uses in diagnosing various cardiac rhythm disturbances and in assessing various therapeutic modalities (Tables 4-1 and 4-2) was presented by Hammill and associates[1] from Rochester, Minnesota.

Wide complex tachycardia

Stewart and associates[2] from Seattle, Washington, assessed the extent and consequence of misdiagnosis of wide complex tachycardia (QRS $\geq$0.12 second; heart rate $\geq$100 beats/minute) presenting emergently: 46 consecutive episodes of wide complex tachycardia were reviewed and their tachycardia mechanisms subsequently established. All 8 episodes of SVT with aberrant conduction were correctly diagnosed, whereas 15 of 38 episodes of VT (39%) were misdiagnosed as SVT at the time initial therapy was given. Ventriculoatrial dissociation was evident in 11 (73%) of the electrocardiograms of misdiagnosed VT. Patients with misdiagnosed episodes had poorer outcomes than those with episodes correctly diagnosed. Verapamil was administered to pa-

TABLE 4-1. *Clinical uses of invasive electrophysiologic testing. Reproduced with permission from Hammill et al.*[1]

PROBLEM	OBJECTIVE OF STUDY
Arrhythmia that cannot be diagnosed from the body surface ECG*	To ascertain the diagnosis, mechanism, prognosis, and appropriate treatment of the arrhythmia
Syncope or near-syncope without apparent neurologic cause	To evaluate sinus node function and atrioventricular conduction; to detect covert atrial or ventricular tachyarrhythmias
Recurrent palpations with normal Holter ECG recording	To search for inducible atrial fibrillation, paroxysmal supraventricular tachycardia, or ventricular tachycardia
Known sinus node dysfunction (sick sinus syndrome)	To ascertain the mechanism and magnitude of dysfunction; to assess the need for pacemaker therapy; to evaluate the efficacy or safety of drug therapy
Atrioventricular conduction defect	To ascertain the site and extent of block, prognosis, and need for pacemaker therapy
Recurrent, sustained supraventricular tachycardia or ventricular tachycardia	To induce the arrhythmia, evaluate its mechanism, and determine effective therapy (medical or surgical)
Survival after cardiac arrest	To ascertain whether inducible ventricular tachycardia or fibrillation is present and to find effective treatment
Wolff-Parkinson-White syndrome	To induce atrial fibrillation or supraventricular tachycardia and ascertain the ventricular rate; to evaluate drug therapy; to ascertain number and location of anomalous atrioventricular connections to guide surgical therapy
Mitral valve prolapse, idiopathic subaortic stenosis, or long QT syndrome, with palpitations or near-syncope	To search for supraventricular tachycardia, anomalous atrioventricular connections, and inducible ventricular tachycardia and to find effective treatment
Asymptomatic, self-limited ventricular tachycardia in patients with coronary artery disease	To search for inducible, sustained ventricular tachycardia and, if present, find effective, safe drug therapy
Uncertain safety of cardioactive drugs (digitalis or antiarrhythmic, tricyclic antidepressant, or antihypertensive drugs) in patients with sinus node or atrioventricular conduction system disease	To search for potential adverse effects on cardiac automaticity and conduction in a controlled environment (acute drug testing for safety)

* ECG = electrocardiogram.

From the Medical Knowledge Self-Assessment Program (MKSAP) VI Syllabus. By permission of the American College of Physicians.

tients in 13 of the 15 episodes of misdiagnosed VT; hemodynamic deterioration occurred in all 13 episodes. Wide complex tachycardia is often incorrectly diagnosed as SVT when, in fact, the 12-lead electrocardiogram strongly suggests VT. Verapamil is often administered in these circumstances and is frequently associated with a poor outcome.

Esophageal electrocardiography

Schnittger and associates[3] from Stanford, California, evaluated the clinical use of an easily swallowed bipolar electrode for recording an esophageal

TABLE 4-2. *Definitions of Electrophysiologic Terms. Reproduced with permission from Hammill et al.*[1]

Antegrade conduction: Conduction that proceeds from the atrium to the ventricle. The conduction can be over the normal atrioventricular conduction system or an accessory atrioventricular pathway

Automatic rhythm: Automatic rhythms can occur throughout the heart and result when cells undergo spontaneous diastolic (phase IV) depolarization and reach the threshold at a rate that is faster than the rate of the normal sinus rhythm

Concealed conduction: The effect of incomplete penetration of an impulse that can result in the following unexpected findings on an electrocardiogram: (1) a spontaneous pacemaker that demonstrates pauses; (2) failure of an impulse to propagate normally, resulting in high-grade block; and (3) prolongation of conduction, resulting in first-degree conduction block

Conduction intervals:

> *HV:* The time from the onset of depolarization of the His bundle to the onset of ventricular activity (usually recorded by an endocardial electrode). The range for the normal HV interval is 35–55 ms
>
> *PP:* The time between two consecutive P waves
>
> *PR:* The time from the onset of the P wave to the onset of the QRS complex
>
> *QT:* The time from the onset of the Q wave to the termination of the T wave
>
> *RP:* The time from the onset of ventricular activity to the onset of atrial activity as manifested by the P wave. This interval is present when there is retrograde conduction from the ventricle to the atrium
>
> *VA:* The time from the onset of ventricular activity to the onset of atrial activity. This measurement is usually obtained by using intracardiac recordings or recordings of atrial activity from the esophagus

Escape complex: Any complex that occurs later than the time of the next expected complex

Mapping: The electrophysiologic procedure used to identify the anatomic location and conduction sequence of supraventricular or ventricular arrhythmias. The procedure is used before or at the time of catheter ablation (fulguration) or surgical procedures to treat tachycardia

Normal atrioventricular conduction system: The atrioventricular node, His bundle, and Purkinje fibers (also referred to as the "specialized conduction system")

Paroxysmal tachycardia: An arrhythmia that is present intermittently and has an abrupt onset and an abrupt termination

Programmed stimulation: The systematic introduction of single or multiple critically timed extrastimuli during a sensed or paced rhythm. Either the atrium or the ventricle is stimulated to stress the sinus node and atrioventricular conduction system or to induce supraventricular or ventricular tachycardia

Reentrant rhythm: Also referred to as a reciprocating rhythm, this rhythm abnormality can occur in multiple locations within the heart. A reentrant circuit consists of two functionally distinct pathways that join proximally and distally to create a closed conduction circuit. A critically timed impulse will encounter this circuit at a time when one of the limbs is refractory to conduction and the other limb is able to maintain conduction (unidirectional block). The conduction proceeds slowly down the unblocked pathway; thus, the previously blocked pathway is granted time to recover its ability to conduct the impulse. As the impulse reaches the distal end of the second pathway, it returns to the proximal common pathway and completes the reentrant circuit. If a single reentrant beat is produced, it is known as a reentrant, echo, or reciprocating beat. If the electrical impulse continues to move around the reentrant circuit, a reentrant tachycardia develops. Reentry may involve a microcircuit that includes a small area within the heart, such as the atrioventricular node or areas of ventricle associated with myocardial infarction, or a macrocircuit that encompasses larger areas of the heart, including the atria, ventricles, or His-Purkinje system

Refractory periods:

> *Effective:* The longest interval between two impulses that fail to be conducted through the tissue
>
> *Functional:* The shortest interval that can be obtained between two consecutively conducted impulses
>
> *Relative:* Prolongation of conduction of a premature impulse marking the end of the full recovery period

Retrograde conduction: Conduction that proceeds from the ventricle to the atrium. The conduction can be over the normal atrioventricular conduction system or an accessory atrioventricular pathway

Supraventricular impulses: Impulses that originate proximal to or within the His bundle

Ventricular impulses: Impulses that originate distal to the His bundle

---

electrocardiogram. Fourteen patients were selected for bedside diagnosis (electrocardiographic group) because of arrhythmias difficult to evaluate using a standard 12-lead electrocardiogram. A second group of 27 nonselected patients scheduled for routine 24-hour ambulatory electrocardiographic recordings (ambulatory electrocardiographic group) had an esophageal electrocardiogram recorded as the "third channel." All 14 patients (100%) in the electrocardiographic group had excellent quality tracings, and the esophageal electrocardiogram was diagnostic in 12 cases (86%). Of 27 patients in the ambulatory electrocardiographic group, 19 (70%) had fairly good to excellent quality 24-hour esophageal pill tracings, with the esophageal electrocardiogram contributing to correct arrhythmia diagnosis in 11 patients (41%). It is concluded that this easily swallowed esophageal electrode provides an excellent quality short-term electrocardiogram and often permits proper arrhythmia diagnosis in selected patients with arrhythmias. Good quality 24-hour esophageal ambulatory electrocardiographic recordings can also be obtained that contribute to arrhythmia diagnosis in a limited number of unselected patients, and should be even more clinically useful in carefully selected patients.

Terminal cardiac electrical activity without apparent structural heart disease

Wang and associates[4] from Taiwan, Republic of China, analyzed terminal electrical events recorded on Holter monitoring in 23 hospitalized adults who died without apparent cardiac disease. Most patients showed a gradual slowing of heart rate with shifting of cardiac pacemaker downward from the sinus node or atria to the AV junction and ventricles, resulting in cardiac asystole. Dominant bradyarrhythmia was more common than ventricular tachyarrhythmia (83% -vs- 17%). Agonal ST-segment elevation was not uncommon (26%). These terminal electrical events became manifest from 1–450 minutes (mean 62) before cessation of cardiac electrical activity. Forty-eight percent of the patients continued to show deteriorating sinus or atrial activity up to the last moment. The mechanism of bradycardiac asystole in patients with no apparent cardiac disease may be attributed to generalized anoxic and toxic depression of the sinus node and subsidiary pacemakers, together with neurogenic suppression of these structures.

ARRHYTHMIAS IN HEALTHY PERSONS

Kantelip and associates[5] from Aurillac, France, recorded 24-hour electrocardiograms in 50 subjects >80 years without cardiovascular disease and with normal standard electrocardiographic responses. During waking and sleeping periods, the mean sinus rates were, respectively, 78 ± 3 and 64 ± 1 beats/minute; heart rate ranged from 43–180 beats/minute over 24 hours. SVT was present in 28% of the subjects. Nocturnal sinus arrhythmia was only noted in 12% of the patients; it was accompanied by sinus pauses of 1.8 to 2 seconds, and 1 woman had a transient pattern compatible with atrioventricular dissociation. Supraventricular ectopic complexes were present in all cases. The frequency was <1 per hour in 25% and >20 per hour in 65%. Serious supraventricular tachycarrhythmias included an episode of ectopic atrial tachycardia (1 subject), a short run of AF (1 subject) and of flutter (1 subject), and several episodes of SVT (2 subjects), all accompanied by >50 ectopic complexes per hour. The number of VPC exceeded 10 per hour in 32%

and were multifocal in 18%. There were couplets in 8% and a run of 6 VPC in 1 subject (2%). In conclusion, sinus pause and AV block are unusual in people >80 years of age without apparent heart disease.

The significance of sinus bradycardia (SB) in clinically healthy, non–endurance-trained, middle-aged and older persons is unknown. From 1,172 normal volunteers, Tresch and Fleg[6] from Baltimore, Maryland, identified SB in 47 subjects aged 58 ± 13 years by rest electrocardiography and compared the group with a group of control subjects matched for age and sex. SB was defined as <50 beats/minute. The prevalence of unexplained SB was approximately 4% and was nearly identical in men and women. At the latest follow-up examination, after a mean follow-up of 5.4 years, the SB group had a higher prevalence of associated conduction abnormalities (first-degree AV block, left-axis deviation, and complete or incomplete right BBB) than the control group (43% -vs- 19%). On maximal treadmill exercise testing, performed in 44 patients within 1 visit of their most recent examination showing SB, maximal heart rate (157 ± 18 beats/minute) did not differ significantly from that of control subjects (163 ± 19 beats/minute); exercise duration, however, was greater in the former group, 11.0 ± 2.8 -vs- 9.7 ± 3.1 minutes. No patients with SB had syncope, high-degree AV block or other manifestation of sick sinus syndrome during follow-up. Angina pectoris, AMI, CHF, or cardiac death occurred in 8% of patients with SB and 11% of control subjects over the observation period. Thus, unexplained SB in apparently healthy, nonathletic subjects >40 years of age is associated with certain abnormalities of AV or intraventricular conduction, but does not signify chronotropic incompetence with exercise and does not appear to adversely influence long-term cardiovascular morbidity or mortality.

ATRIAL FIBRILLATION/FLUTTER

Emboli

Roy and associates[7] from Montreal, Canada, reviewed the medical records of 254 patients with AF to determine the incidence of embolic events in relation to type of cardiovascular disease, duration of AF, and use of anticoagulants. During a total follow-up of 833 patient-years in AF, there were 32 instances of systemic embolism: 21 involved the cerebral circulation and 11 were extracerebral. Thirty of these events occurred during 549 patient-years of follow-up without anticoagulation therapy (5.46 of 100 patient-years), whereas only 2 embolic events occurred during 284 patient-years with anticoagulants (0.7 of 100 patient-years). Thus, the incidence of embolism was 8 times more frequent during the unanticoagulated period of observation in AF. The incidence of embolism during follow-up without anticoagulants was the same regardless of the presence or absence of mitral valve disease and regardless of whether AF was chronic or paroxysmal. The rate of serious hemorrhagic complications with anticoagulants was acceptably low (2.11 of 100 patient-years). It was concluded that in this study population anticoagulant therapy reduced the risk of embolic complications of AF.

Serum magnesium levels

DeCarli and associates[8] from Washington, D.C., in an attempt to study the effect of hypomagnesemia on control of AF determined serum magnesium levels in 45 consecutive patients with symptomatic AF; 20% were hypomagnesemic (serum magnesium level <1.5 mEq/liter). In a blinded treatment protocol, hypomagnesemic patients required twice the amount of intravenous digoxin to effect control of AF. Underlying diagnoses, blood chemistries and the use of other medications that could affect digoxin therapy were similar for the 2 groups. Diuretic therapy before inclusion into the study was not significantly associated with hypomagnesemia. Thus, hypomagnesemia is common among patients with symptomatic AF. Moreover, it appears to interfere with the effect of intravenous digoxin on AF. These results suggest that monitoring of serum magnesium and, where necessary, replacement of magnesium deficiency may be beneficial in patients with symptomatic AF for whom digoxin therapy is being contemplated.

Ambulatory monitoring

Pitcher and associates[9] from Hereford, UK, performed 24-hour ambulatory electrocardiography in 70 patients with chronic AF. None had symptoms suggesting additional arrhythmias, and in all patients the AF was "controlled" in that a change in treatment was not considered necessary. Satisfactory recordings were obtained in 66 patients aged 38–94 years (mean 63): 44 patients had mitral valve disease, including 12 who had MVR, and the remaining patients had various cardiac conditions. Suppressant drugs including digoxin were used in 59 patients, beta blockers in 8, and verapamil in 1. The fastest heart rate occurred during the daytime in all patients and the slowest at night in 63 of the 66 patients. The difference between fastest and slowest rates in individual patients ranged from 35–141 beats/minute (mean 86). Heart rate measured in the clinic correlated poorly with fastest heart rate and slowest heart rate. Only 16 of the 27 patients with ambulatory heart rates >140 beats/minute had heart rates in the clinic >90 beats/minute and in 7 of 23 with rates in the clinic >90 had ambulatory rates that were not >140 beats/minute. Daytime pauses of >2.0 seconds occurred in 16 of the 66 patients. No patient had daytime pauses >2.8 seconds. In the 59 patients taking digoxin, there was no significant relation between serum digoxin concentration and fastest heart rate, slowest heart rate, duration of pauses, or frequency of ventricular arrhythmias. No patient had reported symptoms related to the documented changes in heart rate and arrhythmias.

Diltiazem

Roth and co-investigators[10] in Los Angeles, California, evaluated the efficacy and the safety of medium-dose (240 mg/day) and high-dose (360 mg/day) diltiazem alone and in combination with digoxin when used for control of heart rate in 12 patients with chronic AF. Medium-dose diltiazem was comparable to a therapeutic dose of digoxin at rest (88 -vs- 86 beats/minute) but superior during peak exercise (154 -vs- 170 beats/minute). High-dose diltiazem resulted in better control of heart rate than digoxin both at rest and exercise but was associated with adverse effects in 75% of the patients. Combined therapy of digoxin and diltiazem enhanced the effect of digoxin alone and resulted in significantly better control of heart rate at rest (67 beats/minute with medium-dose and 65 beats/minute with high-dose diltiazem) and during peak exercise (132 and 121 beats/minute, respectively). Reduction of heart rate combined with concomitant effect on BP resulted in a significant decrease in BP–rate product at rest from and during exercise. Continued therapy with digoxin combined with diltiazem, 240 mg/day for 21 days, in 9 patients showed persistent effect on heart rate and BP without any toxic manifestations or change in serum digoxin or plasma diltiazem concentrations. Thus, medium-dose diltiazem when combined with digoxin is an effective and safe regimen for the treatment of patients with chronic AF and enhances digoxin-mediated control of heart rate both at rest and during exercise.

Flecainide -vs- quinidine

Borgeat and associates[11] from Lausanne, Switzerland, compared the effectiveness and safety of flecainide and quinidine for conversion of AF to sinus rhythm. Sixty consecutive patients were treated with either flecainide (up to 2 mg/kg intravenously and then orally) or quinidine (up to 1.2 g orally). There was no statistical difference in age, left atrial size, duration of the arrhythmia, and underlying cardiac diseases between the 2 groups. The overall conversion rate to sinus rhythm was 63% (38 patients): AF was converted in 18 patients (60%) treated with quinidine and 20 (67%) with flecainide. If AF lasted <10 days, the conversion rate was 86% in the flecainide group and 80% in the quinidine group (difference not significant). When AF lasted >10 days the rate was 22% in the flecainide group and 40% in the quinidine group. Adverse effects were more frequent in the quinidine group (27%) (gastrointestinal disturbances) than in the flecainide group (7%) (conduction disturbances), but they were less severe in the quinidine group. Thus, flecainide given intravenously appeared to be as effective as quinidine given orally for conversion of AF of recent onset (within 10 days). However, quinidine should probably remain the preferred drug for conversion of AF of long duration (>10 days) to sinus rhythm. Adverse effects occurred less often with flecainide therapy, but they were more severe.

Amiodarone

AF is a difficult arrhythmia to manage with antiarrhythmic agents. Amiodarone is highly effective in restoring and maintaining normal sinus rhythm in patients with AF. The mechanism and predictors of efficacy of amiodarone in treating AF, however, have not been adequately addressed. Gold and associates[12] from Worcester, Massachusetts, examined various measures of success or failure of amiodarone therapy in 68 patients who had paroxysmal or chronic, established AF refractory to conventional antiarrhythmic agents. The patients were 25–75 years old (mean 59) and mean follow-up was 21 months (range 3 to 56). Maintenance amiodarone dosages were 200–400 mg/day. Overall, amiodarone therapy was effective long term in 54 of the 68 patients (79%). Left atrial diameter, age, gender, and origin of AF were not helpful in predicting success or failure of amiodarone therapy. The presence of chronic AF for >1 year was an adverse factor in maintaining normal sinus rhythm, although the success rate even in this group was relatively high (57%). Thirty-five percent of the patients had adverse effects, which precluded long-term therapy with amiodarone in 10%.

Atrial pacing for conversion

Greenberg and associates[13] from Charlottesville, Virginia, treated 57 episodes of atrial flutter in 46 consecutive medically treated patients (age 60 ± 17 years) by rapid atrial pacing. Thirty-three patients (72%) had structural heart disease. Most pacing trials were conducted in patients receiving digoxin (88%) and antiarrhythmic drugs (77%). In 51 of 57 trials (89%), patients were successfully converted to normal sinus rhythm. Multivariate analysis revealed that patients who had CHF and who were older were more likely to be refractory to pacing. Left atrial size did not influence outcome. Confirmation of local atrial capture with a bipolar atrial electrogram and use of multiple atrial pacing sites enhanced the success rate. Eight patients (17%) demonstrated sinus node suppression after atrial pacing; sinus node disease was previously unsuspected in 4 of these patients. These bradyarrhythmias were easily managed because a pacing catheter was already in place. The only significant complication was femoral vein thrombosis in 1 patient. The authors concluded that atrial pacing is an effective, safe, and convenient method for the elective conversion of atrial flutter in the general population of medically treated patients. This technique is an attractive alternative to transthoracic cardioversion, and may be preferable in many patients.

SUPRAVENTRICULAR TACHYCARDIA WITH OR WITHOUT SHORT PR INTERVAL SYNDROMES

Frequency of symptoms

Milstein and associates[14] from London, Canada, performed electrophysiologic studies in 42 patients with asymptomatic WPW syndrome, mean age 36 years, and thereafter followed them prospectively. They were compared with a matched control group of patients studied within the same period for documented tachycardia associated with the WPW syndrome. Asymptomatic patients had longer anterograde effective refractory periods of the accessory pathway, longer minimum cycle lengths maintaining 1:1 conduction over the accessory pathway, longer minimum RR intervals between consecutive preexcited beats during AF, and longer mean RR intervals during AF than their symptomatic counterparts. Sustained reciprocating tachycardia could not be induced in most patients and induction of AF required rapid atrial pacing in all patients. Nine patients had an anterograde effective refractory period of <270 ms and 17% had minimum cycle length <250 ms during induced AF. Over a follow-up of 29 ± 18 months, 1 patient died of noncardiac causes and the rest remained asymptomatic. Thus, patients with asymptomatic WPW have deficient electrophysiologic substrates to maintain orthodromic reciprocating tachycardia under baseline conditions and do not have atrial vulnerability. Seventeen percent of patients had potentially lethal ventricular rates during induced AF.

Sintetos and associates[15] from Durham, North Carolina, investigated the occurrence of symptomatic paroxysmal SVT in untreated patients and assessed factors that influenced its occurrence in 34 patients with SVT during an observation period in which they received no antiarrhythmic drug therapy for up to 90 days. Recurrence of paroxysmal SVT was documented by telephone transmission of the electrocardiogram. Each patient was allowed to have only 1 episode of SVT before being removed from the study. The authors measured how long patients remained free of their tachycardia (the tachycardia-free period) and heart rate during tachycardia. Twenty-nine of the 34 patients had an attack of symptomatic tachycardia within the 90-day observation period. The proportion of patients who had not had any symptomatic paroxysmal SVT by each day of follow-up was calculated using the Kaplan-Meier method as follows: 75% by day 3, 50% by day 19, 25% by day 36, and 17% by day 90 (Fig. 4-1). Patients with any other heart or lung disease had significantly shorter tachycardia-free periods. The mean heart rate during

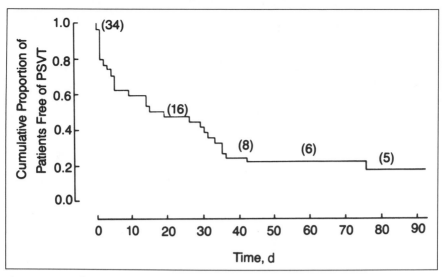

Fig. 4-1.   Cumulative proportion of patients who were still free of paroxysmal supraventricular tachycardia (PSVT) on each day of follow-up. Each step in curve represents day when one or more untreated patients had an attack of tachycardia. Reproduced with permission from Sintetos et al.[15]

spontaneous tachycardia was 204 ± 35 beats/minute (range 142–288 beats/minute). Patients with longer tachycardia-free periods had significantly faster heart rates during tachycardia.

Initiating atrial fibrillation

Paroxysmal SVT and AF are both supraventricular arrhythmias, but their mechanisms are different. Roark and associates[16] from Durham, North Carolina, determined the incidence of symptomatic AF in 39 patients followed closely during routine outpatient care for paroxysmal SVT. The 39 patients with paroxysmal SVT were followed for up to 4 years using telephone transmission of the electrocardiogram to document symptomatic arrhythmias. The cumulative proportion of patients who had AF was calculated using the Kaplan-Meier life-table method. The cumulative proportion of patients who had AF during follow-up was 13% at 3 months, 16% at 6 months, 22% at 1 year, and 29% at 2 years (Fig. 4-2). In most patients the start of AF was documented during an attack of paroxysmal SVT rather than de novo as another primary arrhythmia. Paroxysmal SVT occurred significantly earlier during an observation period without treatment in patients in whom AF developed. The occurrence of AF was not related to age, number of years of paroxysmal SVT, heart rate during tachycardia, or coexistent heart disease.

Inducing cardiomyopathy

Packer and associates[17] from Durham, North Carolina, evaluated 8 patients aged 5–57 years with uncontrolled symptomatic tachycardia for 2.5–41 years (mean 15) and significant LV dysfunction in the absence of other apparent underlying cardiac disease. Incessant tachycardia was present for 0.5–6.0 years (mean 2.1) in 7 patients. One patient had an ectopic atrial tachycardia and 7 patients had an accessory AV pathway that participated in

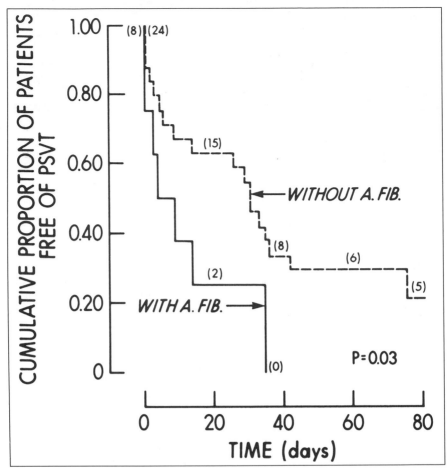

Fig. 4-2. Occurrence of paroxysmal supraventricular tachycardia (PSVT) during an untreated observation period in patients with and without atrial fibrillation (A.FIB.). Eight patients who had atrial fibrillation during follow-up had paroxysmal supraventricular tachycardia significantly earlier than 24 patients who did not have atrial fibrillation (p = 0.03).

reciprocating tachycardia. Six patients underwent surgery; the ectopic focus was ablated in 1 patient and an accessory pathway was divided in 5 patients. One patient underwent open ablation of the His bundle and 1 patient underwent closed-chest ablation of the AV conduction system. Myocardial biopsy specimens were obtained from 5 patients, none of which yielded a specific diagnosis. Pretreatment RNA demonstrated a mean EF of 19 ± 9% (range 10–35%). After tachycardia control a marked improvement in LV function was noted in 6 of 8 patients at rest and in 1 additional patient during exercise. The EF increased to 33 ± 17% (range 16–56%) an average of 8 days after treatment and to 45 ± 15% (range 22–67%) at late follow-up 3.5 ± 40 months (mean 17) later. Seven patients remain asymptomatic 11–40 months (mean 22) after the corrective procedure and have resumed normal activities. These findings suggest that chronic uncontrolled tachycardia may result in significant LV dysfunction, which is reversible in some cases after control of the arrhythmia.

Atrial natriuretic factor

A significant diuretic and natriuretic response occurs during paroxysmal SVT. Although the diuresis may be secondary to suppression of vasopressin secretion, the cause of the natriuresis remains unexplained. Nicklas and colleagues[18] from Ann Arbor, Michigan, determined if atrial natriuretic factor (ANF) could contribute to the polyuric response during SVT. Ten patients were studied: 5 during spontaneous SVT and 5 during simulated SVT produced by rapid simultaneous atrial and ventricular pacing. Plasma immunoreactive ANF levels measured by radioimmunoassay were obtained at baseline (before and/or 24–48 hours after SVT) and after ≥15 minutes of SVT in all patients. During spontaneous and simulated SVT, immunoreactive ANF was significantly elevated (275 ± 68 pmol/liter) compared to baseline (28 ± 7 pmol/liter). Similar increases in immunoreactive ANF were noted during both simulated and spontaneous SVT. To determine if this immunoreactive ANF release was related to the increase in heart rate or the increase in RA pressure during SVT, immunoreactive ANF levels were also measured in 5 patients with sinus tachycardia and in 6 patients with CHF. Immunoreactive ANF was significantly related to RA pressure but not to heart rate. Thus, immunoreactive ANF is elevated during SVT and may contribute to the natriuretic response. The stimulus to immunoreactive ANF secretion during SVT appears to be related to the increase in RA pressure rather than to the increase in heart rate.

Flecainide

Kim and associates[19] from St. Louis, Missouri, studied the electrophysiologic effects and therapeutic efficacy of intravenous and oral flecainide in 15 patients with spontaneous and inducible sustained paroxysmal SVT. Twelve patients had AV reentrance using an accessory pathway for retrograde conduction and 3 had AV nodal reentrance. Fourteen patients received intravenous flecainide (2 mg/kg body weight over 15 minutes) during an initial electrophysiologic study. Nine patients were restudied during oral flecainide administration (200–400 mg/day). After intravenous or oral flecainide therapy, reentrant SVT was noninducible in 6 patients with AV reentrance and in the 3 with AV nodal reentrance. In these 9 patients, intravenous flecainide prevented induction of reentrant SVT by depressing conduction over the retrograde limb of the reentry circuits. In the 6 patients with inducible sustained AV reentrant SVT before and after flecainide therapy, the cycle length of tachycardia increased significantly, mainly as the result of an increase in ventriculoatrial conduction time. There was concordance between the intravenous and the oral effects of flecainide on the mechanism of the SVT. Twelve patients continued oral flecainide treatment for a mean of 16 months (range 5–28). Tachycardia recurred in 3 of 4 patients whose arrhythmia remained inducible after flecainide therapy and in 1 of 8 patients whose SVT was suppressed. It is concluded that flecainide is an effective and convenient antiarrhythmic agent to treat patients who have AV nodal or AV reentrant SVT.

Propafenone

To assess the antiarrhythmic efficacy of intravenous propafenone, Shen and associates[20] from San Francisco, California, treated 20 patients with inducible sustained SVT with 2 mg/kg body weight, or placebo in a double-blind, randomized, crossover study. Three patients had intraatrial reentrant tachycardia, 3 had AV nodal reentrant tachycardia, and 14 had AV-reciprocating tachycardia associated with the WPW syndrome. Termination of SVT occurred in 15 of the 20 patients receiving propafenone but 0 of the 11 patients receiving placebo. Propafenone prolonged refractoriness and slowed conduction of the atrium, the AV node, and accessory AV bypass tracts, and these effects provided antiarrhythmic action to halt tachycardia. No adverse effects were observed in any patient. The authors concluded that intravenous propafenone is safe and effective in the acute treatment of various forms of reentrant SVT.

Esmolol

Efficacy and safety of esmolol in the treatment of SVT was evaluated in this open-label, baseline-controlled, multicenter study conducted by the Esmolol Research Group under the direction of Gray and associates[21] from Los Angeles, California. One hundred sixty patients with SVT received an intravenous infusion of esmolol in doses ranging from 25–300 μg/kg/min for up to 24 hours. All of the 160 patients were evaluated for safety, and 147 of them were eligible for evaluation of therapeutic response. Therapeutic response was defined as $\geq$15% reduction in the average baseline heart rate or conversion to normal sinus rhythm. Seventy-nine percent (116 of 147) of the patients had a therapeutic response. The cumulative percentage response increased significantly with increasing esmolol doses up to 200 μg/kg/min. The mean dose of esmolol producing a therapeutic response was 97 ± 6 μg/kg/min. Among all patients (n = 160), 39% had hypotension. In 58% of these patients, hypotension resolved with or without adjustment of the esmolol dose while the infusion continued; among almost all of the remaining patients, hypotension resolved within 30 minutes after esmolol was discontinued. Most patients at risk for adverse effects during beta blockade (those with diabetes mellitus, CHF, and asthma), tolerated esmolol therapy, and there were no clinically important trends among the reported changes in laboratory variables. The results of this study indicate that esmolol is effective and well tolerated for the treatment of SVT.

Flestolol

Flestolol, a new ultrashort-acting (half-life 6.9 minutes) beta-blocking drug, was administered by intravenous infusion by Steinberg and associates[22] from Bronx, New York, to 18 patients with new-onset AF or flutter and rapid ventricular response ($\geq$120 beats/minute for $\geq$30 minutes). Drug dose of flestolol was progressively increased until at least 1 of 3 endpoints was achieved: 1) $\geq$20% reduction in heart rate from baseline, 2) heart rate $\leq$100 beats/min, or 3) conversion to normal sinus rhythm. Flestolol was then administered as a maintenance infusion up to 24 hours. When flestolol was discontinued, patients were monitored for 1 additional hour. The mean ventricular response at baseline of 133 ± 12 beats/minute decreased to 103 ± 20 beats/minute at the end of flestolol titration. Fourteen patients (78%) achieved defined endpoints. All 14 patients who continued to receive maintenance infusion had a sustained response. When flestolol was discontinued, ventricular response increased 33 ± 23% within 60 minutes. The only adverse effect seen was hypotension in 2 patients. Flestolol is effective in slowing ventricular response in new-onset AF and flutter, maintains a therapeutic effect during continuous infusion, and rapidly loses therapeutic effect when discontinued.

Pindolol + verapamil

Rose and colleagues[23] from Los Angeles, California, and Taipei, Taiwan, evaluated the efficacy of a single oral dose combining 20 mg pindolol and 120 mg verapamil in terminating paroxysmal SVT in 12 patients with recurrent symptomatic tachycardia. All had electrically inducible SVT lasting longer than 30 minutes. Patients were administered placebo or crushed pindolol and verapamil on 2 consecutive days after tachycardia was electrically induced and allowed to sustain for 30 minutes. With placebo, SVT lasted 186 ± 18 minutes; 5 patients converted spontaneously within 121–180 minutes. With pindolol and verapamil, 9 of 12 patients (responders) converted to sinus rhythm within 8–74 minutes. The mean duration of SVT in the 9 responders was 28 ± 8 minutes compared with 168 ± 20 minutes in patients taking placebo. Before termination, tachycardia rate of those taking pindolol and verapamil slowed significantly from 182 ± 5–164 ± 7/minute compared with no significant change in the rate of SVT on placebo. The mean systolic BP during tachycardia was 97 ± 5 mmHg with placebo and 101 ± 7 mmHg with pindolol and verapamil. Serum levels of pindolol and verapamil obtained in 7 patients at time of spontaneous termination of tachycardia were 66 ± 13 and 56 ± 14 ng/ml, respectively. The side effects with pindolol and verapamil included lightheadedness in 1 patient and symptoms of rapid palpitations in 3. A single oral dose of pindolol and verapamil is safe and effective in termination of acute paroxysmal SVT and may be the initial therapy of choice in selected patients.

Intracardiac electrode catheter ablation

Davis and colleagues[24] in San Francisco, California, performed a programmed stimulation, endocardial mapping, and attempted catheter ablation of the arrhythmia focus in 5 patients with chronic or recurrent ectopic SVT unresponsive to drugs. For attempted ablation, an intracardiac electrode catheter was positioned near the exit point of the tachycardia and served as the cathode while a chest wall patch served as the anode. In 2 patients with tachycardia originating near the coronary sinus, discharges of 200 or 400 J each were delivered to 2 electrodes at the earliest area of endocardial activation. These 2 patients with incessant tachycardia remain free of tachycardia for 17 and 11 months, respectively. In 1 patient with tachycardia originating from the RA appendage, both catheter and surgical ablation proved unsuccessful in that a new focus of atrial tachycardia supervened. This patient subsequently underwent successful catheter ablation of the AV junction. Two patients with junctional tachycardia underwent catheter ablation of the AV junction. Complete AV block followed AV junctional ablation and these patients required permanent cardiac pacing. The junctional tachycardia was replaced by sinus rhythm with episodes of unsustained atrial tachycardia. However, after 13 ± 5 months follow-up, neither of the patients require antiarrhythmic drugs. Catheter ablation can be effective for atrial foci near the coronary sinus os, and can be performed with preservation of AV conduction. Arrhythmia ablation is possible in those with AV junctional tachycardia but requires the sacrifice of AV conduction. After ablation, other automatic atrial foci may become operative and complicate use of dual-chamber pacemakers.

VENTRICULAR ARRHYTHMIAS

Without overt heart disease

Since 1974, Deal and co-workers[25] in Chicago, Illinois, evaluated and followed 24 patients aged 1–21 years presenting with VT and without clinical evidence of heart disease. Sixteen (67%) were symptomatic. Clinical episodes of VT were sustained in 18, incessant in 4, and nonsustained in 2 patients. The rate of VT ranged from 130–300 beats/minute. Subtle abnormalities of cardiac size or function were present at cardiac catheterization in 16 of 23 patients (70%). During electrophysiologic studies, spontaneous VT was present in 6 patients. The clinical VT was inducible by programmed stimulation in 13 of 18 patients. The site of origin of the VT based on endocardial mapping in 17 patients was the right ventricle in 14, the ventricular septum in 1, and indeterminate in 2 patients. Seventeen patients were treated based on results of short-term drug testing. During a mean follow-up period of 7.5 years, 3 patients died suddenly. Investigators concluded that in a young population without clinical evidence of heart disease, VT may be the first manifestation of cardiomyopathy. Because at least two-thirds of these patients have abnormalities at cardiac catheterization, without treatment, mortality in this population may be as high as 13% over an 8-year period. Investigators presently recommend treatment of ventricular tachycardia in any symptomatic patient, with therapy guided by electrophysiologic and treadmill testing. In addition, they recommend treatment for any asymptomatic patient with exercise-related VT, since this group appears to be at increased risk for sudden death. Finally, they seriously considered treating any asymptomatic patient in whom sustained monomorphic ventricular tachycardia can be induced by standard programmed stimulation protocols.

Plasma epinephrine and norepinephrine levels

Sokoloff et al[26] in Philadelphia, Pennsylvania, evaluated the relation between plasma norepinephrine levels and the development of VT during exercise in 17 patients. Ten patients had reproducible VT during exercise, recovery, or both. Seven patients had VT only during ambulatory electrocardiographic monitoring. These 2 groups of patients did not differ in age, exercise duration, LVEF at rest, heart rate during exercise or at rest, QT interval, change in QT interval during exercise, the presence of CAD, or exercise-related myocardial ischemia. In addition, there was no difference between the patient groups in plasma norepinephrine levels at rest, peak exercise, or during the recovery period. Beta-blocker therapy with propranolol prevented VT during exercise in 9 of the 10 patients that were retested subsequently. Plasma norepinephrine levels were significantly decreased compared with levels before beta blockade. Therefore, plasma norepinephrine levels do not distinguish patients with exercise-induced VT from otherwise comparable patients. Furthermore, beta blockers, such as propranolol, are highly effective in abolishing exercise-induced VT and this effect is associated with decreased serum norepinephrine levels.

Morady et al[27] in Ann Arbor, Michigan, studied adrenergic activation during electrophysiologic study in 13 patients. Arterial plasma norepinephrine and epinephrine values were measured before, during, at 1, 3, 5, 10, and 15 minutes after VT was induced by programmed stimulation and terminated by a single 100-J external countershock. The mean VT cycle length was

187 ± 30 ms, and the mean duration of VT was 18 ± 4 seconds. Plasma norepinephrine and epinephrine increased, respectively, from a baseline of 286 ± 141 and 119 ± 40 pg/ml to 770 ± 330 (169%) and 597 ± 467 pg/ml (402%), at 1 minute after the countershock. The mean plasma norepinephrine and epinephrine values during VT and at times >1 minute after the shock did not differ significantly from baseline values. Sinus rates increased from a baseline of 74 ± 13 to 103 ± 26/min at 1 minute after the shock and then returned to baseline. RV effective refractory period decreased from a baseline of 236 ± 27 to 212 ± 23 ms and 226 ± 25 ms at 1 and 3 minutes, respectively, after the countershock and then returned to control values. In 6 patients without inducible VT, plasma catecholamine levels did not change during programmed ventricular stimulation. These data indicate that VT induction and termination by countershock cause a major increase in plasma norepinephrine and epinephrine levels that are short-lived, usually less than 3 minutes. However, this increase in adrenergic activation may be sufficient to shorten ventricular refractory periods and affect results of programmed stimulation. A rest period of 15 minutes after VT termination by countershock should avoid these possible effects from adrenergic activation.

Location of site of VPC

To investigate whether gated RNA phase imaging is useful for visually displaying the origin of VPC, Bashore and associates[28] from Columbus, Ohio, studied 82 patients by gating only VPC. The VPC "origin" by the scintigraphic method was defined as the area of earliest phase and was compared with that predicted by 12-lead electrocardiographic criteria in all patients and to invasive electrophysiologic mapping in 10. Separating the right ventricle into 3 and the left ventricle into 4 segments, the phase-imaging method and the electrocardiographic criteria agreed as to ventricle of VPC origin in 69 patients (84%) and segment of origin within each ventricle in 46 (56%). When baseline ventricular wall motion was analyzed, the 2 methods agreed to the ventricle of VPC origin in 31 of 33 patients (94%) with normal wall motion, 20 of 23 (87%) with segmental wall motion abnormalities and 19 of 26 (73%) with diffuse wall motion abnormalities. Agreement between the 2 methods as to specific segmental localization of the arrhythmia focus was noted in 21 of 33 patients (64%) with normal wall motion, 11 of 23 (48%) with segmental wall motion abnormalities, and 12 of 26 (46%) with diffuse hypocontractility. In the 10 patients with endocardial mapping studies, the phase-imaging technique confirmed the segment of VPC origin in all 10; the electrocardiographic method was accurate in 8. Thus, gated radionuclide angiographic phase-imaging methods may be of value in noninvasively defining the origin of spontaneous VPC. The visual format allows ready interpretation of the arrhythmia origin, and there may be an advantage to this approach over electrocardiographic morphometric criteria.

Influence of increased current, pacing site, number of extrastimuli, coupling intervals, and drive cycle length on induction of arrhythmia

Rosenfeld and associates[29] from New Haven, Connecticut, compared 2 stimulation protocols in 47 patients not inducible with double extrastimuli administered during 2 paced cycle lengths at the RV apex. Method I used triple extrastimuli; method II, an abrupt short-to-long change in cycle length, single and double extrastimuli. Clinical arrhythmias included sustained VT or VF (11 patients, group I); nonsustained VT (27, group II); and no documented ventricular arrhythmia (9, group III). Together, methods I and II rendered 21 of 47 patients inducible; 7 were inducible by both methods. No group III patient became inducible. The 2 techniques were equally likely to produce tachycardia in groups I and II, to induce rapid, pleomorphic, or sustained tachycardia, and tachycardia >10 beats. Since both methods can be applied at the RV apex and increase sensitivity without producing tachycardia in patients with a low suspicion for ventricular arrhythmias, they may facilitate serial drug testing with an indwelling catheter, reducing the need for left-sided studies.

Herre and associates[30] from Houston, Texas, and Richmond, Virginia, studied prospectively in 98 patients reproduction of spontaneously occurring VT and induction of previously undocumented VT: 48 patients with documented sustained VT or VF, 25 with nonsustained or exercise-induced VT, and 25 without documented VT. Patients received 1–4 ventricular extrastimuli and ventricular burst pacing at 2 RV sites, first at twice late diastolic threshold, and then at 10 mA using a prospective, tandem study design. Spontaneously occurring VT was reproduced in 37 of 48 patients (77%) at twice late diastolic threshold and in 1 other patient (2%) at 10 mA. VT was reproduced at both RV sites in 17 of 48 patients (35%) and at 1 site in 20 of 48 patients (42%) at twice late diastolic threshold. A previously undocumented VT was induced in 7 of 25 patients (28%) with no documented VT at twice diastolic threshold and in 14 of 25 patients (56%) at 10 mA. A previously undocumented VT was induced in 33 of 73 patients (45%) with a history of sustained or nonsustained VT at twice late diastolic threshold and in 47 of 73 patients (64%) at 10 mA. In patients with documented sustained VT, the use of up to 4 ventricular extrastimuli at multiple RV sites increases the sensitivity of the test. In patients without documented VT, the induction of previously undocumented VT with more than 3 ventricular extrastimuli limits the specificity of the test. Increased current provides only a slight advantage over 4 ventricular extrastimuli at twice late diastolic threshold in terms of reproduction of spontaneously occurring VT, but leads to a marked increase in induction of previously undocumented VT.

The drive cycle length at which programmed ventricular stimulation is performed is a fundamental variable in all stimulation protocols, but the influence of this variable on the ability to induce ventricular arrhythmias has not been systematically analyzed. Estes and associates[31] from Boston, Massachusetts, performed programmed ventricular stimulation with a uniform protocol that incorporated 3 basic drive cycle lengths from the RV apex in 403 patients with prior VT or VF to examine the influence of drive cycle length on the induction of ventricular arrhythmias. The sensitivity of the protocol was 62% for nonsustained VT, 73% for FV, and 89% for sustained VT. Fifty four percent (217 patients) had an arrhythmia induced with programmed ventricular stimulation during ventricular pacing. No arrhythmia was induced in 96 patients (24%), whereas induction was accomplished during sinus rhythm in 61 patients (15%) and rapid ventricular pacing in 29 patients (7%). With this protocol, the sensitivity for single and double extrastimuli during ventricular pacing increases using decremental drive cycle lengths. Although only 2 patients had induction of a ventricular arrhythmia at a drive cycle length of 700–650 ms using a single extrastimulus, 14, 8, and 3 patients had ventricular arrhythmias induced by single extrastimuli at drive cycle lengths of 600–550, 500–450, and 400 ms, respectively. Of 163 patients with arrhythmias induced with double extrastimuli, only 6 had an arrhythmia induced at drive cycle lengths of 700–650 ms. In contrast, 58, 61, and 38 patients had arrhythmia induction with double extrastimuli at drive cycle lengths of 600–550, 500–450, and 400 ms, respectively. Multiple drive cycle lengths over a range of at least 200 ms should be used with single and double extrastimuli before progressing to more provocative and less specific modes of stimulation.

Morady and associates[32] from Ann Arbor, Michigan, compared coupling intervals of extrastimuli that induced 57 previously documented unimorphic VT with coupling intervals that induced 57 episodes of polymorphic VT or VF in patients without a documented or suspected history of polymorphic VT or VF. Programmed stimulation was performed with the patient in the drug-free state, with 1–3 extrastimuli and 2 basic drive cycle lengths (600 or 500 ms, and 400 ms) at 2 RV sites; stimuli were twice diastolic threshold. The mean coupling intervals of the first, second, and third extrastimuli that induced nonclinical VT/VF (241 ± 19, 185 ± 19, and 173 ± 24 ms, respectively, mean ± standard deviation) were significantly shorter than the corresponding coupling intervals that induced the clinical VTs (266 ± 25, 228 ± 32, and 214 ± 27 ms, respectively). Regardless of the basic drive cycle length, the shortest coupling interval required to induce a clinical VT was 180 ms. Depending on the drive cycle length, 29–70% of nonclinical VT/VF induced by 3 extrastimuli required a coupling interval of less than 180 ms to induce. Therefore, a lower limit of coupling intervals may be identified below which only nonclinical VT/VF is induced by programmed stimulation. Restriction of coupling intervals to this lower limit may allow for significant improvement in specificity without compromise in the sensitivity of programmed ventricular stimulation protocols.

Relation between ease of inducibility and response to therapy

Amann and colleagues[33] from Boston, Massachusetts, determined if there was a relation between the number of extrastimuli necessary to induce arrhythmia and the response to antiarrhythmic drugs. A group of 56 patients with sustained VT or VF who were inducible underwent 235 single-drug studies (4.2% per patient). During the control study, 1 extrastimulus provoked an endpoint in 12 patients (group 1) and at least 1 drug was effective in only 2 patients (17%). Of the 18 patients requiring 2 extrastimuli for induction during baseline (group 2), at least 1 drug was effective in 11 patients (61%). At least 1 drug was effective in 20 of 26 patients (77%) who required 3 extrastimuli (group 3). There were no significant differences among the 3 groups with respect to presenting arrhythmia, presence of CAD, or LVEF. When single drugs or a combination of drugs were used, 58% of group 1, 72% of group 2, and 85% of group 3 were rendered noninducible. During a follow-up of 28 to 32 months, yearly recurrence of arrhythmia was 9%, 5%, and 2%, for the 3 groups, respectively.

Mahmud and associates[34] from Milwaukee, Wisconsin, evaluated 718 patients for suspected or documented ventricular arrhythmias, VT was induced in 28 (incidence 4%) by single or double extrastimuli. Nine of the 28 patients had suspected but no clinically documented VT or VF (group 1), 11 had documented VT (group 2), and 8 had out of hospital VF (group 3). In group 1, electropharmacologic control was achieved in 8 patients with the initial agent tested; however, symptoms recurred in 6 patients. In 4 patients the drug was discontinued. After a follow-up of 26 ± 11 months in group 1, no patient had died. In only 2 of 19 patients in groups 2 and 3 were arrhythmias controlled with the initial agent; 15 patients had VT and 2 VF. Control with class I agents was achieved in 9 of 19 patients and none died until the drug regimen was changed empirically in 3 of these 9. Ten patients, all from groups 2 and 3, were treated empirically with amiodarone; 3 died. All patients died either suddenly or during VT. The mortality rate in groups 2 and 3 after a mean follow-up of 24 ± 9 months was 32%. Continued symptoms and no deaths in group 1 suggest a nonclinical nature of induced VF. Control of induced VF on serial drug testing in group 2 and 3 also indicates a false-negative drug efficacy response, as pharmacologic control of emergent VT on subsequent studies appeared essential to their survival despite control of induced VF. Thus, even with single or double premature stimuli, induction of VF can be a nonclinical response, especially in patients without clinical VF.

Reproducibility of VT suppression by antiarrhythmic drugs

Kim and associates[35] from Bronx, New York, studied the value of programmed stimulation in assessing the efficacy of antiarrhythmic agents in 52 patients with sustained VT. All patients in this nonrandomized study had VT inducible by programmed stimulation and also had frequent VPC (≥30 per hour) on Holter monitor recordings before therapy. The efficacy of antiarrhythmic agents was assessed by both programmed stimulation and Holter recordings during serial drug testing. A regimen was deemed effective according to the programmed stimulation criteria in 25 patients (group I). Twenty-seven patients in whom tachycardia could still be induced during programmed stimulation despite extensive drug trials were discharged on a regimen that caused a marked reduction of VPC according to Holter monitoring (group II). In 23 patients no effective drug regimen was identified by either set of efficacy criteria, and these patients were excluded from the present analysis. Follow-up lasted 18.6 ± 13.9 months. Rates of arrhythmia-free survival at 12 and 24 months were 88% and 72%, respectively, in group I and 84% and 75% in group II. The authors concluded that demonstration of antiarrhythmic efficacy by programmed stimulation predicts a good clinical outcome, that inefficacy as shown by the programmed stimulation protocol used in this study may not preclude a good outcome if there is a marked reduction of spontaneous VPC on Holter monitoring, and that randomized trials should be conducted to validate the results of this observational study.

This article was followed by an editorial by Anderson and Mason[36]. These authors emphasized that although the study by Kim and associates did not definitively compare electrophysiologic study with Holter monitoring, it did add to the overall experience by demonstrating that their combined use can reliably predict drug efficacy in patients with unsuppressible, inducible ventricular tachyarrhythmia. This information will be of considerable value to >33% of patients who undergo electrophysiologic study for ventricular tachyarrhythmia or VF. Also, this article sets the stage for more rigorous randomized studies of these 2 important methods of evaluating drug efficacy in patients with malignant, sustained ventricular tachyarrhythmias.

Garan and associates[37] from Boston, Massachusetts, tested the short-term reproducibility of pharmacologic suppression of VT induced by programmed cardiac stimulation in patients with CAD presenting with documented recurrent VT or VF. Sixty-three consecutive patients in whom VT (30 patients) or nonsustained VT (33 patients) was induced by programmed cardiac stimulation without antiarrhythmic drug treatment, and in whom at least 1 oral antiarrhythmic drug regimen suppressed the induced VT during serial electrophysiologic testing, were entered into the study. Programmed cardiac stimulation was repeated after a mean of 37 ± 14 hours during the same antiarrhythmic drug regimen. No VT was induced in 59 of the 63 patients during the second study, resulting in a rate of 94% for short-term reproducibility of pharmacologic suppression of induced VT. Of the remaining 4 patients, programmed cardiac stimulation during the second drug study induced sustained VT in 1 patient and nonsustained VT in 3 patients. There was no significant difference in mean RV effective refractory period and QT interval between the first and second drug study. Thus, in this selected population of patients, pharmacologic suppression of electrically induced VT is a reproducible phenomenon.

Lombardi and associates[38] from Boston, Massachusetts, assessed the reproducibility of electrophysiologic testing on successive days in the absence of antiarrhythmic drug treatment. Forty-two patients, 17 with compromising VT and 25 with VF unrelated to AMI, underwent 2 baseline studies. During the first electrophysiologic study, arrhythmia was induced in 32 of 42 patients (76%); however, during the second study a similar endpoint was reached in only 22 patients (52%). Only 18 of the 32 patients (56%) with induced arrhythmia during the first study had a reproducible result. Reproducibility was not related to presence of CAD, nature of presenting arrhythmia, or endpoint achieved (sustained or nonsustained VT) during electrophysiologic study. Hence, reproducibility of endpoint during electrophysiologic investigation should be ascertained in each patient before initiating serial drug studies.

Procainamide

To assess the ability of procainamide to predict effectiveness of antiarrhythmic agents at programmed electrical stimulation testing, Wynn and associates[39] from Bronx, New York, compared the result of procainamide at programmed electrical stimulation testing with that of all of the other agents studied. One hundred and fifty-three patients underwent programmed electrical stimulation studies because of either sustained or nonsustained VT. Procainamide prevented VT induction in 79 of 153 patients. Seventy-four of the remaining 153 were inducible for VT on procainamide, with 55 of these being protected by another antiarrhythmic agent. If procainamide failed to prevent VT induction, other conventional and experimental agents were equally as likely to be effective in preventing VT induction. Analysis of *flecainide acetate* as a predictor of efficacy was also evaluated. Fifty-five patients received flecainide and 29 of these were protected at programmed electrical stimulation testing; 26 of these patients were also protected with another agent. When VT was inducible in patients who received flecainide, 15 of these 26 patients were protected by another agent, either conventional or experimental. Thus, if procainamide or flecainide prevented VT induction they accurately predicted effectiveness of other drugs; however, when they did not prevent VT induction, they served as a poor predictor of the possible effectiveness of other drugs. Serial drug testing at programmed electrical stimulation studies with multiple conventional and experimental drugs increases the likelihood of finding an effective antiarrhythmic agent.

Flecainide

Roden and Woosley[40] from Nashville, Tennessee, reviewed electrophysiologic effects, hemodynamic effects, clinical pharmacokinetics, drug interactions, clinical efficacy, and adverse effects of the new antiarrhythmic drug, flecainide. It has been shown to be more potent and better tolerated than currently available drugs in patients with nonsustained ventricular arrhythmias and nearly normal LV function. In contrast to treatment with agents such as quinidine, procainamide, or tocainide, treatment with flecainide is characterized by marked prolongation of the duration of PR and QRS intervals and minimal changes in QT intervals. The long elimination half-life of the drug (7–23 hours in normal persons and longer in patients with arrhythmia) makes it suitable for use in twice daily doses, but it also mandates that dosage adjustments not be made at intervals shorter than 4–5 elimination half-lives required for a maintenance regimen to produce a steady-state plasma concentration. The usual dose is 100–200 mg every 12 hours. The range of plasma concentrations that is tentatively associated with efficacy and avoidance of serious side effects is 200–1,000 ng/ml. Provocation of potentially lethal ventricular arrhythmias can occur, particularly in patients with a history of sustained VT and LV dysfunction who are receiving high doses of flecainide.

The development and marketing of flecainide and drugs with similar pharmacologic properties emphasize the fundamental risk-benefit issue in the management of ventricular arrhythmias. Arrhythmias that are not associated with an increased risk of sudden death, such as VPC in patients with normal LV function, can be effectively and conveniently suppressed with flecainide. At the other end of the spectrum, patients with recurrent sustained VT or VF that are associated with a substantial risk of sudden death are at high risk for serious adverse reactions to flecainide. Because of the potential for serious adverse effects, therapy with flecainide and all other antiarrhythmic agents should be undertaken only when the perceived benefit to the patient exceeds the known risk. Measures to minimize the risk associated with flecainide therapy include appropriate patient selection and initiation of therapy in an environment with continuous monitoring of cardiac rhythm, monitoring of plasma flecainide concentrations, and avoidance of plasma levels >1,000 ng/ml. In patients with severe LV dysfunction, both the underlying heart disease and the accumulation of flecainide in plasma due to CHF may contribute to an increased risk of aggrevation of arrhythmia. Patients with highly symptomatic nonsustained arrhythmias may benefit from antiarrhythmic therapy in that it alleviates their symptoms. A cautious trial of flecainide therapy in patients with sustained VT or other highly symptomatic nonsustained ventricular arrhythmias is reasonable if standard drugs are ineffective or poorly tolerated and if LV performance is not severely compromised. The use of flecainide or any other antiarrhythmic treatment drug for the treatment of arrhythmias that produce no symptoms and that represent no known risk to the patient is inappropriate.

The Flecainide Ventricular Tachycardia Study Group[41] from multiple medical centers and headed by Leonard Horowitz from Philadelphia, Pennsylvania, treated 94 patients with VT with flecainide acetate, 49 of whom had sustained and 45 nonsustained VT, and all were refractory to or intolerant of other antiarrhythmic agents. The study was a multicenter open-label one. Most patients had serious cardiac disorders associated with the arrhythmia: 49 patients (52%) had 1 or more conduction disorders on electrocardiography; 43 (46%) had CHF; 30 (33%) had LVEF of ≤30%. Patients were initially treated orally in the hospital with 100 mg twice daily; dosage was titrated upward as needed at 4-day intervals to a maximal dose of 200 mg twice daily. Flecainide plasma level monitoring was performed to ensure plasma levels remained in the therapeutic range of 0.2–1.0 μg/ml. Patients were discharged with flecainide therapy if investigators judged it to be safe and effective. Minimum efficacy requirements included elimination of sustained VT and reduction of other ventricular arrhythmias as determined by ≥1 of the following: 24-hour electrocardiographic monitoring, programmed electrical stimulation, exercise testing, and in-hospital monitoring. Sixty-eight patients (72%) were discharged with flecainide therapy. After a mean follow-up of 8 months, 45 patients (48%) were still taking flecainide, including 22 of 49 (45%) with sustained and 23 of 45 (51%) with nonsustained VT. Nine patients with sustained VT and 1 patient with nonsustained VT had aggravation of arrhythmia. Two patients had third-degree heart block. Nine patients died after discharge from the hospital: 6 from out-of-hospital sudden death and 3 from AMI. Flecainide is an effective antiarrhythmic agent when used for the short- and long-term control of resistant VT.

Morganroth et al[42] in Philadelphia, Pennsylvania, Salt Lake City, Utah, and St. Paul, Minnesota, evaluated 1,330 patients followed for up to 292 ± 393 days to determine the predictive value for cardiovascular safety by which patients were classified according to ventricular arrhythmias on entry, presence or absence of organic heart disease, and drug dose for flecainide acetate. Patients admitted into the study had either 1) VPC only 2) nonsustained VT, and/or 3) sustained VT. In these patients, proarrhythmic events occurred in 7% of patients overall and were serious in 2% and lethal in 1%. Proarrhythmias were highly dependent on arrhythmia class on entry with serious nonlethal proarrhythmic events occurring in 7% of patients with sustained VT, and only 1% of patients with nonsustained VT, and in no patients with VPC only. Proarrhythmic death occurred in 3% of patients with sustained VT, 0.2% with nonsustained VT, and none with VPC only. The risk of proarrhythmias was also associated with the presence of structural heart disease with nonlethal proarrhythmias developing in 2.6% of patients with underlying heart disease compared with 0.4% of those without underlying heart disease. The dosing regimen used with flecainide was also related to the risk of proarrhythmic phenomenon, and the safety of flecainide was increased by a slow, incremental approach to dosing, especially in the high-risk patients.

Lal and associates[43] from St. Louis, Missouri, Milwaukee, Wisconsin, and Houston, Texas, administered flecainide acetate to 32 patients with nonsustained VT after having unsuccessful treatment with a mean of 4 antiarrhythmic drugs. The mean LVEF was 41% in 27 patients. Thirty-one patients had organic heart disease and 22 patients had arrhythmia-related symptoms. Total suppression of VT occurred in 22 patients. Thirty patients were discharged from the hospital receiving flecainide at a mean dosage of 315 ± 76 mg/dl and 26 of these patients attained a mean trough plasma drug level of 567 ± 254 ng/ml. One patient had proarrhythmia and 3 had worsening of CHF. Twenty-two patients remained in the trial for a mean follow-up of 13 ± 7 months. Five patients died (1 suddenly) during the follow-up period. Their data indicate that flecainide suppresses refractory nonsustained VT in 69% of patients who have organic heart disease. Serious adverse effects were minimized by initiation of treatment in the hospital and careful surveillance of electrocardiograms and plasma drug levels.

Encainide

Morganroth and associates[44] in a multicenter 2-week double-blind placebo-controlled parallel group study determined the dose-response relation of encainide administered 3 times daily and also determined its onset of action. To be included in the study, patients with benign or potentially lethal ventricular arrhythmias were required to have an average of ≥30 VPC/hour on 48-hour Holter monitoring after a 48-hour washout period without antiarrhythmic drug treatment. Patients were randomly assigned to receive either placebo or 10, 25, or 50 mg of encainide 3 times daily for 2 weeks. Of the 125 patients who entered the study, 122 were available for efficacy analysis. Efficacy was determined using 24-hour Holter monitoring on days 1, 7, and 14. There was no difference in frequency of VPC or of VT events in the placebo and 10-mg-3 times daily encainide arms. At doses of 25 and 50 mg 3 times daily, encainide was effective in suppressing VPC and in reducing the number of episodes of VT. A positive dose-response relation was identified. The onset of effect of encainide was apparent at 3 hours and lasted for 24 hours with 3 times daily dosing. No difference in on-therapy conditions were found among the 4 study arms. No patients were discontinued from the study because of electrocardiographic changes. In 1 patient an elevated serum glucose level developed. No symptomatic proarrhythmic events occurred and none required discontinuation of study medication. Three patients died, 2 while receiving 50 mg 3 times daily and 1 patient while receiving 10 mg 3 times daily. Encainide's minimal effective dose for suppressing benign or potentially lethal ventricular arrhythmias is 25 mg 3 times daily.

Lorcainide

Somberg and colleagues[45] from Bronx, New York, investigated 38 patients with a prior history of cardiac arrest by programmed electrical stimulation studies and serial drug testing. Lorcainide was tested acutely in all 38 patients and prevented VT or VF induction in 14 patients and failed in 24 (efficacy rate 37%). Procainamide had failed clinically (cardiac arrest or breakthrough VT) in 16 patients, 7 patients had previously severe adverse effects, and thus only 15 were tested with procainamide at programmed electrical stimulation testing with 7 protected. After initial studies, 14 patients were started on lorcainide oral therapy and 24 on other therapy determined effective at programmed electrical stimulation testing (N-acetylprocainamide-2, flecainide-9, bethanidine-3, slow-release procainamide hydrochloride-3, quinidine-2, cibenzoline-1, amiodarone-4). After 29 ± 7 months follow-up, 3 are alive taking lorcainide therapy, 5 discontinued therapy because of adverse effects, 6 died (3 sudden deaths (33%) and 2 cardiac deaths [both AMI]). Twenty of 24 patients are alive who were started on programmed electrical stimulation–predicted effective therapy other than lorcainide; 4 died (3 sudden deaths [13%] and 1 cardiac nonsudden death). Antiarrhythmic therapy guided by programmed electrical stimulation studies gave overall encouraging results in a cardiac arrest group of patients. Lorcainide, however, is not tolerated well and affords less protection against a sudden death recurrence than is noted in a population taking other antiarrhythmic therapy predicted effective at programmed electrical stimulation testing.

Tocainide

Tocainide, an oral congener of lidocaine, has recently been approved for treatment of ventricular arrhythmias. The drug has electrophysiologic properties identical to lidocaine but the usefulness during long-term therapy has not been established. Hohnloser and co-workers[46] in Boston, Massachusetts, administered tocainide to 228 patients referred for treatment of recurrent ventricular tachyarrhythmias that were refractory to therapy with conventional antiarrhythmic drugs. After baseline studies, 1,200 to 2,400 mg of tocainide per day was given for 4 days. Tocainide was effective in 49% of 180 patients evaluated with monitoring and exercise testing and in 35% of 48 patients undergoing electrophysiologic testing. No clinical parameter predicted the response to tocainide, although there was a correlation with the effect of lidocaine. Tocainide was selected for long-term treatment in 73 patients who were followed for an average of 26 months (range 1–92). The incidence of sudden death was 4.3%/year and 2 patients had nonfatal recurrence of arrhythmia. These investigators concluded that tocainide is effective and well tolerated during long-term use if therapy is evaluated carefully and is individualized.

Mexiletine

Kim and associates[47] from Bronx, New York, studied the electrophysiologic effects and clinical efficacy of mexiletine used alone and in combination with class 1A agents in 35 patients with recurrent sustained VT or VF refractory to nonexperimental antiarrhythmic agents. At baseline before therapy, all patients had inducible VT by programmed stimulation (1–3 extrastimuli) and frequent (≥30/hour) VPC during Holter monitoring. Mexiletine therapy was effective by programmed stimulation (VT no longer inducible or ≤15 beats) in 8 and ineffective in 27 patients. Twenty patients were discharged with mexiletine (14 of whom took an additional class 1A agent). The discharge regiment was effective by programmed stimulation in 6 of these 20 patients. In 14 patients the discharge regimen was ineffective by programmed stimulation, but all patients had a marked reduction of ventricular ectopic activity (at least 83% reduction of VPC and abolition of nonsustained VT). During the follow-up period of 18 ± 13 months (mean ± standard deviation), 4 patients had recurrence (3 with an ineffective regimen by programmed stimulation and 1 with an effective regimen by programmed stimulation). Arrhythmia-free survival rates at 12 and 24 months were 86% and 77% as determined by the Kaplan-Meier method, in patients with an ineffective regimen by programmed stimulation, and 80% and 80% in patients with an effective regimen by programmed stimulation. This nonrandomized study suggests that in selected patients with inducible VT and frequent VPC at baseline, persistent induction of VT by programmed stimulation during mexiletine therapy (alone or in combination with class 1A agents) may not preclude good clinical outcome when it is accompanied by a marked reduction of spontaneous ventricular ectopic activity.

Mexiletine -vs- lidocaine

Lui and associates[48] from Davis and San Francisco, California, compared the efficacy and safety of intravenous loading of mexiletine to lidocaine in patients with VPC. Seventeen men and 5 women, average age 63 years, completed this randomized parallel study. Twelve patients received mexiletine intravenously (5–10 mg/minute) until ≥95% VPC suppression was achieved or a total of 450 mg of the drug was given. The average loading dose of mexiletine was 4.4 mg/kg, at an infusion rate of 0.1 mg/kg/min. Ten patients received lidocaine (1 mg/kg) given over 3 minutes, with a second similar bolus given if after 10 minutes of the ≥95% VPC suppression was not achieved. Total VPC were determined for the 60 minutes before drug administration, during drug infusion, and 60 minutes thereafter. Eleven of 12 patients receiving mexiletine were full responders (≥95% suppression) and 1 was a partial responder (≥75% ≤95% suppression). Five of 10 lidocaine patients (50%) were full responders, 3 (30%) were partial responders, and 2 failed to respond. At peak suppression, mexiletine reduced mean VPC from 37 ± 33/5–0.8 ± 0.9/5 minutes (p <0.01) and lidocaine decreased mean VPC from 28 ± 47/5–4.7 ± 2.2/5 minutes (p <0.01). Mexiletine resulted in greater suppression of VPC than lidocaine in terms of mean percent reduction (96% -vs- 68%). All lidocaine patient had therapeutic plasma levels (range 1.6–3.5 μg/ml). In the mexiletine patients, there was 1 subtherapeutic and 1 toxic level observed (mean 1.4 μg/ml, range 0.4–3.2 μg/ml). No significant changes in BP, heart rate, or electrocardiographic intervals were noted for either drug. Three mexiletine and 1 lidocaine patient had transient adverse effects. Intravenous mexiletine was found safe and effective and may be a useful alternative drug in the management of ventricular arrhythmias.

Propafenone

Hammill and associates[49] from Rochester, Minnesota, evaluated the results of therapy with propafenone in 45 patients with complex ventricular arrhythmias that had been refractory to a mean of 3.8 antiarrhythmic drugs. The cardiac diagnoses were CAD (16 patients) cardiomyopathy-type not mentioned (7 patients), MVP (7 patients), idiopathic (6 patients), valvular heart disease (5 patients), and systemic hypertension (4 patients). The frequency of VPC was established after therapy with antiarrhythmic agents had been discontinued. Patients then received propafenone during a dose-ranging protocol. An effective response was defined as a reduction in total VPC of ≥80%. During dose ranging, therapy failed in 4 patients because of side effects, in 8 because of a reduction in VPC ≤80%, and in 3 because of an aggravation of the arrhythmia. Thirty patients had a reduction in total VPC ≥80%. During a mean follow-up of 12.4 months, therapy failed in 1 patient because of sustained VT and in 7 because of intolerable side effects; 22 patients continued to receive propafenone. PR and QRS intervals were significantly prolonged, but the corrected QT interval and the heart rate were unchanged. The mean trough plasma level of propafenone associated with an effective response was 756 ng/ml, and that associated with intolerable side effects was 920 ng/ml. Thus, in patients with refractory VPC, propafenone was effective and well tolerated initially in 67% of patients and during long-term administration in 49%, and toxicity was minor in most patients.

Atenolol

To determine the efficacy and safety of intravenous atenolol in patients with frequent and repetitive benign or potentially lethal ventricular arrhythmias, Morganroth[50] from Philadelphia, Pennsylvania, studied 40 patients who received an open-label, single dose of 10 mg of intravenous atenolol given in aliquots of 2.5 mg every 10 minutes. Twenty-four-hour Holter monitoring was performed on the day before, the day of, and the day after infusion of atenolol. A full 10-mg dose was given to 37 patients; asymptomatic bradycardia developed in 3 patients, and they were not included in the efficacy analysis. A single 10-mg dose of intravenous atenolol was effective rapidly in suppressing ventricular arrhythmias, with peak suppression occurring 1 to 2 hours after infusion and significant suppression lasting for 7 hours. Only 1 patient had symptoms (lightheadedness), plus hypotension lasting 45 minutes after the infusion was concluded. The mean plasma level of atenolol was 231 ng/ml 10 minutes after the infusion, with individual patient values of 148–457 ng/ml. Thus a single intravenous dose of 10 mg of atenolol can significantly reduce the frequency of VPC and VT within the first hour after infusion; suppression can last for 7 hours. Atenolol is well tolerated.

Nadolol

To determine the minimal effective dose of nadolol to suppress frequent VPC, Morganroth and Duchin[51] from Philadelphia, Pennsylvania, studied 23 patients with ≥30 VPC/hour on 2 baseline 24-hour Holter recordings. The initial dose of nadolol was 10 mg/day orally, and this dose was doubled at weekly intervals until arrhythmia suppression was achieved, adverse effects appeared, or a maximal dose of 160 mg/day was reached. After each dose level a 24-hour ambulatory Holter monitor was recorded. A pharmacokinetic trial was conducted in patients who responded to nadolol treatment. Frequent VPC were suppressed ≥75% by nadolol in 11 of 23 patients (48%) and the minimal effective dose was 10 mg/day in 3 patients, 20 mg/day in 4, 40 mg/day in 3, and 80 mg/day in 1 patient. At these doses, minimal steady-state levels of nadolol in serum (Cmin) ranged from 3.9–47.0 ng/ml, and these serum concentrations were proportional to the oral dose of nadolol. No relation, however, was observed between Cmin levels and percent reduction of VPC. Cmin and heart rate changes were comparable between responders and nonresponders, suggesting that the degree of beta blockade was similar between these 2 groups. Adverse reactions were noted in 6 patients, and 2 had an asymptomatic increase in the frequency of VPCs and 1 patient an increase in beats of ventricular tachycardia. This study details the importance of selecting an individualized dose for nadolol for control of ventricular arrhythmias; in more than half of the patients doses of 20 mg/day or less were effective.

Sotalol

Anderson et al[52] in Salt Lake City, Utah; San Diego, California; Bronx, New York; and Evansville, Indiana, studied the effects of sotalol, a nonselective beta blocker, that causes significant repolarization delay to determine its ability to suppress ventricular arrhythmias during a 6-week parallel, placebo-controlled outpatient study of 2 doses (320 and 640 mg/day in 2 divided doses) in 4 hospitals and 56 patients with chronic VPC at a frequency ≥30/hour on ambulatory electrocardiographic recording. During a placebo week, no change in the frequency of arrhythmia occurred. Subsequently, sotalol therapy significantly reduced median arrhythmia frequency in patients receiving both low and high doses compared with that occurring in patients receiving placebo, i.e., by 77% and 83%, respectively as compared to 6%. Twenty-two (59%) of 37 sotalol-treated patients, 11 in each group, reached the prospectively defined criterion of efficacy (≥75% arrhythmia reduction) -vs- 2 (11%) of 19 placebo control patients. Sotalol also reduced the median frequency of VPC couplets by 94% and of runs of VT by 89%. Sotalol reduced heart rates by 17–27% and increased QTcs by 6–9% and PR intervals by 6%. LVEF was unchanged by sotalol. The most common adverse effect was fatigue. No proarrhythmic effects were identified. Thus, sotalol has significant antiarrhythmic activity in doses of 320 and 640 mg/day. It also prolongs the QTc interval, an effect that distinguishes it from other available beta blockers.

Amiodarone

Smith and associates[53] from Auckland, New Zealand, during a 5-year period (from 1979–1983) followed 242 patients who had received amiodarone, 156 for SVT and 86 for ventricular arrhythmias. Five patients were lost to follow-up; the rest were followed to cessation of therapy, death, or recent review for a mean of 24 ± 15 months. Male/female incidence was 1.8:1 and mean age was 58 years (range 4–88). Half the group had impaired LV function. Adverse effects were recorded in 59% of the patients and led to drug withdrawal in 26% of the total group. In contrast, unsuccessful treatment was the cause of drug withdrawal in only 5% of the patients, although an additional 25% stopped taking the drug for various reasons. Actuarial survival for the whole group, and subgroups with SVT and VT/VF were 66%, 74%, and 52%, respectively, at 50 months. For the whole group, the actuarial probability of being alive and continuing with amiodarone therapy was only 19% at 50 months. Thus, although amiodarone was effective, few patients tolerated the drug on a long-term basis. Although amiodarone remains a valuable treatment for patients with VT, its long-term effectiveness for patients with SVT is less certain.

Induction of rapid VT or VF during therapy with amiodarone is associated with an increased risk of sudden death. To determine whether the addition of a type IA antiarrhythmic agent to therapy would improve outcome, Marchlinski and co-workers[54] in Philadelphia, Pennsylvania, randomly assigned 37 patients in whom VT of a cycle length <350 ms was induced after 14 days of amiodarone to therapy with amiodarone alone (group 1, 20 patients) or amiodarone plus type IA agent (group 2, 17 patients). Type IA therapy consisted of procainamide in 13 patients and quinidine in 4 procainamide-intolerant patients. To assess the short-term effects of a type IA agent on inducibility of VT, cycle length, and hemodynamic tolerance, 16 of 20 patients in group 1 and all patients in group 2 underwent repeat programmed stimulation after the intravenous administration of procainamide during amiodarone therapy. Procainamide prevented induction of sustained arrhythmias in only 2 of 33 patients. Procainamide increased the cycle length of induced VT from 283–352 ms. After the addition of procainamide, 16 of 31 patients -vs- 10 of 37 patients taking amiodarone alone had an induced arrhythmia that was tolerated hemodynamically. There were no differences between groups 1 and 2 with respect to patient or arrhythmia characteristics, response to short-term procainamide, or duration of follow-up. The mean follow-up for all patients was 14 ± 10 months. By life-table analysis, outcome did not differ between group 1 and group 2 patients with respect to either development of sudden death or syncope or the development of any arrhythmia event or side effect that required withdrawal of antiarrhythmic therapy. Forty percent of group 2 patients had adverse effects necessitating withdrawal of drug. The investigators conclude that in patients in whom rapid VT is induced with amiodarone 1) type IA agents increase the cycle length and result in improved hemodynamic tolerance but rarely prevent induction of VT, and 2) outcome is not improved by the addition of a type IA agent to therapy.

Veltri and colleagues[55] in Baltimore, Maryland, recently reported a retrospective experience with serial Holter monitoring as a guide to therapy in patients with sustained VT treated with amiodarone. To confirm and substantiate these findings, a prospective study was designed that included baseline 24-hour Holter monitoring and serial Holter monitoring after 1 week of therapy with amiodarone. Fifty-two patients with documented sustained VT who had nonsustained VT on baseline Holter monitoring were treated with amiodarone. Thirty-four patients (group I) had nonsustained VT completely suppressed and 18 patients (group II) had continued nonsustained VT on serial Holter monitoring performed on days 8, 9, and 10 of therapy. At 12 months follow-up, 3 (9%) group I patients and 12 (67%) group II patients had recurrent sustained VT or sudden cardiac death. The sensitivity, specificity, positive and negative predictive value, and predictive accuracy of VT on 24, 48, and 72-hour Holter monitoring over days 8, 9, and 10 for predicting recurrent sustained VT or sudden cardiac death were analyzed. The positive and negative predictive values were 89% and 84%, 69% and 89%, and 67% and 91% for 24-, 48-, and 72-hour Holter monitoring, respectively. Overall predictive accuracy was 85%, 83%, and 83%, respectively. The authors conclude that early Holter monitoring is useful in assessing the clinical efficacy of amiodarone in patients with sustained VT who had nonsustained VT on baseline Holter monitoring.

Kadish and associates[56] from Philadelphia, Pennsylvania, studied 29 patients with recurrent sustained VT or cardiac arrest by baseline, early (after 2 weeks of therapy) and late (after 5 months, mean) electrophysiologic procedures during oral amiodarone therapy. Inducible sustained VT was present in all patients at baseline study, in 21 of 22 at early and in 26 of 29 at late study. The cycle length of induced VT increased from 263 ± 60 ms at baseline to 305 ± 58 ms at early follow-up study and to 318 ± 64 ms at late study. The ventricular effective refractory period increased from 237 ± 22 ms at baseline to 253 ± 26 ms at early and to 268 ± 24 ms at late study. Twenty-four patients had no recurrent VT or cardiac arrest with amiodarone (group 1). Five patients had recurrent arrhythmia (group 2). In group 1, the ventricular effective refractory period increased by 39 ± 19 ms, and in group 2 decreased by 4 ± 27 from baseline to late follow-up study. Similarly, in group 1 the cycle length of induced VT increased by a mean of 75 ± 56 ms and in group 2 decreased a mean of 11 ± 81 ms from baseline to late follow-up study. From these findings it was concluded that 1) chronic electrophysiologic effects of amiodarone are not completely manifest after 2 weeks of oral therapy, and 2) a lack of change of ventricular refractory period and cycle length of induced VT correlates with amiodarone treatment failure.

Torres et al[57] in Bronx, New York, evaluated the influence of amiodarone on the QT interval in 33 patients presenting with cardiac arrest and symptomatic VT in whom no other antiarrhythmic agent was effective in preventing the induction of VT during electrophysiologic studies. There were 30 men and 3 women (mean age 62 ± 10 years). Twenty-three patients were alive after a mean follow-up period of 12 ± 7 months; 10 died, 6 suddenly and 3 of noncardiac causes. Marked prolongation of the QT interval was found in patients remaining alive with amiodarone therapy (Fig. 4-3). There was a significant difference in percent QT prolongation between patients remaining alive and those dying suddenly. There was no difference in the percent change in QRS interval between the 2 groups. The serum levels of amiodarone and its metabolite were not significantly different between the living patients and those who died suddenly. Thus, these data suggest that a prolongation of the QT interval may be a marker of the therapeutic efficacy of amiodarone.

Amiodarone, a drug that has electrophysiologic actions resembling those of hypothyroidism, increases serum levels of T_4 and reverse T_3 (rT_3) and decreased T_3. The drug's long-term effects on thyroid function are poorly defined. Nadémānee and associates[58] from Los Angeles, California, determined serial thyroid hormone indexes in 76 patients given amiodarone for 6–32 months (mean 16) for arrhythmias. Over this period, 68 patients (89%) remained euthyroid; hypothyroidism developed in 6 (8%) and hyperthyroidism developed in 2 (3%). In patients who remained euthyroid, thyroid hormone alterations attained steady-state values at 3 months: T_4 increased 42%, rT_3 increased 172%, and T_3 decreased 16%, without significant effect on thyroid-stimulating hormone. For the euthyroid patients, the 90% tolerance limits (95% confidence) over the follow-up period for T_4 was 5 to 19 $\mu g/dl$ (normal 4–12), for T_3 36 to 163 ng/dl (normal 60–160), for rT_3 22 to 131 ng/dl (normal 15–50) and for thyroid-stimulating hormone 0 to 14 $\mu U/ml$ (normal 1–6). The changes in hormone indexes in hyperthyroid or hypothyroid patients were unrelated to the cumulative dose or duration of drug therapy. The most reliable diagnostic indexes for amiodarone-induced altered thyroid state were: thyroid-stimulating hormone level over 20 μU for

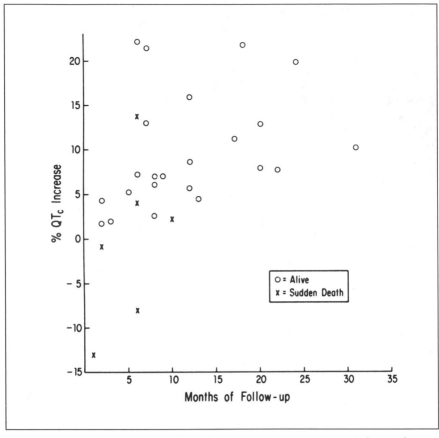

Fig. 4-3. Percent increase in QTc intervals in 33 patients receiving amiodarone therapy. Reproduced with permission from Torres et al.[57]

hypothyroidism and T_4 over 20 ng/dl or high T_3 over 200 ng/dl for hyperthyroidism. All levels were within the 90% tolerance limits derived for these hormones from patients remaining euthyroid taking long-term amiodarone. The data provide the basis for diagnosis of abnormal thyroid function in patients with drug-induced changes in thyroid function tests due to amiodarone and suggest the need for baseline and periodic determinations of thyroid function tests during long-term amiodarone therapy.

Rigas and associates[59] from New Haven and West Haven, Connecticut, and Philadelphia, Pennsylvania, detected amiodarone *hepatotoxicity* on routine biochemical monitoring in 5 patients. Symptoms attributable to hepatotoxicity were minimal or absent; reversible hepatomegaly was seen in 2 patients, whereas 3 patients had signs of nonhepatic amiodarone toxicity before or with hepatotoxicity. Serum aminotransferase levels were elevated in all patients and alkaline phosphatase levels in 4; no patient had hyperbilirubinemia or prolongation of the prothrombin time. Light microscopy showed steatosis, cellular degeneration, and cellular necrosis in the biopsy samples of 4 patients, whereas the fifth patient's sample had a granulomatous injury pattern. These findings suggest that both toxic and hypersensitivity liver injury can occur in response to amiodarone. The presence of phospholipid-laden lysosomal lamellar bodies may help differentiate amiodarone hepatotoxicity from alcoholic liver disease or other causes of hepatic steatosis.

Adverse reactions to antiarrhythmic drugs

Nygaard and associates[60] from Charlottesville, Virginia, analyzed the frequency of adverse reactions to antiarrhythmic drugs in 123 consecutive patients with a history of sustained VT or VF. Blood levels were measured serially and were maintained within the usual therapeutic range. Minor reactions were defined as those that required drug discontinuation or permanent pacing for bradycardia. A total of 237 individual, oral drug trials were evaluated in the 123 patients. Adverse reactions were noted in 79 trials (33%). Fifty-nine (48%) of the 123 patients had ≥1 adverse reaction. Major reactions were noted in 36 patients (29%). Adverse effects occurred during 49% of trials with mexiletine hydrochloride, 44% of trials with amiodarone, 24% of trials with procainamide hydrochloride, and 18% of trials with quinidine sulfate or gluconate. In conclusion, clinically significant adverse reactions are common during drug therapy for ventricular arrhythmias. These observations indicate that with the drugs used in this study, an acceptable risk-benefit ratio will be possible only in patients at a significant risk for a symptomatic arrhythmia. Antiarrhythmic drug therapy in patients at low risk for serious arrhythmia should be discouraged.

Antiarrhythmic drug withdrawl

Selection of an antiarrhythmic drug program by noninvasive means for patients with malignant ventricular arrhythmia has not been demonstrated to be the decisive factor in promoting enhanced long-term survival. Graboys and associates[61] from Boston, Massachusetts, studied 24 patients (16 men, mean age 56 years) with a history of either recurrent VT or noninfarction-induced VF after antiarrhythmic therapy had been discontinued. All patients had been symptom-free on a tailored drug program for a mean of 31 months. Twenty of the 24 patients were hospitalized and underwent systematic drug withdrawal to assess continued need for therapy or because of intolerable side effects. In 4 patients, medication was discontinued either on their own or by their local physician. Recurrence after drug withdrawal was defined as either recurrence of the presenting arrhythmia (VT or VF) (12 patients) or reappearance of repetitive arrhythmia during Holter monitoring or exercise stress testing comparable to pretreatment levels (11 patients). The clinical arrhythmia recurred in 12 patients. Nine patients had a cardiac arrest. These data document the high recurrence rate of malignant ventricular arrhythmia on cessation of a proved antiarrhythmic program. They further support the concept that patients with life-threatening arrhythmia can be protected from recurrence by noninvasive methods of drug selection that are guided by suppression of advanced forms of VPC.

Transvenous catheter ablation

The usefulness of transvenous catheter ablation of the His bundle in 3 patients with recurrent VT, in which the initiating mechanism was recognized during a rapid atrial rhythm was reported by Critelli and associates[62] from Naples, Italy. Tachycardia was refractory to conventional treatment and required transthoracic direct-current shocks in all patients. In patient 1, double tachycardia (atrial flutter and VT) was documented and VT was easily induced by rapid atrial pacing. In patients 2 and 3, initiation of VT during junctional reciprocating and atrial tachycardia, respectively, was observed. Interruption of the His bundle was performed by means of fulguration. Stable AV block was observed in patient 1 after the ablative procedure; patient 2 showed anterograde conduction over a posterior septal accessory pathway with no evidence of conduction over the normal conduction system in both the anterograde and retrograde directions. In patient 3, transient AV block was observed; AV conduction resumed 2 days later and the cardiac rhythm showed persistent ectopic atrial tachycardia with second-degree AV block. Patients 1 and 2 underwent pacemaker implantation, but patient 2 was not pacemaker-dependent. After the procedure, VT no longer occurred in any of the patients (follow-up: 2 years, 5 months, and 6 months).

Surgical ablation

Although subendocardial resection is an effective treatment for patients with CAD and recurrent sustained VT resistant to drug therapy, the extent of endocardium to be removed and the value of preoperative and intraoperative electrophysiologic guidance remains controversial. To determine whether a regional approach for surgery for VT would improve on the results of previously reported endocardial resection, Krafchek and co-workers[63] in Houston, Texas analyzed their surgical experience over a 5-year period. Of 46 consecutive patients operated on for recurrent sustained VT or VF, 39 patients with CAD underwent subendocardial resection or cryoblation, or both. The mean age of the patients was 61 years, the mean LVEF was $32 \pm 11\%$, and the mean number of ineffective antiarrhythmic drugs was 3.8 per patient. In 35 of 39 patients in whom mapping data were obtainable, 56 (86%) tachycardias had earliest sites of activation in the left ventricle and 9 (14%) had earliest sites in the right ventricle. Ten patients had 14 tachycardias mapped to areas outside visible dense scar. Of these 35 patients, 10 underwent localized subendocardial resection and 25 underwent a regional procedure in which all areas activated before the surface QRS during VT were excised or cryoblated or both. In the operative survivors of electrophysiologically guided surgery, 3 of 8 patients with the localized and 1 of 24 patients who underwent the regional procedure had recurrence of VT during a follow-up period of 1–59 (mean 22) months. The favorable outcome of regional surgery was not influenced by the presence of multiple morphologies in 54%, disparate sites of origin in 29%, or inferior wall foci in 46% of patients. The data from this study suggest that 1) some VTs have early sites of activation outside visible dense scar or within the right ventricle, or both, 2) a regional approach to arrhythmia ablation can lead to operative success in >90% of patients, and 3) multiple morphologies, disparate sites, and inferior wall origin are not adverse prognostic factors to success when this approach is used.

Bepridil

To define the efficacy and safety of a new once-a-day calcium antagonist, bepridil, Nestico and associates[64] from Philadelphia, Pennsylvania, performed a 14-day in-patient monitored trial in 21 patients with frequent VPC. After Holter monitoring during placebo administration, patients underwent 2 days of a loading dose of bepridil followed by 12 days of bepridil, 400 mg/day. Holter monitoring during therapy showed that 10 patients (48%) had more than a 70% reduction in VPC frequency and 8 of 16 patients (50%) at least a 95% reduction in frequency of nonsustained VT. Gastrointestinal and central nervous system side effects considered to be mild occurred in 13 patients (62%). One patient had an asymptomatic increase in VPC frequency and another had sustained VT associated with a loading dose of 900 mg of bepridil. Thus, bepridil has moderate antiarrhythmic efficacy in patients with ventricular arrhythmias, but further definition of its potential for causing proarrhythmia must be determined.

Ethmozine

Gear and associates[65] from Tucson, Arizona, treated 20 patients with an average of ≥30 VPC/hour with ethmozine. Eighteen had either not responded or had adverse reactions to ≥1 other antiarrhythmic drug. Patients were treated with 200 to 300 mg 3 times daily (8.25–11.7 mg/kg) and were followed for up to 6 months. Three patients were withdrawn from ethmozine therapy because of unwanted effects before evaluation of efficacy. One patient had sustained VT after a loading dose of ethmozine. Eleven of the remaining 17 patients (65%) had >75% reduction in ventricular ectopic activity. Six patients had a smaller or no decrease in VPC frequency. Eleven of 16 patients (68%) with paired VPC had a >90% reduction in paired VPC frequency. Eleven of 13 patients (84%) with VT events of ≥3 beats had >90% reduction in VT events. Of the 11 patients in whom a >75% reduction in VPC frequency occurred, 1 died suddenly after 133 days of effective drug therapy. Three patients discontinued ethmozine therapy for reasons not related to the drug. Of the 6 patients in whom there was <75% reduction in VPC frequency, 2 patients discontinued treatment, 1 patient because of hyperanxiety and 1 because of drug-related left anterior hemiblock. Ethmozine lengthened PR and QRS intervals but not the JT interval. Thus, ethmozine is effective and clinically useful for suppression of frequent VPC in 50% (10 of 20 patients) of a selected population.

Miura and associates[66] from Bronx, New York, investigated the antiarrhythmic properties of ethmozine in 27 patients with a history of cardiac arrest or symptomatic VT. Programmed electrical stimulation studies were performed in 20 men and 7 women with a mean age of 62 years and a mean LVEF of 43%. All patients had inducible VT by programmed electrical stimulation while taking no antiarrhythmic therapy. Patients were then tested with procainamide if their treatment with this drug orally had not previously failed. Procainamide, 1,000 and 1,500 mg, was administered intravenously, and VT could be provoked in 14 of 18 patients. Ethmozine was given in an oral-loading regimen starting 24–36 hours later. After 500 mg of oral ethmozine, patients were given 15 mg/kg ethmozine every 8 hours for 7–9 doses before drug testing. Ethmozine did not significantly change the baseline heart rate, BP, and corrected QT interval from the initial drug-free values. The PR and QRS intervals were significantly prolonged. Seven patients were protected with oral ethmozine; 14 patients still had VT inducible at programmed electrical stimulation testing, and 6 patients had VT spontaneously with ethmozine and were not tested in the programmed electrical stimulation laboratory. One patient had gastrointestinal complaints and was not discharged with the drug. The 5 patients who tolerated the oral protocol without side effects and who were protected against programmed stimulation induction of VT were discharged with oral therapy. One patient taking long-term therapy appeared to have an allergic reaction to the agent with unexplained fevers and was switched to amiodarone therapy. Chronic therapy with ethmozine appears to be well tolerated in selected patients with control of their VT.

Moricizine

Seals and colleagues[67] from Houston, Texas, evaluated the hemodynamic effects of moricizine in 20 patients with frequent nonsustained VT with a mean LVEF of 39 ± 14% in a prospective single-blind, placebo-controlled study. Hemodynamic measurements were performed at rest and during supine bicycle exercise with placebo and moricizine therapy (10 mg/kg/day). Although 16 of 19 patients experienced no rest or exercise deterioration in hemodynamic parameters[69] during drug dosing, 3 patients had acute deterioration of PA wedge pressure and cardiac index with moricizine. During follow-up of 6 ± 3 months, 2 subgroups were identified: 10 of 19 patients had effective long-term reduction in VT, whereas 9 of 19 patients had poor control of ventricular arrhythmia or CHF and were withdrawn from the trial. Baseline EF and hemodynamic parameters at rest were similar in both patient subgroups. However, protocol dropouts had a hemodynamic response to exercise with moricizine that was significantly depressed compared to patients with a favorable antiarrhythmic outcome. The following hemodynamic profile characterizes patients unlikely to have an antiarrhythmic response to moricizine: 1) an increase in cardiac index of <1.0 liters/min/m^2, and 2) no increase in LV stroke work index during supine exercise.

Cibenzoline

Rothbart and Saksena[68] from Newark, New Jersey, evaluated the electrocardiographic and electrophysiologic effects, clinical efficacy, and safety of oral cibenzoline therapy using a twice-daily dosing regimen in patients with refractory VT. Twenty patients underwent electrophysiologic studies in the control (drug-free) state and after cibenzoline therapy using an incremental dose-titration protocol. Oral cibenzoline (1.4–5.8 mg/kg/day) was administered in doses of 130, 160, or 190 mg at 12-hour intervals. Electrocardiographic and electrophysiologic variables, 24-hour ambulatory electrocardiographic monitoring and programmed electrical stimulation studies were obtained in the control state and after 11 ± 4 days of cibenzoline therapy. Cibenzoline therapy prolonged the mean PR interval (from 179 ± 29–201 ± 36 ms), the mean QRS duration (from 107 ± 21–130 ± 25 ms), and the mean QTc interval (from 422 ± 25–460 ± 42 ms). It increased the mean HV interval (from 50 ± 17–65 ± 20 ms) and mean RV effective refractory period (from 245 ± 24–266 ± 27 ms). After cibenzoline therapy, 5 patients (25%) had suppression of inducible sustained VT during programmed electrical stimulation. High-degree AV block occurred in 2 patients. Chronic cibenzoline therapy (mean follow-up 24 ± 3 months) remained effective in long-term suppression of VT in 4 patients. Two patients had to discontinue therapy because of gastrointestinal intolerance. Cibenzoline is effective in suppression of refractory VT in selected patients using a twice-daily dosing schedule.

Automatic cardiodefibrillator

Platia and associates[69] from Baltimore, Maryland, and Washington, D.C., planted an automatic cardiodefibrillator in conjunction with endocardial resection in 28 patients with drug refractory ventricular arrhythmias, all of whom had had previous AMI and between 1 and 5 cardiac arrests. There were 3 perioperative deaths. During follow-up of 8–18 months (mean 25), 4 of the 25 survivors had recurrences of hypotensive VT, which in all instances were automatically terminated by the implanted device. One patient, whose automatic cardioverter defibrillator was not functional, died suddenly. The authors concluded that patients undergoing mapping-directed endocardial resection can be provided with additional protection against recurrent ventricular tachyarrhythmias or sudden death by implantation of an automatic cardioverter defibrillator.

CARDIAC ARREST

Definitions and causes

Roberts[70] from Bethesda, Maryland, reviewed causes of sudden cardiac death and emphasized that this term is relatively imprecise and if death is due to coronary atherosclerotic disease, a preferred term would be sudden coronary death (Fig. 4-4).

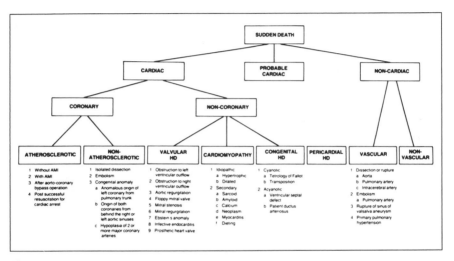

Fig. 4-4

Risk factors

Beard and associates[71] from Rochester, Minnesota, conducted a case-controlled study of unexpected death as the initial manifestation of CAD in young women <60 years of age. Risk factors among the 15 cases identified during the years 1960 through 1974 were compared with those in 2 control groups—a population group of 60 (4 age-matched controls per case) and the 59 cases of AMI diagnosed in women <60 years of age in Rochester during the same period. By using Miettinen's matched analysis for comparison of sudden death cases and matched controls, the relative risks for the accepted CAD risk factors of ever smoking and systemic hypertension were 9 and 6, respectively. In a comparison of sudden death cases and AMI cases by using the Mantel-Haenszel procedure and stratifying by 5 age groups, the odds ratios were 1 for ever smoking and 0.8 for hypertension. Six of the 15 sudden death cases had a diagnosis of alcoholism compared with 2 of the 60 controls and 4 of the 59 AMI cases; thus, the relative risks were 12 and 5, respectively. Ever married sudden death cases were nulliparous or had fewer children more often than the controls or the AMI cases. The combination of major psychiatric diagnosis and major tranquilizer use occurred with greater frequency among sudden death cases than among controls, whereas comparison of sudden death cases and AMI cases for this variable resulted in a relative risk of 0.7.

Sudden infant death

Sudden infant death syndrome (SIDS) is made by excluding known causes of death. The assessment of circumstances surrounding the sudden death of an infant, however, is often minimal. Bass and associates[72] from Brooklyn, New York, conducted death-scene investigations in 26 consecutive cases in which a presumptive diagnosis of SIDS was made and the infants thereafter were brought to the emergency room of the county hospital. In 6 cases, the authors observed strong circumstantial evidence of accidental death. In 18 other cases, the authors discovered various possible causes of death other than SIDS, including accidental asphyxiation by an object in the crib or bassinet, smothering by overlying while sharing a bed, hyperthermia, and shaken baby syndrome. This study suggests that many sudden deaths of infants have a definable cause that can be revealed by careful investigation of the death scene and that the extremely high rate of SIDS (4.2/1,000 live births) reported in the population of low socioeconomic status served by their county hospital should be questioned. This article was followed by an editorial by Bradley P. Thach[73] entitled "Sudden Infant Death Syndrome—Old Causes Rediscovered?"

Symptoms preceding arrest

Goldstein and associates[74] from Detroit and Ann Arbor, Michigan, examined prodromal symptoms and cardiac history in 227 patients with CAD who were successfully resuscitated after out-of-hospital cardiac arrest. Cardiac arrest was sudden—<1 hour in 71% of the patients. Nonsudden death—death occurring after >1 hour of symptoms—occurred in 29% of the patients. A history of cardiovascular disease was present in 85% of patients with sudden cardiac arrest and in 83% with nonsudden arrest (Fig. 4-5). Cardiac arrest occurred without symptoms in 38% of the patients with sudden cardiac arrest and was the first expression of CAD in 4% of the entire study group. This study indicates that cardiac arrest usually occurs with symptoms and almost always in the setting of a history of cardiovascular disease.

In Air Force recruits

Phillips and associates[75] from San Antonio, Texas, and Washington, D.C., reviewed clinical and necropsy records of 19 sudden cardiac deaths that occurred among 1,606,167 U.S. Air Force healthy, medically screened recruits aged 17 to 28 years during a 42-day basic training period. Sixteen (all men) died suddenly of underlying structural heart disease and in the other 3 no anatomic cause of death was identified. During the same period, 32 nonsudden, noncardiac deaths occurred, and only 2 had structural heart disease. Strenuous physical exertion was associated with sudden death in 17 of the 19 cases. The cause of the sudden cardiac death is shown in Table 4-3.

In Southeast Asian refugees

Sudden death during sleep has occurred among previously healthy Southeast Asian male refugees, but autopsies have not determined the cause of death in any case. Kirschner and associates[76] from Chicago, Illinois, and Atlanta, Georgia, reported the first systematic attempt to define the cardiac abnormalities associated with this syndrome. Among 18 hearts examined, 14 showed slight to significant cardiomegaly, characteristic of increased cardiac

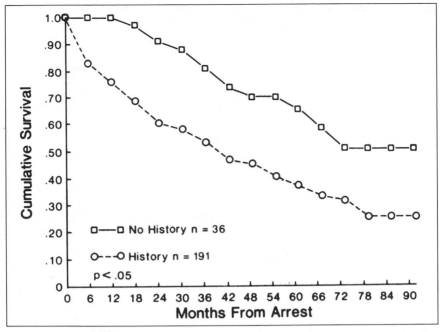

Fig. 4-5. Cumulative survival of resuscitated out-of-hospital cardiac arrest victims related to history of cardiac history before arrest.

work load. The reasons for the cardiomegaly remain unexplained. Conduction system anomalies were present in all but 1 heart. These included persistent fetal dispersion of the atrioventricular node or bundle of His, or both, present in 14 hearts; accessory conduction fiber connections found in 13 cases; and congenital heart block observed in 1 case. These abnormalities were associated with variations in the structure of the cardiac base, suggesting a common aberrant developmental process. Although the functional sig-

TABLE 4-3. *Cardiac deaths in recruits: etiology. Reproduced with permission from Phillips et al.*[75]

	NO. OF DEATHS
Sudden deaths	19
Myocarditis	
Nonrheumatic	4
Vaccinia	1*
Rheumatic	3
Coronary anomalies	3
Hypertrophic cardiomyopathy	2
Floppy mitral valve	1
Shone's syndrome	1
Focal subendocardial fibrosis and calcification with normal	
coronary arteries	1
No etiologic diagnosis	3
Nonsudden deaths	2
Myocardial infarction with normal coronary arteries	1
Myocardial infarction with atherosclerotic coronary arteries	1

* Vaccinia virus in blood was confirmed by electron microscopy.

nificance of these findings has not been established, the conduction system anomalies may be the substrate for sleep-related cardiac arrhythmias and sudden death.

Cardiopulmonary resuscitation

The June 6, 1986, issue of the JAMA was devoted to standards and guidelines for cardiopulmonary resuscitation and emergency cardiac care.[77] The article summarizes a conference held in Dallas in July 1985. Previous national conferences on this subject were held in 1966, 1973, and 1979. The objectives of all these conferences were to define the standards and guidelines. These standards and guidelines have been called by some the most important medical document ever published because of their content, distribution, and widespread acceptance. Reprints of the 1974 and 1980 JAMA standards exceed 5 million copies, and virtually all public and professional training in cardiopulmonary resuscitation and emergency cardiac care has been guided by the outcome of these conferences and the subsequent publication of the standards and guidelines. The conference in 1985 marked the silver anniversary of contemporary cardiopulmonary bypass. The conference was sponsored by the American Heart Association, the American Red Cross, the American College of Cardiology, and the National Heart, Lung, and Blood Institute. Also, representatives from 22 foreign countries actively participated in the meeting. The changes noted between the publication of the 1980 standards and the publication of the present 1986 standards are the following: Because it is an incontrovertible fact that early defibrillation of cardiac arrest victims is associated with survival, the new guidelines recommend that emergency medical technicians traditionally trained only in basic life support also be trained to recognize VF and to learn the skills of defibrillation. This recommendation is couched in the context of strict medical control. Specifically, in the treatment of out-of-hospital VF, 3 immediate and consecutive energy discharges should be administered as soon as the equipment is available in contrast to the 1980 standards that recommended 2 consecutive defibrillation attempts. In the advanced cardiac life support section sufficient data have disproved the efficacy of calcium chloride and isoproterenol in the routine treatment of cardiac arrest and thus their use has been eliminated in this setting. Calcium chloride is still indicated, however, in specific situations such as cardiac arrest related to hyperkalemia, hypocalcemia, or toxic reaction to calcium antagonists. The new standards also markedly modify the use of sodium bicarbonate during cardiac arrest. Instead, other avenues of treatment such as defibrillation, ventilatory support (endotracheal intubation), chest compressions, epinephrine, and antiarrhythmics should be used first, before administering sodium bicarbonate. New drugs have been added to the CPR pharmacy: intravenous nitroglycerin, verapamil, and amrinone. To facilitate drug delivery to the heart, the 1986 guidelines suggest that intravenous lines be inserted only in the antecubital fossa of the arm or in a central vein. If circulation is not readily restored with a peripheral line, then a central line should be inserted by an experienced operator. Ventilations in the intubated cardiac arrest victim no longer have to be synchronized with chest compressions and should be performed at a rate of 12–15/minute. The Adult Basic Life Support section has also been revised. To avoid confusion and simplify teaching, lay persons will be taught only 1-rescuer CPR. Medical professionals, however, will continue to be trained in the 2-rescuer sequence. In addition, lay persons will be taught only the head tilt/chin lift method of opening the airway because of considerations of safety, efficacy, and ease in learning and performing.

A major change in the new standards involved a rethinking of the physiology and application of mouth-to-mouth ventilation to a respiratory arrest victim. The rescuer should now administer 2 initial ventilations of about 1.5 seconds each, instead of previously taught 4 quick, full breaths. For the single rescuer CPR sequence, the compression ventilation ratio remains the same, 15:2, but the number of chest compressions is increased from 60–80/minute to 80–100/minute. In the 2-rescuer sequence, the compression ratio remains 5:1 but the frequency of compressions has been increased from 60/minute to 80–100/minute. Additionally, there is a 1.5-second pause with each ventilation to allow adequate delivery of oxygen.

Regarding foreign body airway obstruction, 2 notable items have been changed. The Heimlich maneuver is designated as a preferred method to dislodge foreign matter from the airway; that is, back blows have been virtually eliminated.

The other revisions include a new subsection that addresses the special needs of the hypothermic arrest victim. The subsection on the near drowning victim discusses the need for Heimlich maneuver to clear the lower airway of water before initiating CPR. The pediatric advanced life support section has been added as a new feature to the 1986 standards. A major change in the neonatal resuscitation guidelines is the elimination of 2 drugs, calcium and atropine, since neither has been shown to be effective during the acute phase of resuscitation. The use of sodium bicarbonate is recommended only during prolonged resuscitation to treat documented metabolic acidosis and is discouraged for brief arrest and episodes of bradycardia. This issue is well worth a thorough reading by all physicians.

Weil and associates[78] from North Chicago, Illinois, investigated the acid-base condition of arterial and mixed venous blood during cardiopulmonary resuscitation (CPR) in 16 critically ill patients who had arterial and PA catheters in place at the time of cardiac arrest. During CPR, the arterial blood pH averaged 7.41, whereas the average mixed venous blood pH was 7.15. The mean arterial partial pressure of carbon dioxide (PCO_2) was 32 mmHg, whereas the mixed venous PCO_2 was 74 mmHg. In a subgroup of 13 patients in whom blood gases were measured before, as well as during, cardiac arrest, arterial pH, PCO_2, and bicarbonate were not significantly changed during arrest. However, mixed venous blood demonstrated striking decreases in pH and increased in PCO_2. The authors concluded that mixed venous blood most accurately reflects the acid-base state during CPR, especially the rapid increase in PCO_2. Arterial blood does not reflect the marked reduction in mixed venous (and therefore tissue) pH, and thus arterial blood gases may fail as appropriate guides for acid-base management in this emergency.

This article was followed by an editorial entitled "Blood Gases" Arterial or Venous? by Relman.[79] Relman concluded that henceforth to monitor during CPR appropriately mixed venous pH and PCO_2 must be measured to determine the acid-base condition of the tissues.

Bachman and associates[80] from Rochester and Duluth, Minnesota, examined 583 cardiac arrests occurring from December 31, 1982–December 31, 1984, in 35 communities in rural areas in northeastern Minnesota. For 9 months before and during the first 3 months of the study, 11 courses in advanced cardiac life support were taught to 225 persons (registered nurses and physicians in the 35 communities). By July 1, 1983, the region had 52 instructors and 311 trained providers of advanced cardiac life support. These authors found that advanced cardiac life support and defibrillation and community programs in cardiopulmonary resuscitation (CPR) had limited success in resuscitating patients with cardiac arrest in the 35 communities. Factors associated with survival included advanced cardiac life support within 16 minutes, ambulance traveling <1 mile (<1.6 km), use of para-medics, CPR within 4 minutes, and a call for help within 2 minutes. The use of technicians trained in defibrillation was associated with a statistically significant increase in hospital admissions, but not in survivors. The study failed to confirm the findings of previous studies of resuscitation in some rural areas. It was consistent, however, with reports that associated poor survival in rural areas with poor response times. No victims of unwitnessed arrests survived. Of the hospital deaths, 80% were due to neurologic causes and overall survival was low.

Survivors after resuscitation

Weaver et al[81] in Seattle, Washington, evaluated patients with witnessed cardiac arrest due to VF to determine factors associated with the likelihood of survival to hospital discharge. The period from collapse until initiation of basic life support and the duration of basic life support before delivery of the first defibrillation shock were shorter in patients surviving compared with those who died (3.6 ± 2.5 -vs- 6.1 ± 3.3 minutes and 4.3 ± 3.3 -vs- 7.3 ± 4.2 minutes). In 942 patients discovered in VF, a linear regression model based on emergency response times was used to estimate expected survival times when the first-responding rescuers were equipped and trained in resuscita-tion procedures, including defibrillation. Expected survival rates were higher with early defibrillation (38 ± 3%) than the observed rate (28 ± 3%). These data suggest that factors affecting response times should be carefully exam-ined by all emergency care systems and improved as much as possible.

Dunn and associates[82] from Belfast, Northern Ireland, carried out an investigation on factors determining survival to leave hospital from VF. In 125 consecutive patients with 173 cardiac arrests due to VF, 53 survived to leave the hospital. At the initial arrest and using univariate analysis, those who had primary VF, had VF <24 hours from the onset of symptoms, re-ceived the first DC shock <1 minute after the onset of VF, who required <4 shocks to terminate the VF, whose first established rhythm within the first minute of correction of VF was AF, sinus rhythm or paced rhythm, or who were not receiving prior antiarrhythmic agents, had a significantly improved survival to leave hospital. To predict survival to leave the hospital using dis-criminant function analysis, the most significant factors ranking in order of importance at the time of the initial arrest were: ≤5 shocks to correct VF, no prior antiarrhythmic therapy, primary VF, and time from onset of VF to first shock <1 minute. For the last arrest, the most significant factors were: no prior cardiac arrest, ≤5 shocks to correct VF, no prior antiarrhythmic ther-apy, and primary VF. The most significant factors measured at the time of the last arrest provided a better prediction of survival to leave the hospital (sensitivity 77%, specificity 75%) than did similarly defined factors for the initial arrest (sensitivity 59%, specificity 89%).

Chadda and associates[83] from New Hyde Park, New York, performed a post–hospital follow-up system based on predetermined antiarrhythmic strategies and telephone transmitters used to record electrocardiograms in managing the post-hospital course and improved survival in patients with a history of out-of-hospital sudden death. All patients underwent therapy guided by serial electrophysiologic testing. Of the 47 patients, 19 used the telephone transmitter system and 28 did not. During follow-up, residual symptomatic and silent ventricular arrhythmia was documented in 78% of patients using telephone transmitters. VT was transmitted in 2 patients—all survived. During an average 15-month follow-up, 1 of 19 patients using the telephone transmitter system died -vs- 12 deaths among the 28 patients who did not use the system (Fig. 1). These results were independent of EF, presence of CHF, amiodarone therapy, and the outcome on electrophysiologic therapy. Thus, patients with a history of out-of-hospital sudden death, discharged after electrophysiologic-guided therapy, require repeated antiarrhythmic dose titration for adverse effects or residual ventricular arrhythmia. Prompt diagnosis and treatment of potentially fatal arrhythmia is crucial and feasible, especially with regular electrocardiographic checks through telephone transmission.

Hallstrom and associates[84] from Seattle, Washington, obtained information about cessation of cigarette smoking in 310 survivors of out-of-hospital cardiac arrest who had been habitual cigarette smokers at the time of the arrest. Patients with CAD were stratified according to mortality risk on the basis of recognized criteria. The expected first-year rate of recurrent arrest ranged from 2–40% among the strata. Life-table analyses showed that reformed smokers had a lower incidence of recurrent arrest than patients who continued to smoke (19 -vs- 27% at 3 years; by 1-sided test adjusted across strata). This effect occurred to varying degrees in all but the highest risk stratum. No differences in survival were observed for mortality due to other causes. It is possible that continued smoking in these patients led to acceleration of an ongoing atherosclerotic process, but the differences in early survival suggest that smoking may also act in the short term to enhance vulnerability to cardiac arrest.

Skale and associates[85] from Indianapolis, Indiana, studied 62 patients aged 15–75 years resuscitated from at least 1 cardiac arrest unrelated to AMI. No patient was taking antiarrhythmic drugs at the time of the initial cardiac arrest. Thirty-five patients had CAD and 27 did not. Before drug therapy, control electrophysiologic studies induced VT in 43 of 58 patients (74%) (30 of 35 with CAD and 17 of 27 without CAD) (Fig. 4-6). At control continuous electrocardiographic monitoring for ≥48 hours, only 19 of 62 patients (31%) had spontaneous VT, 5 of whom had no VT induced at control electrophysiologic study (Fig. 4-6). Mean follow-up was 22 months. Fourteen of 41 patients, 8 of 25 with and 6 of 16 without CAD, had VT suppressed with drugs during serial electrophysiologic testing, and none had a recurrent arrhythmic event. VT was suppressed in 12 of 14 patients receiving conventional drugs. Of 27 patients with VT induced during all drug studies, 6 died from cardiac arrest and 4 had recurrent VT. Drug efficacy in 20 patients was guided by continuous electrocardiographic monitoring, and 4 of 9 patients in whom VT and ventricular pairs were suppressed by drug therapy, as documented by continuous electrocardiographic monitoring for ≥48 hours, died of cardiac arrest. Overall, 26 patients were discharged receiving amiodarone therapy, 5 died of cardiac arrest, and 3 had recurrent sustained VT. It is concluded that in survivors of cardiac arrest, suppression of inducible VT during electrophysiologic testing predicts a favorable outcome, whereas suppression of spontaneous VT and repetitive beats during continuous electrocardiographic monitoring often is associated with recurrence of cardiac arrest. Further, the risk of recurrent cardiac arrest or sustained VT is substantial if VT is initiated at electrophysiologic study, even during amiodarone therapy.

Effect of therapy on prevention

Holmes and participants[86] in the Coronary Artery Surgery Study in Rochester, Minnesota, examined the effect of medical and surgical treatment on subsequent cardiac death in 13,476 patients in the study registry who had significant CAD, operable arteries, and no significant valvular disease. Pa-

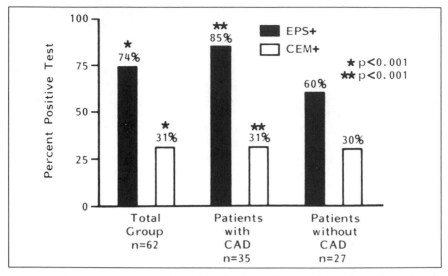

Fig. 4-6. Identification of ventricular tachycardia during the control period. For the total study group and for the group of patients with coronary artery disease (CAD), ventricular tachycardia was induced more often (p <0.001) at control electrophysiologic study (EPS) than it was identified during at least 48 hours of control continuous electrocardiographic monitoring (CEM). EPS$^+$ = ventricular tachycardia induced at EPS; CEM$^+$ = ventricular tachycardia during 48 hours or more of CEM.

tients were assigned to medical or surgical therapy on the basis of clinical judgment and not according to a randomized scheme; therefore, biases associated with unknown variables could not be evaluated. Sudden cardiac death occurred in 452 patients (3.4%) during a mean follow-up of 4.6 years (Fig. 4-7). Five-year survival free of sudden death for medically treated patients was 94%, and that for surgically treated patients was 98%. Twelve baseline clinical, electrocardiographic, and angiographic variables were significantly

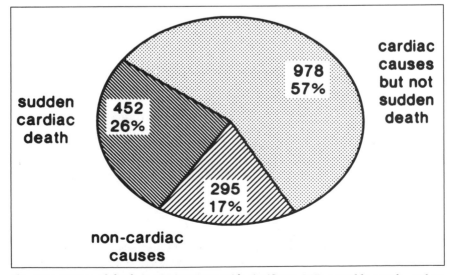

Fig. 4-7. Causes of death in 1725 patients with significant CAD, operable vessels, and no significant valvular heart disease. Reproduced with permission from Holmes et al.[86]

different between patients alive at the last follow-up and those having cardiac death. Data on these variables were available for 11,508 patients. Sudden death occurred in 257 (4.9%) of 5,258 medically treated and 101 (1.6%) of 6,250 surgically treated patients. In a high-risk patient subset with 3-vessel CAD and a history of CHF, 91% of surgically treated patients had not died suddenly compared with 69% of medically treated patients. After Cox survival analysis was used to correct for baseline variables, surgical treatment had an independent effect on sudden death. This reduction was most pronounced in high-risk patients.

Blevins and associates[87] from Detroit, Michigan, studied 33 patients with CAD and frequent, complex ventricular arrhythmias to evaluate factors related to sudden death. Patients with malignant ventricular arrhythmias (sustained VT, resuscitated sudden death, or AMI) were excluded. Baseline data included angiographic EF, segmental wall motion, and Holter evidence of frequent (>30/hour) and complex (repetitive) VPC. Control of ventricular arrhythmias was attempted with conventional or experimental agents and was defined as ≥70% reduction in VPC, ≥90% reduction in couplets, and abolition of nonsustained VT on 2 consecutive Holter tapes. After 24 ± 15 months of follow-up on the single most effective agent, 18 patients survived while 15 patients died suddenly. There was no difference between these groups with respect to age, sex, or baseline ventricular arrhythmias. Survivors had a higher EF (51% -vs- 34%), fewer dyskinetic segments (0.05 -vs- 1.0), and better ventricular arrhythmia control (83% -vs- 40%) than nonsurvivors. By analysis of variance, ventricular arrhythmia control was not independent of EF. The 1-, 2-, and 3-year survival rates were 90%, 90%, and 82% for patients with EF ≥40%, and 22%, 11%, and 11% for those with EF <40% and uncontrolled ventricular arrhythmias. It was concluded that LV function and ventricular arrhythmia control are dependent determinants of sudden death, and this "intermediate" risk group consists of 1) low-risk patients with EF ≥40% (Fig. 4-8), in whom a multicenter placebo-controlled trial

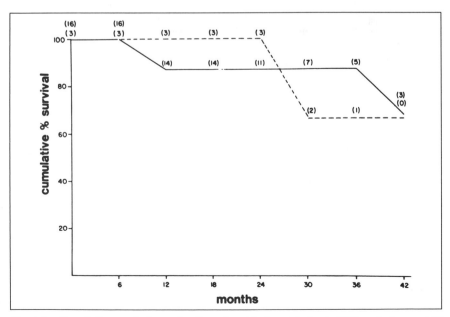

Fig. 4-8. Cumulative survival as a function of ventricular arrhythmia (VA) control among 19 patients with left ventricular ejection fraction ≥40%. *Solid line* = VA controlled; *dashed line* = VA uncontrolled. Survival rates were not significantly different at any 6-month interval. Reproduced with permission from Blevins et al.[87]

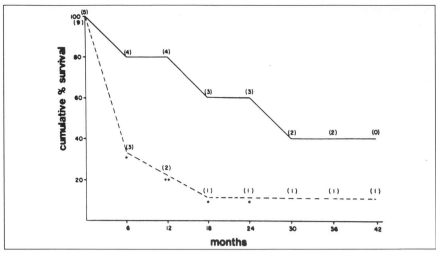

Fig. 4-9. Cumulative survival as a function of ventricular arrhythmia (VA) control among 14 patients with left ventricular ejection fraction <40%. *Solid line* = VA controlled; *dashed line* = VA uncontrolled. *p <0.05 and **p <0.005 by comparison of survival at 6-month intervals. Reproduced with permission from Blevins et al.[87]

may be justified, and 2) high-risk patients with EF <40% (Fig. 4-9) for whom no effective agent can be identified by noninvasive means and in whom a more aggressive approach may be needed.

LONG QT INTERVAL SYNDROME

Moss[88] from Rochester, New York, reviewed causes of the prolonged QT-interval syndrome and strategies for the prevention and treatment of malignant arrhythmias in this population (Table 4-4).

The Romano-Ward prolonged QT syndrome is associated with an abnormality of ventricular recovery, rendering the patients susceptible to life-

TABLE 4-4. *Etiology of prolonged QT interval syndromes. Reproduced with permission from Moss.[88]*

Congenital long QT syndrome
    Hereditary form
        Jervell-Lange-Nielsen syndrome
        Romano-Ward syndrome
    Sporadic type
Acquired long QT syndrome
    Drug induced
        Antiarrhythmic agents
        Phenothiazines
        Tricyclic antidepressants
        Lithium carbonate
    Metabolic/electrolyte abnormalities
    Very-low-energy diets
    Central and autonomic nervous system disorders
    Miscellaneous
        Coronary heart disease
        Mitral valve prolapse

threatening ventricular arrhythmias. The pathophysiology has not been clearly defined. It has been proposed that the syndrome involves disparity of right and left cardiac sympathetic activity, with the left side dominant. This could be the result of left-sided overactivity or right underactivity. The right-sided nerves contain the chronotropic fibers that affect heart rate. A deficiency of the effect of the right-sided nerves might, therefore, be manifest by slower heart rates. Vincent[89] from Salt Lake City, Utah, examined the heart rates at rest of 58 Romano-Ward syndrome patients compared with those of 255 age-matched normal controls. A significant difference in heart rate at rest was observed between the Romano-Ward syndrome patients and the normal controls in newborns and children up through age 3 years. No difference was present in older children or in adults. The data are consistent with right-sided sympathetic deficiency manifest by a slower heart rate at birth and during early years of life, when sympathetic tone is high and contributes to heart rate at rest, but not in older children or in adults in whom heart rate at rest is principally under parasympathetic control.

Quinidine therapy is 1 of the most common causes of the acquired long QT syndrome and torsades de pointes. In reviewing clinical data in 24 patients with the quinidine-associated long QT syndrome, 20 of whom had torsades de pointes, Roden and colleagues[90] from Nashville, Tennessee, delineated several heretofore unreported or underemphasized features: 1) This adverse drug reaction occurred either in patients who were being treated for frequent nonsustained ventricular arrhythmias or for AF or atrial flutter. 2) In patients being treated for AF, torsades de pointes occurred only after conversion to sinus rhythm. 3) Although most patients had the syndrome within days of starting quinidine, 4 had torsades de pointes during long-term quinidine therapy, usually in association with hypokalemia. 4) Because of the large experience with this entity at their institution, they were able to estimate the risk as at least 1.5% per year. 5) Twenty of the 24 patients had at least 1 major, easily identifiable, associated risk factor including serum potassium below 3.5 mEq/liter (4 patients); serum potassium between 3.5 and 3.9 mEq/liter (9 patients); high-grade AV block (4 patients); and marked underlying, (unrecognized) QT prolongation (2 patients). Plasma quinidine concentrations were low, being at or below the lower limit of the therapeutic range in half of the patients. The electrocardiographic features typically included absence of marked QRS widening, marked QT prolongation (by definition), and a stereotypic series of cycle length changes just before onset of torsades de pointes. Torsades de pointes started after the T wave of a markedly prolonged QT interval that followed a cycle that had been markedly prolonged (usually by a postectopic pause). It was concluded that the quinidine-associated long QT syndrome that can be accompanied by a potentially lethal ventricular tachyarrhythmia is a common adverse drug reaction with a distinctive spectrum of plasma quinidine concentrations, electrocardiographic manifestations, and associated conditions. Based on these data, the investigators advocate close attention to serum potassium concentrations and to QT intervals, particularly following abrupt decreases in heart rate; and suggest initiation of quinidine therapy on an inpatient basis only.

BUNDLE BRANCH BLOCK

Liao et al[91] in Chicago, Illinois, studied 1,960 white men, aged 40–56 years, without apparent heart disease and with 11 years of annual rest electrocardiograms and 20-year mortality data. Incomplete right BBB was found in 134 men (7%) at entry. During follow-up, 222 men had incomplete right BBB, an incidence rate of 14%. Left-axis deviation of −30° or less was more frequent in men with than in those without incomplete block at entry (8.2 -vs- 2.4%). Men with left-axis deviation had a higher incidence of incomplete right BBB and men having incomplete right BBB had a significantly greater risk of developing left-axis deviation. Men with incomplete right BBB also had a greater likelihood of having complete right BBB. The 11-year incidence rate of complete block was 5% for men with baseline incomplete block and 0.7% for those without incomplete block. Complete right BBB developed in 2 of 220 incident cases of incomplete block, but in none of 440 control men matched by age and duration of follow-up. Thus, these data suggest that incomplete right BBB is frequently a manifestation of a primary abnormality of the cardiac conduction system in middle-aged men.

ATRIOVENTRICULAR BLOCK

The long-term prognosis of first-degree heart block in the absence of organic heart disease has not been clearly defined. Mymin and associates[92] from Winnipeg, Canada, addressed the question in a 30-year longitudinal study of 3,983 healthy men. These authors identified 52 cases that were present on entry into the study and 124 incident cases during follow-up. The incidence increased steadily after age 40 and was 1.13/1,000 person-years over the entire period. Two-thirds of the cases had only moderate prolongation of the PR interval (0.22–0.23 second). They compared 4 age-matched controls with each case for histories of scarlet fever, rheumatic fever, diphtheria, smoking, BP, and body-mass index. No significant differences were found. Likewise, mortality from all causes did not differ between cases and controls. Although somewhat higher rates of morbidity and mortality from ischemic heart disease were observed in the cases than in the controls, the differences were not significant. Progression to higher grades of heart block occurred in only 2 cases. In view of the prognostic findings and the rare occurrence of advanced degrees of heart block, the authors concluded that primary first-degree heart block with moderate PR prolongation is a benign condition. This conclusion may not apply, however, to persons with more marked prolongation of the PR interval, a very rare condition.

The clinical, electrocardiographic, and electrophysiologic findings of 35 consecutive patients with second- and third-degree intra-His block with normal QRS complexes were examined in a study by Mangiardi and associates[93] from Torino, Italy. The follow-up period varied between 12 and 120 months (mean 45). Underlying heart disease was present in 43% of patients. Electrocardiograms were characterized by both second-degree type I and type II AV block, normal, or slightly prolonged PR interval of the conducted beats or of the first conducted beat of a Wenckebach sequence, and by subtle changes in the initial forces of the QRS complexes of the escape beats. Electrophysiologic study showed normal sinus and AV node function and normal infra-His conduction in all patients. In 4 patients repetitive bradycardia-dependent intra-His block was induced. Thirty-two patients were permanently paced soon after the initial evaluation and 3 during the follow-up period. Total long-term mortality rate was 23%. No patient had BBB.

Alpert et al[94] in Columbia, Missouri, determined whether survival after permanent ventricular demand (VVI) pacing differs from survival after permanent dual chamber (DVI or DDD) pacing in patients with chronic high-degree AV block (Mobitz II or trifascicular block) in 132 patients receiving a

VVI pacemaker (group 1) and 48 patients who received a DVI or DDD pacemaker (group 2) who were followed for 1–5 years. The predicted cumulative survival rate at 1, 3, and 5 years was 89, 76, and 73%, respectively, for patients in group 1 and 95, 82, and 70%, respectively for patients in group 2. In patients with preexisting CHF, the predicted cumulative survival rate at 1, 3, and 5 years was 85, 66, and 47%, respectively, for group 1 (n = 53) and 94, 81, and 69%, respectively, for group 2 patients (n = 20). The 5-year predicted cumulative survival rate was lower in group 1 patients with preexisting CHF than in group 2 patients with the same condition (p <0.02). There was no difference in 5-year cumulative survival rates between group 1 and 2 patients without CHF. Thus, permanent dual chamber pacing enhances survival to a greater extent than does permanent ventricular demand pacing in patients with high-degree AV block and CHF.

SYNCOPE FROM CAROTID SINUS HYPERSENSITIVITY

Sugrue et al[95] in Rochester, Minnesota, evaluated 56 consecutive patients with carotid sinus hypersensitivity and syncope in whom 24-hour ambulatory monitoring and intracardiac electrophysiologic study revealed no other cause for the syncope. Mean duration of symptoms was 44 months and a mean number of episodes was 4.0 (range 1–20). Syncope recurred in 3 of 13 patients who received no therapy, in 2 of 23 patients receiving a pacemaker, and in 4 of 20 patients taking anticholinergic drugs. Thus, the incidences for recurrent syncope at follow-up were 27, 9, and 22%, respectively, during a follow-up period of 6–120 months (median 40 months). Two-thirds of the patients receiving no treatment were asymptomatic as were all 9 patients with syncope associated with cardioinhibitory response to carotid sinus massage who received AV sequential pacemakers. Thus, although pacing was effective in abolishing syncope, its use should be reserved for recurrent episodes of syncope and syncope associated with a cardioinhibitory response to carotid sinus massage because of the high rate of spontaneous remission of symptoms.

PACEMAKERS AND CARDIOVERTERS

Mechelen and associates[96] from Rotterdam, The Netherlands, performed electrophysiologic studies before DDD pacemaker implantation in 50 patients with symptomatic heart block. The patients were separated into 2 groups. Group I consisted of patients with intact retrograde conduction and group II consisted of patients with blocked retrograde conduction. After pacemaker implantation, postventricular atrial refractory periods in patients in group I were programmed at 50–100 ms, in excess of the retrograde conduction times measured during electrophysiologic studies. In group II patients, postventricular atrial refractory periods were routinely programmed at 300 ms. During follow-up, patients visited the outpatient clinic at 3-month intervals for noninvasive assessment of the prevalence of retrograde conduction, and to test the inducibility of pacemaker-mediated tachycardias. The mean follow-up of group I (15 patients) was 27 ± 10 months, whereas the mean follow-up of group II (35 patients) was 19 ± 9 months. The mean number of noninvasive tests performed during follow-up was 8 ± 3 per patient for group I and 5 ± 3 per patient for group II. In group I, retrograde conduction remained intact in 12 patients. In 29 of 31 patients in group II, retrograde conduction remained absent. In 4 patients in group II, chronic AF occurred during follow-up. Chronic AF did not occur in any patient in group I. During serial electrophysiologic testing, no pacemaker-mediated tachycardias could be induced in any patient in group I or II. These results suggest that electrophysiologic studies performed before pacemaker implantation reliably predict the prevalence of retrograde conduction during follow-up of patients with symptomatic heart block and that adjusted atrial refractory periods of the pulse generator at implantation prevent the induction of pacemaker-mediated tachycardias during serial electrophysiologic testing.

Palomo and associates[97] from Miami, Florida, analyzed data retrospectively from 518 consecutive cardiac catheterizations to test the value of prophylactic pacemaker insertion during coronary angiography and to compare the frequency of arrhythmic complications in patients with and without pacemakers. In patients without pacing, 1 episode of VF occurred, which responded promptly to defibrillation. Sinus bradycardia (<30 beats/minute for 10 seconds) was recorded in 74 patients (27%) and required treatment in 30 (11%). No patient required or would have benefited from pacemaker placement. Of the 245 patients with prophylactic pacemakers, there was an increased incidence of all ventricular (9 -vs- 1) and supraventricular (5 -vs- 0) arrhythmias. Pacemaker-associated induction of VF occurred in 2 patients and was clearly related to electrical stimulation during a normally nonvulnerable period of the cardiac cycle. In conclusion, routine prophylactic pacemaker insertion during coronary angiography is not warranted in patients with normal sinus rhythm and normal AV conduction. More information is needed to determine if pacing is needed in patients with conduction system disease.

Miles and colleagues[98] in Indianapolis, Indiana, followed 11 patients from 5–27 months (mean 15) after implantation of a permanent transvenous low-energy synchronized *cardioverter* to evaluate both long-term reproducibility of VT induction via noninvasive programmed electrical stimulation with the cardioverter and efficacy of cardioversion. Induction and termination of VT were attempted at implantation and approximately every 3 months thereafter. All patients had CAD and were receiving antiarrhythmic drug therapy (amiodarone in 8). VT cycle length, morphology, and mode of induction were reproducible on multiple occasions in 9 patients; clinical VT was induced inconsistently in 2 patients. Multiple VT episodes in 5 patients had one morphology, whereas 2 morphologies occurred in 6 patients. Synchronization of the shock within the QRS complex and RV effective refractory periods determined via the cardioverter remained constant over the follow-up period. VT was terminated on every occasion in 9 patients and in 8 of 9 occasions in 1 patient. Tachycardia was accelerated on 3 of 5 occasions in 1 patient. Consistently effective cardioversion energy (0.2–2.0 J) increased modestly in 4 patients. The investigators concluded that 1) patients with inducible monomorphic VT usually have sustained VT with similar characteristics inducible over a period of time and 2) cardioversion and sensing functions of the cardioverter remain relatively stable over time.

Saksena and associates[99] from Newark, New Jersey, evaluated the Cordis Omni-Orthocor model 234A, an *implantable antitachycardia system*, in 13 patients. Two patients had recurrent sustained SVT and 11 had VT. The system was used for SVT or VT termination (group 1: SVT, 2 patients; VT, 4 patients) or for demand pacing and noninvasive electrophysiologic studies for tachycardia induction and serial electrophysiologic testing alone (group 2: VT, 7 patients). The overdriver was used successfully in 4 of 6 patients in group 1 for repeated tachycardia termination (SVT and VT) during a mean follow-up period of 18 months. One patient had 1 sustained VT episode unresponsive to pacing and 1 patient had no recurrence of tachycardia. Tachycardia termination zones varied when using the system in 2 patients receiving long-term amiodarone therapy. Eighteen noninvasive electrophysiologic studies for serial drug testing were performed, 4 in group 1 and 14 in group 2. Clinical tachycardia was induced and successfully terminated by use of the overdriver in 12 studies. It was concluded that implantable antitachycardia systems can be used successfully for noninvasive tachycardia induction and termination and for reliable serial electrophysiologic studies. Such systems provide improved patient safety and acceptability and are reasonable in cost.

Marchlinski and associates[100] from Philadelphia, Pennsylvania, inserted an *automatic implantable cardioverter-defibrillator* in 26 patients with refractory ventricular arrhythmias. A patch lead only was placed during arrhythmia surgery in 7 other patients. During 13 ± 6 months, the device discharged in 10 patients because of a sustained ventricular arrhythmia. No sudden deaths occurred. There were 31 complications in 17 patients, including postoperative refractory CHF, coronary artery erosion, subclavian vein thrombosis, postoperative stroke after conversion of AF, atelectasis with pneumonia, symptomatic pleural effusions, and infection at the generator site. The cardioverter-defibrillator discharged in 9 asymptomatic patients, failed to terminate VF during postoperative testing in 3 patients, and had premature battery failure in 4 patients. Tachycardia slowing during chronic amiodarone therapy and unipolar ventricular pacing during VF precluded or delayed arrhythmia sensing. Thus, the cardioverter-defibrillator can be life-saving, but its potential complications and interactions with antiarrhythmic drugs and pacemakers must be considered at patient selection.

Weaver and associates[101] from Seattle, Washington, treated 260 patients in cardiac arrest with an *automatic external defibrillator* by first-responding firefighters before arrival of paramedics. On average, first responders arrived 5 minutes before paramedics. Of 118 patients with ventricular fibrillation, 91 (77%) were administered shocks, 21 (23%) of whom had return of pulse and BP by the time paramedics arrived. Fifty-six (62%) were admitted to the hospital and 30 (33%) survived. The survival rate for all 118 victims discovered with VF was 27%. The device correctly classified the initial and all subsequent rhythms in 92 patients with asystole, 46 with electromechanical dissociation, and 22 others with presumed respiratory arrest; it did not deliver any inappropriate shocks to patients or to the rescuers using the device. An automatic external defibrillator can be used by first responders as an adjunct to basic life support, and its use may improve survival by shortening the time to defibrillation.

An initial experience with the use of the *automatic implantable cardioverter-defibrillator* was described by Thurer and colleagues[102] from Miami, Florida. Twelve patients received the device, 1 death occurred during a mean follow up of 15 months, and it was due to causes other than arrhythmias. Appropriate device discharge that terminated a malignant arrhythmia occurred in 9 patients. The observed survival (92%) far exceeds that to be expected in survivors of sudden death treated by conventional means. There have been no operative deaths, morbidity has been minimal, although 3 reoperations were required in 2 patients because of lead dislodgement. The authors recommend median sternotomy for placement of the required leads and patches. They suggest that the 2-patch configuration is superior to the intravenous superior vena cava spring-LV patch configuration. Bipolar sensing was noted on 1 occasion. The authors stress the possible complications when concomitant pacing is necessary. These problems are potentially more common when unipolar pacing is used because of the magnitude of the pacemaker stimulus artifact. Sensing leads of the defibrillator should be placed at some distance from the pacing leads.

External noninvasive cardiac pacing offers a rapid and simple method of pacing the heart during an emergency. It has been suggested that early use of cardiac pacing for bradycardia or asystole may improve survival in patients who have cardiac arrest. To investigate this possibility, Knowlton and Falk[103] from Boston, Massachusetts, studied 58 consecutive episodes of cardiac arrest occurring on medical wards or emergency room. Twenty-six episodes underwent external noninvasive pacing or bradycardia or asystole refractory to standard drugs. Only 2 patients survived, and survival could be directly attributed to pacing in only 1 of them. Of the 32 episodes not undergoing pacing, 23 had transient asystole or bradycardia, 13 of which rapidly responded to medications. The 17 cases (53%) not undergoing pacing survived. In conclusion, when bradycardia or asystole during cardiac arrest fails to respond to standard pharmacologic measures, it is an indicator of severe myocardial damage, and attempts at cardiac pacing rarely improve survival.

Nishimura and associates[104] from Osaka, Japan, determined the optimal mode of *transesophageal atrial pacing* by clinical electrophysiologic studies in 15 healthy adult volunteers. The point at which the unipolar atrial electrogram was biphasic and largest in amplitude (35.4 ± 1.6 cm from the incisors) was considered the best stimulation site for atrial pacing. The stimulation threshold on bipolar pacing (using the proximal pole as cathode and the distal pole as anode) at this site was 27 ± 7 mA, which was significantly lower than that on unipolar cathodal stimulation (41 ± 8 mA). Although the stimulation threshold tended to be higher with a No. 10Fr electrode catheter (30 ± 5 mA) than with a No. 6Fr catheter (27 ± 7 mA), the difference was statistically insignificant. When the interpolar distance in bipolar stimulation was varied in 5 steps from 12–80 mm, the threshold was lowest at the distance of 24 mm. Of the 10 pulse durations tested, ranging from 0.25–128 ms, 8 ms appeared most desirable in minimizing the total amount of current and chest discomfort accompanying the pacing. With the optimal site, interpolar distance and pulse duration, transesophageal atrial pacing was successfully performed in all patients, without producing significant complications such as chest pain. Transesophageal atrial pacing is noninvasive, technically simple and efficient, and may be valuable in the diagnosis and treatment of various cardiac arrhythmias.

Despite the apparent lack of biologic effects of *magnetic resonance imaging* (MRI), the safety of performing MRI in patients with implanted electrical devices such as pacemakers has not been convincingly demonstrated. Specifically, the function of a variety of more advanced *DDD pacemakers* and the effect of higher magnetic and radio frequency field strengths has not been reported. Erlebacher and associates[105] from New York and Bronx, New York, tested 4 different DDD pacemakers (Cordis 233F, Intermedic 283-01, Medtronic 7000A, and Pacesetter 283) in a saline phantom under several conditions and with various imaging sequences. Pacemaker output was monitored using electrocardiographic telemetry. All units paced normally in the static magnetic field. However, during imaging, all units malfunctioned, with total inhibition of atrial and ventricular output in 3 of the pacemakers. In the fourth pacemaker, ventricular backup pacing was activated at high radio frequency pulse repetition rates. However, the MRI scanner could trigger atrial output in this pacemaker at rates of up to 800/minute. All malfunctions were a result of radio frequency interference, whereas gradient and static magnetic fields had no effect. Thus, despite magnetic field strengths adequate to close pacemaker reed switches, radio frequency interference during MRI may cause total inhibition of atrial and ventricular output in

DDD pacemakers, and can also cause dangerous atrial pacing at high rates. MRI should be avoided in patients with these DDD pacemakers.

The inability of cardiac pacemakers to selectively reject retrograde P waves limits the usefulness of *dual-chamber pacemakers* (because of the possibility of endless loop tachycardias) and of antitachycardia devices that use a dual-chamber-sensing algorithm. Pannizzo and associates[106] from Bronx, New York, determined selective sensing parameters, amplitude, slew rate, and configuration of anterograde and retrograde atrial electrograms in 34 patients undergoing dual-chamber pacemaker implant—31 with unipolar and 3 with bipolar units. All anterograde and retrograde pairs were measurably different. All 34 cases had measurable anterograde/retrograde amplitude differences; 30 of the unipolar cases (96.8%) and all bipolar cases displayed anterograde/retrograde amplitude differences of at least 0.25 mV. Thirty of the unipolar cases (96.8%) and 2 bipolar cases had measurable slew rate differences. Configuration differed in 14 of 31 (45.2%) of unipolar and in 2 bipolar cases. A combined criterion with 0.25 mV sensitivity steps (available in at least 2 presently available pacemakers) and 0.5 V/s slew rate gradations (through the use of externally programmable filters) would allow the discrimination of retrograde from anterograde depolarizations in all 34 cases. With the use of amplitude and slew rate differences, it is therefore possible to reject retrograde P waves while sensing anterograde P waves with current technology.

References

1. HAMMILL SC, SUGRUE DD, GERSH BJ, PORTER CJ, OSBORN MJ, WOOD DL, HOLMES DR: Clinical intracardiac electrophysiologic testing: Technique, diagnostic indications, and therapeutic uses. Mayo Clin Proc 1986 (June); 61:478–503.

2. STEWART RB, BARDY GH, GREENE HL: Wide complex tachycardia; misdiagnosis and outcome after emergent therapy. Ann Intern Med 1986 (May); 104:766–771.

3. SCHNITTGER I, RODRIGUEZ IM, WINKLE RA: Esophageal electrocardiography: A new technology revives an old technique. Am J Cardiol 1986 (Mar 1); 57:604–607.

4. WANG F, LIEN W, FONG T, LIN J, CHERNG J, CHEN J, CHEN J: Terminal cardiac electrical activity in adults who die without apparent cardiac disease. Am J Cardiol 1986 (Sept 1) 58:491–495.

5. KANTELIP JP, SAGE E, DUCHENE-MARULLAZ P: Findings on ambulatory electrocardiographic monitoring in subjects older than 80 years. Am J Cardiol 1986 (Feb 15); 57:398–401.

6. TRESCH DD, FLEG JL: Unexplained sinus bradycardia: clinical significance and long-term prognosis in apparently healthy persons older than 40 years. Am J Cardiol 1986 (Nov 1); 58:1009–1013.

7. ROY D, MARCHAND E, GAGNÉ P, CHABOT M, CARTIER R: Usefulness of anticoagulant therapy in the prevention of embolic complications of atrial fibrillation. Am Heart J 1986 (Nov); 112:1039–1043.

8. DECARLI C, SPROUSE G, LAROSA JC: Serum magnesium levels in symptomatic atrial fibrillation and their relation to rhythm control by intravenous digoxin. Am J Cardiol 1986 (Apr 15); 57:956–959.

9. PITCHER D, PAPOUCHADO M, JAMES MA, REES JR: Twenty-four hour ambulatory electrocardiography in patients with chronic atrial fibrillation. Br Med J 1986 (Mar); 292:594.

10. ROTH A, HARRISON E, MITANI G, COHEN J, RAHIMTOOLA SH, ELKAYAM U: Efficacy and safety of medium- and high-dose diltiazem alone and in combination with digoxin for control of heart rate at rest and during exercise in patients with chronic atrial fibrillation. Circulation 1986 (Feb); (73:2):316–324.

11. BORGEAT A, GOY J, MAENDLY R, KAUFMANN U, GRBIC M, SIGWART U: Flecainide versus quinidine for conversion of atrial fibrillation to sinus rhythm. Am J Cardiol 1986 (Sept 1); 58:496–498.

12. Gold RL, Haffajee CI, Charos G, Sloan K, Baker S, Alpert JS: Amiodarone for refractory atrial fibrillation. Am J Cardiol 1986 (Jan 1); 57:124–127.
13. Greenberg ML, Kelly TA, Lerman BB, DiMarco JP: Atrial pacing for conversion of atrial flutter. Am J Cardiol 1986 (July 1); 58:95–99.
14. Milstein S, Sharma AD, Klein GJ: Electrophysiologic profile of asymptomatic Wolff-Parkinson-White Pattern. Am J Cardiol 1986 (May 1); 57:1097–1100.
15. Sintetos AL, Roark SF, Smith MS, McCarthy EA, Lee KL, Pritchett ELC: Incidence of symptomatic tachycardia in untreated patients with paroxysmal supraventricular tachycardia. Arch Intern Med 1986 (Nov); 146:2205–2209.
16. Roark SF, McCarthy EA, Lee KL, Pritchett ELC: Observations on the occurrence of atrial fibrillation in paroxysmal supraventricular tachycardia. Am J Cardiol 1986 (Mar 1); 57:571–575.
17. Packer DL, Bardy GH, Worley SJ, Smith MS, Cobb FR, Coleman E, Gallagher JJ, German LD: Tachycardia-induced cardiomyopathy: a reversible form of left ventricular dysfunction. Am J Cardiol 1986 (Mar 1); 57:563–570.
18. Nicklas JM, DiCarlo LA, Koller PT, Morady F, Diltz EA, Shenker Y, Grekin RJ: Plasma levels of immunoreactive atrial natriuretic factor increase during supraventricular tachycardia. Am Heart J 1986 (Nov); 112:923–928.
19. Kim SS, Lal R, Ruffy R: Treatment of paroxysmal reentrant supraventricular tachycardia with flecainide acetate. Am J Cardiol 1986 (July 1); 58:80–85.
20. Shen EN, Keung E, Huycke E, Dohrmann ML, Nguyen N, Morady F, Sung RJ: Intravenous propafenone for termination of reentrant supraventricular tachycardia: a placebo-controlled, randomized, double-blind, cross-over study. Ann Intern Med 1986 (Nov); 105:655–661.
21. The Esmolol Research Group. Intravenous esmolol for the treatment of supraventricular tachyarrhythmia: results of a multicenter, baseline-controlled safety and efficacy study in 160 patients. Am Heart J 1986 (Sept); 112:498–505.
22. Steinberg JS, Katz RJ, Somberg JC, Keefe D, Laddu AR, Burge J: Safety and efficacy of flestolol, a new ultrashort-acting beta-adrenergic blocking agent, for supraventricular tachyarrhythmias. Am J Cardiol 1986 (Nov 1); 58:1005–1008.
23. Rose JS, Bhandari A, Rahimtoola SH, Wu D: Effective termination of reentrant supraventricular tachycardia by single dose oral combination therapy with pindolol and verapamil. Am Heart J 1986 (Oct); 112:759–765.
24. Davis J, Scheinman M, Ruder MA, Griffin JC, Herre JM, Finkebeiner WE, Chin MC, Eldar E: Ablation of cardiac tissues by an electrode catheter technique for treatment of ectopic supraventricular tachycardia in adults: Circulation (Nov); 74:1044–1053.
25. Deal BJ, Miller SM, Scagliotti D, Prechel D, Gallastegui JL, Hariman RJ: Ventricular tachycardia in a young population without overt heart disease. Circulation 1986 (June); 73(6):1111–1118.
26. Sokoloff NM, Spielman SR, Greenspan AM, Rae AP, Porter S, Lowenthal DT, Hakki AH, Iskandrian AS, Kay HR, Horowitz LN. Plasma norepinephrine in exercise-induced ventricular tachycardia. J Am Coll Cardiol 1986 (July); 8:11–17.
27. Morady F, DiCarlo LA Jr, Halter JB, de Buitleir M, Krol RB, Baerman JM: The plasma catecholamine response to ventricular tachycardia induction and external countershock during electrophysiologic testing. J Am Coll Cardiol 1986 (Sept); 8:584–591.
28. Bashore TM, Rasor T, Rolfe SJ, Schaal SF, Stine RA, Diblasio GH, Hatton PA, Shaffer P: Localization of the site of ventricular premature complexes by radionuclide angiographic phase imaging. Am J Cardiol 1986 (Sept 1); 58:503–511.
29. Rosenfeld LE, McPherson CA, Kennedy EE, Stark SI, Batsford WP: Ventricular tachycardia induction: comparison of triple extrastimuli with an abrupt change in ventricular drive cycle length. Am Heart J 1986 (May); 111:868–874.
30. Herre JM, Mann DE, Luck JC, Magro SA, Figali S, Breen T, Wyndham CRC: Effect of increased current, multiple pacing sites and number of extrastimuli on induction of ventricular tachycardia. Am J Cardiol 1986 (Jan 1); 57:102–107.
31. Estes NAM, Garan H, McGovern B, Ruskin JN: Influence of drive cycle length during programmed stimulation on induction of ventricular arrhythmias: analysis of 403 patients. Am J Cardiol 1986 (Jan 1); 57:108–112.
32. Modray F, DiCarlo LA, Baerman JM, Buitleir M: Comparison of coupling intervals that induce clinical and nonclinical forms of ventricular tachycardia during programmed stimulation. Am J Cardiol 1986 (June 1); 57:1269–1273.

33. AMANN FW, BLATT CM, PODRID PJ, LOWN B: Relationship between ease of inducibility of arrhythmia with electrophysiologic testing and response to antiarrhythmic therapy. Am Heart J 1986 (Apr); 111:625–631.

34. MAHMUD R, DENKER S, LEHMANN MH, TCHOU P, DONGAS J, AKHTAR M: Incidence and clinical significance of ventricular fibrillation induced with single and double ventricular extrastimuli. Am J Cardiol 1986 (July 1); 58:75–79.

35. KIM SG, SEIDEN SW, FELDER SD, WASPE LE, FISHER JD: Is programmed stimulation of value in predicting the long-term success of antiarrhythmic therapy for ventricular tachycardias? N Engl J Med 1986 (Aug 7); 315:356–362.

36. ANDERSON JL, MASON JW: Testing the efficacy of antiarrhythmic drugs. N Engl J Med 1986 (Aug 7); 315:391–393.

37. GARAN H, STAVENS CS, MCGOVERN B, KELLY E, RUSKIN JN: Reproducibility of ventricular tachycardia suppression by antiarrhythmic drug therapy during serial electrophysiologic testing in coronary artery disease. Am J Cardiol 1986 (Nov 1); 58:977–980.

38. LOMBARDI F, STEIN J, PODRID PJ, GRABOYS TB, LOWN B: Daily reproducibility of electrophysiologic test results in malignant ventricular arrhythmia. Am J Cardiol 1986 (Jan 1); 57:96–101.

39. WYNN J, TORRES V, FLOWERS D, MIZRUCHI M, KEEFE D, MIURA D, SOMBERG J: Antiarrhythmic drug efficacy at electrophysiology testing: predictive effectiveness of procainamide and flecainide. Am Heart J 1986 (Apr); 111:632–638.

40. RODEN DM, WOOSLEY RL: Flecainide. N Engl J Med 1986 (July 3); 315:36–41.

41. FLECAINIDE VENTRICULAR TACHYCARDIA STUDY GROUP: Treatment of resistant ventricular tachycardia with flecainide acetate. Am J Cardiol 1986 (June 1); 57:1299–1304.

42. MORGANROTH J, ANDERSON JL, GENTZKOW GD: Classification by type of ventricular arrhythmia predicts frequency of adverse cardiac events from flecainide. J Am Coll Cardiol 1986 (Sept); 8:607–615.

43. LAL R, CHAPMAN PD, NACCARELLI GV, SCHECHTMAN KB, RINKENBERGER RL, TROUP PJ, KIM SS, DOUGHERTY AH: Flecainide in the treatment of nonsustained ventricular tachycardia. Ann Intern Med 1986 (Oct); 105:493–498.

44. MORGANROTH J, POOL P, MILLER R, HSU PH, LEE I, CLARK DM, ENCAINIDE RESEARCH GROUP: Dose-response range of encainide for benign and potentially lethal ventricular arrhythmias. Am J Cardiol 1986 (Apr 1); 57:769–774.

45. SOMBERG JC, LAUX B, WYNN J, KEEFE D, MIURA DS: Lorcainide therapy in a cardiac arrest population. Am Heart J 1986 (Apr); 111:648–653.

46. HOHNLOSER SH, LANGE HW, RAEDER EA, PODRID PJ, LOWN B: Short- and long-term therapy with tocainide for malignant ventricular tachyarrhythmias. Circulation 1986 (Jan); 73(1):143–149.

47. KIM SG, FELDER SD, WASPE LE, FISHER JD: Electrophysiologic effects and clinical efficacy of mexiletine used alone or in combination with class 1A agents for refractory recurrent ventricular tachycardias or ventricular fibrillation. Am J Cardiol 1986 (Sept 1); 58:485–490.

48. LUI HK, HARRIS FJ, CHAN MC, LEE G, MASON DT: Comparison of intravenous mexiletine and lidocaine for the treatment of ventricular arrhythmias. Am Heart J 1986 (Dec); 112:1153–1158.

49. HAMMILL SC, SORENSON PB, WOOD DL, SUGRUE DD, OSBORN MJ, GERSH BJ, HOLMES DR: Propafenone for the treatment of refractory complex ventricular ectopic activity. Mayo Clin Proc 1986 (Feb); 61:98–103.

50. MORGANROTH J: Intravenous atenolol for ventricular arrhythmias. Am J Cardiol 1986 (Sept 1) page 499–502.

51. MORGANROTH J, DUCHIN KL: Effectiveness of low-dose nadolol for ventricular arrhythmias. Am J Cardiol 1986 (Aug 1); 58:273–278.

52. ANDERSON JL, ASKINS JC, GILBERT EM, MILLER RH, KEEFE DL, SOMBERG JC, FREEDMAN RA, HAFT LR, MASON JW, LESSEM JN: Multicenter trial of sotalol for suppression of frequent, complex ventricular arrhythmias: a double-blind, randomized, placebo-controlled evaluation of two doses. J Am Coll Cardiol 1986 (Oct); 8:752–762.

53. SMITH WM, LUBBE WF, WHITLOCK RM, MERCER J, RUTHERFORD JD, ROCHE AH: Long-term tolerance of amidarone treatment for cardiac arrhythmias. Am J Cardiol 1986 (June 1); 57:1288–1293.

54. MARCHLINSKI F, BUXTON A, MILLER MM, VASALLO JA, FLORES BT, JOSEPHSON ME: Amiodarone versus amiodarone and a type IA agent for treatment of patients with rapid ventricular

tachycardia. Circulation 1986 (Nov); 74:1037–1043.

55. VELTRI EP, GRIFFITH LSC, PLATIA EV, GUARNIERI T, REID PR: The use of ambulatory monitoring in the prognostic evaluation of patients with sustained ventricular tachycardia treated with amiodarone: Circulation 1986 (Nov); 74:1054–1060.

56. KADISH AH, MARCHLINSKI FE, JOSEPHSON ME, BUXTON AE: Amiodarone: correlation of early and late electrophysiologic studies with outcome. Am Heart J 1986 (Dec); 112:1134–1140.

57. TORRES V, TEPPER D, FLOWERS D, WYNN J, LAM S, KEEFE D, MIURA DS, SOMBERG JC: QT prolongation and the antiarrhythmic efficacy of amiodarone. J Am Coll Cardiol 1986 (Jan); 7:142–147.

58. NADEMANEE K, SINGH BN, CALLAHAN B, HENDRICKSON JA, HERSHMAN JM: Amiodarone, thyroid hormone indexes, and altered thyroid function: long-term serial effects in patients with cardiac arrhythmias. Am J Cardiol 1986 (Nov 1); 58:981–986.

59. RIGAS B, ROSENFELD LE, BARWICK KW, ENRIQUEZ R, HELZBERG J, BATSFORD WP, JOSEPHSON ME, RIELY CA: Amiodarone hepatoxicity: a clinicopathologic study of five patients. Ann Intern Med 1986 (Mar 1); 104:348–351.

60. NYGAARD TW, SELLERS TD, COOK TS, DIMARCO JP: Adverse reactions to antiarrhythmic drugs drug therapy for ventricular arrhythmias. JAMA 1986 (July 4); 256:55–57.

61. GRABOYS TB, ALMEIDA EC, LOWN B: Recurrence of malignant ventricular arrhythmia after antiarrhythmic drug withdrawal. Am J Cardiol 1986 (July 1); 58:59–62.

62. CRITELLI G, SCHERILLO M, MONDA V, D'ASCIA C, MUSUMECI S, ANTIGNANO A: Transvenous catheter ablation of the His bundle in ventricular tachycardia. Am Heart J 1986 (June); 111:1106–1112.

63. KRAFCHEK J, LAWRIE GM, ROBERTS R, MAGRO SA, WYNDHAM CRC: Surgical ablation of ventricular tachycardia: improved results with a map-directed regional approach. Circulation 1986 (June); 73(6):1239–1247.

64. NESTICO PF, MORGANROTH J, HOROWITZ LN, MULHERN C: Bepridil hydrochloride for treatment of benign or potentially lethal ventricular arrhythmias. Am J Cardiol 1986 (Nov 1); 58:1001–1004.

65. GEAR K, MARCUS FI, HUANG SK, FENSTER PE, APPLETON C, MOELLER V, RENAUD G, SEROKMAN R: Ethmozine for ventricular premature complexes. Am J Cardiol 1986 (Apr 15); 57:947–949.

66. MIURA DS, WYNN J, TORRES V, LAUX B, KEEFE D, SOMBERG JC: Antiarrhythmic efficacy of ethmozine in patients with ventricular tachycardia as determined by programmed electrical stimulation. Am Heart J 1986 (Apr); 111:661–666.

67. SEALS AA, ENGLISH L, LEON CA, WIERMAN AW, YOUNG JB, ZOGHBI W, QUINONES MA, MAHLER SA, ROBERTS R, PRATT CM: Hemodynamic effects of moricizine at rest and during supine bicycle exercise: results in patients with ventricular tachycardia and left ventricular dysfunction. Am Heart J 1986 (July); 112:36–43.

68. ROTHBART ST, SAKSENA S: Clinical electrophysiology, efficacy and safety of chronic oral cibenzoline therapy in refractory ventricular tachycardia. Am J Cardiol 1986 (Apr 15); 57:941–946.

69. PLATIA EV, GRIFFITH LSC, WATKINS L, MOWER MM, GUARNIERI T, MIROWSKI M, REID PR: Treatment of malignant ventricular arrhythmias with endocardial resection and implantation of the automatic cardioverter-defibrillator. N Engl J Med 1986 (Jan 23); 314:213–216.

70. ROBERTS WC: Sudden cardiac death: definitions and causes. Am J Cardiol 1986 (June 1); 58:1410–1413.

71. BEARD CM, GRIFFIN MR, OFFORD KP, EDWARDS WD: Risk factors for sudden unexpected cardiac death in young women in Rochester, Minnesota, 1960 through 1974. Mayo Clin Proc 1986 (Mar); 61:186–191.

72. BASS M, KRAVATH RE, GLASS L: Death-scene investigation in sudden infant death. N Engl J Med 1986 (July 10); 315:100–105.

73. THACH BT: Sudden infant death syndrome: old causes rediscovered? N Engl J Med 1986 (July 10); 315:126–128.

74. GOLDSTEIN S, MEDENDORP S, LANDIS JR, WOLFE RA, LEIGHTON R, RITTER, G, VASU CM, ACHESON A: Analysis of cardiac symptoms preceding cardiac arrest. Am J Cardiol 1986 (Dec 1); 58:1195–1198.

75. PHILLIPS M, ROBINOWITZ M, HIGGINS JR, BORAN KJ, REED T, VIRMANI R: Sudden cardiac death in Air Force recruits: a 20-year review. JAMA 1986 (Nov 21); 256:2696–2699.

76. KIRSCHNER RH, ECKNER FAO, BARON RC: The cardiac pathology of sudden, unexplained nocturnal death in Southeast Asian refugees. JAMA 1986 (Nov 21); 256:2700–2705.

77. Standards and guidelines for cardiopulmonary resuscitation and emergency coronary care. JAMA 1986 (June 6); 255:2905–2992.

78. WEIL MH, RACKOW EC, TREVINO R, GRUNDLER W, FALK JL, GRIFFEL MI: Difference in acid-base state between venous and arterial blood during cardiopulmonary resuscitation. N Engl J Med 1986 (July 17); 315:153–156.

79. RELMAN AS: "Blood gases": Arterial or venous? N Engl J Med 1986 (July 17); 315:188–189.

80. BACHMAN JW, McDONAD GS, O'BRIEN PC: A study of out-of-hospital cardiac arrests in northeastern Minnesota. JAMA 1986 (July 25); 256:477–483.

81. WEAVER WD, COBB LA, HALLSTROM AP, FAHRENBRUCH C, COPASS MK, RAY R: Factors influencing survival after out-of-hospital cardiac arrest. J Am Coll Cardiol 1986 (Apr); 7:752–757.

82. DUNN HM, McCOMB JM, MacKENZIE G, ADGEY AAJ: Survival to leave hospital from ventricular fibrillation. Am Heart J 1986 (Oct); 112:745–751.

83. CHADDA KD, HARRINGTON D, KUSHNIK H, BODENHEIMER MM: The impact of transtelephonic documentation of arrhythmia on morbidity and mortality rate in sudden death survivors. Am Heart J 1986 (Dec); 112:1159–1165.

84. HALLSTROM AP, COBB LA, RAY R: Smoking as a risk factor for recurrence of sudden cardiac arrest. N Engl J Med 1986 (Jan 30); 314:271–5.

85. SKALE BT, MILES WM, HEGER JJ, ZIPES DP, PRYSTOWSKY EN: Survivors of cardiac arrest: prevention of recurrence by drug therapy as predicted by electrophysiologic testing or electrocardiographic monitoring. Am J Cardiol 1986 (Jan 1); 57:113–119.

86. HOLMES DR, DAVIS KB, MOCK MB, FISHER LD, GERSH BJ, KILLIP T, PETTINGER, M: The effect of medical and surgical treatment on subsequent sudden cardiac death in patients with coronary artery disease: a report from the Coronary Artery Surgery Study. Circulation 1986 (June); 73(6):1254–1263.

87. BLEVINS RD, KERIN NZ, FRUMIN H, FAITEL K, JARANDILLA R, GARFINKEL C, RUBENFIRE M: Arrhythmia control and other factors related to sudden death in coronary disease patients at intermediate risk. Am Heart J 1986 (Apr); 111:638–643.

88. MOSS AJ: Prolonged QT-interval syndromes. JAMA 1986 (Dec 5); 256:2985–2987.

89. VINCENT GM: The heart rate of Romano-Ward syndrome patients. Am Heart J 1986 (July); 112:61–64.

90. RODEN DM, WOOSLEY RL, PRIMM RK: Incidence and clinical features of the quinidine-associated long QT syndrome: implications for patient care. Am Heart J 1986 (June); 111:1088–1093.

91. LIAO Y, EMIDY LA, DYER A, HEWITT JS, SHEKELLE RB, OGLESBY P, PRINEAS R, STAMLER J: Characteristics and prognosis of incomplete right bundle branch block: an epidemiologic study. J Am Coll Cardiol 1986 (Mar); 7:492–499.

92. MYMIN D, MATHEWSON FAL, TATE RB, MANFREDA J: The natural history of primary first-degree atrioventricular heart block. N Engl J Med 1986 (Nov); 315:1183–1187.

93. MANGIARDI LM, RONZANI G, GAITA F, PRESBITERO P, CONTE MR, DI LEO M, COMMODO E, BRUSCA A: Clinical and electrocardiographic features and long-term results of electrical therapy in patients with isolated His bundle disease. Am Heart J 1986 (Dec); 112:1183–1191.

94. ALPERT MA, CURTIS JJ, SANFELIPPO JF, FLAKER GC, WALLS JT, MUKERJI V, VILLARREAL D, DATTI SK, MADIGAN NP, KROL RB: Comparative survival after permanent ventricular and dual chamber pacing for patients with chronic high degree atrioventricular block with and without preexistent congestive heart failure. J Am Coll Cardiol 1986 (Apr); 7:925–932.

95. SUGRUE DD, GERSH BJ, HOLMES DR, WOOD DL, OSBORN MJ, HAMMILL SC: Symptomatic "isolated" carotid sinus hypersensitivity: natural history and results of treatment with anticholinergic drugs or pacemaker. J Am Coll Cardiol 1986 (Jan); 7:158–162.

96. MECHELEN R, RUITER J, VANDERKERCKHOVE Y, BOER H, HAGEMEIJER F: Prevalence of retrograde conduction in heart block after DDD pacemaker implantation. Am J Cardiol 1986 (Apr 1); 57:797–801.

97. PALOMO AR, SCHWARTZ AM, TROHMAN RG, CHAHINE RA, MYERBURG RJ, KESSLER KM: Cardiac arrhythmias associated with prophylactic pacing during coronary angiography. Am J Cardiol 1986 (July 1); 58:100–103.

98. MILES WM, PRYSTOWSKY EN, HEGER JJ, ZIPES DP: The implantable transvenous cardioverter: long-term efficacy and reproducible induction of ventricular tachycardia. Circulation 1986 (Mar); 74:518–524.

99. SAKSENA S, PANTOPOULOS D, PARSONNET V, ROTHBART ST, HUSSAIN SM, GIELCHINSKY I: Usefulness of an implantable antitachycardia pacemaker system for supraventricular or ventricular tachycardia. Am J Cardiol 1986 (July 1); 58:70–74.

100. MARCHLINSKI FE, FLORES BT, BUXTON AE, HARGROVE WC, ADDONIZIO VP, STEPHENSON LW, HARKEN AH, DOHERTY JU, GROGAN EW, JOSEPHSON ME: The automatic implantable cardioverter-defibrillator: efficacy, complications, and device failures. Ann Intern Med 1986 (Apr); 104:481–488.

101. WEAVER WD, COPASS MK, HILL DK, FAHRENBRUCH C, HALLSTROM AP, COBB LA: Cardiac arrest treated with a new automatic external defibrillator by out-of-hospital first responders. Am J Cardiol 1986 (May 1); 57:1017–1021.

102. THURER RJ, LUCERI RM, BOLOOKI H: Automatic implantable cardioverter-defibrillator: techniques of implantation and results. Ann Thorac Surg 1986 (Aug); 42:143–147.

103. KNOWLTON AA, FALK RH: External cardiac pacing during in-hospital cardiac arrest. Am J Cardiol 1986 (June 1); 57:1295–1298.

104. NISHIMURA M, KATOH T, HANAI S, WATANABE Y: Optimal mode of transesophageal atrial pacing. Am J Cardiol 1986 (Apr 1); 57:791–796.

105. ERLEBACHER JA, CAHILL PT, PANNIZZO F, KNOWLES RJR: Effect of magnetic resonance imaging on DDD pacemakers. Am J Cardiol 1986 (Feb 15); 57:437–440.

106. PANNIZZO F, AMIKAM S, BAGWELL P, FURMAN S: Discrimination of antegrade and retrograde atrial depolarization by electrogram analysis. Am Heart J 1986 (Oct); 112:780–786.

Systemic Hypertension

Measuring blood pressure

The British Hypertension Society developed an article prepared by Petrie and associates[1] for recommendations on BP measurement. This 5-page highly illustrated article is worth the reading of all physicians. BP measurement is one of the most commonly performed procedures in clinical medicine and it should not be done carelessly. Defective or inappropriate equipment should not be used. All those who measure BP should be assessed on the practical aspects of the procedure.

Automated ambulatory blood pressure monitoring

The Health and Public Policy Committee of the American College of Physicians, a committee whose report was authored by Constance Monroe Winslow[2], assessed the usefulness of automated ambulatory BP monitoring for identifying and managing patients with systemic hypertension. The committee concluded that it is not known at present whether treatment based on readings from ambulatory monitors result in a lower frequency of subsequent hypertensive complications. It is not known which of the possible measurements are most important—home or work environment readings, percentage of time above certain levels, or average BP readings—and whether these differ with type of end-organ damage (stroke, cardiovascular, peripheral vascular disease, or renal disease). Once these questions are answered, the fundamental question will remain of whether automated BP monitoring offers sufficient advantage over office or manual home BP measurements to justify its expense and inconvenience.

To assess the discrepancy between casual (office) and home BP readings in patients performing home BP monitoring, White[3] from Farmington, Connecticut, analyzed office, home, and 24-hour ambulatory BP and heart rates in 19 patients in a prospective 4-week study. After the month of study, the average difference between mean office and manual home BP in this office hypertensive group was 30 ± 17/20 ± 6 mmHg. The BP taken in the office was substantially greater than the 24-hour average and ambulatory BP during work or while at home (awake). An analysis of the automatic monitor readings while in the doctor's office and at 15-minute intervals after leaving the office showed a progressive reduction in BP and heart rate during the first hour after leaving the office. A mean 24-hour BP of <130/80 mmHg was found in 13 (68%) patients. These data suggest that patients with office hypertension are usually normotensive but may have a persistent and recurrent pressor response in a medical care setting. Ambulatory BP monitoring provides confirmation of not only the office-home disparity, but also suggests that stress other than office visits fails to elicit a hypertensive response.

Impact of hypertension control program in rural community

Kentucky is a predominantly rural state with relatively high death rates from systemic hypertension and cardiovascular disease. Kotchen and associates[4] from Lexington, Kentucky, examined a community-based high BP control educational program in 2 rural counties of southeastern Kentucky. In the intervention counties, systolic and diastolic BP of both men and women decreased despite the 5-year increase in age; moreover, hypertension was better controlled after the program, and substantial decreases in deaths due to cardiovascular disease were seen. These differences were greater among men in the 2 regions than among women. The results of this program suggest that, in sparsely populated rural areas, existing resources and programs can be successfully utilized in a community-wide cardiovascular disease risk reduction educational program.

Heart rate

Borderline hypertensives who have tachycardia have a tendency toward the development of essential hypertension. However, the documentation of tachycardia in previous studies has been generally based on brief periods of observation. Mehta and associates[5] from Cleveland, Ohio, measured heart rates through a 24-hour period in 16 ambulatory mildly hypertensive subjects (aged 5–23 years). When compared with normal matched controls, significantly higher heart rates were observed during the waking periods (99 ± 9 -vs- 90 ± 11) and sleep periods (72 ± 12 -vs- 62 ± 7). Similar observations also were made for 24 hours (90 ± 8 -vs- 79 ± 8). In addition, hypertensives also had thickened (during diastole) LV posterior wall (0.96 ± 0.17 -vs- 0.85 ± 0.13 cm) and ventricular septum (0.98 ± 0.17 -vs- 0.84 ± 0.19 cm). It was suggested that tachycardia was an early manifestation of borderline hypertension in children.

In the elderly

Research indicates that isolated systolic and diastolic hypertension, is associated with increased morbidity and mortality in people over age 65 years. According to data from the 1976–1980 National Health and Nutrition Examination Survey, the prevalence of these combined types of hypertension (≥140/90 mmHg) is estimated to be 64% in persons aged 65 to 74 years, with an even higher prevalence in blacks (76%) than in whites (63%). Although a number of studies have demonstrated the benefits of antihypertensive therapy in elderly patients, many questions unique to this population remain unanswered. This article addresses several of these issues and presents recommended guidelines on topics such as the pressure at which treatment should be initiated, goal pressure for people over age 65, antihypertensive drugs of choice, and appropriate dosages, the accuracy of indirect measurements, side effects specific to elderly patients, and the effect of treatment on the quality of life.[6]

Left ventricular mass and function

It has been suggested that the heart plays an active role in the pathogenesis of arterial hypertension. If this is true, there must be early cardiac involvement in young normotensive subjects in whom hypertension develops later in life; differences in cardiac morphology or function may exist between young normotensive subjects with different risks of hypertension developing. Thus, Radice and colleagues[7] from Milan, Italy, performed M-mode echocardiography in 51 normotensive male adolescents with at least 1 hypertensive parent. These subjects were compared with 55 normotensive sons of normotensive parents and with 25 adolescents with borderline hypertension. Control groups were matched for sex and age. The following morphologic parameters were significantly greater in the persons with 1 hypertensive parent than in the normotensive persons with normotensive parents: ventricular septum $(0.54 \pm 0.08$ -vs- 0.49 ± 0.09 cm/m^2) and posterior wall $(0.54 \pm 0.11$ -vs- 0.50 ± 0.08 cm/m^2) thickness, LV mass $(125 \pm 29$ -vs- 109 ± 25 gm/m^2), and cross-sectional area $(9.9 \pm 1.8$ -vs- 8.9 ± 1.6 cm^2/m^2); no significant differences between subjects with 1 hypertensive parent and those with borderline hypertension were observed. Excursion of LV posterior wall was significantly higher in the borderline hypertensive group; no differences were observed between those subjects with 1 hypertensive parent and those with normotensive parents. These data show that the same kinds of changes in cardiac morphology are present in normotensive subjects with a family history of hypertension and in subjects with borderline hypertension, suggesting that cardiac involvement may precede elevation of BP.

Boudoulas and associates[8] from Columbus, Ohio, Detroit, Michigan, and Denver, Colorado, performed a study to define the relation between the extent of LV hypertrophy and ventricular systolic performance in 90 patients with chronic systemic hypertension compared with 41 normal control subjects determined by angiography. The mass was estimated from the M-mode echocardiogram. Patients were separated into 3 groups: those with LV mass of <2 (group I, n = 58), 2–4 (group II, n = 21), and >4 (group III, n = 11) standard deviations above mean normal. The ratio of PEP/LVET, percent shortening of the echocardiographic internal diameter (%ΔD) and velocity of circumferential shortening (Vcf) were used as indexes of LV systolic performance. The frequency of abnormality, expressed as percent of patients in groups I, II, and III, was 33%, 55%, and 85% for PEP/LVET, 15%, 35%, and 72% for %ΔD, and 0%, 15%, and 55% for Vcf. For each group PEP/LVET was the most frequently abnormal measure and Vcf was the least frequent abnormality. Calculation of peak and end-systolic wall stress was used as an index of the adequacy of LV hypertrophy. This index was significantly reduced in group I, did not differ from control in group II, and was significantly increased in group III, indicating that hypertrophy was appropriate to wall tension in groups I and II. It is concluded that the occurrence of LV dysfunction with increasing LV mass in patients with moderate LV hypertrophy (group I and II) reflects a deficiency in intrinsic contractile performance of the hypertrophied myocardium. With a marked increase in LV mass (group III), inadequacy in LV hypertrophy relative to wall tension may also contribute to LV dysfunction.

To assess whether echocardiographic and electrocardiographic detection of LV hypertrophy could predict cardiovascular morbid events in patients with uncomplicated systemic hypertension, Casale and associates[9] from New York, New York, followed 140 men a mean of 5 years. Initial echocardiographic measurements of LV mass were normal (<125 g/m^2 body surface area) in 111 patients and revealed hypertrophy in 29 patients. Morbid events occurred in more patients with hypertrophy on echocardiography (7 of 29, 4.6/100 patient-years) than with normal ventricular mass (7 of 111, 1.4/100 patient-years). Electrocardiography showed hypertrophy in too few patients to be of predictive value. Multiple logistic regression analysis showed that LV mass index had the highest independent relative risk for future events and that systolic and diastolic pressures and age had slightly lower relative risks. In men with mild uncomplicated hypertension, LV hypertrophy detected by echocardiography identifies patients at high risk for cardiovascular morbid events and is a significant risk factor for future morbid events independent of age, BP, or ventricular function at rest.

Relation of left ventricular mass to renal hemodynamics

To assess the relation between early clinically detectable involvement of hypertensive vascular disease in heart and kidneys, Kobrin and associates[10] from New Orleans, Louisiana, obtained systemic and renal hemodynamics in M-mode echocardiographic measurements in 65 patients with essential hypertension. The results indicate that patients with and without LV hypertrophy had similar renal hemodynamic findings. In contrast, patients with altered renal hemodynamics (reduced renal distribution of cardiac output and absolute renal flow with increased renal vascular resistance) and increased serum uric acid levels also had increased LV posterior and septal wall thicknesses and mass index. Moreover, these data also demonstrated that in patients with altered renal hemodynamics, the lower the renal distribution of cardiac output and the higher the serum uric acid levels, the greater were the indexes of cardiac enlargement. These results demonstrated that the pathophysiologic and hemodynamic effects of essential hypertension in the heart precede those in the kidneys.

Sodium reabsorption by proximal renal tubules

Weder[11] from Ann Arbor, Michigan, investigated the rate of sodium reabsorption by the proximal renal tubules by a lithium clearance test and red-cell countertransport in 14 patients with untreated essential hypertension and in 31 controls. As a group the hypertensive patients had a higher average rate of red-cell countertransport (0.378 ± 0.030 mmol of lithium per liter of cells per hour) and a lower renal fractional lithium clearance (13.96 ± 0.69%) than normotensive subjects (0.317 ± 0.015 mmol of lithium per liter of cells per hour and 17.75 ± 0.81%, respectively). Within the normotensive group, subjects with hypertension in at least 1 first-degree relative had significantly lower fractional lithium clearances than subjects with no hypertensive relatives (15.37 ± 0.84% -vs- 19.06 ± 1.07%). The author concluded that hypertensive patients have heightened proximal tubular reabsorption of sodium and that red-cell countertransport is a marker of the renal abnormality. Enhanced proximal tubular sodium reabsorption may precede the development of essential hypertension.

Relation of plasma renin activity and sodium metabolism to calcium-regulating hormones

Resnick and associates[12] from New York, New York, analyzed circulating levels of calcium-regulating hormones, calcitonin, calcitriol, and parathyroid hormone in relation to plasma renin activity in 10 persons with normal BP and in 51 persons with essential hypertension. Calcitriol and parathyroid hormone levels were elevated in hypertensives with low-renin activity, whereas calcitonin levels were higher in patients with high-renin activity, compared with normotensive controls and other hypertensive patients. Continuous relations were observed between calcitriol levels and plasma renin activity in all patients and between parathyroid hormone levels and urinary sodium excretion in hypertensive patients with low-renin activity. Together, these results support a linkage between calcium metabolism and renin-sodium factors in essential hypertension. Calcium-regulating hormones and the renin-aldosterone system may coordinately mediate the BP effects of differing dietary calcium and sodium intakes at the cellular level by altering cellular handling of monovalent and divalent ions.

Atrial natriuretic factor

Sagnella and associates[13] from London, England, measured plasma levels of immunoreactive atrial natriuretic peptides (ANP) in 28 hypertensive subjects and found them to be higher than in 24 normotensive subjects (17 ± 14 pg/ml -vs- 8 ± 4 pg/ml). All subjects were studied while taking their normal dietary sodium intake. In the normotensive subjects ANP levels were significantly correlated with age but not with BP, whereas in the hypertensive subjects ANP levels were significantly correlated with systolic BP but not with age. These findings may indicate a compensatory reaction to a diminished renal capacity for sodium excretion, in response to increasing age in normotensive subjects and to higher BP in hypertensive subjects.

Relation of blood pressure to insulin levels

Fournier and associates[14] from Miami, Florida, examined the relation of BP to fasting (basal) insulin in glycosylated hemoglobin (hemoglobin A_1) in 248 nondiabetic subjects. No subject was taking hypertensive medicines. There were statistically significant associations of systolic and diastolic BP with insulin levels and with hemoglobin A_1 levels in the 137 women. These BP indexes also were related to insulin levels in men. In a multiple regression analysis, the association between BP and insulin level was diminished with an allowance for adiposity; however, it remains statistically significant. These data indicate that BP is related to insulin levels in nondiabetic subjects and suggest that insulin may be a physiologic determinant of BP.

Effect of meals

Fagan and associates[15] from Charleston, South Carolina, examined the effects of a standardized mixed meal, a self-selected meal, and a sham meal on heart rate, arterial BP, cardiac output, total systemic resistance and echocardiographic indexes of LV performance in 8 male volunteers. Supine heart rate and cardiac output increased after the meals, but not after the sham meal. Supine diastolic BP and total systemic resistance decreased after the meals but not after the sham meal. EF and mean velocity of circumferential fiber shortening increased after the standard meal and tended to increase after the self-selected meal, but did not increase after the sham meal. Meals of normal size may induce splanchnic vasodilation and a decrease in total systemic resistance. Ingestion of food also significantly affects heart rate, BP, cardiac output, and echocardiographic indexes of LV performance. Patients should not eat during short-term evaluation of cardiovascular interventions because the cardiovascular effects of a meal may compromise interpretation of the cardiovascular effects of the primary intervention. The hemodynamic effects of food may also interact with the effect of cardiovascular disease processes.

Effect of obesity and weight loss

Weight loss, of course, has a role in the treatment of essential hypertension. Cohen and Flamenbaum[16] from New York, New York, studied 129 patients with essential hypertension who fulfilled the following criteria: 1) morbid obesity defined as body weight ≥25% calculated ideal body weight; and 2) essential hypertension defined as 2 diastolic BP measurements ≥90 mmHg, or medical records indicating the use of antihypertensive medicines. The 129 patients were separated into 2 groups on the basis of the use of antihypertensive medications: 30 subjects not receiving medication (Table 5-1) and 99 subjects receiving medication (Table 5-2). With the use of a medically supervised protein-sparing supplemented fast and a behavioral program, the changes in BP as a result of weight loss were examined. The diet consisted of a regimen of 5 feedings per day of RF 045, a powder providing a daily intake of 300 calories from the following constituents: 45 g of protein, 30 g sucrose, 1 g fat, and 1,000 mg sodium. The powder was blended with any cold, noncholoric beverage, water, or diet soda. Additionally, each patient received 20 mEq/day of potassium and 1 multivitamin tablet. The results are displayed in Tables 1 and 2.

Extracellular and interstitial fluid volume

Raison and associates[17] from Paris, France, investigated fluid volumes and cardiac and renal hemodynamics in 44 obese men, 22 with normal BP, and 22 with sustained essential hypertension. For the same degree of obesity,

TABLE 5-1. *Weight and blood pressures in untreated hypertensive subjects at baseline and at conclusion of the supplemented fast**

	BASELINE (N = 30)	CONCLUSION OF SUPPLEMENTED FAST (N = 30)
Weight (lbs)	238 ± 48	194 ± 40†
% Overweight	57 ± 25	28 ± 25†
Systolic BP (mm Hg)	143 ± 10	123 ± 15
Diastolic BP (mm Hg)	95 ± 6	77 ± 10

* The data are presented as mean ± SD
† p = 0.0001 versus baseline

TABLE 5-2. *Weight, blood pressures, and number of medications used at baseline and at conclusion of the supplemented fast in the group receiving medication**

	BASELINE (N = 30)	CONCLUSION OF SUPPLEMENTED FAST (N = 30)
Weight (lbs)	225 ± 48	186 ± 40†
% Overweight	54 ± 30	27 ± 25†
Systolic BP (mm Hg)	140 ± 18	127 ± 16
Diastolic BP (mm Hg)	89 ± 10	82 ± 10
Number of medications	2 ± 1	0.4 ± .7

* The data are presented as mean ± SD
† p = 0.0001 versus baseline

hypertensive patients had a higher value in extracellular and interstitial fluid volumes than normotensive subjects, whereas plasma volume, total body water, body cellular water, cardiac output, renal blood flow, and glomerular filtration rate were similar. For the same level of BP, the expansion of extracellular and interstitial fluid volume paralleled the degree of obesity. Thus, obese patients with hypertension have an absolute increase in extracellular and interstitial fluid volumes. The increase was related both to the degree of overweight and to the mechanisms of hypertension.

Effect of habitual alcoholism

Because systemic hypertension is observed in one-third of persons with habitual alcoholism, Friedman and associates[18] from Brooklyn, New York, analyzed the relation of this finding to LV function in 66 alcoholics (26 with BP of ≥160/95 mmHg) 4–5 days after alcoholic withdrawl. Hypertensive alcoholics had a more abnormal ratio of PEP/ET (0.398 ± 0.01 -vs- 0.35 ± 0.01) than normotensive alcoholics (matched normal 0.290 ± 0.01). Hypertensive alcoholics (transitory hypertension) with BP of 120/80 mmHg or less at the time of study also had more abnormal PEP/LVET than matched normotensive alcoholics (0.415 ± 0.03 -vs- 0.331 ± 0.01). In both hypertensive 77 ± 6 dynes/cm^2 × 10^3) and normotensive alcoholics (67 ± 4 dynes/cm^2 × 10^3) LV stress was elevated (normal 46 ± 3 dynes/cm × 10^3). However, LV mass was not increased (hypertensive 96 ± 4 g/m^2 -vs- normotensive 100 ± 4 g/m^2; (normal 92 ± 5 g/m^2), resulting in a markedly increased stress-to-mass ratio (hypertensive 0.8 ± 0.06; normal 0.5 ± 0.05). Hypertensive alcoholics also had LV "hyperfunction," with an increased stress/LV end-systolic volume ratio (1.7 ± 0.1 -vs- 1.3 ± 0.1 dynes/cm^2 × 10^3/ml). Thus, hypertensive alcoholics, even those with transitory hypertension, have more abnormal cardiac function than normotensive alcoholics. Presence of hypertension with hyperdynamic LV features may be a prelude to CHF.

Although a number of population studies have almost unanimously shown an empiric link between regular use of alcoholic beverages and systemic hypertension, the absence of a proved mechanism for the alcohol-hypertension relation prevents general acceptance of a causal association. In a new study controlled for many factors, Klatsky and co-workers[19] in Oakland, California, reconfirmed the relation of higher BP to alcohol use. The relation was stronger in men, whites, and persons ≥55 years of age. A slight increase in BP appeared in men who drank 1 to 2 drinks daily, and a continued increase occurred at all higher drinking levels among white men who had constant drinking habits. For women, an increase occurred only at ≥3 drinks daily. The data suggest complete regression beginning within days of alcohol-associated hypertension on abstinence. BP showed minor differences with beverage preference: those who preferred liquor had higher adjusted mean BP than those preferring wine or beer. The results of this study contribute to the likelihood that the alcohol–BP association is causal. Smoking, coffee use, and tea use showed no association with higher BP. Systolic BP showed a positive relation to total serum calcium and an inverse relation to serum potassium, but diastolic BP showed little relation to these blood constituents. Because alcohol associated hypertension might be controlled by omitting the offending agent instead of adding antihypertensive drugs, investigators emphasize that the public health implications are substantial.

MacMachon and Norton[20] from Bethesda and Rockville, Maryland, reviewed the evidence suggesting that alcohol consumption raises systemic arterial BP. At least 30 studies since 1977 concerning BP and alcohol consumption have been conducted. With few exceptions, these studies have indicated that among persons whose reported average alcohol consumption was 3 to 4 drinks per day (1 drink being defined as the equivalent of 8 to 10 g of ethanol), systolic BP was 3–4 mmHg greater and diastolic BP was 1–2 mmHg greater than in nondrinkers. In persons consuming 5–6 drinks per day, systolic BP was 5–6 mmHg greater and diastolic BP was 2–4 mmHg greater than in nondrinkers. Thus, these studies provide evidence of a typical dose-response relation between alcohol consumption and BP at levels of consumption of >2 drinks per day. An association of moderate to heavy alcohol consumption with high BP also has been observed in at least 4 prospective observational studies. Heavier consumers had greater increases in BP during follow-up than did nondrinkers. Whether the BP of lighter drinkers is different from that of nondrinkers is not clear. In 7 of the 30 cross-sectional studies reviewed by these 2 authors, the BP of drinkers consuming <3 drinks per day was greater than that of nondrinkers. In 11 studies there was no difference in BP between light drinkers and nondrinkers, and in remaining 12 studies, the BP of drinkers consuming <3 drinks per day was lower than that of nondrinkers. Data on the prevalence of hypertension at various levels of alcohol consumption has been reported in several cross-sectional studies. Compared with rates in nondrinkers, the prevalence was approximately 50% greater in persons consuming 3–4 drinks per day and 100% greater in those consuming 6–7 drinks per day. These results suggest that in men, at least, interventions to reduce alcohol consumption to ≤2 drinks per day may produce an important preventive or therapeutic effect in systemic hypertension. Stronger evidence is provided by a few randomized, controlled, crossover trials that have sought to evaluate the effect on BP of interventions to reduce alcohol consumption. In 1 study, complete withdrawal of alcohol in a group of hypertensive men who usually consumed 6–8 drinks per day resulted in a decrease of both systolic (13 mmHg) and diastolic (5 mmHg) BP over 3–4 days. These short-term results are encouraging and suggestive of therapeutic benefit in hypertensive persons and preventive benefit in normotensive persons. In addition to the potentially beneficial effects on BP levels, reduced alcohol consumption in hypertensive patients also may improve responsiveness to antihypertensive drug therapy and increase adherence to drug treatment regimens. Lowering alcohol consumption also may reduce the risk of stroke, the risk of which is increased in both hypertensive persons and in heavy drinkers (independent of BP levels). In summary, the available evidence suggests that the consumption of 3 drinks or more per day is associated with higher BP; as much as 11% of hypertension in men but a much smaller proportion in women may be due to consumption at this level. In persons consuming 3 drinks or more per day, whether hypertensive or normotensive, the total withdrawal of alcohol or its restriction is likely to result in decreases in BP at least in the short term.

Parathyroid gland hypertension

Diamond and associates[21] from Johannesburg, South Africa, retrospectively studied 75 patients who were surgically cured of primary hyperparathyroidism from 1976–1984 to evaluate the BP and metabolic responses to the surgery. The overall prevalence of systemic hypertension before surgery was 47% compared with 23% in the general population. Systemic hypertension was most frequent in patients >60 years of age (62% -vs- 39% expected). Renal insufficiency was found in 13 of 35 hypertensive and in 2 of 40 normotensive patients. The frequency of urolithiasis and mean levels of serum and urine calcium and phosphate were similar in normotensive and hypertensive patients. Parathyroidectomy resulted in a substantial decrease in both mean systolic and mean diastolic BP in 54% of the hypertensive subjects, unrelated to improvement in renal function (Table 5-3).

The calcium deficiency hypothesis

Kaplan and Messe[22] of Dallas, Texas, reviewed the hypothesis that primary (essential) hypertension was related to calcium deficiency rather than to excess. The evidence used to support this hypothesis includes surveys showing lesser dietary intake of calcium, lower levels of ionized calcium in the blood, and reduction of blood pressure with calcium supplements. This

TABLE 5-3. *Calcium and phosphate responses to parathyroidectomy in normotensive and hypertensive patients with PHPT.* Reproduced with permission from Diamond et al.[21]*

	PREOPERATIVE VALUES	POSTOPERATIVE VALUES	P
Normotensive patients†			
MSBP, mm Hg	126.9 ± 2.2	122.6 ± 1.7	<.01
MDBP, mm Hg	77.3 ± 1.2	78.0 ± 1.2	NS
Calcium, mg/dL (8.42–10.62)	12.02 ± 0.16‡	9.02 ± 0.12	<.001
(mmol/L) (2.1–2.65)	(3.0 ± 0.04)	(2.25 ± 0.03)	
Phosphate, mg/dL (2.51–4.21)	2.48 ± 0.12	3.69 ± 0.12	<.001
(mmol/L) (0.81–1.30)	(0.80 ± 0.04)	(1.19 ± 0.04)	
Creatinine, mg/dL (0.68–1.24)	1.20 ± 0.14	1.21 ± 0.19	NS
(μmol/L) (60–110)	(106.3 ± 12.3)	(107.1 ± 16.9)	
Hypertensive patients			
MSBP, mm Hg	158.6 ± 3.3	148.7 ± 3.2	<.001
MDBP, mm Hg	94.5 ± 1.5	87.7 ± 1.8	<.001
Calcium, mg/dL	12.75 ± 0.28	9.46 ± 0.12	<.001
(mmol/L)	(3.18 ± 0.07)	(2.36 ± 0.03)	
Phosphate, mg/dL	2.39 ± 0.12	3.72 ± 0.09	<.001
(mmol/L)	(0.77 ± 0.04)	(1.20 ± 0.03)	
Creatinine, mg/dL	1.51 ± 0.15	1.44 ± 0.13	NS
(μmol/L)	(133.2 ± 13.6)	(127.0 ± 11.6)	

* Hypertensive patients were receiving treatment. BP indicates blood pressure; MSBP, mean systolic BP; MDBP, mean diastolic BP; PHPT, primary hyperparathyroidism; and NS, not significant.
† Parenthetical values in this column represent normal ranges.
‡ Significantly different from preoperative values in hypertensive group (p <.05).

critique examines each of these points and the theoretical construct used to explain the hypothesis. The authors concluded that the theoretical construct is based on the use of only a portion of available experimental data and the clinical evidence remains inconclusive. Until the hypothesis is supported further, calcium deficiency should not be accepted as a mechanism responsible for hypertension and calcium supplements should be used with caution.

Management by fee-for-service physicians -vs- management by large prepaid groups

To examine the influence of method of payment on ambulatory testing by internists, Epstein and associates[23] from Boston, Massachusetts, compared the rate at which patients with uncomplicated systemic hypertension were tested by 10 doctors practicing in large fee-for-service groups compared to that by 17 doctors in large prepaid groups. After correcting for the patient's age, sex, duration of disease, and severity of disease as measured by pretreatment BP, and for the doctor's year of medical school graduation, the authors found that 50% more electrocardiograms were obtained among patients in fee-for-service practices (0.69 per patient per year -vs- 0.45) and 40% more chest radiographs (0.49 -vs- 0.35). Fee-for-service doctors believe that both tests were associated with high profit and cost. These results suggest that the use of certain high-profit, high-cost tests is higher in large fee-for-service groups than in large prepaid groups. Although the generalizability of conclusions based on this limited study must be considered tentative, the findings suggest that it may be appropriate to consider changing the payments for tests as part of a more general reform of the fee schedules.

TREATMENT

Major clinical trials

Wilcox and associates[24] from Nottigham, UK, reviewed the results of 9 trials comparing patients treated with various antihypertensive agents to those not treated. More than 50,000 patients participated in these 9 trials. The treatment regiments are displayed in Tables 5-4, 5-5 and 5-6 and in Figure 5-1. Table 5-6 summarizes the main results of the trials. The authors of this review concluded their review with the following 6 suggestions: 1) Clearly, patients with malignant (accelerated) hypertension need treatment. 2) There is no evidence that any particular level of *systolic* pressure should be treated, and, therefore, there is no reason to treat patients with isolated systolic hypertension. 3) BP varies considerably and in an appreciable proportion of patients with diastolic BP up to 115 mmHg. Some will revert to normal values over a few months. Therefore, it is prudent to check the BP on several occasions before deciding whether to treat and also to measure it yearly in any patient found at any time to have a diastolic BP >100 mmHg. 4) It is probably more important to stop a patient from smoking cigarettes than it is to treat his mildly raised BP, because any pharmaceutical treatment causes side effects. Nonpharmaceutical methods to lower BP should always be considered. Weight control may be enough to control a raised BP. 5) There is no evidence that a different treatment policy is needed in any particular race, sex, or age group, although the effects of different treatments in very elderly patients have not been adequately studied. 6) There is no evidence that any particular form of drug treatment is superior to any other, except for

TABLE 5-4. *Type of patient, blood pressure, and number of patients included in major trials of reduction of blood pressure. Reproduced with permission from Wilcox et al.[24]*

TRIAL	PATIENTS	BLOOD PRESSURE (MM HG)	NO. OF PATIENTS
Veterans Administration	Men in hospital	Diastolic >90	523
Gothenburg	Men aged 47–54	Systolic >175 or diastolic >115	635
Hypertension detection and follow up programme	Men and women aged 30–69	Diastolic >90	10 940
Oslo	Men aged 40–49	150–179/ > 100	785
Australian	Men and women aged 30–69	Diastolic 95–109	3 437
Multiple risk factor interventions trial	"High risk" men aged 35–59	Diastolic 90–115	12 866
European	Men and women over 60	Diastolic 90–119	940
International prospective primary prevention study	Men and women aged 40–69	Diastolic 100–125	6 357
MRC	Men and women aged 35–60	Diastolic 90–109	17 354
Total			53 827

TABLE 5-5. *Treatment regimen and trial design in hypertension studies. Reproduced with permission from Wilcox et al.[24]*

TRIAL	RANDOMISED	DOUBLE BLIND	SINGLE BLIND	PLACEBO	ACTIVE TREATMENT
Veterans Administration	+	+		+	1 Hydrochlorothiazide + reserpine + hydralazine
Gothenburg					*1 β blocker 2 Thiazide diuretic 3 Hydralazine 4 Spironolactone or bethanidine or high dose frusemide
Hypertension detection and follow up programme	+				*1 Chlorthalidone or triamterene or spironolactone 2 Reserpine or methyldopa 3 Hydralazine 4 Guanethidine ± 2 or 3 5 Others
Oslo	+				*1 Hydrochlorothiazide 2 Methyldopa or propranolol 3 Others
Australian	+		+	+	*1 Chlorothiazide 2 Methyldopa or propranolol or pindolol 3 Hydralazine or clonidine
Multiple risk factor interventions trial	+				*1 Hydrochlorothiazide or chlorthalidone 2 Reserpine or hydralazine or guanethidine or others
European	+	+		+	*1 Hydrochlorothiazide or triamterene 2 Methyldopa
International prospective primary prevention study	+	+		+	*1 Slow release oxprenolol 2 Other non-β blockers
MRC	+		+	+	*1 Bendrofluazide or propranolol 2 Methyldopa

* Step care treatment.

TABLE 5-6. *Summary of principal results of trials. Parentheses indicate that results should be interpreted with caution. Reproduced with permission from Wilcox et al.*[24]

| | | HEART ATTACK | | STROKE | |
TRIAL	TOTAL MORTALITY	FATAL	TOTAL	FATAL	TOTAL
Veterans Administration (combined)	(+)				(+)
Gothenburg	(+)		(+)		
Hypertension detection and follow up programme	(+)			(+)	(+)
Oslo					+
Australian	(+)				+
Multiple risk factor interventions trial					
European		+	(+)		
International prospective primary preventive study					
MRC					+

+ =Effect significant, p <0.05.

a suggestion that beta blockers are less effective in preventing the complications of high BP in cigarette smokers. The choice of initial treatment, therefore, depends mainly on the expected side effects, which dictate patient compliance, and on cost. These authors recommended on all counts that initial drug treatment should be bendrofluazide. A dose of 2.5 mg/day is as effective as higher doses, and although this low dose has not been tested in a large-scale trial designed to evaluate its effect on mortality, it would seem logical not to use the high doses, which probably carry a high risk of unwanted effects.

Amery and associates[25] from the *European Working Party on High Blood Pressure in the Elderly* (EWPHE) Trial analyzed the data in relation to age,

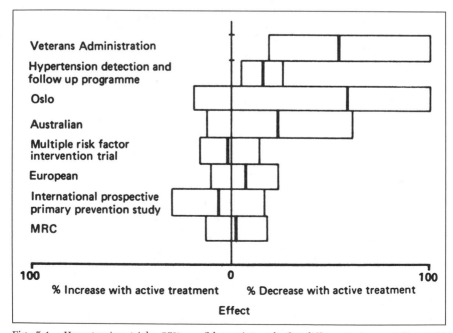

Fig. 5-1. Hypertension trials: 95% confidence intervals for differences in mortality. Bold vertical bars indicate mean reduction (or increase). Reproduced with permission from Wilcox et al.[24]

sex, BP, and previous cardiovascular disease. Cardiovascular mortality and cardiovascular study-terminating events were significantly and independently related to treatment, age, cardiovascular complications at randomization, and systolic but not diastolic BP (Figs. 5-2, 5-3, and 5-4). The benefits of treatment observed in the trial seemed to be independent of entry BP and the presence or absence of cardiovascular complications at entry. There was

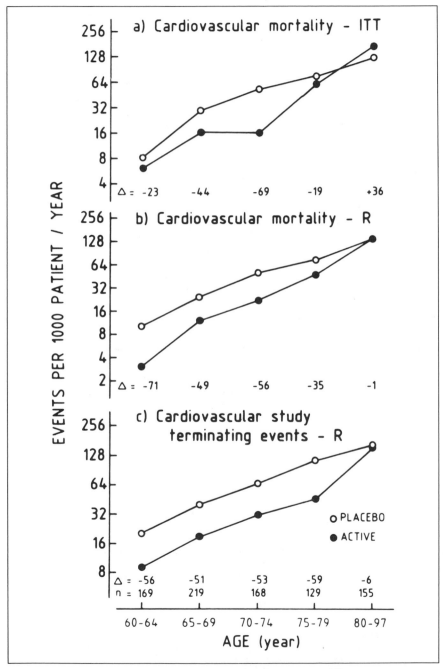

Fig. 5-2. Event rates. Reproduced with permission from Amery et al.[25]

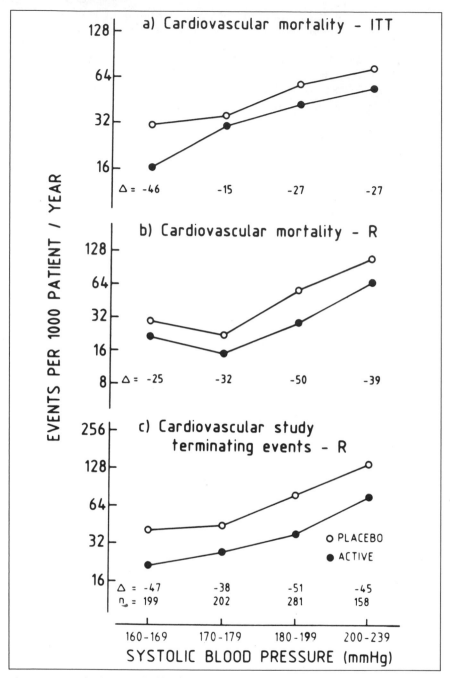

Fig. 5-3. Data for four systolic blood pressure related subgroups. Reproduced with permission from Amery et al.[25]

some evidence that treatment effect decreases with advancing age. Little or no benefit from treatment could be demonstrated in patients >80 years of age, most of whom were women.

In a supplement to Progress in Cardiovascular Disease, the results of the largest hypertension trial held in the USA, namely *The Hypertension Detection and Follow-Up Program* (HDFP), are brought together in a single publication

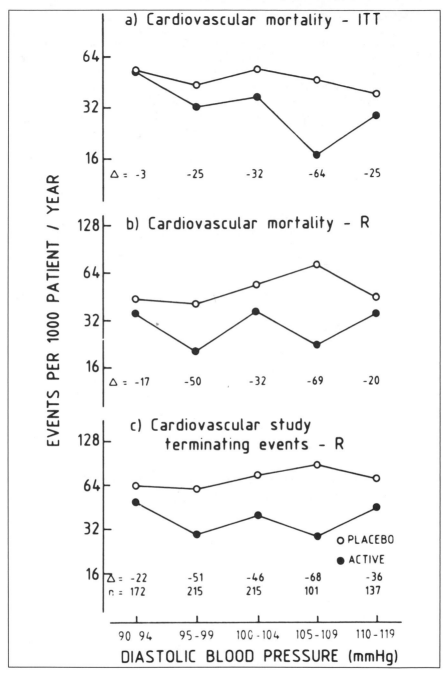

Fig. 5-4. Data for five diastolic blood pressure related subgroups. Reproduced with permission from Amery et al.[25]

guest edited by M. Donald Blaufox. Most important and significant results of the HDFP study are included in this supplement. In addition, Cressman and Gifford and MacMahon and associates provide 2 additional articles giving outsiders prospective of the significance of the HDFP study and its relation to other clinical trials of hypertension throughout the world. This is a superb collection of 8 articles.[26–33]

Hypertensive emergencies

Ferguson and Vlasses[34] from Reno, Nevada, and Philadelphia, Pennsylvania, summarized recommendations for treatment of hypertensive emergencies and urgencies. The authors defined *emergencies* as situations in which greatly elevated BP must be lowered within 1 hour to reduce actual patient risk, and *urgencies* as situations where severe elevations in BP are not causing immediate in-organ damage, but should be controlled within 24 hours to reduce potential patient risk (Tables 5-7 and 5-8).

Houston[35] from Nashville, Tennessee, reviewed findings in a total of 101 patients who had been reported in whom oral clonidine was used to control BP in a hypertensive crisis (Table 5-9). The average total dose of clonidine hydrochloride used was 0.36 mg, the average decrease in systolic BP was 56 mmHg; in diastolic BP, 25 mmHg; and in mean arterial pressure, 38 mmHg. The average time to maximum reduction in BP was 2.75 hours, and the average response rate was 93%. In all patients studied, there was no apparent

TABLE 5-7. *Hypertensive emergencies -vs- urgencies. Reproduced with permission from Ferguson and Vlasses.*[34]

Emergencies
  Blood pressure should be reduced within 1 hr
    Hypertensive encephalopathy
    Severe malignant hypertension accompanied by
      Acute left ventricular failure
      Acute myocardial infarction or unstable angina pectoris
      Dissecting aortic aneurysm
      Stroke or head trauma
      Progressing renal insufficiency
      Eclampsia with convulsions or fetal distress
      Postoperative bleeding
      Extensive burns
Urgencies
  Blood pressure should be reduced within 24 hr
    Severe or accelerated hypertension without evidence of end-organ dysfunction
    Perioperative hypertension, including patients requiring emergency surgery

TABLE 5-8. *Drugs recommended for hypertensive emergencies and urgencies. Reproduced with permission from Ferguson and Vlasses.*[34]

Emergencies
  Parenteral therapy required
    Sodium nitroprusside
    Diazoxide
    Trimethaphan camsylate
    Nitroglycerin
    Labetalol
    Hydralazine
    Captopril*
Urgencies
  Oral therapy preferred
    Clonidine
    Nifedipine
    Captopril
    Labetalol

* Renal crisis of scleroderma.

TABLE 5-9. *Hypertensive emergencies. Reproduced with permission from Ferguson and Vlasses.*[34]

Cerebrovascular accidents (CVAs), including intracranial hemorrhage, thrombotic CVA, or subarachnoid hemorrhage
Hypertensive encephalopathy
Acute dissection of aorta
Acute pulmonary edema and severe congestive heart failure
Eclampsia
Pheochromocytoma with hypertensive crisis
Grade III or IV Keith-Wagener funduscopic changes (exudates, hemorrhages, papilledema)
Acute renal insufficiency secondary to hypertension
Myocardial insufficiency syndromes (angina pectoris, accelerated angina pectoris, acute myocardial infarction)

Hypertensive Urgencies

Severe blood pressure elevation (diastolic blood pressure >120 mm Hg), minimal end-organ damage with no evidence of conditions listed in Table I
Grade I or II Keith-Wagener changes
Postoperative hypertension
Preoperative uncontrolled or untreated hypertension

relation between baseline mean arterial pressure and the dose of clonidine necessary to achieve a successful response, and no clinical characteristics predicted which patients would and would not respond. A rapid, graded reduction in BP started 30–60 minutes after an oral dose, with peak blood levels at 90 minutes, a maximum clinical effect at 2–4 hours, and a duration of 8–12 hours. This gradual reduction in BP allows for careful titration to a BP level that does not decrease below the critical profusion pressure for vital organs.

Tricyclic antidepressant use in hypertensive patients

Little information exists on the epidemiology of central nervous system side effects in patients taking antihypertensive medications. Avorn and associates[36] from Boston, Massachusetts, examined prevalence rates of tricyclic antidepressant (TCA) use among a random sample of 143,253 Medicaid recipients. The TCA use was compared for patients taking any of 7 antihypertensive agents and for those prescribed insulin or oral hypoglycemic agents. Use of TCA was significantly higher in patients taking beta-blockers (23% over 2 years) (Fig. 5-5) than for patients taking hydralazine or hypoglycemics (both 15%) or methyldopa or reserpine (both 10%). Prevalence rate ratios revealed a risk of being prescribed a TCA of 1.5 for patients receiving beta blockers relative to patients receiving hydralazine or hypoglycemics. Beta-blocker use may be an important cause of iatrogenic depression among hypertensive patients.

Effects of nonsteroidal anti-inflammatory drugs in patients taking beta blockers or diuretics

The adverse effects of nonsteroidal anti-inflammatory drugs (NSAIDs) on renal function has been attributed partly to inhibition of renal synthesis of vasodilator prostaglandins such as prostacyclin and prostaglandin E_2.

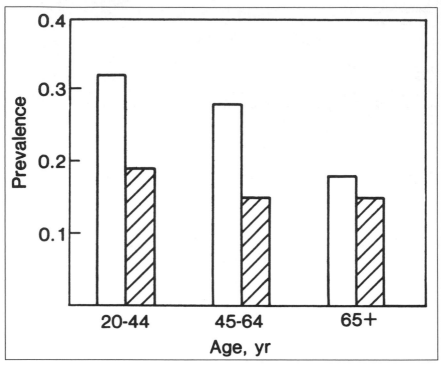

Fig. 5-5. Antidepressant use among patients receiving β-blockers. Two-year prevalence by age. Solid bars indicate women; slashed bars, men. Reproduced with permission from Avron et al.[36]

NSAIDs are reported to cause fluid retention and systemic hypertension, and may impair BP control in hypertensive patients treated with beta blockers. Because sodium deprivation exacerbates the renal effects of NSAIDs, these drugs might be expected to impair BP control in hypertensive patients being treated with diuretics and beta blockers. In a hypertension clinic population of >2,000 referred patients, most of whom have resistant hypertension, Wong and associates[37] from London, Canada, observed such an interaction in about 1% of patients annually. Because hypertension is common and because NSAIDs are used frequently, the authors explored the interaction between NSAIDs, namely, *sulindac*, and antihypertensive therapy, and they determined whether any NSAID is less likely to effect BP control in patients taking antihypertensive drugs. These authors compared the effect of sulindac on renal function and BP with those of placebo, *piroxicam*, and *naproxen* in 20 patients with primary systemic hypertension being treated with a diuretic and a beta blocker. Although the 3 NSAIDs did not differ in their effect on renal function or on serum thromboxane and plasma 6-keto prostaglandin $F_1\alpha$ (6-keto $PGF_1\alpha$), BP was significantly lower with sulindac than with placebo, piroxicam, or naproxen. These differences were associated with less renal cyclooxygenase inhibition by sulindac than by other NSAIDs. These findings suggest that BP differences reflect vasodilation due to differences in the balance between systemic and renal effects of the NSAIDs.

Antihypertensive Therapy in Chronic Obstructive Pulmonary Disease

Hill[38] from Boston, Massachusetts, reviewed choices of drugs for treatment of systemic hypertension in patients with chronic obstructive lung disease (Table 5-10). He suggested the following: "Thiazide diuretics have no adverse effect on airway function and are the agents of choice for initial therapy. B-Antagonists are usually considered first-line agents in antihypertensive therapy, but even relatively cardioselective ones may increase airway resistance in patients with obstructive lung diseases, and they should be used with caution, if at all, in such patients. Although potassium-wasting diuretics are the preferred agents for treating hypertension in patients with chronic obstructive lung disease, they may worsen carbon dioxide retention in hypoventilating patients and potentiate hypokalemia in those receiving corticosteroids. In addition, B-agonists may substantially lower serum potassium levels in patients already rendered hypokalemic by diuretics. Patients with chronic obstructive lung disease receiving potassium-wasting diuretics who have chronic respiratory acidosis or are receiving corticosteroids or B-agonists should undergo close monitoring of electrolyte levels and be considered for therapy with potassium supplements or, preferably, potassium-sparing agents."

Vegetarian diet

Margetts and associates[39] from Nedlands and Perth, Australia, allocated in a randomized crossover trial 58 subjects aged 30–64 years with mild untreated systemic hypertension either to a control group eating a typical omnivorous diet or to 1 or 2 groups eating an ovolactovegetarian diet for 1 of 2 6-week periods. A decrease in systolic BP of about 5 mmHg occurred during the vegetarian diet periods, with a corresponding increase on resuming a meat diet. The main nutrient changes with the vegetarian diet included an increase in the ratio of polyunsaturated to saturated fats and intake of fibre, calcium, and magnesium and a decrease in the intake of protein and vitamin B_{12}. There were no consistent changes in urinary sodium or potassium excretion or body weight. In untreated subjects with mild hypertension, changing to a vegetarian diet may bring about a worthwhile decrease in systolic BP.

Weight reduction -vs- metoprolol

MacMahon and associates[40] from Sydney, Australia, compared the effects of weight reduction, metoprolol, and placebo on M-mode echocardiographic measurements of LV thickness and mass in a 21-week, randomized-controlled trial that enrolled 41 young, overweight patients with systemic

TABLE 5-10. *Diuretics commonly used for antihypertensive therapy. Reproduced with permission from Hill.*[38]

	THERAPEUTIC DOSE, MG/DAY	ESTIMATED MONTHLY COST, $*	MAJOR SIDE EFFECTS
Potassium-wasting diuretics			Hypokalemia, hypomagnesemia,
Thiazides			hyperglycemia, hyperuricemia,
Hydrochlorothiazide	25–200	1–4	hyperlipidemia, and hypercalcemia
Chlorthalidone	25–100	3–6	
Loop diuretics: furosemide	20–200	2–15	Same as thiazides, plus hypercalciuria and possibly deafness
Potassium-sparing diuretics			Gynecomastia (spironolactone only);
Spironolactone	50–200	12–44	nausea, headaches, dizziness;
Triamterene	100–200	7–14	hyperkalemia possible with renal
Amiloride	5–20	8–28	insufficiency or high potassium intake

* Based on 1985 prices from New England Medical Center Pharmacy, Boston.

hypertension. At the end of the follow-up period, the patients in the weight reduction group had lost an average of 8.3 kg, and their BP had decreased by an average of 14/13 mmHg, compared with 12/8 mmHg in the metoprolol group and 9/4 mmHg in the placebo group. In the weight reduction group, interventricular septal and posterior wall thickness decreased by 14% and 11%, respectively, and LV mass decreased by 20% (16% when adjusted for body-surface area). Decreases in ventricular septal and posterior wall thickness and in LV mass in the weight reduction group were significantly greater than those in the placebo group. The changes in thickness of the ventricular septum and LV mass in the weight reduction group were also greater than those in the metoprolol group. Changes in weight, independent of changes in BP were directly associated with changes in LV mass. The authors concluded that weight reduction decreases LV mass in overweight hypertensive patients and that control of obesity is important not only for the treatment of hypertension but also for the prevention of LV hypertrophy. This article was followed by an editorial entitled "Cardiomyopathy of Obesity—A Not So Victorian Disease" by Franz Messerli.[41]

Physical activity

Nelson and associates[42] from Prahran, Australia, assessed the long-term effect of exercise on BP in 13 untreated patients with essential hypertension. After a 6-week run-in period the levels of activity studied were 1) sedentary, 2) 45-minute bicycling at 60–70% of maximum work capacity (Wmax) 3 times per week (3/week), and 3) 45-minute bicycling 7 times per week (7/week), each for 4 weeks. The order differed between subjects in accordance with a Latin square. Supine BP, 48 hours after each phase, averaged 148/99 mmHg with 3/week exercise, and by 16/11 mmHg with 7/week exercise. With increasing activity total peripheral resistance decreased and the cardiac index increased. Plasma noradrenaline concentration decreased below values in the sedentary phase by 21% and 33% after 3/week and 7/week exercise. Body weight and 24-hour sodium excretion remained constant. Moderate regular exercise lowers BP and seems to be an important nonpharmacologic method of treating hypertension.

Calcium supplementation

In a double-blind trial, Grobbee and Hofman[43] from Rotterdam, The Netherlands, randomly assigned 90 mildly hypertensive subjects ages 16–29 years 1 g/day of calcium, or placebo. Calcium supplementation did not affect systolic BP, but at 6 and 12 weeks diastolic BP had decreased by 3·1 and 2·4 mmHg, respectively, more in the calcium group than in the placebo group. Subjects with a baseline plasma parathyroid hormone higher than the median showed a 6·1 mmHg greater decrease in diastolic BP after 6 weeks and 5·4 mmHg after 12 weeks than did the placebo group. The decrease in diastolic BP was greater in the calcium group than in the placebo group in subjects with a lower than median serum total calcium and in those with a large body weight. Calcium supplementation may lower BP in young people with mildly raised BP, particularly in those with high plasma parathyroid hormone or low serum total calcium, or both.

Fish oil

MaxEPA is an oil derivative of marine fish rich in o3 polyunsaturated fatty acids eicosapentaenoic acid (20:5o3) and docosahexaenoic acid (22:6o3), which significantly reduce systolic BP in both normal volunteers and patients undergoing hemodialysis. No data exist on the effect of dietary supplementation with fish oil in patients with systemic hypertension. To fill this void, Norris and associates[44] from London, England, studied 8 men and 8 women, aged 45–74 years, in whom the supine diastolic BP was 90–110 mmHg and systolic pressure <200 mmHg. After a 2-month run-in period without treatment they were randomly assigned to double-blind treatment with Max EPA 16, 5 g/day, or indistinguishable placebo capsules. Patients crossed over to the alternate treatment after 6 weeks. The mean BP before randomization was 160/94 mmHg. Mean BP after 6 weeks of placebo treatment was 161/95 mmHg and after 6-weeks treatment with Max EPA 151/93 mmHg (Fig. 5-6). Lying systolic BP was lower after treatment with MaxEPA than treatment

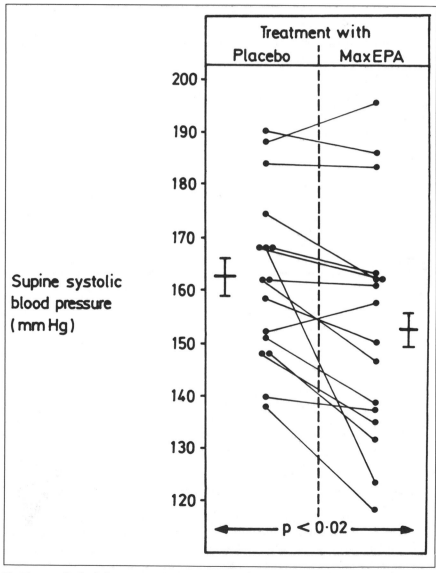

Fig. 5-6. Individual changes in supine systolic blood pressure between sixth week of placebo and sixth week of MaxEPA treatment. Bars represent means and SEM. Reproduced with permission from Norris et al.[44]

with placebo by a mean of 6% and standing systolic BP was a mean 6% lower after MaxEPA. The mechanism of antihypertensive action of fish oil in unclear.

Hydrochlorothiazide -vs- acebutolol

Wahl and associates[45] from Los Angeles, California, compared oral acebutolol (n = 182) with hydrochlorothiazide (n = 178) in the treatment of mild-to-moderate essential hypertension (diastolic BP 95–114 mmHg). Both agents produced significant and comparable reductions in systolic, diastolic, and mean BP of 16, 15, and 15 mmHg with acebutolol, and 15, 13, and 12 mmHg with hydrochlorothiazide. Acebutolol induced a significant reduction in heart rate at rest of 9 beats/minute from baseline. The mean effective doses of acebutolol and hydrochlorothiazide were 757 and 68 mg, respectively. Significantly fewer patients taking acebutolol had arrhythmia, anorexia, and flatulence, although an equal number of patients in each group discontinued therapy prematurely because of side effects (14 patients). More hydrochlorothiazide-treated patients had abnormalities in the levels of serum glucose, uric acid, blood urea nitrogen, serum potassium, and chloride. No clinically significant trends in laboratory parameters were seen with acebutolol, although a small number of patients (11 taking acebutolol and 3 taking hydrochlorothiazide) had asymptomatic positive antinuclear antibody tests of low titer. The data show that acebutolol is as effective as hydrochlorothiazide in the treatment of hypertension, is as well as tolerated, and produces fewer biochemical abnormalities.

Hydrochlorothiazide -vs- metroprolol

Wikstrand and associates[46] in an international multicenter study, compared in a randomized, double-blind study involving 562 patients, a traditional treatment schedule starting antihypertensive treatment in elderly patients, aged 60–75 years, with 25 mg of hydrochlorothiazide once daily. If a satisfactory response was not achieved the dose was doubled to 100 mg of metoprolol once daily, adding 12.5 mg of hydrochlorothiazide for patients whose response was not satisfactorily achieved with metoprolol alone. Systolic and diastolic BP was significantly reduced with both regimens. The frequency rates of responders (diastolic BP ≤95 mmHg) in the metoprolol group and the hydrochlorothiazide group were 50% and 47% after 4 weeks and 65% and 61% after 8 weeks, respectively. There were no significant differences in total symptom score or single symptoms between the regimens, but significantly more patients had hypokalemia and hyperuricemia with the hydrochlorothiazide regimen. Thus, the authors concluded that beginning antihypertensive treatment with 100 mg of metoprolol once daily and adding a small dose of hydrochlorothiazide (12.5 mg) in patients whose response is not satisfactory with metoprolol alone appears to be effective and safe in elderly hypertensive patients.

Hydrochlorothiazide -vs- atenolol -vs- enalapril

Helgeland and associates[47] from 3 centers in Norway, compared enalapril, atenolol, and hydrochlorothiazide in a double-blind, randomized parallel study in general practice: 436 patients with mild-to-moderate systemic hypertension (sitting diastolic BP 95–120 mmHg for patients aged <60 years and 100–120 mmHg for patients over age 60 years after ≥3 initial recordings) (Fig. 5-7). A 2-week placebo run-in period was followed by 16 weeks of monotherapy. The initial doses were enalapril 20 mg, atenolol 50 mg, and

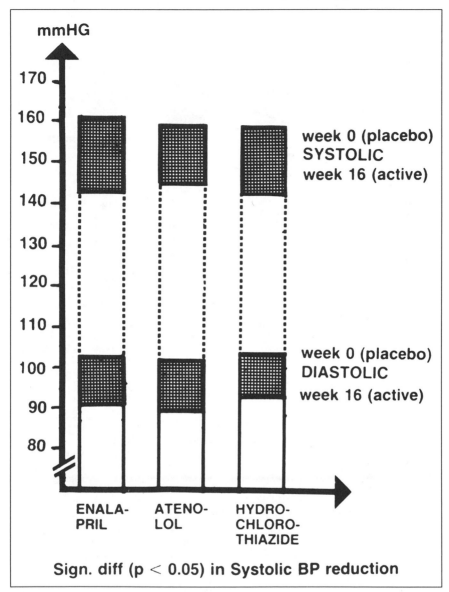

Fig. 5-7. Blood pressure after placebo (week 0) and active treatment (week 16). Reproduced with permission from Helgeland et al.[47]

hydrochlorothiazide 25 mg. These were doubled if treatment was not effective after 4 weeks. Adverse reactions were the main reason for withdrawal from the study (9 taking enalapril, 19 taking atenolol, and 8 taking hydrochlorothiazide) (Fig. 5-8). Systolic and diastolic BP was significantly reduced in all 3 groups. The reduction in systolic BP was greater with enalapril than with atenolol. Serum potassium was reduced and uric acid increased with hydrochlorothiazide. Fasting blood sugar increased with atenolol but decreased with enalapril. The frequency of adverse reactions was acceptable in all 3 groups. After 16 weeks of treatment, significantly more adverse reactions were recorded in the atenolol group than in the enalapril group. Enalapril is effective and well tolerated in patients with mild-to-moderate hypertension.

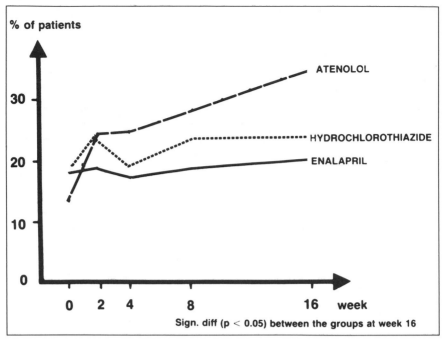

Fig. 5-8. Number of patients with adverse reactions. Reproduced with permission from Helgeland et al.[47]

Diuretic + nadolol + minoxidil

Spitalewitz and associates[48] from Brooklyn, New York, tested a once-a-day antihypertensive regimen using minoxidil, nadolol, and a diuretic in 55 patients with resistant systemic hypertension. Forty-seven patients had evidence of end-organ damage. Twelve had mild renal insufficiency (serum creatinine concentration, 2.5 ± 0.3 mg/dl). In 34 patients, treatment with nadolol and a diuretic was started with minoxidil added 1 to 4 weeks later. In the remaining patients, minoxidil, nadolol, and a diuretic were begun simultaneously because of severe hypertension. Initial supine and standing BP in the 55 patients were $186 \pm 4/111 \pm 2$ and $180 \pm 4/108 \pm 2$ mmHg, respectively. After 7 ± 1 weeks, BP was controlled in 46 patients (84%) with supine and standing BP reduced to $140 \pm 3/80 \pm 1$ and $134 \pm 3/80 \pm 1$ mmHg, respectively. In 6 patients, BP was controlled but intolerable side effects occurred, making the regimen therapeutically successful in 40 patients (73%). The BP remained controlled during a follow-up of 43 ± 5 weeks. In 31 patients, BPs measured 24 hours after the last dose were not different from random measurements. Mean serum creatinine levels remained stable in the 12 patients with renal insufficiency.

Pindolol

van den Meiracker and colleagues[49] from Rotterdam, The Netherlands, administered pindolol, a beta blocker with considerable partial agonist activity, to 10 hypertensive patients. The maximal decrease in mean arterial pressure was seen 3 to 4 hours after oral dosing with 10 mg of pindolol ($-15 \pm 3\%$). This was caused by reduction in total peripheral resistance, which amounted to $25 \pm 4\%$ after 24 hours. Cardiac output increased by $16 \pm 5\%$. Cardiac filling pressures and PA pressure did not change. Increasing the dose of pindolol from 5 mg twice a day to 15 mg twice a day over a 3-week period, caused no further change in mean arterial pressure. After 3 weeks, the decrease in mean arterial pressure ($-11 \pm 2\%$) was maintained by reduced total peripheral resistance ($-26 \pm 6\%$), whereas cardiac output and stroke volume were increased by $16 \pm 6\%$ and $26 \pm 6\%$. Renal blood flow and glomerular filtration rate did not change. Beta blockers devoid of partial agonist activity lower cardiac output, whereas the elevated total peripheral resistance in hypertension is unchanged. The hemodynamic profile of pindolol essentially differs from that of beta blockers devoid of partial agonist activity.

Propranolol -vs- verapamil

Cubeddu and associates[50] from multiple medical centers in the USA compared verapamil and propranolol for monotherapy of systemic hypertension. Verapamil lowered BP more effectively than propranolol in both black and white patients (Fig. 5-9). Verapamil was equally effective in blacks and whites, whereas propranolol was more effective in whites. Heart rate was reduced by 6 beats/minute with verapamil, and by 14 beats/minute with propranolol. In blacks, verapamil lowered systolic BP 17 -vs- 8 mmHg for propranolol; verapamil reduced diastolic BP 13 -vs- 9 mmHg for propranolol. In whites, verapamil lowered systolic BP 19 -vs- 13 mmHg for propranolol; verapamil reduced diastolic BP 17 -vs- 12 mmHg for propranolol. Increases in systolic BP were observed in 22% and 3% of patients receiving propranolol and verapamil, respectively. The PR interval was increased from 164–175 ms for verapamil -vs- 160–164 ms for propranolol. Constipation (15%) and headaches (10%) were most frequent complaints for verapamil -vs- fatigue (18%) and dizziness (7%) for propranolol. Changes in blood biochemistry values were of small magnitude. The authors concluded that verapamil monotherapy is a safe and effective means of achieving BP control in patients with essential hypertension.

Propranolol -vs- methyldopa -vs- captopril

Croog and associates[51] from several medical centers, conducted a multi-center randomized double-blind clinical trial among 626 men with mild-to-moderate systemic hypertension (a median diastolic BP in the seated position of 92–109 mmHg on 3 determinations within 5 minutes) to determine the effects of captopril, methyldopa, and propranolol on their *quality of life*. Hydrochlorothiazide was added if needed to control BP. After a 24-week treatment period, all 3 groups had similar BP control, although fewer patients taking propranolol required hydrochlorothiazide. Patients taking captopril alone or in combination with a diuretic were least likely to withdraw from treatment because of adverse effects (8% -vs- 20% for methyldopa and 13% for propranolol). The treatment groups were similar in scores for sleep dysfunction, visual memory, and social participation. However, patients taking captopril, compared with patients taking methyldopa, scored significantly higher on measures of general well-being, had fewer side effects, and had better scores for work performance, visual-motor functioning, and measures of life satisfaction. Patients taking propranolol also reported better work performance than patients taking methyldopa. Patients taking captopril reported fewer side effects and less sexual dysfunction than those taking propranolol and had greater improvement on measures of general well-being. The findings show that antihypertensive agents have different effects on the quality of life and that these can be meaningfully assessed with available psychosocial measures. This article was followed by an editorial by

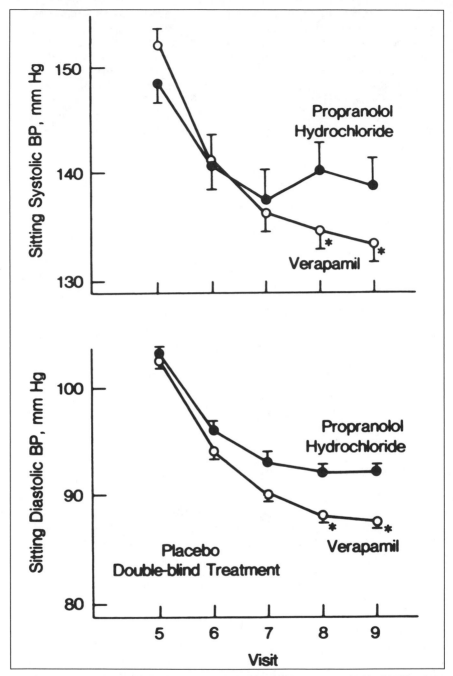

Fig. 5-9.   Comparative antihypertensive effects of verapamil and propranolol hydrochloride in patients with mild to moderate essential hypertension. Shown are means ± SD of sitting systolic and diastolic blood pressure (BP) in patients receiving propranolol (n = 59) or verapamil (n = 60) during last week of placebo run-in period (week 5) and four weeks of treatment period (weeks 6 through 9). Asterisks indicate significantly different from propranolol at p <.01. Reproduced with permission from Cubeddu et al.[50]

Chobanian.[52] Chobanian pointed out that the goal of antihypertensive therapy should be not only to reduce morbidity and mortality, i.e., to reduce the BP level, but also to do so without adverse effects on the functional well-being of patients.

Atenolol -vs- nifedipine

Daniels and Opie[53] from Capetown, South Africa, used 3 therapies to treat 35 patients with mild-to-moderate systemic hypertension: 1) the cardio-selective beta-adrenoceptor blocker atenolol, 2) the calcium antagonist nifedipine, and 3) combination therapy for those who failed to reach the target diastolic BP of <90 mmHG with monotherapy. After an initial run-on placebo period, when the mean supine diastolic BP was 102 ± 1 mmHg (mean ± standard error of the mean), patients were randomized (double-blind) to atenolol, 100 mg, as a single daily dose of nifedipine (slow-release form), 20 mg twice daily, then to a washout dummy placebo period before crossover. Each period lasted 4 weeks. Supine, erect, and exercise BP were recorded. Atenolol and nifedipine, in the same fixed doses but in combination, were given to 20 patients in whom either supine or erect diastolic BP exceeded 90 mmHg after the period of monotherapy. Atenolol monotherapy reduced the erect diastolic BP to <90 mmHg in 14 patients (40%); of the remaining patients, 1 responded only to fixed-dose nifedipine and 11 to combination therapy, yielding a total success rate of 74%. The combination gave enhanced control, as shown by a further decrease in supine and erect BP and by better control of exercise BP; these effects were achieved without an increased incidence of adverse effects. The mean reductions in supine diastolic BP were: atenolol, 9 ± 2 mmHg; nifedipine, 6 ± 2 mmHg; and combination therapy, 16 ± 2 mmHg. Corresponding reductions in erect BP were: atenolol, 12 ± 2 mmHg; nifedipine 5 ± 2 mmHg; and combination therapy, 21 ± 2 mmHg. Thus, fixed-dose atenolol-nifedipine combination gave enhanced control of BP, resulting in mean diastolic values close of 90 mmHg in patients who did not respond to monotherapy.

Diltiazem

Amodeo and co-workers[54] from New Orleans, Louisiana, evaluated the immediate effects of intravenous diltiazem and short-term effects (4 weeks) of the oral drug on systemic and regional hemodynamics, cardiac structure, and humoral responses by previously reported methods in 9 patients with mild-to-moderate essential hypertension and in 1 patient with primary aldosteronism. Diltiazem was first administered in 3 intravenous doses of 0.06, 0.06, and 0.12 mg/kg, respectively; patients were then treated for 4 weeks with daily doses ranging from 240 to 360 mg. Intravenous diltiazem immediately reduced mean arterial pressure from 115–96 mmHg through a decrease in total peripheral resistance index from 37–23 U/m^2 that was associated with an increase in heart rate from 66–77 beats/minute; and cardiac index from 3.3–4.3 liters/min/m^2. These changes were not associated with changes in plasma levels of catecholamines or aldosterone or in plasma renin activity. After 4 weeks the significant decrease in mean arterial pressure persisted and there were still no changes in the humoral substances or plasma volume. Renal blood flow index increased from 368–462 ml/min/m^2 and renal vascular resistance index decreased from 0.37–0.26 U/m^2; splanchnic hemodynamics did not change. LV mass significantly decreased from 242–217 g.

Thus, the decrease in arterial BP produced by diltiazem was associated with improved renal hemodynamics and reduced LV mass without expansion of intravascular volume or alterations in circulating humoral substances.

Pool and associates[55] from San Francisco and Duarte, California, carried out a multicenter, randomized, placebo-controlled parallel group study of diltiazem in essential hypertension in 77 patients (40 diltiazem, 37 placebo) with stable supine diastolic BP between 95 and 110 mmHg. Patients were withdrawn from previous antihypertensive therapy for ≥ 4 weeks, titrated to the optimal dose, and followed for a total of 12 weeks during therapy. A diltiazem dose of 360 mg/day was required in 85% of the patients. Average BP in all positions was significantly reduced by diltiazem compared with placebo. With diltiazem, average supine BP decreased from 156/100 mmHg at baseline to 141/87 mmHg at end titration and 145/90 mmHg at week 12, whereas average standing BP decreased from 152/101–136/90 and 143/91 mmHg, respectively, at those times. There was no significant change in heart rate at week 12. Diltiazem tended to be more effective in older patients, but caused no increase in orthostatic BP reduction. There were no statistically significant changes in BP in the placebo group. Two patients receiving placebo and 1 patient receiving diltiazem discontinued therapy as a result of adverse effects, and overall, side effects were only slightly more common with diltiazem treatment. Thus, diltiazem was effective and well-tolerated single therapy for mild-to-moderate systemic hypertension and appears to compare favorably to most agents being used.

Yamauchi and associates[56] from Nagoya, Japan, evaluated the effects of diltiazem on exercise-induced changes in cardiovascular response, plasma renin activity, platelet function and blood coagulability with multistage treadmill exercise in 20 patients who had systemic hypertension. Heart rate, BP, and BP–heart rate product at rest, at peak exercise, and in the recovery period were significantly reduced after 4 weeks of diltiazem administration, 180 mg/day. Plasma renin activity tended to increase after the medication. However, platelet adenosine diphosphate-induced aggregation sensitivity, prothrombin time, activated partial thromboplastin time, plasma fibrinogen concentration, and antithrombin III activity did not change significantly. The authors concluded that diltiazem could ameliorate the hyperresponsiveness of heart rate and BP to exercise in hypertensive patients without affecting blood coagulability.

Nifedipine

Nifedipine is known to reduce BP both acutely and chronically. However, the following questions remain to be answered: 1) Can nifedipine be given acutely and safely to patients with severe hypertension in an outpatient setting? 2) Would its efficacy be retained with long-term therapy? and 3) Is nifedipine safe in the presence of cardiomegaly? Jennings and colleagues[57] from Cape Town, South Africa, gave nifedipine (10-mg capsules sublingually) to 46 outpatients with severe or apparently refractory hypertension; 19 were followed up for 18 months and 18 for 24 months. Nifedipine reduced BP acutely and safely in 43 of 46 outpatients (mean control diastolic pressure 137 mmHg) irrespective of prior treatment regimen. BP levels after 2–24 months of twice-daily oral nifedipine (10 mg) were similar to 20-minute levels, showing that tolerance did not occur. In a separate series of 37 patients, who had radiologic cardiomegaly in addition to hypertension, the control EF was 62%. Nifedipine, when used acutely, slightly increased EF to 65%. These studies show that in outpatients with severe hypertension, sublingual nifedipine is an antihypertensive agent that acts swiftly and safely, without causing a decrease in EF when used for acute BP reduction; and that subsequent therapy with oral nifedipine results in a predictive long-term hypotensive effect.

Adler and associates[58] from Philadelphia, Pennsylvania, administered nifedipine sublingually perioperatively to 19 patients ≥60 years of age undergoing ophthalmologic surgery. All patients had a systolic BP >200 mmHg or diastolic BP of 110 mmHg and 18 patients had both. Average (mean ± standard deviation) systolic BP decreased from 225 ± 14–155 ± 19 mmHg, whereas average diastolic BP decrease from 122 ± 12–78 ± 11 mmHg. Mean time to onset of response to nifedipine was 9 ± 4 minutes, whereas the maximum antihypertensive response occurred at 35 ± 10 minutes. A prompt antihypertensive response was obtained without any serious side effects. This is the first study demonstrating the efficacy and safety of sublingual nifedipine for the management of perioperative hypertension.

Ferlinz[59] from Chicago, Illinois, nicely reviewed the uses and abuses of nifedipine for a variety of cardiovascular disorders.

Verapamil

Frishman and associates[60] from Bronx, New York, evaluated the antihypertensive effect of twice-daily administration of verapamil hydrochloride in 21 adult patients with mild-to-moderate essential hypertension. After 4 weeks of placebo therapy, verapamil was given for 4 weeks with a treatment goal of sitting diastolic BP of <90 mmHg, or to a maximum dose of 160 mg twice daily. Sitting and standing BP, heart rate, and verapamil plasma levels were determined weekly, 10–12 hours after dose administration. At the maximal dose (mean 154 ± 19.2 mg), heart rate was not affected, side effects were minimal, and sitting diastolic BP was significantly reduced from placebo baseline, with 12 of 21 patients having a decrease in sitting diastolic BP of ≥10 mmHg or to <90 mmHg. A trough verapamil plasma level of >80 ng/ml was associated with a good hypotensive response. These data indicate the safety and utility of twice-daily verapamil administration for the treatment of essential hypertension and suggest the value of obtaining verapamil plasma levels as a guide to dosage determination.

Nifedipine -vs- verapamil

Agabiti-Rosei et al[61] in Perugia, Italy, studied the short- and long-term effects of 2 calcium channel blocking agents, verapamil and nifedipine, on BP, heart rate, plasma catecholamines, plasma renin activity, plasma volume, and cardiac performance in patients with essential hypertension and normal subjects. Verapamil, 160 mg orally, reduced BP within 60 minutes in 22 hypertensive patients, but not in 12 normal subjects. Nifedipine, 10 mg sublingually, reduced BP within 15 minutes in 19 hypertensive patients, but not in 7 normotensive subjects. Plasma norepinephrine was significantly increased both in normal subjects and in hypertension patients only after nifedipine was administered. Verapamil, 80 mg, 3 times a day initially and nifedipine, 10 mg, 3 times a day thereafter or in a reverse order were administered to 12 hospitalized hypertensive patients on a fixed sodium and potassium diet (Fig. 5-10). The drugs produced similar BP reductions, but heart rate and plasma catecholamines were increased only after nifedipine. Thus, BP is effectively reduced by both verapamil and nifedipine in patients with sys-

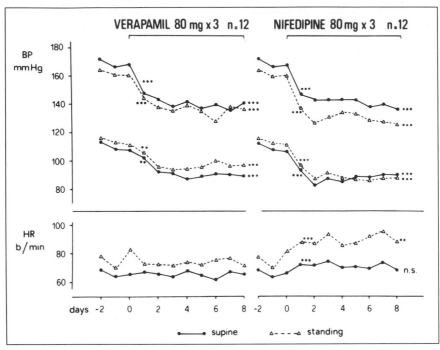

Fig. 5-10. Daily average values of blood pressure (BP) and heart rate (HR) in 12 hypertensive patients treated with verapamil (80 mg three times a day) and nifedipine (10 mg three times a day). Statistical significance is given only for the first and the eighth day of treatment. **p <0.01; ***p <0.001. Reproduced with permission from Agabiti-Rosei et al.[61]

temic arterial hypertension, but an important adrenergic stimulation may be caused by nifedipine but not usually by verapamil.

Captopril

To evaluate the role of regional hemodynamics in mediating the long-term depressor effect of the converting enzyme inhibitor, captopril, at a low dose (37.5 mg/day) for 2 weeks, its systemic, renal, and forearm circulatory actions were determined in 12 patients with mild-to-moderate essential hypertension by Ando and associates[62] from Ibaraki, Japan. After administration of captopril, there was a significant decline in mean BP (average −12 ± 2%) accompanied by a decrease in systemic vascular resistance (−9 ± 3%), but cardiac output did not change. Although forearm vascular resistance was not altered, renal vascular resistance decreased considerably (−17 ± 5%). Moreover, there was a highly significant correlation between the changes in mean BP and renal vascular resistance. Plasma renin activity increased after therapy as plasma aldosterone decreased, while plasma norepinephrine slightly increased. The change in renal vascular resistance significantly correlated with the pretreatment level of plasma renin activity. These findings suggest that suppression of the renin-angiotensin system in essential hypertension induces selective vasodilation in the renal vasculature, which may play an important role in the long-term antihypertensive effect of the converting enzyme inhibitor. This renal vasodilator action appears to be the feature that distinguishes the converting enzyme inhibitor from conventional vasodilator drugs.

Enalapril

Reams and Bauer[63] from Columbia, Missouri, examined the effect of the angiotensin-converting enzyme inhibitor, enalapril maleate, on BP, renal function, protein excretion, and potassium homeostasis in 9 patients with systemic hypertension (diastolic BP >90 mmHg) and moderate-to-severe renal dysfunction (creatinine clearance <70 ml/min/1.73 m²). The initial inulin clearance for the 9 patients was 48 ml/min/1.73². Six patients were treated with enalapril monotherapy and 3 with combination enalapril/furosemide therapy. Systolic and diastolic BP was well controlled. Supine plasma renin activity was stimulated; the supine plasma aldosterone level was suppressed, with a resultant increase in the serum potassium level. Clinical hyperkalemia was not observed. Glomerular filtration rate, assessed by inulin and creatinine clearances, was not significantly changed. Effective renal plasma flow, assessed by para-aminohippurate clearance was significantly increased, with a resultant decrease in filtration fraction. Importantly, urinary protein excretion was markedly reduced. These results suggest that enalapril therapy produces efferent arteriolar dilitation with preservation of the glomerular filtration rate. Enalapril therapy may also blunt the effects of anglotensin II on transglomerular passage of protein, as demonstrated by reduced proteinuria. These findings suggest that interruption of the renin-angiotensin system in patients with preexisting renal disease may have renal protective effects.

Clonidine

Popli and associates[64] from Hines, Illinois, treated 30 patients with mild essential hypertension, (diastolic BP from 90–105 mmHg) with clonidine from a skin patch reservoir designed to release medication at a constant rate for 7 days. After a 4-week washout period of former antihypertensive medications, patients were randomized double-blindly into a clonidine- or a placebo-treated group. Clonidine or placebo was then given for 5 weeks, followed by a 2-week washout period to assess withdrawal from treatment. BP was controlled in 11 of 15 clonidine-treated patients but in only 4 of 15 placebo-treated patients. The clonidine-treated group evidenced larger decreases in both systolic and diastolic BP. In the clonidine-treated group, BP and plasma clonidine levels were stable throughout a representative 7-day period. Besides mild skin irritation with both clonidine and placebo patches, few side effects were observed. After discontinuation of clonidine administration, plasma levels declined in a non-log linear manner. There was no rebound hypertension. The results suggest that clonidine delivered transdermally is safe and effective for control of mild essential hypertension.

Aspirin

Pregnancy-induced hypertension and pre-eclampsia appear to be associated with increased production of thromboxane A₂ (TXA₂), a potent vasoconstrictor and stimulator of platelet aggregation, by the placenta and by platelets. TXA₂ has been put forward as an etiologic factor for the vasoconstriction, platelet hyperactivity, and uteroplacental arterial thrombosis that characterize pregnancy-induced hypertension and pre-eclampsia. A daily dose of aspirin as low as 1–2 mg/kg effectively inhibits platelet cyclo-oxygenase and synthesis of TXA₂ by platelets, and therefore may have a favorable effect. Accordingly, Wallenburg and associates[65] from Rotterdam, The Netherlands, investigated in a randomized, placebo controlled, double-blind trial the effect of low-dose aspirin, taken daily from 28 weeks' gestation until delivery, on development of pregnancy-induced hypertension and pre-eclampsia in normotensive primigravidae judged to be at risk of hypertension because of an increased BP response to intravenous angiotensin II. An exaggerated sensitivity to angiotension II in normotensive pregnant women is a sensitive predictor of pregnancy-induced hypertension or pre-eclampsia later in pregnancy. To ensure maximum patient compliance, the trial was kept simple and only BP and proteinuria were taken as endpoints. This article was followed by an unsigned editorial entitled Aspirin in Pre-Eclampsia.[66]

Withdrawal of antihypertensive therapy

Alderman and associates[67] from Bronx, New York, and Mineola, New York, conducted a study of a patient group originally drawn from a screened population of union members to determine the fraction of all persons with systemic hypertension who could be successfully withdrawn from antihypertensive medication. Of the 157 patients, 88 (56%) met preestablished BP criteria for drug interruption, and 66 (75%) actually had medication withdrawn (Fig. 5-11). Of these 66 patients, 70% and 55% followed up for 1 and 2

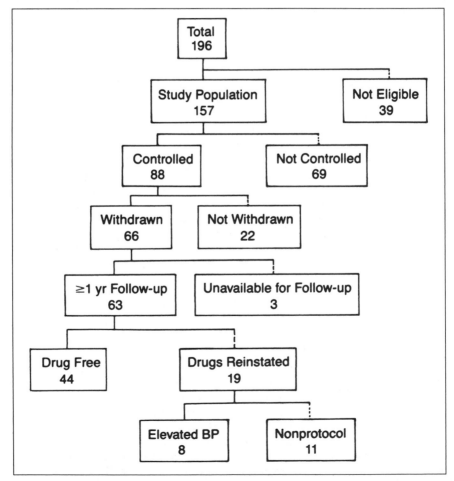

Fig. 5-11. Follow-up of withdrawal study population. BP indicates blood pressure. Reproduced with permission from Alderman et al.[67]

years, respectively, remained normotensive. Patients requiring reintroduction of antihypertensive therapy were distinguished from those remaining drug free by increased systolic BP (141 ± 13-vs-132 ± 9 mmHg) after 1 month. Extrapolation of the finding that 28% of the study population remained normotensive 1 year after drug therapy withdrawal suggests the possibility that as many as 5 million Americans currently taking antihypertensive drugs could have therapy interrupted for at least 1 year and thus avoid both the hazards and costs of drug therapy.

Members of the Medical Research Council Working Party on Mild Hypertension[68] chaired by Professor Sir Stanley Peart randomly allocated a series of 1,418 men and 1,347 women with mild hypertension (diastolic pressure 90–109 mmHg), aged 35–64 years, who had either had long-term antihypertensive treatment with *bendrofluazide* or *propranolol* or taken placebo tablets for a similar period into 2 groups in which their tablets were either stopped or continued. The course of BP and of biochemical variables was followed up for 2 years. Mean BP increased rapidly after the withdrawal of active treatment, and between 9 and 12 months after stopping treatment the antihypertensive effect had almost disappeared. The effect persisting longer than this, and possibly due to resetting of the baroreceptors or of other BP control mechanisms, was very small, and as the increase in mean pressure was due to an upward movement in general distribution there was no evidence of a

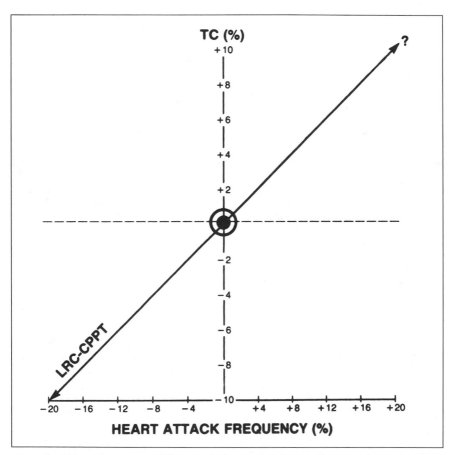

Fig. 5-12. Effect of increasing or decreasing plasma total cholesterol (TC) level on heart attack frequency. LRC-CPPT = Lipid Research Clinics Coronary Primary Prevention Trial. Reproduced with permission from Roberts.[69]

subgroup in whom these mechanisms had been permanently reset to a clinically important extent. After withdrawal of propranolol the increase in pressure was more rapid in younger than in older people. After discontinuing bendrofluazide, pressure increased more rapidly in men who had had higher pressures before and during treatment; this effect was not seen in women. Disturbances in biochemical variables associated with drug treatment had largely resolved by the end of 2 years after withdrawal. Discontinuing placebo tablets made no consistent difference to BP.

Effects of antihypertensive drugs on blood lipids

Roberts[69] from Bethesda, Maryland, reviewed the effects of various antihypertensive drugs on blood lipid levels. It is essential to know that for every 1% drop in the plasma total cholesterol level, the frequency of heart attack (fatal coronary artery disease or non-fatal AMI) drops 2%. Conversely, for every 1% the serum total cholesterol level rises, the heart attack frequency rises by 2% (Fig. 5-12). Diuretics and beta blockers without intrinsic sympathetic activity (ISA) adversely affect blood lipid levels. Beta blockers with ISA, calcium antagonists, and converting-enzyme inhibitors do not adversely affect blood lipid levels.

References

1. Petrie JC, O'Brien ET, Littler WA, Swiet M: Recommendations on blood pressure measurement. Br Med J 1986 (Sept 6); 293:611–615.
2. Health and Public Policy Committee, American College of Physicians: Automated ambulatory blood pressure monitoring. Ann Intern Med 1986 (Feb); 104:275–278.
3. White WB: Assessment of patients with office hypertension by 14-hour noninvasive ambulatory blood pressure monitoring. Arch Intern Med 1986 (Nov); 146:2196–2199.
4. Kotchen JM, McKean HE, Jackson-Thayer S, Moore RW, Straus R, Kotchen TA: Impact of a rural high blood pressure control program on hypertension control and cardiovascular disease mortality. JAMA 1986 (Apr 25); 2177–2182.
5. Mehta SK, Bahler RC, Hanson R, Walsh JT, Rakita L: Relative tachycardia in ambulant children with borderline hypertension. Am Heart J 1986 (Dec); 112:1257–1263.
6. The Working Group on Hypertension in the Elderly: Statement on hypertension in the elderly. JAMA 1986 (July 4); 256:70–74.
7. Radice M, Alli C, Avanzini F, Di Tullio M, Mariotti G, Taioli E, Zussino A, Folli G: Left ventricular structure and function in normotensive adolescents with a genetic predisposition to hypertension. Am Heart J 1986 (Jan); 111:115–120.
8. Boudoulas H, Mantzouratos D, Sohn YH, Weissler AM: Left ventricular mass and systolic performance in chronic systemic hypertension. Am J Cardiol 1986 (Feb 1); 57:232–237.
9. Casale PN, Devereux RB, Milner M, Zullo G, Harshfield GA, Pickering TG, Laragh JH: Value of echocardiographic measurement of left ventricular mass in predicting cardiovascular morbid events in hypertensive men. Annals Intern Med 1986 (Aug); 105:173–178.
10. Kobrin I, Frohlich ED, Ventura HO, Messerli FH: Renal involvement follows cardiac enlargement in essential hypertension. Arch Intern Med 1986 (Feb); 146:272–276.
11. Weder AB: Red-cell lithium-sodium counter-transport and renal lithium clearance in hypertension. N Engl J Med 1986 (Jan 23); 314:198–201.
12. Resnick LM, Muller FB, Laragh JH: Calcium-regulating hormones in essential hypertension: Relation to plasma renin activity and sodium metabolism. Ann Intern Med 1986 (Nov); 105:649–654.
13. Sagnella GA, Shore AC, Markandu ND, MacGregor GA: Raised circulating levels of atrial natriuretic peptides in essential hypertension. Lancet 1986 (Jan 25); 179–181.

14. FOURNIER AM, GADIA MT, KUBRUSLY DB, SKYLER JS, SOSENKO JM: Blood pressure, insulin, and glycemia in nondiabetic subjects. Am J Med 1986 (May); 80:861–870.

15. FAGAN TC, SAWYER PR, GOURLEY LA, LEE JT, GAFFNEY TE: Postprandial alterations in hemodynamics and blood pressure in normal subjects. Am J Cardiol 1986 (Sept 15); 58:636–641.

16. COHEN N, FLAMENBAUM W: Obesity and hypertension: Demonstration of a "floor effect". Am J Med 1986 (Feb); 80:177–181.

17. RAISON J, ACHIMASTOS A, ASMAR R, SIMON A, SAFAR M: Extracellular and interstitial fluid volume in obesity with and without associated systemic hypertension. Am J Cardiol 1986 (Feb 1); 57:223–226.

18. FRIEDMAN HS, VASAVADA BC, MALEC AM, HASSAN KK, SHAH A, SIDDIQUI S: Cardiac function in alcohol-associated systemic hypertension. Am J Cardiol 1986 (Feb 1); 57:227–231.

19. KLATSKY AL, FRIEDMAN GD, ARMSTRONG MA: The relationships between alcoholic beverage use and other traits to blood pressure: a new Kaiser Permanente study. Circulation 1986 (April); 73(4):628–636.

20. MACMAHON SW, NORTON RN: Alcohol and hypertension: Implications for prevention and treatment. Ann Intern Med 1986 (July); 105:124–126.

21. DIAMOND TW, BOTHA JR, WING J, MEYERS AM, KALK WJ: Parathyroid hypertension: a reversible disorder. Arch Intern Med 1986 (Sept); 146:1709–1712.

22. KAPLAN NM, MEESE RB: The calcium deficiency hypothesis of hypertension: a critique. Ann Intern Med 1986 (Dec); 105:947–955.

23. EPSTEIN AM, BEGG CB, MCNEIL BJ: The use of ambulatory testing in prepaid and fee-for-service group practices: relation to perceived profatability. N Engl J Med 1986 (Apr 24); 314:1089–94.

24. WILCOX RG, MITCHELL JRA, HAMPTON JR: Treatment of high blood pressure: should clinic practice be based on results of clinical trials? Br Med J 1986 (Aug 16); 293:433–437.

25. AMERY A, BRIXKO R, CLEMENT D, DE SCHAEP-DRYVER A, FAGARD R, FORTE J, HENRY JF, LEONETTI G, O'MALLEY K, STRASSER T, BIRKENHAGER W, BULPITT C, DERUYTTERE M, DOLLERY C, FORETTE F, HAMDY R, JOOSSENS JV, LUND-JOHANSEN P, PETRIE JC, TUOMILEHTO J: Efficacy of antihypertensive drug treatment according to age, sex, blood pressure, and previous cardiovascular disease in patients over the age of 60. Lancet 1986 (Sept 13); 589–594.

26. THE HYPERTENSION DETECTION AND FOLLOW-UP PROGRAM COOPERATIVE GROUP: Implications of the hypertension detection and follow-up program. Prog Cardiovasc Dis 1986 (Nov/Dec); 29, No. 3, Suppl 1:3–10.

27. DAVIS BR, FORD CE, REMINGTON RD, STAMLER R, HAWKINS CM: The hypertension detection and follow-up program design, methods, and baseline characteristics and blood pressure response of the study population. Prog Cardiovasc Dis 1986 (Nov/Dec); 29, No. 3, Suppl 1:11–28.

28. LANGFORD HG, STAMLER J, WASSERTHEIL-SMOLLER S, PRINEAS RJ: All-cause mortality in the hypertension detection and follow-up program: findings for the whole cohort and for persons with less severe hypertension, with and without other traits related to risk of mortality. Prog Cardiovasc Dis 1986 (Nov/Dec); 29, No. 3, Suppl 1:29–54.

29. BORHANI NO, BLAUFOX MD, OBERMAN A: Incidence of coronary heart disease and left ventricular hypertrophy in the hypertension detection and follow-up program. Prog Cardiovasc Dis 1986 (Nov/Dec); 29, No. 3, Suppl 1:55–62.

30. DAUGHERTY SA, BERMAN R, ENTWISLE G, HAERER AF: Cerebrovascular events in the hypertension detection and follow-up program. Prog Cardiovasc Dis 1986 (Nov/Dec); 29, No. 3, Suppl 1:55–62.

31. CURB JD, MAXWELL MH, SCHNEIDER KA, TAYLOR JO, SHULMAN NB: Adverse effects of antihypertensive medications in the hypertension detection and follow-up program. Prog Cardiovasc Dis 1986 (Nov/Dec); 29, No. 3, Suppl 1:73–88.

32. CRESSMAN MD, GIFFORD RW: Clinicians' interpretation of the results and implications of the hypertension detection and follow-up program. Prog Cardiovasc Dis 1986 (Nov/Dec); 29, No. 3, Suppl 1:89–98.

33. CUTLER JA, FURBERG CD, PAYNE GH: The effects of drug treatment for hypertension on morbidity and mortality from cardiovascular disease: a review of randomized controlled trials. Prog Cardiovasc Dis 1986 (Nov/Dec); 29, No. 3, Suppl 1:99–118.

34. FERGUSON RK, VLASSES PH: Hypertensive emergencies and urgencies. JAMA 1986 (Mar 28); 255:1607–1613.

35. HOUSTON MC: Treatment of hypertensive emergencies and urgencies with oral clonidine

loading and titration. Arch Intern Med 1986 (Mar); 146:586–589.

36. AVORN J, EVERITT DE, WEISS S: Increased antidepressant use in patients prescribed B-blockers. JAMA 1986 (Jan 17); 255:357–360.

37. WONG DG, LAMKI L, SPENCE JD, FREEMAN D, McDONALD JW: Effect of non-steroidal anti-inflammatory drugs on control of hypertension by beta-blockers and diuretics. Lancet 1986 (May 3); 997–1001.

38. HILL NS: Fluid and electrolyte considerations in diuretic therapy for hypertensive patients with chronic obstructive pulmonary disease. Arch Intern Med 1986 (Jan); 146:129–133.

39. MARGETTS BM, BEILIN LJ, VANDONGEN R, ARMSTRONG BK: Vegetarian diet in mild hypertension: a randomized controlled trial. Br Med J 1986 (Dec 6); 293:1468–1471.

40. MACMAHON SW, WILCKEN DEL, MACDONALD GJ: The effect of weight reduction on left ventricular mass: A randomized controlled trial in young, overweight hypertensive patients. N Engl J Med 1986 (Feb 6); 314:334–339.

41. MESSERLI FH: Cardiomyopathy of obesity—a not so victorian disease. N Engl J Med 1986 (Feb 6); 314:378–379.

42. NELSON L, ESLER MD, JENNINGS GL, KORNER PI: Effect of changing levels of physical activity on blood-pressure and hemodynamics in essential hypertension. Lancet 1986 (Aug 30); 473–476.

43. GROBBEE DE, HOFMAN A: Effect of calcium supplementation on diastolic blood pressure in young people with mild hypertension. Lancet 1986 (Sept 27); 703–706.

44. NORRIS PG, JONES CJH, WESTON MJ: Effect of dietary supplementation with fish oil on systolic blood pressure in mild essential hypertension. Br Med J 1986 (July 12); 293:104–105.

45. WAHL J, SINGH BN, THODEN WR: Comparative hypotensive effects of acebutolol and hydrochlorothiazide in patients with mild to moderate essential hypertension: a double-blind multicenter evaluation. Am Heart J 1986 (Feb); 111:353–362.

46. WIKSTRAND J, WESTERGREN G, BERGLUND G, BRACCHETTI D, VAN COUTER A, FELDSTEIN CA, MING KS, KURAMOTO K, LANDAHL S, MEANEY E, PEDERSEN EB, RAHN KH, SHAW J, SMITH A, WAAL-MANNING H: Antihypertensive treatment with metoprolol or hydrochlorothiazide in patients aged 60 to 75 years: report from a double-blind international multicenter study. JAMA 1986 (Mar 14); 255:1304–1310.

47. HELGELAND A, HAGELUND CH, STROMMEN R, TRETLI S: Enalapril, atenolol, and hydrochlorothiazide in mild to moderate hypertension: A comparative multicenter study in general practice in Norway. Lancet 1986 (Apr 19) 872–875.

48. SPITALEWITZ S, PORUSH JG, REISER IW: Minoxidil, nadolol, and a diuretic: once-a-day therapy for resistant hypertension. Arch Intern Med 1986 (May); 146:882–886.

49. VAN DEN MEIRACKER AH, MAN IN 'T VELD AJ, RITSEMA VAN ECK HJ, SCHALEKAMP MADH: Systemic and renal vasodilation after beta-adrenoceptor blockade with pinodolol: a hemodynamic study on the onset and maintenance of its antihypertensive effect. Am Heart J 1986 (Aug); 112:368–374.

50. CUBEDDU LX, ARANDA J, SINGH B, KLEIN M, BRACHFELD J, FREIS E, ROMAN J, EADES T: A comparison of verapamil and propranolol for the initial treatment of hypertension: racial differences in response. JAMA 1986 (Oct 24); 256:2214–2221.

51. CROOG SH, LEVINE S, TESTA MA, BROWN B, BULPITT CJ, JENKINS CD, KLERMAN GL, WILLIAMS GH: The effects of antihypertensive therapy on the quality of life. N Engl J Med 1986 (Jun 26); 314:1657–1664.

52. CHOBANIAN AV: Antihypertensive therapy in evolution. N Engl J Med 1986 (Jun 26); 314:1701–1702.

53. DANIELS AR, OPIE LH: Atenolol plus nifedipine for mild to moderate systemic hypertension after fixed doses of either agent alone. Am J Cardiol 1986 (Apr 15); 57:965–970.

54. AMODEO C, KOBRIN I, VENTURA H, MESSERLI F, FROHLICH E: Immediate and short-term hemodynamic effects of diltiazem in patients with hypertension. Circulation 1986 (Jan); 73(1):108–113.

55. POOL PE, MASSIE BM, VENKATARAMAN K, HIRSCH AT, SAMANT DR, SEAGREN SC, GAW J, SALEL AF, TUBAU JF, VOLLMER C, WALKER S, SKALLAND ML: Diltiazem as monotherapy for systemic hypertension: a multicenter, randomized, placebo-controlled trial. Am J Cardiol 1986 (Feb 1); 57:212–217.

56. YAMAUCHI K, FURUI H, TANIGUCHI N, SOTOBATA I: Effects of diltiazem hydrochloride on cardiovascular response, platelet aggregation and coagulating activity during exercise testing in systemic hypertension. Am J Cardiol 1986 (Mar 1); 57:609–612.

57. JENNINGS AA, JEE LD, SMITH JA, COMMERFORD PJ, OPIE LH: Acute effect of nifedipine on blood pressure and left ventricular ejection fraction in severely hypertensive outpatients: predictive effects of acute therapy and prolonged efficacy when added to existing therapy. Am Heart J 1986 (Mar); 111:557–563.

58. ADLER AG, LEAHY JJ, CRESSMAN MD: Management of perioperative hypertension using sublingual nifedipine: experience in elderly patients undergoing eye surgery. Arch Intern Med 1986 (Oct); 146:1927–1930.

59. FERLINZ J: Nifedipine in myocardial ischemia, systemic hypertension, and other cardiovascular disorders. Ann Intern Med 1986 (Nov); 105:714–726.

60. FRISHMAN W, CHARLAP S, KIMMEL B, SALTZBERG S, STROH J, WEINBERG P, MONUSZKO E, WIEZNER J, DORSA F, POLLACK S, STROM J: Twice-daily administration of oral verapamil in the treatment of essential hypertension. Arch Intern Med 1986 (Mar) 146:561–565.

61. AGABITI-ROSEI E, MUIESAN ML, ROMANELLI G, CASTELLANO M, BESCHI M, COREA L, MUIESAN G: Similarities and differences in the antihypertensive effect of two calcium antagonist drugs, verapamil and nifedipine. J Am Coll Cardiol 1986 (Apr); 7:916–924.

62. ANDO K, FUJITA T, ITO Y, NODA H, YAMASHITA K: The role of renal hemodynamics in the antihypertensive effect of captopril. Am Heart J 1986 (Feb); 111:347–352.

63. REAMS GP, BAUER JH: Effect of enalapril in subjects with hypertension associated with moderate to severe renal dysfunction. Arch Intern Med 1986 (Nov); 146:2145–2148.

64. POPLI S, DAUGIRDA JT, NEUBAUER JA, HOCKENBERRY B, HANO JE, ING TS: Transdermal clonidine in mild hypertension: a randomized, double-blind, placebo-controlled trial. Arch Intern Med 1986 (Nov); 146:2140–2144.

65. WALLENBURG HCS, MAKOVITZ JW, DEKKER GA, ROTMANS P: Low-dose aspirin prevents pregnancy-induced hypertension and pre-eclampsia in angiotensin-sensitive primigravidae. Lancet 1986 (Jan 4); 1–3.

66. UNSIGNED: Aspirin and pre-eclampsia. Lancet 1986 (Jan 4) 18–20.

67. ALDERMAN MH, DAVIS TK, GERBER LM, ROBB M: Antihypertensive drug therapy withdrawal in a general population. Arch Intern Med 1986 (July); 146:1309–1311.

68. MEDICAL RESEARCH COUNCIL WORKING PARTY ON MILD HYPERTENSION: Course of blood pressure in mild hypertensives after withdrawal of long term antihypertensive treatment. Br Med J (Oct 18); 293:988–992.

69. ROBERTS WC: Effects of antihypertensive therapy on blood lipid levels. Am J Cardiol 1986 (Feb 1); 57:379–380.

Valvular Heart Disease

Morphologic studies

Hutchins and associates[1] from Baltimore, Maryland, examined 900 hearts at necropsy of adults and 25 (3%) had typical MVP: in 23 (92%) the mitral anulus fibrosus showed disjunction, i.e., a separation between the LA wall–mitral valve junction and the LV attachment. In 42 other hearts (5%) there was mitral anulus disjunction but no MVP. Two hearts had MVP, but no disjunction of the anulus; both of them had healed infarcts involving a LV papillary muscle. These authors concluded that MVP is significantly associated with disjunction of the mitral anulus fibrosus. Significance of this observation is unclear.

Frequency in relatives

Devereux and co-workers[2] from New York, New York, evaluated patients with MVP to determine the "true" spectrum of the syndrome. They studied clinical findings in 88 patients with echocardiographic evidence of MVP and compared them with findings in 81 of their adult first-degree relatives with MVP and in 2 control groups without MVP, including 172 first-degree relatives and 60 spouses. These studies demonstrated that relatives with and without MVP had true associations between MVP and clicks or murmurs, or both (67 -vs- 9%), thoracic bony abnormalities (41 -vs- 16%), systolic BP <120 mmHg (53 -vs- 31%), body weight ≤90% of ideal (31 -vs- 14%) and palpitations (40 -vs- 24%). Relatives with MVP had no significant increase over normal relatives or spouses without MVP in prevalence of chest pain, dyspnea, panic attacks, high anxiety or repolarization abnormalities, but all of these features were more common in women than in men. Therefore, the true spectrum of the MVP syndrome includes a midsystolic click and late systolic murmur, thoracic bony abnormalities, low body weight and BP, and palpitations. Several additional previously suggested clinical features of the MVP syndrome, including nonanginal chest pain, dyspnea, panic attacks, and electrocardiographic abnormalities are probably more related to female sex than to the MVP syndrome per se.

Relation to symptoms

To determine whether symptoms and functional impairment are related to MVP, Retchin and associates[3] from Chapel Hill and Durham, North Carolina, studied 274 outpatients referred to an echocardiography laboratory for suspicion of MVP. The age, sex, and symptoms at the time of echocardiography were similar among patients with and without evidence of MVP. After 14 to 36 months, 158 patients were interviewed. There was a high rate of dysfunction, but echocardiographic evidence of MVP was not associated with disability, health care utilization, or reported symptoms. These results suggest that symptoms and dysfunction are not related to the presence of MVP by echocardiography. The functional impairment that is seen in patients suspected of MVP may be caused by other factors.

Progression

Little information is available concerning the progression of mild to severe MR in patients with MVP. Kolibash and associates[4] from Columbus, Ohio, studied 86 patients, average age 60 years, who presented with cardiac symptoms, precordial systolic murmurs, severe MR, and a high frequency of MVP on echocardiography (57 of 75 [75%]) and left ventriculography (61 of 84 [73%]). Seventy-five surgically excised mitral valves appeared grossly enlarged and floppy. Histologic studies showed extensive myxomatous changes throughout the leaflets and chordae. Eighty patients had had precordial murmurs first described at average age 34 years, but the average age at which symptoms of cardiac dysfunction appeared was 59. However, once symptoms developed, mitral valve surgery was required within 1 year in 67 of 76 patients who had undergone surgery. AF, present in 48 of 86 patients (56%), or ruptured chordae tendineae, present in 39 of 76 patients (51%), may have contributed to this rapid progression and deterioration. Additionally, 13 patients had a remote history of documented infective endocarditis. Twenty-eight patients had at least 1 type of serial clinical evaluation that indicated progressive MR in all 28 patients on the basis of changing auscultatory findings (24 of 26), progressive radiographic cardiomegaly (24 of 25), echocardiographic LA enlargement (4.3–5 cm in 11 patients) and angiographically worsening MR (14 of 15). Twenty-four of these patients had evidence of MVP on at least 1 of their initial studies. Thus, mild MR due to MVP and myxomatous mitral valves is a progressive disease in some patients with MVP.

Severity of mitral regurgitation

Panidis et al[5] in Philadelphia, Pennsylvania, used Doppler echocardiography in 80 consecutive patients with MVP diagnosed by 2-D echocardiography to evaluate the severity of MR. Among the 80 patients, 16 (20%) were asymptomatic and 11 (14%) had no click or precordial murmur. The M-mode echocardiogram was negative for MVP in 11 patients (14%) and equivocal or nondiagnostic in 19 patients (24%). MR was evaluated using pulsed mode

Doppler echocardiography and quantified by the mapping technique as minimal or mild when a holosystolic regurgitant jet was recorded just below the MV into the left atrium, and as moderate or severe, when the jet was detected at the mid or distal portions of the left atrium. Fifty-five patients (69%) had MR. The MR was minimal or mild in 47 patients (59%) and moderate or severe in 8 (10%). In 20 of the 55 patients with MR by Doppler measurement, a systolic murmur was not detected and each of these patients had only mild MR. The 8 patients with moderate or severe MR were all men and 6 were more than 50 years of age. The MVP was holosystolic and involved both leaflets in these patients. Thus, these data suggest that 1) MR as assessed by Doppler echocardiography is common in patients with MVP, but usually mild and not always associated with an audible murmur; and 2) significant MR occurs in 10% and usually in older men.

Frequency of complications in men -vs- women and in older persons

To determine factors influencing the strength of association between MVP and MR, ruptured chordae tendineae and infective endocarditis, Devereux and associates[6] from New York, New York, compared the prevalence of MVP in patients with disease with both clinical and population control groups. The prevalence of MVP was 4% among population and clinical control groups (8 of 196 and 84 of 2,146, respectively) and was significantly higher in patients with infective endocarditis (11 of 67, 16%), MR (17 of 31, 55%), and ruptured chordae (27 of 43, 63%). Odds ratios for complications in persons with MVP ranged from 5 for infective endocarditis to 41 for ruptured chordae in overall analyses, and from 7 for infective endocarditis to 53 for ruptured chordae based on age- and sex-matched control triplets. All complications occurred disproportionately in men with MVP in whom odds ratios ranged from 3 to 7 compared with an additional control group of unselected subjects with MVP (Table 6-1). Compared with this control group, patients with MVP and infective endocarditis were slightly more likely to have a previously known precordial murmur (odds ratio 3.2) but significantly more likely to have murmurs at the time of evaluation (odds ratio 8.5). Patients with MVP and MR and ruptured chordae tendineae were also significantly older than the unselected subjects with MVP (48 ± 14 and 55 ± 16 -vs- 38 ± 14 years). The concentration of risk of infective endocarditis in men

TABLE 6-1. *Sex of subjects with complicated and uncomplicated mitral prolapse*

	PATIENTS WITH MITRAL PROLAPSE			CONTROL GROUP
	INFECTIVE ENDOCARDITIS	MITRAL REGURGITATION	RUPTURED CHORDAE TENDINEAE	RELATIVES WITH PROLAPSE
Number	11	17	27	81
Male (percent)	8 (73)	9 (53)	20 (74)†	25 (31)
Female (percent)	3 (27)	8 (47)	7 (26)	56 (69)
Odds ratio versus relatives with mitral prolapse	6.0*	2.5	7.4†	—

Statistical significance: * p <0.01; † p <0.001.

TABLE 6-2. *Frequency of complications in 145 patients with mitral valve prolapse*

	NO. OF PTS	M:F	AGE (YR)
Infective endocarditis	7	4:3	66
Stroke	5†	1:4	67
Transient ischemic attacks	8†	4:4	70
Ruptured chordae tendineae	37	25:12	68‡
Severe CHF requiring mitral valve surgery	11	6:5	67

* Mean age at time of the complication.
† No cause other than mitral valve prolapse was identified in 2 of 5 patients with strokes and in 2 of 8 patients with transient ischemic attacks.
‡ Mean age at the time of echocardiographic evidence for ruptured chordae tendineae was noted. Chordal rupture may have antedated the echocardiographic study. In 33, patients ruptured chordae tendineae were spontaneous and in 4 were associated with infective endocarditis.
CHF = congestive heart failure; M:F = male:female.

with MVP and patients with antecedent murmur suggests that antibiotic prophylaxis is warranted in these groups but not in women without a murmur of MR.

Naggar and associates[7] from Burlington, Massachusetts, studied 145 patients (74 women and 71 men) aged 60 years or older with echocardiographically documented MVP. One hundred sixteen patients had precordial systolic murmurs, 20 of whom were suspected of having MVP before the echocardiographic study. Infective endocarditis occurred in 7 patients, cerebral ischemic events in 13, and spontaneous rupture of chordae tendineae in 37 (Table 6-2). Four other patients had ruptured chordae tendineae associated with infective endocarditis. CHF was present in 35 patients, 11 of whom had undergone mitral valve surgery.

In anorexia nervosa and in bulimia

Myers and associates[8] from Omaha, Nebraska, examined 28 consecutive women who met the diagnostic criteria for anorexia nervosa: weight loss of more than 25%, refusal to maintain weight, intense fear of obesity, distorted body image, and absence of organic disease causing weight loss. Twenty-eight women of normal weight served as controls. Patients and controls were matched by age (mean 22 ± 6 years) and height (158 ± 6 cm). Two independent observers performed dynamic cardiac auscultation. Criteria for MVP included a mobile apical systolic click heard by both examiners or both an echocardiographically determined MVP and an apical systolic murmer. MVP was found in 9 of the 28 patients with anorexia nervosa and in 2 of 28 controls. Of the 9 anorexic patients with MVP, 7 had systolic clicks and echocardiographic evidence of MVP, 1 had a murmur and echocardiographic evidence of MVP, and 1 had an isolated click only. The 2 controls with prolapse had both systolic clicks and echocardiographic evidence of MVP. No patient had symptoms attributable to MVP. Uncomplicated MVP, found transiently during recurrent periods of very low weight in one-third of the patients with anorexia nervosa, resolved after weight gain. Thus, MVP and anorexia nervosa is at least in part due to a weight-loss-induced reduction in LV size that results in a size disproportion between mitral valve and the LV cavity.

Johnson and associates[9] from Lexington, Kentucky, studied 43 consecutive persons with anorexia nervosa and/or bulimia for the presence of MVP and/or cardiac arrhythmias by physical examination. M-mode and 2-D echocardiograms, and 24-hour continuous electrocardiographic monitoring was performed. Ten of the 23 patients had MVP on rest precordial auscultation. Echocardiographic evaluation confirmed the diagnosis of MVP in these 10 patients and also in 6 other patients, giving an overall frequency of 37% (16 of 43). Similar echocardiographic findings were present in only 4% (1/23) of control subjects. Cardiac arrhythmias other than benign isolated premature extrasystoles were noted in 5 patients with an eating disorder; all 5 also had echocardiographic findings of MVP. The incidence of MVP appears to be increased in patients with eating disorders. In addition, the arrhythmogenic effects of MVP may present an additional risk factor in these patients.

In psoriatic arthritis

Pines and associates[10] from Tel Aviv, Israel, studied 25 patients with psoriatic arthritis by echocardiography: 15 men and 10 women, mean age 47 ± 15 years. Twenty-two patients had peripheral disease and 3 also had axial involvement. None had abnormal aortic valves by echocardiography. MVP was detected, however, in 14 patients (56%), 9 men and 5 women. The mean age, mean duration of psoriasis, and mean duration of arthritis were similar in patients with and without MVP. HLA tissue typing, which was done in 9 patients with MVP, revealed only 1 patient with HLA-B27. There was no predominance of any of the typical antigens found in psoriasis (HLA-B13, HLA-Cw6). In a control group of 32 psoriatic patients without arthritis, only 2 (6%) had MVP.

Ring valvuloplasty

Kreindel and associates[11] from Cleveland, Ohio, described findings in 45 patients with severe MR who underwent mitral valvuloplasty with insertion of a semirigid Carpentier ring. No patient had echocardiographic evidence of systolic anterior motion (SAM) preoperatively, whereas 5 patients had this echocardiographic finding postoperatively. All 5 had MVP as their underlying disease process and SAM developed at varying intervals after valvuloplasty. The development of SAM is related to insertion of the semirigid ring, persistence of a redundant anterior mitral leaflet, narrowing of the LV outflow tract and the Venturi effect. LV and aortic pressure measurements with simultaneous Doppler echocardiography have confirmed the presence of a significant LV outflow tract gradient in these patients. Although all 5 patients are functionally improved after mitral valvuloplasty, the long-term implications of SAM after valvuloplasty are unknown.

MITRAL REGURGITATION

Quantitation by Doppler

Miyatake et al[12] in Suita, Osaka, Japan, used real-time 2-D Doppler flow imaging in 109 patients undergoing left ventriculography to determine whether MR may be detected and its severity evaluated semiquantitatively. Using Doppler flow imaging, Doppler signals resulting from blood flow in the cardiac chambers are processed using a high-speed autocorrelation technique so that the direction, velocity, and turbulence of the intracardiac blood flow are displayed in a color-coded mode on a monochrome B-mode echo in real time. MR flow was imaged as a jet spurting up from the mitral orifice in to the LA cavity (Fig. 6-1). The sensitivity of this approach in the detection of MR was 86% compared with left ventriculography. MR in the falsely negative cases was usually mild. The severity of MR was graded on a 4-point scale on the basis of the distance reached by the regurgitant flow signal from the mitral orifice and the results were compared with those of angiography. There was a significant correlation between Doppler imaging and angiography in the evaluation of the severity of MR. A similar result was obtained when the evaluation was based on the area covered by the regurgitant signals in the LA cavity. These data are encouraging as regards the future ability of noninvasive semiquantitative evaluation by real-time 2-D Doppler flow imaging to detect and estimate the severity of MR.

Blumlein and co-workers[13] in San Francisco, California, described a new Doppler echocardiographic method that measures the regurgitant fraction and compares it with angiographic and scintigraphic methods. A total of 27 patients with MR were evaluated by echocardiography and either cardiac catheterization or scintigraphy. With 2-D echocardiography, diastolic and systolic volumes were measured to derive the LV stroke volume. Forward SV was obtained from the product of M-mode-derived aortic valve area and ascending aortic flow velocity integral assessed by continuous-wave Doppler. Regurgitant fraction was calculated as follows: (LVSV − Forward SV)/LVSV. Comparisons showed that regurgitant fraction calculated by Doppler echocardiography correlated with regurgitant fraction determined by both cardiac catheterization and by scintigraphy. There was, however, an important interobserver variability within each method: 10%, 13%, and 11% for Doppler echocardiography, angiography, and scintigraphy, respectively. In conclusion, Doppler echocardiography can be used to quantitate MR. Serial noninvasive determinations of regurgitant fraction may be useful in the evaluation of therapy and in the follow-up of patients with MR.

Ventricular function

To determine objective predictors of survival after MVR, 53 patients with chronic, hemodynamically severe MR underwent rest and exercise radionuclide cineangiography, echocardiography, treadmill exercise testing, and ambulatory echocardiographic monitoring before prospective follow-up, by Hockreiter and co-investigators[14] in New York, New York. At entry, symptom status correlated best with radionuclide-based RV EF and LA size, while treadmill exercise tolerance correlated best with RVEF during exercise. Correspondingly, in 23 patients who underwent cardiac catheterization, PA systolic and wedge pressures were significantly inversely related to RVEF. On the 24 hour ambulatory electrocardiogram, nonsustained VT was present in 29% of patients, most frequently when both RVEF and LVEF were subnormal. Since entry, 35 patients have been managed without surgery for 9–57 months (average 28); 3 who subsequently underwent operation also are among the 21 patients who have undergone MVR. During the average 28 months of observation under medical treatment 5 of 35 nonoperated patients have died; all 5 were among the 6 nonoperated patients with RVEF ≤30% at entry, a descriptor that significantly identified those at high mortality risk -vs- patients with RVEF >30%. All 5 also were among the 8 nonoperated patients with LVEF ≤45%, a descriptor that also significantly predicted mortality. Three of the 21 patients who had MVR died, all late. Among operated patients, only age was a predictor of postoperative survival. A trend toward improved survival was found in the patients with depressed RVEF or LVEF who underwent MVR compared with those who did not.

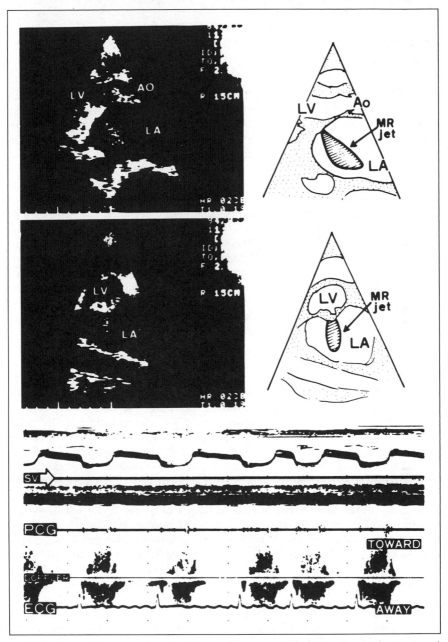

Fig. 6-1. Mitral regurgitant flow in a 42 year old woman with rheumatic mitral stenosis and insufficiency. Top left panel, Blue signals or a mosaic of blue and yellow signals were recorded spreading from the mitral orifice into the left atrial (LA) cavity indicating the mitral regurgitant (MR) flow. These signals spread from the mitral orifice in a teardrop shape in this parasternal long-axis view. The schematic drawing is shown on the right. Middle left panel, Regurgitant signals spreading from the center of the mitral orifice directed toward the left atrial (LA) posterior wall (short-axis view). The schematic drawing is shown on the right. Bottom panel, Regurgitant signals recorded as a bidirectional wide-band spectrum by pulsed Doppler spectogram. Ao = aorta; ECG = electrocardiogram; LV = left ventricle; PCG = phonocardiogram; SV = sample volume. Reproduced with permission from Miyatake et al.[12]

MITRAL STENOSIS

Mitral calcific deposits

Rahko and associates[15] from Pittsburgh, Pennsylvania, determined the relation between the degree of leaflet calcium in a stenotic mitral valve and several parameters of valve mobility, hemodynamics, and clinical signs in 105 patients with relatively pure MS. The amount of mitral valve calcific deposits was determined by grading cineangiograms. Compared to 71 patients with no or minimal valvular calcium, the 23 patients with heavy valve leaflet calcium were significantly older, more likely to be men and more likely to have AF. These patients also had a significant reduction of valve mobility in that their M-mode measurements of valve excursion and rate of valve opening were significantly reduced compared to those of patients without heavy valvular calcium. Two-D echocardiograms also documented a significant reduction in valve mobility and progressive restriction in doming of the anterior mitral leaflet as the level of calcium increased. The prevalence of an opening snap was significantly decreased in patients with heavy -vs- no or light valvular calcium, and patients without an opening snap had reduced valve mobility. However, a considerable number of patients with moderate to heavy valve calcium retained an opening snap.

Importance of "atrial kick"

AF with a rapid ventricular response in patients with MS is often accompanied by pulmonary congestion and reduced cardiac output owing to a diminished diastolic filling period and the loss of the end-diastolic LV pressure increment. To test the hypothesis that loss of atrial contraction (atrial kick) also results in a decrease in effective mitral valve orifice area, Nicod and associates[16] from Dallas, Texas, studied 6 patients with pure isolated MS and sinus rhythm during atrial pacing and simultaneous AV pacing. Atrial pacing at 140 beats/minute caused no significant change from baseline in cardiac output or mitral valve area, but there was a decrease in LV end-diastolic volume and EF and an increase in LA pressure and mean diastolic gradient. Simultaneous atrioventricular pacing (to eliminate atrial kick) induced a decrease in cardiac output (4.4 ± 0.9 -vs- 5.2 ± 0.8 liters/min at 110 beats/minute, 4.2 ± 0.9 -vs- 5.1 ± 0.9 liters/minute at 140 beats/minute) and LV end-diastolic volume (77 ± 27 -vs- 93 ± 29 ml at 110 beats/minute, 54 ± 17 -vs- 65 ± 19 ml at 140 beats/minute), an increase in LA pressure (28 ± 3 -vs- 20 ± 5 mmHg at 110 beats/minute, 30 ± 4 -vs- 25 ± 5 mmHg at 140 beats/minute), and a decrease in mitral valve area (1.2 ± 0.4 -vs- 1.4 ± 0.4 cm^2 at 140 beats/minute). Thus, loss of atrial kick may cause pulmonary congestion and reduced cardiac output in patients with MS, partly because of a decrease in effective mitral valve area.

Effect of atrial fibrillation and regurgitation on mitral valve area

Bryg and associates[17] from St. Louis, Missouri, studied 49 patients with MS by Doppler echocardiography and 2-D echocardiography to assess the ability of Doppler ultrasound to accurately measure mitral valve orifice area and to assess whether AF or MR affected calculation. Twenty-four patients underwent cardiac catheterization. Mitral valve area by Doppler was determined by the pressure half-time method. Mean mitral valve area of all 49 patients by Doppler and 2-D echocardiography correlated well. There was good correlation between Doppler and 2-D echocardiography in patients with pure MS in sinus rhythm, in patients with MR and in patients with AF. In the 7 patients with pure MS in sinus rhythm, there was good correlation between Doppler, 2-D echocardiography, and cardiac catheterization. In patients with either MR or AF, cardiac catheterization appeared to underestimate mitral valve orifice compared with both Doppler and 2-D echocardiography. Doppler echocardiography can estimate valve area in patients with MS regardless of the presence of MR or AF.

Comparison of 2-dimensional and Doppler echocardiography for assessing severity

Smith and co-investigators[18] in Lexington, Kentucky, compared the accuracies of the 2-D echocardiographic and Doppler pressure half-time methods for the noninvasive estimation of cardiac catheterization measurements of mitral valve area in patients with "pure" MS both with and without a previous commissurotomy. Data were retrospectively obtained from 74 consecutive patients who underwent cardiac catheterization within a 30-month period for evaluation of MS, and who had 2-D echocardiography performed before catheterization. Continuous-wave Doppler echocardiographic examinations were attempted in 45 patients and adequate measurements of pressure half-times were obtained in all patients studied. Mitral valve area by 2-D echocardiography was measured as the planimetered area along the inner border of the smallest mitral orifice visualized during short-axis scanning, while pressure half-time was calculated as the interval between the peak transmitral velocity and velocity/2 as measured from the envelope of the Doppler spectral signal. Calculations from catheterization represented the minimal valve area at rest as derived from the Gorlin formula with the use of pressure gradients and thermodilution measurements of cardiac output. Thirty-seven patients had a previous mitral commissurotomy a mean of 11 years before while the remaining 37 patients did not. Mean valve area as determined at catheterization for the total group of patients ranged from $0.37–2/30 \text{ cm}^2$. Linear regression analysis of data from the group of 33 previously unoperated patients revealed a good correlation between 2-D echocardiography and catheterization measurements of mitral valve area. Similarly, the correlation between Doppler measurements of mitral valve area were also good. However, in the group of 35 patients who had undergone commissurotomy, the Doppler pressure half-time correlated much better with catheterization measurements than with 2-D echocardiographic estimates. Reproducibility was similar for the 2 noninvasive methods, with a mean error of 0.14 cm^2 for 2-D echocardiographic planimetry and of 0.15 cm^2 for Doppler pressure half-time. Thus, these data show that both 2-D echocardiography and Doppler pressure half-time methods provide accurate noninvasive estimates of mitral orifice area in patients who have not undergone surgery. However, the Doppler pressure half-time is superior to 2-D echocardiography in estimating mitral valve area in patients who have undergone commissurotomy.

Intracardiac flow

Khandheria and associates[19] from Rochester, Minnesota, used Doppler color flow imaging, a new noninvasive technique for mapping of intracardiac blood flow, to visualize and characterize the blood flow jet in 42 patients with MS. Color flow imaging provided information about the direction of blood flow, its velocity, and the presence of turbulence. Although these authors found various jet configurations, most frequently the jet was centrally and apically directed and had a "candle flame" appearance (a central blue zone surrounded by hues of yellow and orange). The blood flow jet could be used to guide the positioning of the continuous-wave Doppler beam parallel to the blood flow, thus enhancing the accuracy of the Doppler data.

Electrocardiographic criteria for right ventricular hypertrophy

Current electrocardiographic criteria for diagnosing RV hypertrophy have low sensitivity. Butler and associates[20] from Durham, North Carolina, developed maximally specific and sensitive electrocardiographic criteria for RV hypertrophy due to MS that incorporated the principles derived from spatial changes in the QRS complex observed on the vectorcardiogram and any existent electrocardiographic criteria that supplement the diagnostic capability of the criteria derived from the vectorcardiogram. The standard 12-lead electrocardiograms of a control group of 500 consecutively selected subjects with 50 women and 50 men in each decade between ages 20 and 69 years were compared with the electrocardiograms of a study population of 50 patients with RV hypertrophy due to MS. Inclusion criteria were a diagnosis of MS by catheterization, normal coronary arteriographic and left ventriculographic findings, and no other valvular abnormalities. It was hypothesized that patients with RV hypertrophy resulting from MS would have QRS forces that are maximally anterior (A) and rightward (R) and minimally posterolateral (PL); thus, the A + R − PL value in the study group would be greater than that in the control group. The subsequently derived formula criterion (A + R − PL $\geq$ 0.7 mV) and 2 additional criteria, R 0.2 mV in lead 1 and P 0.25 mV in leads II, III, aVF, V_1 or V_2, were tested in both groups. The specificity and sensitivity of each individual criterion was determined; when combined, the criteria yielded 94% specificity and 64% sensitivity. Moderate-to-severe RV hypertrophy due to MS was detected in two-thirds of the patients using the proposed criteria.

Coronary arterial narrowing

Mattina and associates[21] from Manhasset and New York, New York, retrospectively analyzed 96 consecutive patients older than 40 years of age with severe MS to determine the relation of angina pectoris and coexistent CAD. Of the 96 patients, 27 (28%) had angiographically significant CAD, 10 (37%) with angina pectoris and 17 (63%) without angina pectoris (Fig. 6-2). Of the 96 patients, 21 had angina pectors, 10 (48%) with angiographically significant CAD and 11 (52%) without (CAD). Of 75 patients without angina pectors, 17 (23%) had angiographically significant CAD. Angina pectoris had a specificity of 84% and a sensitivity of 37% in its ability to detect significant CAD. The PA systolic, diastolic, and mean pressures and the pulmonary vascular resistance did not differ between patients with and those without angina pectoris. It was concluded that coexistent CAD is commonly found in patients older than age 40 with severe MS, and is usually clinically silent.

Although several studies have described the status of the coronary arteries by angiography in patients with MS, few necropsy studies of the coronary arteries in these patients are available. Reis and Roberts[22] from Bethesda, Maryland, described in detail the amounts of narrowing by atherosclerotic

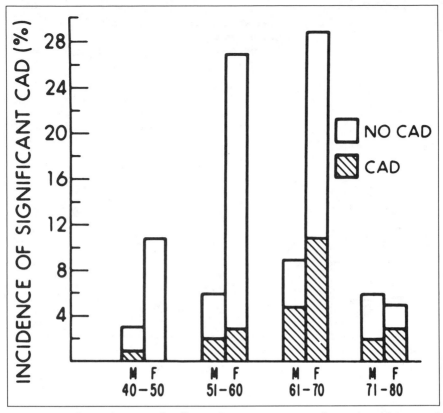

Fig. 6-2. Incidence of angiographically significant coronary artery disease (CAD) by age and sex in patients with severe mitral stenosis. M = male; F = female. The *absciss* lists patients according to age (years) and sex and the *ordinate* the incidence of angiographically significant CAD as a percentage of the total study group.

plaque of the 4 major epicardial arteries in 76 necropsy patients, aged 31 to 79 years (mean 53) with clinically isolated MS (with or without associated MR but without aortic valve dysfunction). Of the 76 patients, ≥1 major coronary artery was narrowed >75% in cross-sectional area (XSA) in 38 (50%) and in 10 of the 38 patients ≥1 major coronary artery was totally occluded or nearly so (>95% XSA narrowing) (Fig. 6-3). A higher percent of the 29 men had significant (>75% XSA) coronary narrowing than did the 47 women (62 -vs- 44%) and the men had more major coronary arteries significantly narrowed compared with the women (31 of 116 arteries [27%] -vs- 33 of 188 arteries [18%]). The 4 major coronary arteries in the 76 patients were divided into 5-mm segments and examined histologically: of the 3,124 segments (41 per patient), 620 segments (20%) were narrowed 0–25% in XSA, 1,826 (58%) were narrowed 26–50%, 470 (15%) were narrowed 51–75%, 188 (6%) were narrowed 76–95%, and 20 segments (1%) were narrowed 96–100% in XSA. The percent of segments narrowed >75% in XSA was 9% in the men and 5% in the women. The percent of segments narrowed >75% in XSA was highly variable in the 38 patients with significant narrowing, ranging from 2–59% (mean 13%). Grossly visible LV scars were present in 11 patients and in each they involved the posterior (inferior) wall; 8 of the 11 patients had significant coronary narrowing and 3 did not. Angina pectoris was present in 13 patients, 8 (62%) had significant coronary narrowing and 5 (38%) did not.

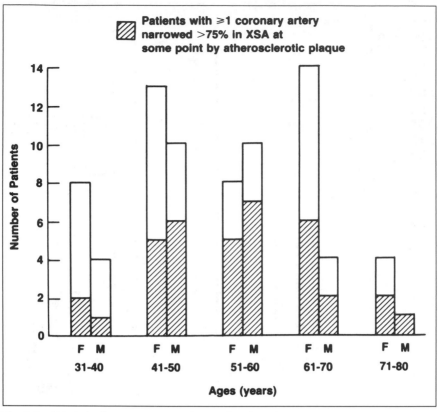

Fig. 6-3.   Number of necropsy patients by age decade and sex with clinically isolated mitral stenosis, with or without associated mitral regurgitation, in whom ≥1 major epicardial coronary artery was narrowed 76 to 100% in cross-sectional area at some point by atherosclerotic plaque.

Cardioversion after commissurotomy

Sato and associates[23] from Osaka, Japan, determined during a 7-year period cardiac rhythm before and after mitral valve open commissurotomy for MS in 106 patients with AF. Forty-three patients reverted to sinus rhythm after primary or secondary direct-current cardioversion after surgery and maintained it until discharge from the hospital. Thirty patients maintained sinus rhythm for 3 months to 7.2 years (mean 2.5 years) after surgery. The actuarial maintenance rate of sinus rhythm was 50% at 7 years after surgery in these 43 patients (Fig. 6-4). The duration of AF, preoperative left atrial dimension by M-mode echocardiogram, and pathologic classification of the mitral valve were factors supposedly influencing the maintenance of sinus rhythm for a long period after direct-current cardioversion. In 30 patients who reverted back to sinus rhythm and maintained sinus rhythm late postoperatively, the preoperative duration of AF was up to 5 years, and 35% of the patients had had AF for >1 year. Also, in 40% of these 30 patients, the preoperative cardiothoracic ratio was >60%. The authors concluded that sinus rhythm is restored by direct-current cardioversion before discharge from hospital after open mitral commissurotomy, it has a 50% chance of being maintained for 7 years after surgery. Long duration of AF and large cardiothoracic ratio should probably not dissuade one from attempting secondary direct-current cardioversion in these patients.

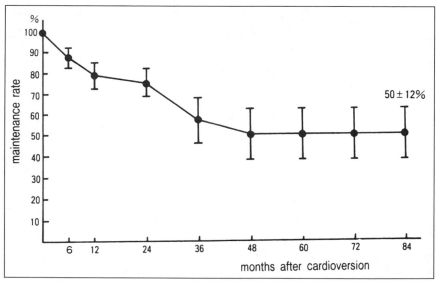

Fig. 6-4.   Actuarial maintenance rate of sinus rhythm in 43 patients who reverted to sinus rhythm after primary or secondary direct-current cardioversion after surgery and maintained it until discharge from hospital. The rate was 50 ± 12% at 7 years after surgery.

Percutaneous transarterial balloon valvuloplasty

Zaibag and associates[24] from Rayadh, Kingdom of Saudi Arabia, performed percutaneous transatrial mitral valvotomy with a double-balloon technique in 9 patients with severe MS and produced striking symptomatic improvement in 7 of them (Table 6-3). In 7 patients the mitral valve area (Gorlin formula) increased significantly and the mitral end-diastolic gradient decreased significantly. Similar improvements were noted in follow-up hemodynamic studies at 6 weeks. There were no procedure-related complications. Percutaneous double-balloon mitral valvotomy appears to be an alternative to surgical treatment of MS.

Babic and associates[25] from Beograd, Yugoslavia, performed percutaneous transarterial balloon valvuloplasty in 3 patients with moderate MS. The balloon catheter was inserted percutaneously from the left femoral artery over a long guidewire introduced into the right femoral artery and advanced transeptally through the Brockenbrough catheter to the left ventricle and drawn out of the body through the left femoral artery using an intravascular retriever set. After the procedure, the mean diastolic pressure gradient across the mitral valve was reduced and left ventriculography revealed no resultant MR in any patient (Table 6-4). There were no complications.

AORTIC VALVE STENOSIS

Clinical variables indicative of severity

To determine the predictors of surgically correctable AS in patients with systolic precordial murmurs, Hoagland and associates[26] from Boston, Massachusetts, evaluated 231 patients. Five variables (carotid upstroke timing, carotid upstroke volume, aortic valve calcium on chest radiography, single or absent second heart sound, and a murmur with its maximal intensity at the

TABLE 6-3. *Hemodynamic echocardiographic, and phonocardiographic results in 9 patients before (B), immediately after (A), and 6 weeks after (F) valvotomy. Reproduced with permission from Zaibag et al.*[24]

PATIENT NO	AGE/SEX	HEART-RATE (BEATS/MIN)	CARDIAC INDEX (L/MIN M²)	LA/LV (END DIASTOLIC)	LA/LV MEAN	PULMONARY ARTERY SYSTOLIC PRESSURE (MM HG)	AORTIC SYSTOLIC PRESSURE (MM HG)	MVA (GORLIN)	MVA (ECHO)	A2-OS (PHONO)	MR (ANGIO)
1	26 M	B 75	2·2	17	20	80	125	0·5	0·7	..	None
		A 82	2·2	13	16	70	120	0·7	0·7	..	None
		F :	..	..	..	..	..	..	..		
2	39 F	B 86	3·0	15	20	50	96	0·7	0·8	..	None
		A 78	2·9	18	15	50	110	0·8	0·8	..	None
		F :	..	..	..	..	..	..	..		
3	17 M	B 75	3·7	10	15	40	125	1·0	1·0	..	None
		A 93	4·8	0	9	32	120	2·0	1·5	100	None
		F115	4·8	2	10	30	118	2·0	1·7	70	None
4	20 F	B 55	2·2	10	12	52	100	0·6	0·6	..	None
		A 64	3·4	2	4	30	100	2·0	1·4	100	Trace
		F 60	3·2	2	5	37	98	1·5	1·4	70	Trace
5	22 F	B 95	2·4	15	17	45	100	0·7	0·8	70	¼
		A100	2·4	5	7	34	130	1·4	1·5	80	Trace
		F 76	3·6	15	12	33	120	1·4	1·5	90	Trace
6	33 M	B 63	2·5	20	20	45	118	0·7	0·7	70	Trace
		A 69	2·3	0	1	27	110	3·5	1·7	120	Trace
		F 55	2·3	6	8	30	140	1·1	1·3	100	Trace
7	26 F	B 65	2·2	17	18	70	120	0·5	0·6	80	None
		A 78	3·2	2	3	40	90	2·3	1·8	110	None
		F 63	2·3	4	6	50	120	1·2	1·5	120	Trace
8	16 F	B 65	2·8	11	15	42	102	0·6	0·8	80	None
		A 56	3·3	2	5	25	95	1·4	1·1	80	Trace
		F 65	2·6	7	12	33	100	1·2	1·1	70	¼
9	24 F	B 65	2·4	7	10	35	90	0·8	0·6	55	Trace
		A 60	3·0	2	3	38	88	1·4	1·6	100	Trace
		F 60	3·0	0	3	28	120	1·5	1·4	95	¼
Total (mean ± SD)		B 69 ± 13	2·6 ± 0·5	13 ± 4·6	15 ± 3·5	47 ± 11	108 ± 13	0·7 ± 0·2	0·7 ± 0·2	71 ± 9	
		A 74 ± 17	*3·0 ± 0·9	§1·9 ± 1·7	¶4·6 ± 2·7	‡32 ± 5·5	105 ± 16	‡2·0 ± 0·8	¶1·5 ± 0·2	‡98 ± 18	
		F 71 ± 21	‡3·2 ± 0·9	‡5·1 ± 5·0	§8·0 ± 3·5	‡34 ± 7·5	117 ± 14	‡1·4 ± 0·3	¶1·4 ± 0·2	‡96 ± 15	

Statistical calculations apply to patients 3–9. LA/LV = left-atrial/left-ventricular pressure gradient. MVA = mitral valve area. A2-OS = interval between aortic closure and opening snap. MR = angiographic mitral regurgitation. * Not significant; † p <0·01; ‡ p <0·005; §p <0·001; ¶p <0·0005.

TABLE 6-4. *Hemodynamic summary before and immediately after balloon mitral valvuloplasty*

CASE	AGE (YR) & SEX	CARDIAC RHYTHM	BEFORE VALVULOPLASTY					AFTER VALVULOPLASTY		
			HR (BEATS/ MIN)	CO (LITERS/ MIN)	MVA (CM²)	MEAN LAP (MM HG)	MVG (MM HG)	HR (BEATS/ MIN)	MEAN LAP (MM HG)	MVG (MM HG)
1	34M	AF	98	8.1	1.8	22	19	115	11	5
2	37F	SR	83	5.1	1.5	15	11	120	11	6
3	63M	AF	89	7.3	1.4	26	21	115	20	15

AF = atrial fibrillation; CO = cardiac output; HR = heart rate; LAP = left atrial pressure; MVA = mitral valve area; MVG = mitral valve gradient; SR = sinus rhythm.

right upper sternal border) were significant multivariate correlates. Two echocardiographic factors (a maximal aortic valve leaflet separation of ≤7 mm and thickening of the posterior wall of the left ventricle to ≥12 mm) and 1 systolic time interval factor (a rate-corrected ejection time of >340 ms) added significant incremental information. When prospectively tested on an independent set of 86 patients with suspected aortic outflow obstruction, the combined clinical and noninvasive information correctly placed 10 patients (12%) into a low-risk group in which catheterization may not be indicated and 15 patients (17%) into a high-risk group in which it might be avoided or limited to coronary arteriography.

Quantification of valve area by Doppler echocardiography

Smith and associates[27] from Lexington, Kentucky, compared estimates of pressure gradients obtained from continuous-wave Doppler recordings with direct pressure measurements derived from cardiac catheterization in 40 patients with AS. The patient underwent cardiac catheterization for evaluation of AS and were prospectively studied with continuous-wave Doppler spectral recordings of the aortic valve before catheterization. Thirty-three patients underwent a second Doppler examination simultaneously with pressure recordings in the catheterization laboratory. Nineteen patients had catheterization pressures measured using high-fidelity, micromanometer-tip catheters. Doppler and pressure tracings were digitized using a microprocessor-based computer with a software program that allowed for calculation of maximal instantaneous, mean, and peak-to-peak gradients, plus ejection and acceleration times. Maximal instantaneous gradient by continuous-wave Doppler showed an excellent correlation with maximal instantaneous catheterization gradient (9 mmHg). The correlation of maximal instantaneous Doppler gradient with peak-to-peak catheterization gradient was also linear (12 mmHg), but there was a consistent overestimation of peak-to-peak gradient in 38 of 40 cases (mean = 17 mmHg). Mean gradient as calculated by the 2 techniques correlated best of all measurements performed (6 mmHg). When patients were grouped into subsets of mild (0–25 mmHg), moderate (25–50 mmHg), and severe (>50 mmHg) levels of AS, the correlation of maximal instantaneous Doppler and peak-to-peak catheterization gradients were r = 0.22, 0.44, and 0.77, respectively. Doppler and catheterization maximal instantaneous gradients correlated better in the 19 patients who had micromanometer recordings than in the 21 patients in whom fluid-filled systems were used. The correlation also was better for Doppler studies performed before, rather than simultaneously with cardiac catheterization. The data indicate that Doppler spectral signals accurately reflect instantaneous catheterization pressure gradients, and that mean systolic pressure can be calculated using planimetry methods. However, the peak-to-peak catheterization gradient is consistently overestimated by Doppler maximal instantaneous gradient, especially in mild and moderate degrees of AS. In addition, certain technical factors such as types of catheter pressure recording systems and the timing of Doppler studies in relation to catheterization, may be important in the accuracy of continuous-wave Doppler predictions of hemodynamic parameters.

Laminar flow through a conduit is equal to the mean velocity times the cross-sectional area of the orifice. Volume is equal to the time-velocity interval multiplied by the cross-sectional area. In AS, flow in the stenotic jet is laminar and the aortic valve area should be equal to the volume of blood ejected through the valve divided by the time-velocity integral of the aortic jet velocity recorded by continuous-wave Doppler echocardiography. To test whether this concept can be used to determine accurately aortic valve area noninvasively by the Doppler method, 39 patients underwent pulsed Doppler by Zoghbi and co-workers[28] in Houston, Texas, combined with 2-D echocardiography for measurement of stroke volume at the aortic, pulmonic, and mitral anulus and continuous-wave Doppler recording of the aortic jet. Aortic valve area determined at cardiac catheterization by the Gorlin equation ranged from $0.4–2.07$ cm^2. The Doppler-derived valve area, determined with the stroke volume value from either the aortic, pulmonic, or mitral anulus, correlated well with the area determined at cardiac catheterization. A simplified method for measuring aortic valve area derived as the cross-sectional area of the aortic anulus times peak velocity just proximal to the aortic valve divided by peak aortic jet velocity correlated well measurements obtained at cardiac catheterization (Fig. 6-5). An excellent separation between critical and noncritical aortic stenosis was seen using either one of the Doppler methods. Thus, combined pulsed and continuous-wave Doppler accurately measures valve area in adult patients with aortic stenosis.

Otto et al[29] in Seattle, Washington, used Doppler echocardiography in 48 adults (mean age 67 years) undergoing cardiac catheterization to evaluate the severity of AS. The maximal Doppler systolic gradient correlated with peak-to-peak pressure and mean Doppler gradient correlated with mean pressure gradient. However, LV dysfunction was present in 33% of the patients studied and 6 of the 32 patients with an aortic valve area ≤ 1.0 cm^2 at catheterization (19%) had a peak Doppler gradient <50 mmHg. The influence of volume flow across the aortic valve was incorporated into the noninvasive estimates of aortic valve area in subsequent studies so that aortic valve area was calculated as stroke volume, measured simultaneously by thermodilution, divided by the Doppler systolic velocity integral in the aortic jet. The aortic valve areas calculated in this manner were compared with results of catheterization in the total group and in the patients without significant aortic insufficiency, closer agreement of valve area by Doppler with catheterization was noted (n = 14) (Fig. 6-6). A simple index, derived as the ratio of the systolic velocity integral in the LV outflow tract to that in the aortic jet, provided even better identification of patients with severe AS (sensitivity = 97%) than did the Doppler pressure gradient alone (sensitivity = 81%). These data indicate that the noninvasive estimation of aortic valve area using Doppler echocardiography is feasible and potentially useful clinically for identifying patients with severe AS, especially when low transaortic valve flow is suspected.

Ohlsson and Wranne[30] in Linkoping, Sweden, evaluated a noninvasive

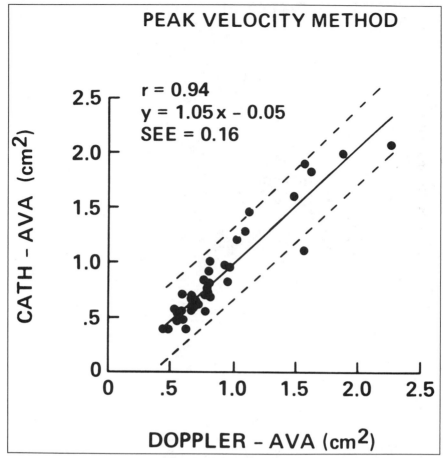

PEAK VELOCITY METHOD

r = 0.94
y = 1.05x – 0.05
SEE = 0.16

CATH – AVA (cm^2)

DOPPLER – AVA (cm^2)

Fig. 6-5. Correlation between aortic valve areas determined by cardiac catheterization and those derived by the simplified peak velocity method. The broken lines indicate the 95% confidence limit of the regression. AVA = aortic valve area; CATH = catheterization. Reproduced with permission from Zobhdi et al.[28]

method for quantification of aortic orifice area in patients with valvular AS and compared the results with cardiac catheterization data in 24 patients with a mean age of 67 years. A continuous-wave 2-MHz Doppler ultrasound instrument was used to measure the maximal velocity of the aortic jet and time-averaged pressure reduction was obtained by planimetry from the maximal velocity spectral recording using a simplified Bernoulli equation. LV ejection time was also measured from the spectral recording. Stroke volume was determined from a carbon dioxide-rebreathing method.

The aortic valve area determined noninvasively with the continuous-wave 2-MHz Doppler ultrasound instrument showed a close correlation of the aortic valve areas determined at cardiac catheterization, but mean pressure gradients measured noninvasively were significantly higher than those determined at cardiac catheterization leading to an underestimation of valve area with the Doppler method, especially when the valve areas were large. However, all patients with an aortic valve area <1 cm^2 at cardiac catheterization, also had an aortic valve area <1 cm^2 by Doppler evaluation.

Over a 1-year period Yeager and associates[31] from Stanford, California, performed cardiac catheterization in 58 patients, mean age 66 years, who had elevated aortic blood flow velocity (>1.7 m/s) by continuous-wave Dopp-

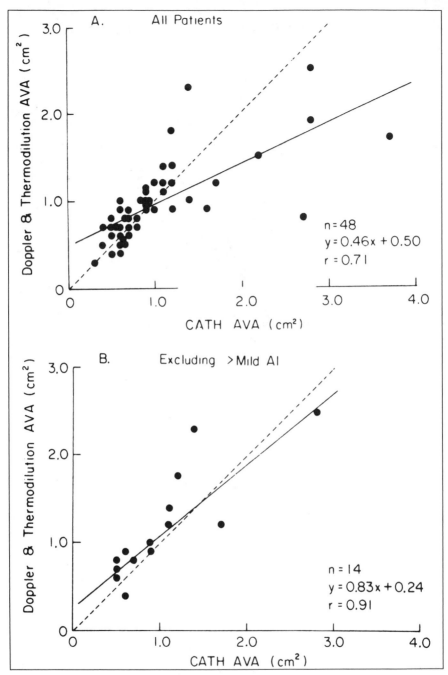

Fig. 6-6. Aortic valve area (AVA) calculated using the thermodilution stroke volume and Doppler aortic jet signal is compared with aortic valve area at catheterization (CATH) in the total group (A) and the subgroup (B) with no or only mild aortic insufficiency (AI). Reproduced with permission from Otto et al.[29]

ler echocardiography. Doppler echo signals were initially judged acceptable for quantitative analysis in 95% of patients, usually from the apical transducer position. Cardiac catheterization was performed within a mean of 8 days (60% within 1 day) of the Doppler echocardiographic study. The aortic valve mean pressure gradients at catheterization ranged from 0–93 mmHg.

The linear correlation coefficient between the mean pressure gradient deter-mined by Doppler echocardiography and catheterization was 0.87. The cor-relation was maintained in 15 patients with AR and in 16 patients with significant CAD. In the 16 patients with reduced cardiac output (mean 3.1 liters/minute, range 2.2 to 3.9) the correlation was 0.81. A strategy for using the Doppler echo-calculated pressure gradient to manage patients with val-vular AS was derived by investigating the relation of the Doppler echocardio-graphic gradient to the aortic valve area in 35 patients with no AR detected at catheterization. All 12 patients with a Doppler echo mean gradient of <30 mmHg had an aortic valve area of >0.75 cm^2 and all 11 patients with a Doppler echo mean gradient <50 mmHg had an aortic valve area >0.75 cm^2. Nine patients with an aortic valve area >0.75 cm^2 and 3 patients with an aortic valve area >0.75 cm^2 had a Doppler echo mean gradient between 30 and 50 mmHg. The data suggested that Doppler echocardiography is useful for distinguishing subgroups of patients with critical (mean gradient >50 mmHg) and noncritical (mean gradient <30 mmHg) AS. When the mean gradient is intermediate (30–50 mmHg), additional data are necessary for accurate noninvasive assessment of AS.

Panidis and associates[32] from Philadelphia, Pennsylvania, performed continuous-mode Doppler ultrasound and cardiac catheterization within 1.4 ± 2.0 days in 70 patients, aged 26 to 84 years (mean 67 ± 11), with suspected AS. Optimal Doppler spectral display signal was recorded from the apical window in 43% of the patients, the second or third right parasternal area in 34%, and from the suprasternal notch view in 20% of the patients. Aortic valve gradients by Doppler ultrasound were calculated by the simpli-fied Bernoulli equation: pressure gradient = 4 × velocity^2. There was an overall fair correlation between the peak gradient by Doppler technique and both the maximal instantaneous and peak-to-peak aortic pressure gradient obtained at catheterization, and a good correlation between mean gradient by Doppler technique and catheterization. These correlation coefficients improved significantly in the last 51 patients compared to the initial 19 pa-tients of the study. Of the last 51 patients, correlation was better in those in normal sinus rhythm than in those in AF, and in patients with no or insignifi-cant coexistent AR compared to those with ≥2+ AR. The age of the patient and the status of cardiac output did not significantly affect the accuracy of correlations. The authors concluded that measurements of aortic valve gradi-ent by continuous-mode Doppler ultrasound may not correlate closely with those by catheterization when the experience with the Doppler technique is limited and when patients in AF or with significant coexistent AR are stud-ied.

Teirstein et al[33] in Stanford, California, evaluated 30 adult patients with AS by Doppler echocardiography within 1 day of cardiac catheterization. Noninvasive measurement of the mean transaortic pressure gradient was calculated by applying the simplified Bernoulli equation to the continuous-wave Doppler transaortic velocity recording. Stroke volume was measured noninvasively by multiplying the systolic velocity integral of flow in the LV outflow tract (obtained by pulsed Doppler ultrasonography) by the cross-sectional area of the LV outflow tract (measured by 2-D echocardiography). Noninvasive measurement of aortic valve area was calculated by 2 methods. In method 1, the Gorlin equation was applied using Doppler-derived mean pressure gradient, cardiac output, and systolic ejection period. Method 2 used the continuity equation. These noninvasive measurements were compared with the invasive ones using linear regression analysis, and mean pressure gradients correlated well. Aortic valve area by noninvasive method also cor-related well with cardiac catheterization values. The sensitivity of Doppler detection of critical AS was 0.86, with a specificity of 0.88 and a positive predictive value of 0.86. Doppler echocardiography may distinguish critical from noncritical AS with a high degree of accuracy. Measurement of aortic valve area aids in the interpretation of Doppler-derived mean pressure gradient data when the gradients are in an intermediate range, i.e., 30–50 mmHg.

Diastolic filling dynamics

Although myocardial hypertrophy is an important adaptive mechanism to cope with abnormal loading conditions, inadequate hypertrophy or depressed myocardial contractility can lead to deterioration of ejection performance in patients with AS or systemic hypertension. Murakami and co-workers[34] in Zurich, Switzerland, investigated LV filling dynamics in 24 patients with AS. Biplane angiography was performed with simultaneous micromanometry in these 24 patients and in 6 control subjects. Twelve patients with AS had moderate hypertrophy with a LV muscle mass index of <180 g/m^2 (AS1 group) and 12 had severe hypertrophy with an index of ≥180 g/m^2 (AS2 group). Filling dynamics also were evaluated postoperatively in 8 patients in the AS1 and 6 patients in the AS2 group. Preoperatively, end-diastolic and end-systolic volume indexes were larger and EF was lower in the AS2 group than in the control or AS1 group. Peak filling rate in the first half of diastole (%V1) was higher in the AS2 than in the control or in the AS1 group, whereas peak filling rates in the second half of diastole (PFR2) was considerably greater in the ASI group than in the other 2 groups. The time constant of LV pressure decline, an index of the rate of relaxation, was prolonged in the AS2 group. In contrast, mitral valve opening pressure was significantly higher in this group than in the other 2 groups. After surgery, in patients in the AS1 group, preoperatively reduced %V in the first half of diastole had increased and preoperatively enhanced PFR2 had decreased. In patients in the AS2 group, excluding 1 with a persistent low EF after surgery, preoperatively enhanced PFR1 decreased in association with a decrease in mitral valve opening pressure. Thus, LV filling dynamics vary in patients with AS depending on the degree of LV hypertrophy and systolic function. In patients with AS and moderate hypertrophy, early diastolic filling is slightly reduced but is compensated for by a forceful atrial contraction. In those with severe hypertrophy and systolic dysfunction, increased driving pressure allows early diastolic filling to remain within normal limits despite prolonged LV relaxation and diastolic elastic recoil. Both changes in LV filling dynamics tend to normalize after surgery in association with a reduction in LV hypertrophy or improvement of systolic function, or both.

Although an increase in LV diastolic pressure has been repeatedly observed during angina in patients with CAD and regional demand ischemia, the role of relaxation abnormalities -vs- LV segmental dyssynchrony is controversial. Since angina due to AS is likely to have diffuse rather than segmental ischemia, these patients may provide an alternative model for examining the diastolic physiology of angina. Thus, Fifer and co-investigators[35] in Boston, Massachusetts, examined the hemodynamic manifestations of angina in 8 patients with AS without significant CAD. Angina was induced by pacing tachycardia, and hemodynamic and echocardiographic variables were measured in the control period and during angina in the beats immediately after cessation of pacing. Heart rate and LV peak systolic pressure were similar in the control and postpacing angina periods. LV end-diastolic pressure was significantly higher during postpacing angina. The time constant of LV pressure decline during isovolumetric relaxation increased as did the time constant derived from the slope of a linear fit of dP/dt -vs- pressure. The LV diastolic pressure-volume relation and pressure-wall thickness relation obtained from 2-D-targeted M-mode echocardiograms in the controlled and postpacing periods were shifted upward during angina in these patients. Investigators concluded that angina in patients with AS is accompanied by substantial and reversible increase in LV end-diastolic pressure, and this increase appears to be due in part to an impairment of diastolic distensibility of the left ventricle and LV relaxation. These observations, which are similar to those observed during pacing-induced angina in patients with CAD, suggest that the increase in LV end-diastolic pressure that occurs during angina is a manifestation of demand ischemia per se, and does not depend on the presence of dyssynergistic contraction of ischemic and nonischemic regions.

Percutaneous transluminal valvuloplasty

To assess the safety and efficacy of percutaneous balloon valvuloplasty in calcific AS, McKay and co-workers[36] in Boston, Massachusetts, performed balloon dilatation of critically stenosed, calcific aortic valves in 5 postmortem hearts, in 5 patients intraoperatively before AVR, and in 2 elderly patients percutaneously at the time of diagnostic catheterization. The etiology of AS in the 12 cases was rheumatic in 2, congenital bicuspid calcific stenosis in 1, and senile calcific degenerative stenosis in the remaining 9. Prevalvuloplasty examination in the 10 postmortem and intraoperative cases revealed rigid valve cusps with commissural fusion in 3 valves and extensive nodular calcific deposits in 7. Subsequent balloon dilatation with 15–18-mm valvuloplasty balloons resulted in decreased cusp rigidity and increased mobility of valve leaflets in all cases, without evidence of tearing of valve cusps, disruption of valve ring, or liberation of calcific or valvular debris. In the 3 valve specimens with commissural fusion, balloon dilatation resulted in partial or complete separation of leaflets along fused commissures. In 2 cases with extensive nodular calcific deposits, balloon dilatation resulted in a fracture of a calcified leaflet that was evident on both gross and radiologic examinations. After postmortem and intraoperative studies, percutaneous catheter valvuloplasty was performed at the time of diagnostic catheterization in 2 elderly patients (93- and 85-year-old women) with calcific AS. Balloon dilatation with 12–18-mm balloons resulted in significant decreases in aortic gradients and significant increases in cardiac index and aortic valve area in both patients. Percutaneous valvuloplasty in both patients resulted in a mild increase in AR and no evidence of embolic phenomena. Investigators concluded that balloon valvuloplasty is possible in elderly patients with calcific AS and can result in significant improvement in LV and valvular function without the production of life-threatening complications.

Cribier and associates[37] from Rouen, France, performed percutaneous transluminal balloon catheter aortic valvuloplasty in 3 patients, aged 68, 77, and 79 years, with severe AS. In the first patient the transvalvular peak systolic gradient decreased by balloon inflation from 90–40 mmHg (Fig. 6-7). In the second patient the transvalvular peak systolic gradient decreased from 80–30 mmHg, and in the third patient from 60–30 mmHg. In the second and third patients the aortic valve area, calculated by Gorlin's formula, increased from 0.46–0.96 cm^2 and from 0.50–0.75 cm^2, respectively. Subsequent clinical course in all 3 patients showed a pronounced functional improvement. Thus, this procedure appears to be a good alternate to AVR in elderly patients.

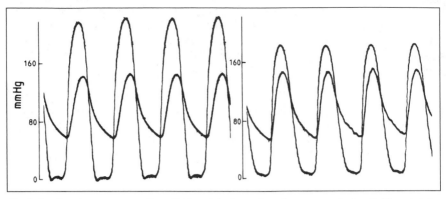

Fig. 6-7. Simultaneous recording of left ventricular and aortic pressures before (left) and at the end of PTAV (right) in case 1. Reproduced with permission from Cribier et al.[37]

Operative decalcification

In an effort to avoid prosthetic AVR and its attendant risk of thromboembolism and anticoagulation, King and colleagues[38] from Rochester, Minnesota, reviewed an experience between 1978 and 1984 dealing with decalcification of the aortic valve. Decalcification was performed in 8 patients, all of whom were undergoing CABG. Preoperative gradients of between 30 and 80 mmHg were abolished after operation. To determine the long-term outcome of decalcification, the records of 84 additional patients who had undergone that procedure between 1959 and 1978 were reviewed (Fig. 6-8). Follow up was 98% complete and ranged from 6 months to 22 years. AVR subsequently was required in 25 patients. Freedom from reoperation at 1, 5, 10, and 15 years was 98, 75, 43, and 26%, respectively, for patients with rheumatic valves compared to 97, 76, 57, and 51% for those with bicuspid valves (Fig. 6-9). Causes of late death were valve related in 30%, CHF in 27%, and AMI in 24%. The authors concluded that aortic valve decalcification is not as successful as current mitral reparative procedures; however, with proper selection, decalcification may be an acceptable alternative to AVR in some patients.

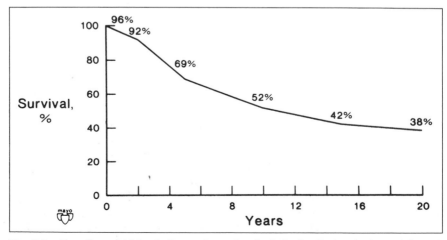

Fig. 6-8. Overall survival (excluding perioperative deaths) of patients who have undergone mechanical decalcification of the aortic valve. Reproduced with permission from King et al.[38]

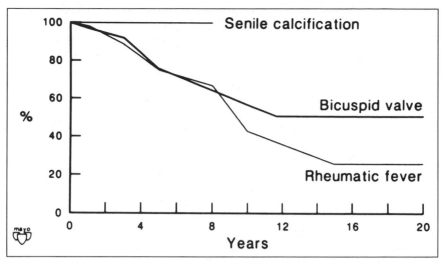

Fig. 6-9. Freedom from reoperation of patients with rheumatic fever, bicuspid aortic valves, and senile calcification who have undergone aortic valve decalcification. Reproduced with permission from King et al.[38]

AORTIC REGURGITATION

Usefulness of echocardiography

To determine the relative sensitivity and specificity of noninvasive methods for detecting AR, Grayburn and associates[39] from Lexington, Kentucky, compared the accuracy of auscultation, echocardiography, and pulsed Doppler echocardiography in detecting AR in 106 patients in whom the presence or absence of AR were shown by supravalvular aortography. The sensitivity and specificity for the diagnosis of AR was 96% and 96% for pulsed Doppler echocardiography, 73% and 92% for auscultation, 43% and 91% for 2-D echocardiography, 46% and 81% for anterior mitral leaflet flutter, and 9% and 96% for ventricular septal flutter, respectively. Auscultation was more sensitive than either M-mode or 2-D echocardiography in the diagnosis of AR. Pulsed Doppler echocardiography was significantly more sensitive than auscultation and was positive in 19 patients in whom no murmur was found. Thus, pulsed Doppler echocardiography is the optimal noninvasive marker for AR.

Parameswaran and associates[40] from Philadelphia, Pennsylvania, assessed LV diastolic filling using digitized M-mode echocardiography in 12 patients with AR and in 10 normal subjects. Ten patients with AR were asymptomatic and 2 patients had CHF. LV chamber dimensions, fractional shortening and the rate of change of LV dimensions during systole and diastole were determined. In addition, the timing of the rate of change of LV dimensions in diastole (peak dD/dt, 50% peak dD/dt and 20T peak dD/dt) was also measured. Patients with AR had a significant reduction in dD/dt (12 ± 4 cm/s in patients with AR -vs- 16 ± 2 cm/s in normal subjects) and a delay in the timing of peak dD/dt (160 ± 35 ms in patients with AR -vs- 86 ± 18 ms in normal subjects) from the minimum LV dimension. These diastolic abnormalities were present in patients with symptomatic and those with asymptomatic AR, occurred even when the fractional shortening and peak systolic emptying rate (peak −dD/dt) were normal, and showed no correlation with the calculated LV mass. The delay in the diastolic filling velocities (peak dD/dt, 50% and 20% peak dD/dt) was associated with a decreased rate of change of LV dimension in diastole, suggesting delayed early LV filling. These findings indicate an abnormality of LV diastolic filling in patients with symptomatic as well as asymptomatic AR and suggest that diastolic abnormalities may precede echocardiographic indexes of systolic LV dysfunction.

Teague et al[41] in Oklahoma City, Oklahoma and Durham, North Carolina, studied 86 patients with AR to determine whether the severity of AR can be quantified using continuous-wave Doppler ultrasound. The Doppler velocity half-time was defined as the time required for the diastolic AR velocity profile to decrease by 29%, and cardiac catheterization-determined pressure half-time was calculated as the interval required for transvalvular pressure to decrease by 50%. Doppler velocity and catheterization pressure half-times were linearly related. Doppler velocity half-times were inversely related to regurgitant fraction. Angiographic severity (1+ = mild to 4+ = severe) was also related inversely to pressure and velocity half-times; the Doppler half-time threshold of 400 ms distinguished mild from significant AR with specificity and good predictive value. In these studies, the Doppler velocity half-time was independent of pulse pressure, mean arterial pressure, EF, and LV end-diastolic pressure. These data suggest that an estimation of transvalvular aortic pressure half-time utilizing continuous-wave Doppler ultrasound is a reliable and accurate method for the noninvasive evaluation of the severity of AR.

Labovitz et al[42] in St. Louis, Missouri, determined the usefulness of continuous-wave Doppler echocardiography in the evaluation of AR. The aortic regurgitant flow velocity pattern obtained with continuous-wave Doppler examination was compared with the results of aortography and conventional pulsed Doppler techniques in 25 patients with AR. The diastolic deceleration slope as measured from the continuous-wave tracing was significantly different among subgroups of patients with mild (1.6 ± 0.5 m/s^2), moderate (2.7 ± 0.5 m/s^2), and severe (4.7 ± 1.5 m/s^2) AR as determined from aortography. Deceleration slopes greater than 2 m/s^2 separated those with moderate and severe AR from those with mild AR. Similar findings were found when comparing the pressure half-time methods of diastolic velocity decay with the more severe grades of AR exhibiting the shortest pressure half-times. There was a strong correlation between the deceleration slope measured by continuous-wave Doppler and the degree of AR as assessed by pulsed Doppler echocardiography. End-diastolic velocities correlated poorly with catheter-measured end-diastolic pressure difference between the aorta and the left ventricle. These data indicate that the AR flow pattern may be quantitated by continuous-wave Doppler echocardiography in a manner that is useful for identifying the severity of AR by assessing the rate with which aortic and LV pressures equilibrate during diastole.

Response to exercise

Fifteen patients with symptomatic mild-to-moderate and severe chronic AR performed supine bicycle exercise while measurements of rest and exercise hemodynamics and LV function were obtained by Kawanishi and co-workers[43] in Los Angeles, California. A continuous Doppler method was used to determine the change in distribution of total LV stroke volume between forward stroke volume and regurgitant volume (RgV) with exercise. The PA wedge pressure was lower in the mild-to-moderate AR group than in the severe AR group at rest and during exercise. In all patients there were increases in heart rate, forward stroke volume, and the cardiac index despite a decrease in total LV stroke volume index. The systemic vascular resistance decreased with the exercise and the RgV and regurgitant fraction both decreased with exercise. LVEF increased with exercise from 0.51–0.55 for the group, but either decreased or failed to increase by at least 0.05 in 7 of 13 patients. The change in EF on exercise was directly related to the change in systemic vascular resistance. These investigators concluded that: 1) in patients with mild-to-moderate AR, the PA wedge pressure is generally normal at rest and exercise, 2) in most of those with severe AR, the PA wedge pressure is elevated at rest and increases significantly with exercise, which is the likely mechanism for dyspnea on exertion in these patients, 3) the cardiac index in both groups is normal at rest and increases during exercise, 4) the increase in cardiac output results from both an increased heart rate and forward stroke volume, 5) the increase in forward stroke volume results from reductions of RgV and RgF, 6) the RgV and RgF are decreased due to a decreased systemic vascular resistance, and 7) the EF response to exercise is variable and correlates best with changes in systemic vascular resistance with exercise.

Shen and associates[44] from Sydney, Australia, assessed in 31 patients with AR (20 asymptomatic, 11 symptomatic) and in 10 control subjects the relation between systolic loading conditions at rest and LV functional response to exercise. Peak and end-systolic wall stress determined from echocardiography and cuff systolic BP at rest were used as indirect measures of LV systolic loading and were compared with LVEF response to handgrip and bicycle exercise by radionuclide ventriculography. Both peak and end-systolic wall stress were significantly higher in both asymptomatic (164 ± 33 and $90 \pm 25 \times 10^3$ dynes/cm^2) and symptomatic (196 ± 33 and $134 \pm 17 \times 10^3$ dynes/cm^2) patients with AR than in the control subjects (125 ± 22 and $61 \pm 14 \times 10^3$ dynes/cm^2), and correlated inversely with the changes in LVEF during handgrip and bicycle exercise. In patients with AR, resting systolic loading conditions closely reflect LV functional reserve during exercise.

Diagnostic guidelines for syphilis

Although the frequency of primary syphilis continues to be high, the frequency of cardiovascular syphilis appears to be diminishing. Nevertheless, syphilis remains one of the more frequent causes of AR in older persons. Hart[45] from Adelaide, Australia, provided diagnostic guidelines for diagnosis of syphilis. Specificity of the VDRL (Venereal Disease Research Laboratory) and treponemal tests is high in healthy persons but less in elderly and ill persons. Sensitivity of the VDRL test is high in secondary and early latent syphilis but reduced in primary and late syphilis or in cerebrospinal fluid evaluations. Primary syphilis should be diagnosed by darkfield microscopy, with VDRL confirmation for atypical lesions. Screening of asymptomatic persons with the VDRL test, followed by treponemal test confirmation on positive sera is recommended for all pregnant women, contacts of persons with infectious syphilis, and other high-risk groups. Quantitative VDRL assessment of 3, 6, and 12 months after treatment should be used to assess the adequacy of treatment for both late latent and early syphilis. Cerebrospinal fluid VDRL assessment and cell count should be restricted to seropositive persons with a high risk of neurosyphilis.

Ankylosing spondylitis

Thomsen and associates[46] from Graasten, Denmark, performed ambulatory 24-hour monitoring in 54 patients with ankylosing spondylitis, 48 of whom were HLA B27 positive. Of these 48 HLA B27 positive patients, 12 had electrocardiographic abnormalities on monitoring. The frequency of AV block and atrial tachycardia was significantly higher in this group of patients than that found in similar studies of healthy adults.

Coronary artery disease

Pathak and associates[47] from Manhasset and New York, New York, studied 78 patients with isolated severe AR retrospectively to determine the prevalence of angiographically significant CAD and its relation to angina pectoris. Angiographically significant CAD was present in 29 of 78 patients (37%), and 36 patients (46%) had angina pectoris. Twenty-one of 36 patients (58%) with and 8 of 42 patients (19%) without angina pectoris had angiographically significant CAD. Angina pectoris as a predictor of significant CAD had a sensitivity of 73%, specificity of 69%, and a risk ratio of 3:1. The predictive accuracy of detecting CAD in the absence of angina pectoris was 81%. The benefit from concomitant CABG at the time of AVR for AR has not been clearly demonstrated; therefore, routine coronary angiography is still recommended for all AR patients >40 years undergoing AVR.

Hydralazine treatment

Kleaveland and associates[48] from Philadelphia, Pennsylvania, studied 17 patients with chronic asymptomatic AR to determine whether 6 months of hydralazine therapy could reduce the severity of AR or reverse LV enlargement and hypertrophy. Echocardiography, radionuclide angiography at rest and during exercise, and maximal treadmill exercise with respiratory gas analysis were performed at intake and after a 6-month double-blind treatment period. After dose titration with hydralazine, patients were randomized to their maximal tolerated hydralazine dose or to placebo. At intake, hydralazine and placebo groups were similar. Six patients taking hydralazine and 8 taking placebo completed the study protocol. One patient taking placebo died and 2 patients taking hydralazine withdrew with drug-related adverse effects. The mean titrated dose of hydralazine was 96 ± 9 mg, but the mean treatment dose was 63 ± 21 mg administered 3 times daily because of drug intolerance. After 6 months, mean systolic BP with hydralazine therapy decreased from 136–125 mmHg, and end-systolic posterior wall thickness increased from 1.58–1.70 cm, resulting in a significant reduction in M-mode meridional end-systolic stress (from 104–80 kdynes/cm^2). M-mode fractional shortening increased from 0.28–0.31 with hydralazine, but mean LV echocardiographic dimensions were unchanged. LV mass increased from 383–434 with hydralazine, primarily because of an increase in end-diastolic wall thickness. In the placebo group, there was no change in any of the hemodynamic or echocardiographic parameters at 6 months. Treadmill exercise variables, radionuclide EF, and regurgitant fraction at rest were unchanged in either group at 6 months; however, in patients taking hydralazine, the EF during exercise increased from 64 ± 12–$72 \pm 9\%$. It is concluded that 6 months of hydralazine therapy in maximal tolerated doses does not alter the severity of regurgitation or reduce LV enlargement and hypertrophy in chronic severe AR, although systolic function may be improved.

Timing valve replacement

Hoshino and Gaasch[49] from Boston, Massachusetts, reviewed studies concerning timing of AVR in patients with chronic pure AR. These authors suggested the following: Asymptomatic patients with normal LV function are not surgical candidates, but AVR should be performed in most patients with LV dysfunction, even if symptoms are absent. The short-term administration of vasodilators is generally beneficial, but there is meager evidence that the hemodynamic benefits are maintained. Therefore, the wide application of these agents should be postponed until well designed clinical trials document a long-term benefit.

Operative treatment of the Marfan syndrome

The life expectancy of patients with Marfan syndrome is reduced by complications caused by dilatation of the ascending aorta. Because operative therapy with a composite graft may alter this natural history, Gott and associates[50] from Baltimore, Maryland, analyzed the preoperative and long-term postoperative status of 50 consecutive patients who received such a graft. At surgery (Fig. 6-10), the patients had a mean age of 32 years and a mean aortic diameter of 7 cm (range, 5–10). Dissection of the ascending aorta was present in 14 patients and was acute in 5. None of the 44 patients who underwent elective repair, and only 1 of the 6 patients who had emergency surgery died in the hospital; thus, the overall hospital mortality was 2%. Five of the 49 survivors died during a follow-up period of up to 8 years (10% late mortality) (Fig. 6-11). During the most recent 4 years of evaluation of this series (38 patients), no postoperative deaths due to intrathoracic problems occurred. Actuarial survival was 87% at both 2 and 5 years. Composite-graft repair of the ascending aorta in patients with the Marfan syndrome can be performed with low operative and long-term mortality. Because of the unfavorable natural history of the Marfan syndrome and the potential for dissection in moderately dilated aortic roots, the authors recommended prophylactic repair when the aneurysm reaches a diameter of 6 cm.

INFECTIVE ENDOCARDITIS

Prophylaxis

Kaye[51] from Philadelphia, Pennsylvania, summarized the recent update of the American Heart Association recommendations for prevention of bacterial endocarditis (Tables 6-5, 6-6, 6-7, and 6-8). The major changes are less emphasis on administration of parenteral agents and a reduction of the period of prophylaxis. The simplified new recommendations should make compliance easier and should be assiduously implemented by dental and medical practitioners. However, several changes are suggested for possible consideration: Because of the relatively low risk, prophylaxis may not be needed for persons with MVP (unless there is a holosystolic murmur) or for most gastrointestinal endoscopic procedures. Consideration should be given to using a single oral 3-g dose of amoxicillin for dental procedures in all patients at risk and for genitourinary and gastrointestinal tract procedures in patients at risk who have natural cardiac valves. Vancomycin should probably be the agent of choice for prophylaxis in cardiac valve surgery.

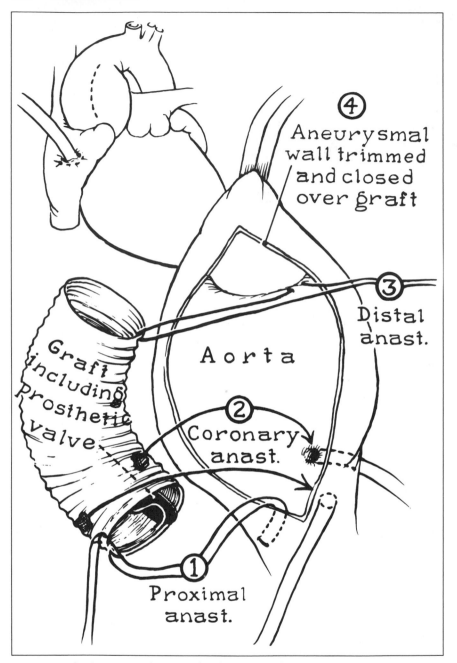

Fig. 6-10.   The four principal steps in the placement of the composite-graft valve.

Vegetation size

Robbins and associates[52] from Bronx, New York, evaluated the prognostic value of echocardiographically determined vegetation size in 23 episodes of *right-sided valvular endocarditis* in 21 patients. Right-sided vegetations were visualized in 19 of 23 episodes (83%). Of these, a vegetation ≥1.0 cm was found in 11. No patient with an echocardiographically determined vegetation size of <1.0 cm required surgery, whereas 4 of 11 (36%) of those episodes in

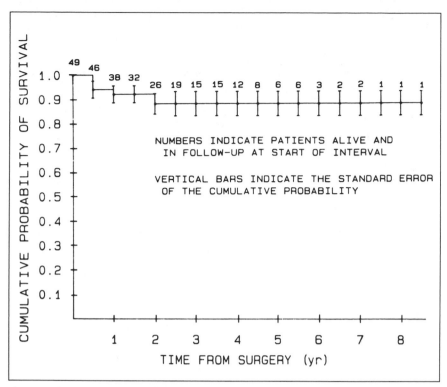

Fig. 6-11. Actuarial survival curve for 49 patients with the Marfan syndrome who were discharged from the hospital after composite-graft repair of the ascending aorta.

which the vegetation size was ≥1.0 cm required surgery for persistent pyrexia. In all patients requiring surgery, a bioprosthetic tricuspid valve was placed at the time of initial surgery and in no patient did early reinfection occur. This study reconfirms the "benign" prognosis of right-sided valvular endocarditis.

Although 2-dimensional echocardiography is considered the most sensi-

TABLE 6-5. *Cardiac conditions for which endocarditis prophylaxis is recommended.* Reproduced with permission from Kaye.[51]

Endocarditis prophylaxis recommended
    Prosthetic cardiac valves (including biosynthetic valves)
    Most congenital cardiac malformations
    Surgically constructed systemic-pulmonary shunts
    Rheumatic and other acquired valvular dysfunction
    Idiopathic hypertrophic subaortic stenosis
    Previous history of bacterial endocarditis
    Mitral valve prolapse with insufficiency†
Endocarditis prophylaxis not recommended
    Isolated secundum atrial septal defect
    Secundum atrial septal defect repaired without a patch 6 or more months earlier
    Patent ductus arteriosus ligated and divided 6 or more months earlier
    Postoperatively after coronary artery bypass graft surgery

---

* Adapted from Shulman and colleagues (1).
† Definitive data to provide guidance in management of patients with mitral valve prolapse are particularly limited. In general, such patients are clearly at low risk of development of endocarditis, but the risk-benefit ratio of prophylaxis in mitral valve prolapse is uncertain.

TABLE 6-6. *Procedures for which endocarditis prophylaxis is indicated.* Reproduced with permission from Kaye.[51]*

Oral cavity and respiratory tract
  All dental procedures likely to induce gingival bleeding (not simple adjustment of orthodontic
    appliances or shedding of deciduous teeth)
  Tonsillectomy or adenoidectomy
  Surgical procedures or biopsy involving respiratory mucosa
  Bronchoscopy, especially with a rigid bronchoscope†
  Incision and drainage of infected tissue
Genitourinary and gastrointestinal tracts
  Cystoscopy
  Prostatic surgery
  Urethral catheterization (especially in the presence of infection)
  Urinary tract surgery
  Vaginal hysterectomy
  Gallbladder surgery
  Colonic surgery
  Esophageal dilatation
  Sclerotherapy for esophageal varices
  Colonoscopy
  Upper gastrointestinal tract endoscopy with biopsy
  Proctosigmoidoscopic biopsy

* Adapted from Shulman and colleagues (1).
† The risk with flexible bronchoscopy is low, but the necessity for prophylaxis is not yet defined.

TABLE 6-7. *Summary of recommended antibiotic regimens for adults having dental or respiratory tract procedures.* Reproduced with permission from Kaye.[51]*

Standard regimen
  For dental procedures that cause gingival bleeding, and oral or respiratory tract surgery — Penicillin V, 2.0 g orally, 1 hour before, then 1.0 g 6 hours later. For patients unable to take oral medications, 2×10^6 U of aqueous penicillin G intravenously or intramuscularly 30 to 60 minutes before a procedure and 1×10^6 U 6 hours later may be substituted.

Special regimens
  Parenteral regimen for use when maximal protection is desired, for example, for patients with prosthetic valves — Ampicillin, 1.0 to 2.0 g intramuscularly or intravenously, plus gentamicin, 1.5 mg/kg body weight intramuscularly or intravenously, 0.5 hours before procedure, followed by 1.0 g of oral penicillin V 6 hours later. Alternatively, the parenteral regimen may be repeated once 8 hours later.
  Oral regimen for patients allergic to penicillin — Erythromycin, 1.0 g orally 1 hour before, then 500 mg 6 hours later.
  Parenteral regimen for patients allergic to penicillin — Vancomycin, 1.0 g intravenously, slowly over 1 hour, starting 1 hour before. No repeat dose is necessary.

* Adapted from Shulman and colleagues (1).

tive method for detecting vegetations in infective endocarditis, the independent clinical significance of these vegetations continues to be debated. To further examine this, Buda and associates[53] from Ann Arbor, Michigan, identified 74 patients who were diagnosed over a 54-month period as having infective endocarditis. The 50 patients who underwent 2-D echocardiographic examination form the basis of this report. Definite vegetations were present in 21 (42%) patients and measured 1.2 ± 0.2 cm^2. The vegetation was localized to the aortic valve in 10 patients, mitral valve in 8, and tricus-

TABLE 6-8. *Summary of recommended regimens for adults having gastrointestinal or genitourinary tract procedures.* Reproduced with permission from Kaye.[51]*

Standard regimen	
For genitourinary and gastrointestinal tract procedures listed in Table 2	Ampicillin, 2.0 g intramuscularly or intravenously, plus gentamicin, 1.5 mg/kg body weight intramuscularly or intravenously, given 0.5 to 1 hour before the procedure. One follow-up dose may be given 8 hours later.
Special regimens	
Oral regimen for minor or repetitive procedures in low-risk patients	Amoxicillin, 3.0 g orally, 1 hour before procedure and 1.5 g 6 hours later.
Patients allergic to penicillin	Vancomycin, 1.0 g intravenously, given slowly over 1 hour, plus gentamicin, 1.5 mg/kg body weight intramuscularly or intravenously, given 1 hour before procedure. May be repeated once 8 to 12 hours later.

* Adapted from Shulman and colleagues (1).

pid valve in 3. A major complication, defined as death, new-onset CHF, major arterial embolus, or valve surgery occurred in 86% of the patients with vegetative endocarditis compared to 62% of those without vegetations. Among those patients with vegetations, death occurred in 24%, CHF in 38%, arterial embolus in 48%, and surgery in 43%. This compared to 7%, 21%, 21%, and 24%, respectively, in those patients without vegetations. These data support the concept that 2-D echocardiographic detection of a vegetation defines a high-risk subgroup of patients with infective endocarditis in whom careful monitoring and aggressive management are warranted.

Conduction abnormalities

Dinubile and associates[54] from Boston, Massachusetts, reviewed 211 episodes of native cardiac valve active infective endocarditis treated in their hospital between 1975 and 1983. The aortic (36%) and mitral (33%) valves were most frequently involved, but in 21% of the cases the site of infection could not be localized. Streptococcal (50%) and staphylococcal (35%) species were the most frequently isolated pathogens. New or changing ("unstable") conduction abnormalities developed in 9% of the patients, while an additional 7% had conduction abnormalities of "indeterminate" age. Unstable conduction block was more likely to develop in patients with aortic valve infective endocarditis than in those with mitral infection. Surgery was performed in 23% of the patients. Unstable conduction abnormalities were significantly associated with valve replacement, but in a multivariate analysis, this effect could be explained by the site of valvular infection. The mortality rate was 20%. Patients with unstable conduction abnormalities had a significantly higher mortality rate, even after other significant predictors of death (age, type of causative organism) were taken into account. Patients whose conduction changes persisted had a worse prognosis than those with transient conduction abnormalities. Although more hemodynamically compromised, patients with unstable conduction block who underwent valve replacement did at least as well as those given medical therapy alone. Patients with native valve active infective endocarditis in whom persistent, unstable conduction abnormalities develop without other identifiable cause, especially in the presence of aortic valve infection, should be considered for valve replacement.

Fever during therapy

Douglas and associates[55] from London, UK, reviewed 83 episodes of culture-positive infective endocarditis of a native valve, and fever persisted or recurred in 42 (50%) despite appropriate bactericidal antibiotics (Table 6-9). The most frequent cause of fever was extensive infection of the valve ring and adjacent structures, even when the infecting organisms were *viridans streptococci*; urgent surgery was required. Less frequent causes were systemic and pulmonary emboli and drug hypersensitivity. Infected intravenous access sites were seldom responsible. In no case was fever due to antibiotic resistance of the infecting organism. In patients with a definite microbiologic diagnosis who have been given appropriate antibiotics, the temptation to alter antibiotic therapy because of persistent or recurrent fever should be resisted unless there are features of drug hypersensitivity. When fever persists or recurs during treatment of IE, the opinions of a cardiologist and cardiac surgeon should be obtained as soon as possible; delay in valve replacement may prove fatal in patients with extensive infection.

Operative treatment

The timing of surgery in patients with severe AR and LV failure, particularly when associated with active infective endocarditis, is of utmost importance. From July 1982 to May 1984, Sareli and associates[56] from Johannesburg, South Africa, performed aortic valve surgery in 34 patients, aged 15–60 years, who had severe AR from infective endocarditis. All patients were in New York Heart Association class IV for LV failure. Eighteen patients had right-sided CHF. Decision for immediate surgery was based on the echocardiographic demonstration of diastolic closure of the mitral valve or of vegetations on the aortic valve. Premature closure of the mitral valve was demonstrated echocardiographically in 17 patients, 13 of whom had diastolic crossover of LV and left atrial pressure tracings recorded at surgery. Infective endocarditis of the aortic valve was confirmed at surgery in 29 patients, 27 of whom had vegetations on echocardiography. Seven patients required replacement of both aortic and mitral valves. Antibiotic therapy for infective endocarditis was started immediately after blood cultures were taken and continued for 4 to 6 weeks postoperatively. The mortality rate within 30 days of surgery was 6% for the group as a whole and 7% for those with infective endocarditis. Mean follow-up period for the 32 survivors was 10.6 months. There were 2 late deaths. No patient had periprosthetic regurgitation or persistence of endocarditis. Procrastination in referral for surgery of these extremely ill patients is not justified and is likely to be associated with higher risks of morbidity and mortality.

Tricuspid valve excision for tricuspid endocarditis in *addicts* is recommended to avoid early reinfection, continued sepsis, and late reinfection because of the resumption of intravenous drug abuse. Valvectomy is allegedly well tolerated hemodynamically by some, but it leads to CHF in at least a third of patients. Stern and associates[57] from Bronx, New York, examined the records of 10 addicts in whom staphylococcal endocarditis had failed to respond to antibiotic therapy and tricuspid valve replacement was done. All 10 patients left the hospital free of infection and free of CHF. Resumption of drug addiction in 3 patients led to septic death, but not necessarily to tricuspid reinfection. Two patients returned to jobs requiring a high level of physical labor and tolerated this without difficulty. The authors found no need to follow the practice of tricuspid valve excision for tricuspid endocarditis in

TABLE 6-9. *Sites of infection. Reproduced with permission from Douglas.*[55]

GROUP	MITRAL NO (%)	AORTIC NO (%)	AORTIC AND MITRAL NO (%)	TRICUSPID NO (%)	VSD NO (%)
Afebrile (n = 41)	22 (54)	24 (32)	3 (7)	2 (5)	1 (2)
Febrile (n = 42)	12 (29)	12 (29)	11 (26)	6 (14)	1 (2)
Total (n = 83)	34 (41)	25 (30)	14 (17)	8 (10)	2 (2)

VSD = ventricular septal defect.

addicts. Those who refrained from drug abuse are well served by valve replacement. Those who do not are doomed with or without a tricuspid valve.

Prosthetic valve endocarditis

Calderwood and associates[58] from Boston analyzed 116 patients with prosthetic valve endocarditis (PVE) treated between 1975 and 1983 (Fig. 6-12). Complicated PVE was defined as the presence of a new or changing heart murmur, new or worsening CHF, new or progressive cardiac conjunction abnormalities, or prolonged fever during therapy. Complicated PVE was present in 64% of the patients. Factors associated with complicated PVE included aortic valve infection and onset of endocarditis within 12 months of cardiac operation. Mortality rate for PVE was 23%. Patients with complicated PVE had a higher mortality than patients with uncomplicated infection. Surgical therapy was more common in patients with complicated PVE and in patients infected with coagulase-negative staphylococci. Survival after initially successful therapy for PVE was adversely affected by the presence of moderate or severe CHF at hospital discharge. The presence of complicated PVE is a central variable in assessing prognosis and planning therapy. Most patients with complicated PVE are best treated by medical-surgical therapy. Those who are not treated surgically during their hospitalization are at high risk for progressive prosthetic dysfunction and require careful follow up.

MISCELLANEOUS TOPICS

Regurgitant flow patterns in normal valves

Although Doppler echocardiography allows recording of regurgitant turbulent flow patterns in normal persons, sparse information is available concerning the incidence, characteristics, and mechanism of these flow patterns. Accordingly, Kostucki and associates[59] from Brussels, Belgium, recorded pulsed Doppler echocardiograms in 25 normal persons to detect regurgitation. A regurgitant turbulent flow pattern was recorded at the pulmonic valve in 23 subjects (92%), covered up to 81% of the diastole, and could never be recorded in early diastole. An early to midsystolic regurgitant flow pattern was recorded at the mitral valve in 10 subjects (40%) and covered up to 60% of systole. A similar regurgitant flow was recorded at the tricuspid valve in 11

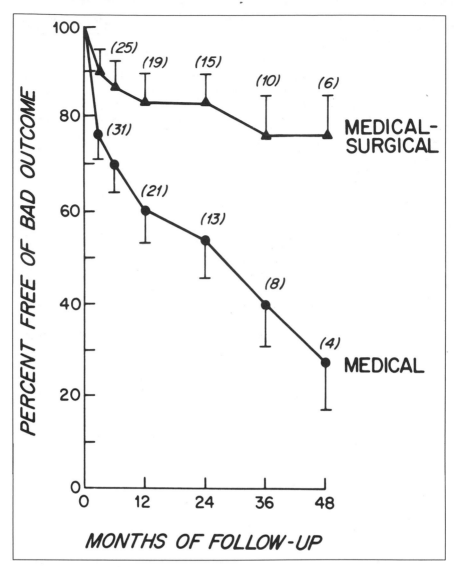

Fig. 6-12. Percent of patients free of bad outcome after medical versus medical-surgical therapy for PVE. *Data points* are mean values ±1 standard error of the mean. Figures in *parentheses* refer to the number of patients in each group being followed up at the start of the subsequent interval. Reproduced with permission from Calderwood et al.[58]

subjects (44%) and was holosystolic in 1 subject. An early diastolic regurgitant flow with low maximal velocities and rapid decrease in velocities was recorded at the aortic valve in 8 subjects (33%) and covered up to 26% of the diastole. In no person could those flows be recorded farther than 1 cm proximal to the valve closure. Whatever the still-debated mechanisms of those regurgitant flow patterns in normal subjects, one should be aware of their existence and characteristics when assessing valvular function by Doppler.

Origin of Still's murmur

Seventy normal children and young adults, 29 with Still's murmur and 49 with no murmur were studied by pulsed Doppler and 2-D echocardiography to evaluate possible etiology by Schwartz and associates[60] from Tucson, Arizona. There was no difference between the 2 groups in terms of TR, ventricular bands, pulmonary velocity, and magnitude of spectral widths. Mean ascending aortic diameter relative to body surface area was smaller for the group with Still's murmur and the average peak ascending velocity was significantly higher than the group without a murmur. These authors provide interesting new data in regard to possible origin of Still's murmur. This well-known musical murmur, which tends to disappear with increasing age, has never been satisfactorily explained as to etiology. These data are suggestive that it may be due to vibrations in the ascending aorta rather than blood turbulence.

Detection of tricuspid regurgitation by Doppler

Suzuki and associates[61] from Kyoto, Japan, studied 27 patients (18 with suspected TR and 9 normal subjects) to detect and evaluate regurgitant flow in TR with a newly developed, real-time, 2-D, color-coded, Doppler flow imaging system (Doppler 2-D echocardiography) and compared the findings with those obtained using contrast 2-D echocardiography and right ventriculography. In 16 of 18 patients with suspected TR, Doppler 2-D echocardiography easily visualized the color-coded regurgitant flow in the right atrium and estimated the severity of TR from the distance of the visible TR jet. On the basis of the QRS synchronized appearance of contrast in the inferior vena cava by the subxiphoid approach or of the negative contrast effect above the tricuspid valve just after the contrast entered the right ventricle with its subsequent back-and-forth movements across the tricuspid valve, Doppler 2-D echocardiography was more sensitive and specific in detecting TR (100% and 100%) than contrast 2-D echo (75% and 82% in the subxiphoid view, 56% and 100% in the 4-chamber view) when the fast Fourier transformation frequency analysis was used as the standard of TR, and it was more sensitive in detecting TR (85%) than contrast 2-D echo (69% in the subxiphoid approach, 46% in the 4-chamber view) when right ventriculography was used as the standard of TR. Additionally, the severity of TR as shown by Doppler 2-D echocardiography correlated fairly well with that shown by right ventriculography. Thus, Doppler 2-D echocardiography is clinically useful for detecting and evaluating TR.

Use of blood pressure cuff to increase intensity of left-sided regurgitant murmur

Lembo and associates[62] from San Antonio, Texas, transiently produced arterial occlusion of both arms with BP cuffs inflated to 20–40 mmHg above systolic BP for 20 seconds in 30 patients and found that the intensity of left-sided regurgitant murmurs caused by AR, MR, and VSD increased in intensity (Fig. 6-13). These authors compared this new maneuver with handgrip exercise, squatting, and amyl nitrite inhalation in 30 patients with left-sided regurgitant murmurs and in 30 patients with murmurs not caused by left-sided regurgitation. Transient arterial occlusion increased the intensity of left-sided regurgitant murmurs more than squatting and did not statistically differ from isometric handgrip exercise and amyl nitrite inhalation in ability to identify the presence of these murmurs. A false-positive diagnosis of left-sided regurgitant murmur was less likely when using transient arterial occlusion than when using handgrip exercise and squatting. Thus, transient arterial occlusion works as well as or better than other standard bedside maneuvers for diagnosing or excluding left-sided regurgitant murmurs and can be applied to all patients.

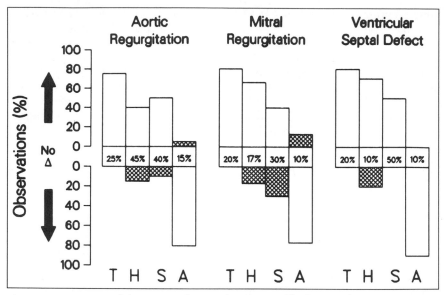

Fig. 6-13. Percentage of observations that noted an increase (↑), decrease (↓), or no change (*no* Δ) in murmur intensity of aortic regurgitation, mitral regurgitation, and ventricular septal defect using transient arterial occlusion (*T*), handgrip exercise (*H*), squatting (*S*), and amyl nitrite inhalation (*A*). Open bars indicate expected correct observations; cross-hatched bars, observations that were opposite to those expected, or incorrect. Reproduced with permission from Lembo et al.[62]

Heart and aorta in osteogenesis imperfecta

Although aortic root dilatation and valvular dysfunction have been well documented in osteogenesis imperfecta, the nature and extent of cardiovascular involvement in these patients have not been clearly delineated. Hortop and co-workers[63] in Montreal, Canada, undertook a clinical and echocardiographic study involving 109 subjects with various nonlethal osteogenesis imperfecta syndromes from 66 separate families. Clinical discernible valvular dysfunction was encountered in only 4 of the 109 persons (AR in 2, AS in 1, and MVP in 1), none of whom were related. Aortic root dilatation was recognized echocardiographically in 8 (12%) of 66 patients comprising a subset of the sample in which each family was represented by a single subject. The extent of the aortic root dilatation was mild and unrelated to the age of the subject. Dilatation was seen in each of the different osteogenesis imperfecta syndromes but was strikingly segregated within certain families. In the same subset of 66 subjects, MVP was encountered in 2 or 7% of the 29 subjects aged ≥15 years in whom adequate studies were obtained. This observed frequency was not different from that seen in a normal adult population. Aortic root dilatation appears to represent a distinct phenotypic trait in patients with osteogenesis imperfecta that is nonprogressive and occurs in about 12% of affected persons.

Echocardiographic evaluation of aortic valvular and mitral anular calcium in older persons

Aronow and associates[64] from Bronx, New York, performed M-mode and 2-D echocardiography in a blinded prospective study in 565 unselected elderly persons older than 62 years in a long-term health care facility. An aortic systolic murmur was heard in 265 of 565 persons (47%) and in 220 of 473 persons (47%) in whom technically adequate M-mode and 2-D echocardiograms of the aortic valves were recorded. An aortic systolic murmur was heard in 71 of 73 persons (97%) with calcified aortic cusp and decreased excursion, in 20 of 22 persons (91%) with calcified aortic cusps and normal excursion, and in 47 of 50 persons (94%) with thickened aortic cusps and decreased excursion, in 69 of 96 persons (72%) with thickened aortic cusps or root and normal excursion, and in 13 of 232 persons (6%) with normal aortic cusps and root. AS was present in 123 of 473 elderly persons (26%). Mitral anular calcium was present in 80 of 95 persons (84%) with calcified aortic cusps compared with 102 of 146 persons (70%) with thickened aortic cusps or root and compared with 76 of 232 persons (33%) with normal aortic valve cusps and root.

CARDIAC VALVE REPLACEMENT

Flow characteristics of mechanical valves

Rashtian and associates[65] from Los Angeles, California, and Atlanta, Georgia, reviewed the *in vivo* and *in vitro* fluid dynamic performance of 4 mechanical heart valves: 1) Starr-Edwards silicon-rubber ball valves (models 1200/1260 aortic and 6120 mitral valves); 2) Björk-Shiley tilting disc valves (standard spherical model, modified and unmodified convexo-concave [60° and 70°C-C] models); 3) the Medtronic-Hall (Hall-Kaster) tilting disc valve; and 4) the St. Jude Medical bileaflet valve. These valves were chosen because of their past or present popularity in clinical use and because they encompass most of the basic mechanical valve designs used during the past 2 decades. The flow measurements reported include *in vivo* and *in vitro* mean pressure drop, cardiac output or cardiac index, regurgitant volume, effective orifice area, and performance index.

Echocardiographic evaluation of prosthetic and bioprosthetic valves

Panidis et al[66] in Philadelphia, Pennsylvania, used Doppler echocardiography in 136 patients with a normally functioning prosthetic valve in the aortic (n = 59), mitral (n = 74), and tricuspid (n = 3) positions. These included patients with St. Jude, Björk-Shiley, Beall, Starr-Edwards, or tissue valves. Peak and mean pressure gradients across the prostheses were measured using a simplified Bernoulli equation. The prosthetic valve orifice only in the mitral position was calculated using the equivalent: PVO = 220/pressure half-time. In the aortic position, the St. Jude valve had a lower peak velocity, peak gradient, and mean gradient than the other valves. In the mitral position, the St. Jude valve had the largest orifice (3.0 ± 0.6 cm^2, range 1.8 to 5.0). Insignificant regurgitation was commonly found by pulsed Doppler technique in patients with a St. Jude or Björk-Shiley valve in the aortic or mitral position and in patients with a Starr-Edwards or tissue valve in the aortic position. In 17 other patients with a malfunctioning prosthesis (4 St. Jude, 2 Björk-Shiley, 4 Beall, and 7 tissue valves) proved by cardiac catheterization, surgery or autopsy, Doppler echocardiography correctly identified the complication (significant regurgitant or obstruction) in all but 2 patients with a Beall valve. Thus, it appears that 1) the St. Jude valve has the most optimal hemodynamic characteristics; 2) mild MR may be detected by the Doppler echocardiographic technique in normally functioning St. Jude and Björk-Shiley valves in the aortic and mitral positions and in the Starr-Edwards and tissue valves in the aortic position; and 3) Doppler echocardiography is a useful method for the detection of prosthetic valve malfunction, especially when the St. Jude, Björk-Shiley, and tissue valves are involved.

Ryan and associates[67] from Indianapolis, Indiana, used Doppler echocardiography to evaluate 40 patients with porcine mitral valves implanted 0.5–99 months before examination. Three parameters of porcine mitral valvular flow were assessed: maximum diastolic LV inflow velocity (V_{max}), pressure half-time, and presence or absence of MR. Normally functioning porcine mitral valves (n = 29) were characterized by V_{max} ≤180 cm/s and pressure half-time ≤160 ms. Within this group, pressure half-time was not correlated significantly with the age of the patient or with prosthesis size. Doppler correctly identified all 10 patients with MR. Among these 10 patients, V_{max} was 206 ± 53 cm/s, significantly higher than the mean observed in normally functioning prostheses (136 ± 24 cm/s). In 8 patients with stenosis of the porcine mitral valve, mean pressure half-time was 220 ± 63 ms, and in 7 of 8 it was ≥180 ms. It was concluded that: 1) V_{max} ≤180 cm/s, pressure half-time ≤160 ms, and absence of systolic turbulence in the left atrium characterize normally functioning porcine mitral valves; 2) pressure half-time ≥180 ms identifies patients with stenosis of the porcine mitral valve; and 3) Doppler echocardiography can detect MR and separate MR from TR.

Sagar et al[68] in Richmond, Virginia, and Milwaukee, Wisconsin, used Doppler echocardiography to study Hancock and Björk-Shiley valve prostheses in the mitral and aortic positions in 50 patients whose valve function was considered normal and in 46 patients with suspected malfunctions of their valves who also underwent cardiac catheterization. Mean pressure gradients were estimated for both mitral (Fig. 6-14) and aortic valve (Fig. 6-15) pros-

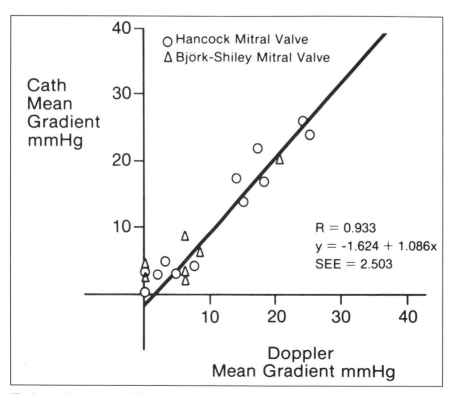

Fig. 6-14. Comparison of the mean transprosthetic mitral pressure gradient of Hancock (open circles) and Björk-Shiley (open triangles) valves in 19 patients with normal function or obstruction obtained with Doppler echocardiography and cardiac catheterization (Cath). Reproduced with permission from Sagar et al.[68]

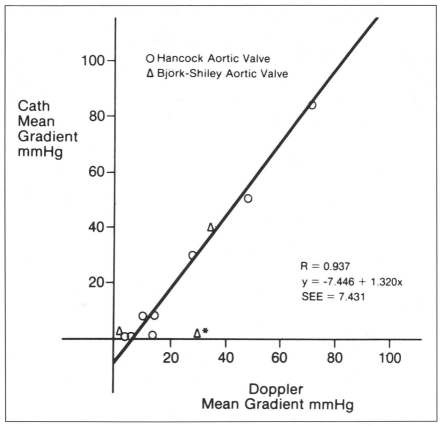

Fig. 6-15. Comparison after Doppler echocardiography and cardiac catheterization (Cath) of the mean transprosthetic aortic gradient of Hancock (open circles) and Björk-Shiley (open triangles) valves in 11 patients with normal function or obstruction. Note that Doppler echocardiography overestimated the gradients at lower levels of obstruction. See the text for details on the patient indicated by the triangle and asterisk. Reproduced with permission from Sagar et al.[68]

theses and valve areas were calculated for the mitral valve prostheses. The Doppler estimates of prosthetic valve gradient and function demonstrated good correlations with values obtained at cardiac catheterization for both types of prosthetic valves (Figs. 1 and 2). Doppler echocardiography overestimated the mean gradient at lower degrees of obstruction, but regurgitant lesions across the Hancock and Björk-Shiley prostheses in the mitral and aortic positions were correctly diagnosed. These data suggest that Doppler echocardiography is a reliable method for evaluating normal and abnormal prosthetic valve function with these specific prostheses.

Wilkins and co-workers[69] in Boston, Massachusetts, recorded simultaneous continuous-wave Doppler flow profiles and transvalvular manometric gradients in 12 catheterized patients in whom all atrial and ventricular pressures were directly measured (transseptal LA catheterization and transthoracic ventricular puncture were performed where necessary). A total of 13 prostheses were studied: 11 mitral (7 porcine, 3 Starr-Edwards, and 1 Björk-Shiley) and 2 tricuspid (1 porcine and 1 Björk-Shiley). The Doppler-determined mean gradient was calculated as the mean of the instantaneous gradients ($\Delta P = 4v^2$) at 10-ms intervals throughout diastole. The correlation of simultaneous Doppler and manometric mean gradients for the whole group demonstrated a highly significant correlation. This correlation was equally good for porcine valves alone and for mechanical valves alone. In a subset of patients without regurgitation, prosthetic valve areas were estimated by 2 Doppler methods originally described by Holen and Hatle, as well as by the invasive Gorlin method. As expected from theoretical considerations, a close correlation was not demonstrated between results of the Gorlin method and those of either Hatle's Doppler method or Holen's method. These results suggest that in patients with disk-occluder, ball-occluder, and porcine prosthetic valves, Doppler estimates of transvalvular gradients are virtually identical to those obtained invasively.

Patient-related determinants of prosthetic or bioprosthetic valve performance

Mitchell and associates[70] at Stanford, California, using a time-dependent multivariate discriminate analysis, allowed an opportunity to identify patient-related factors that portend a higher likelihood of risk for various morbid events after prosthetic valve replacement. Accordingly, a Cox model univariate and multivariate analysis was performed in a patient population with various types of prosthetic or bioprosthetic valves and the interactions among patient-related, disease-related, operation-related, time-related, and valve-related variables were interpreted in terms of long-term patient prognosis. A total of 2,871 patients survived either AVR or MVR between 1968 and 1980. AVR was performed in 1,456 patients, 439 of whom received Starr-Edwards model 1260 mechanical prostheses, and 1,017 either Hancock or Carpentier-Edwards porcine xenograft prostheses. MVR was performed in 1,315 patients, 503 of whom received either Starr-Edwards model 6120 mechanical valves and 812 tissue valves. For AVR patients, valve type was the most significant determinant for thromboembolism anticoagulant-related hemorrhage and fatal valve failure, and was the second most powerful predictor of decreased late survival. Functional class, however, was a significant determinant for 5 of 7 valve-related events, reaffirming the clear relation between a patient's degree of preoperative functional impairment and the likelihood of these complications. Functional class was the most significant determinant for late survival. In this study also, valve lesion had a marked negative influence on late survival. The lack of adverse influence of some other variables on morbid and fatal events was noted. These included prior operation, endocarditis, and AF. For patients undergoing MVR, valve type was the most significant variable, portending an increased likelihood of thromboembolism, anticoagulant-related hemorrhage, fatal valve failure, and all valve-related morbidity and mortality, and valve type was also highly significant for late survival. For MVR, younger age was the strongest determinant of reoperation. Hypertension significantly increased the risk of valve failure and reduced the probability of late survival. AF had no significant effect on any of the complications. In addition, for MVR, the preoperative presence of CHF, previous heart operation, and prior thromboembolism also independently increased the risk of thromboembolism.

Performance of patient and prosthesis

From 1975 to 1979, Bloomfield and colleagues[71] in Edinburgh, Scotland entered 540 patients undergoing valve replacement into a randomized trial and the patients received either a Björk-Shiley (273 patients) or a porcine heterograft prosthesis (initially a Hancock valve [107 patients] and later a Carpentier-Edwards prosthesis [160 patients]). Two hundred and sixty-two patients had MVR, 210 required AVR, 60 required MVR and AVR, and 8 also had tricuspid valve replacement. Analysis of 34 preoperative and operative variables showed the treatment groups to be well randomized. In-hospital mortality was not significantly different among patients receiving the 3 prostheses for AVR (8% overall) and MVR plus AVR (10% overall), but there was a higher in-hospital mortality for patients undergoing MVR with the Carpentier-Edwards prosthesis (16% compared with 9%). Actuarial survival after MVR was 57% at 7 years, that after AVR was 70% at 7 years, and that after MVR plus AVR 63% at 7 years. There was no significant difference in actuarial survival of patients receiving the 3 prostheses within the MVR, AVR, and MVR plus AVP groups, nor was there a difference when these groups were amalgamated. Thirty-seven patients required reoperation for valve failure (15 with Björk-Shiley, 12 with Hancock, and 10 with Carpentier-Edwards valves) and 11 died at reoperation (overall operative mortality 30%). Up to 7 years after surgery, there was no significant difference in the incidence of thromboembolism in patients with the different prostheses undergoing MVR or AVR. There were too few patients undergoing MVR plus AVR for meaningful comparison. There was no significant beneficial effect of anticoagulant therapy in patients undergoing MVR or AVR with procine prostheses, but patients were not randomly allocated to anticoagulant therapy. All patients with Björk-Shiley prostheses received anticoagulant therapy. Multivariate analysis of factors associated with embolism identified AF with MVR and age <65 years and a rheumatic cause of valvular disease with AVR. The risks of anticoagulation were low with an overall incidence of complications of approximately 1 per 100 years treatment. To date, no significant advantage of any of the 3 prostheses has been observed, but the investigators concluded that further follow-up is necessary because important differences may yet emerge.

The use of the St. Jude Medical (SJM) prosthesis for routine valve replacement has gained increasing support. Duncan and colleagues[71A] from Houston, Texas, report on 736 patients who had valve replacement with the SJM device. There were 478 aortic valve patients, 188 mitral valve patients, 63 double valve patients, and 7 tricuspid valve replacement only patients. Mean age at the time of operation was 47 years for patients having AVR and 49 years for those having MVR. Follow-up totaled 1,116 patient-years (range 4–82 months). Patients undergoing reoperation or having associated procedures comprised 49% of the AVR and 54% of the MVR groups. Early mortality for the entire series was 7.3%. It was lowest in the group of patients undergoing isolated MVR (2.3%) and AVR (3.7%). The number of early deaths increased in all groups when associated procedures were performed and was highest with MVR (16%) and AVR plus MVR (27%). Early mortality for patients having AVR and CABG was 10%, whereas MVR and CABG carried an operative mortality of 9%. There were 37 late deaths. All patients were advised of the need for long-term anticoagulation with warfarin. Seven patients with AVR, 1 patient with MVR, and 1 patient with double valve replacement had suspected or confirmed episodes of systemic thromboembolism, a linearized incidence of 1% per patient-year for AVR, 0.36% per patient-year for MVR, and 1% per patient-year for double valve replacement (Table 6-10) (Fig. 6-16). There were no instances of structural valve failure.

Lindblom and associates[72] from Stockholm, Sweden, reported their experience after implantation of 3,334 Björk-Shiley valves over a 15-year period. There was a 99.2% follow-up covering 17,511 patient-years (mean follow up 6.3 years). Nineteen cases of mechanical failure were documented. There were no mechanical failures among the standard Delrin valves (n = 217), the aortic standard Pyrolyte valve (n = 739), or the Monostrut valve (n = 377). One of 430 initial standard Pyrolyte valves fractured. Among the 1,461 con-

TABLE 6-10. *Linearized morbidity and mortality rates.[a,b] Reproduced with permission from Duncan et al.[71]*

VARIABLE	AVR	MVR	AVR + MVR
Mechanical failure	0.00	0.00	0.00
Systemic embolism	0.99 (7)	0.36 (1)	0.98 (1)
Infective endocarditis	1.13 (8)	0.00	0.00
Perivalvular leak	0.28 (2)	1.08 (3)	0.00
Anticoagulant-related complications	1.13 (8)	0.00	0.00
Late death	3.20 (23)	4.26 (12)	1.94 (2)

[a] Data are shown as percent per patient-years.
[b] Numbers in parentheses are numbers of patients.
AVR = aortic valve replacement; MVR = mitral valve replacement.

vexo-concave valves, 18 fractured. The actuarial incidence of mechanical failure at 5 years was 0.6% for the 60-degree convexo-concave valve and 2.8% for the 70-degree convexo-concave valve. Two groups of valves were especially affected by strut fracture. The 23-mm aortic 60-degree convexo-concave valve and the 29–31-mm mitral 70-degree convexo-concave valve. (The manufacturer has recalled all convexo-concave Björk-Shiley valves in the United States inventory). Management of patients with a suspected mechanical failure (strut fracture) to be effective should be based on clinical symptoms, a plain chest x-ray, and emergency operation. Invasive investigations have no place. Prophylactic rereplacement of patients asymptomatic with the convexo-concave Björk-Shiley device cannot generally be recommended; however, the authors suggest that with a decreasing hazard function for mechanical failure in the mitral valve or a constant, but low, hazard function for mechanical failure in the aortic valve, one should probably refrain from

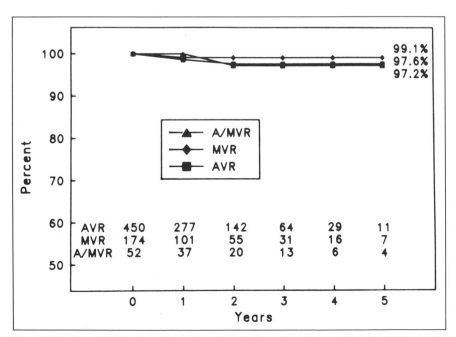

Fig. 6-16. Actuarial freedom from thromboembolism by valve position (excluding early deaths). (AVR = aortic valve replacement; MVR = mitral valve replacement.) Reproduced with permission from Duncan et al.[71]

elective rereplacement. The authors argue that there are many complications which are valve related and patient related that occur especially in the first year after valve replacement. Strut fracture is only one of them and is the only probable complication that would be averted by elective rereplacement within the first year.

Gallo and colleagues[73] from Santander, Spain, provide important information on the degeneration potential of the Hancock bioprosthesis. From June 1972 through June 1978, 547 porcine xenografts were inserted in 459 selected patients. There were 299 mitral, 239 aortic, 8 tricuspid, and 1 pulmonic valve inserted. There were 92 instances of primary tissue valve degeneration in 82 patients. Of patients who underwent surgery 10 years ago, 28% of valves implanted in the mitral position and 33% in the aortic position failed. None of the tricuspid or pulmonary valves has failed. The rate of valve survival without primary degeneration was $70 \pm 6\%$ for the mitral and $69 \pm 7\%$ for the aortic prosthesis at 10 years of follow-up. The authors believe that these data allow comparison of different types of bioprostheses, but especially they provide information suggesting that, at 10 years, an individual patient has a 30% chance of tissue valve explantation for degeneration. Additional information from this study suggests that there is a breakpoint in the degeneration curve at about age 40 years (Fig. 6-17). Thus, degeneration was significantly higher in the subdivision of the population age <40 years compared with those aged >40 years. In this study, the porcine bioprosthesis in the mitral position did not fail more frequently than did those in the aortic position, compared with failure modes reported in other studies.

Ferrazzi and colleagues[74] from Birmingham, Alabama, analyzed patients undergoing isolated or combined mitral valve replacement, 1975 to 1979 (n = 478), and compared those results with a later era, July 1979 to July 1983 (n = 341). Patients in the later era were older, had a higher LV end-diastolic pressure, a higher prevalence of ischemic mitral disease, and a lower prevalence of rheumatic disease. Patients who underwent surgery in the later era had, on the average, longer and more extensive operations. Patients in the later era had a slightly, but inconclusively, lower 2-week and 4.5 year survival than those in the earlier era. The hazard functions for survival were similar in each era. A higher proportion of the deaths in the later era was due to chronic CHF. Neither the era nor the specific year in which a patient underwent operation was a risk factor for death in a multivariate analysis. By contrast to this study, in many subsets of patients with congenital heart disease and CAD, the risks have been shown to be lower in the current era. Contemporary risk for isolated MVR is 2%. Contemporary risk for MVR in ischemic MR with CABG is 14%. These results are not significantly different from the risk in an earlier era, 2.6% and 18%. The authors suggest that if there is to be improvement in the results of MVR, delay in advising mitral valve operation must be reversed and imperfections in the methods of myocardial protection must be improved.

Christakis and colleagues[75] from Toronto, Canada, assessed results of AVR over the past 15 years. Operative mortality was 10 to 33% between 1969 and 1975. The mortality is <5% at present. This study addresses the factors that predict postoperative morbidity and mortality contemporaneously, with the attempt to develop alternative strategies for high-risk patients to decrease the present 5% figure. A total of 277 consecutive patients undergoing isolated AVR between 1982 and 1984 were evaluated; 37 clinical and 13 preoperative hemodynamic variables were analyzed by univariate and multivariate statistics to determine the risk factors for postoperative morbidity and mortality. The operative mortality during this period was 3%, the incidence of postoperative low cardiac output was 12%, and the incidence of perioperative AMI, 5%. A multivariate, logistic regression analysis found that age was the only

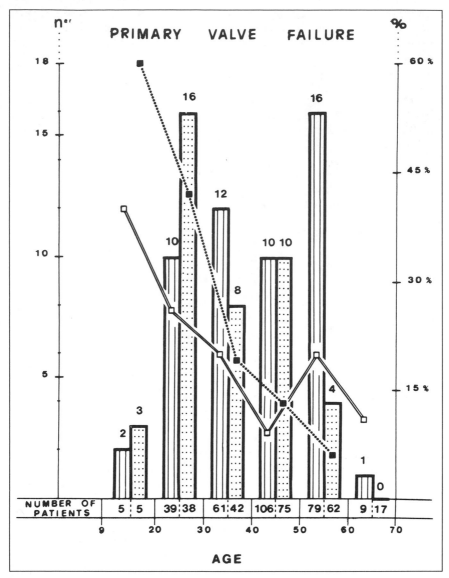

Fig. 6-17. Percentage of valve failures related to patient's age at time of implantation. Reproduced with permission from Gallo et al.[73]

independent predictor of mortality. Three factors independently predicted postoperative low cardiac output: age, CAD, and the peak systolic gradient in patients with AS. AS was accompanied by a higher incidence of postoperative ventricular dysfunction than mixed valvular disease or AR. The incidence of perioperative AMI was higher in patients with 3-vessel CAD and those with LM stenosis than in patients with 1- or 2-vessel CAD. Because of the higher risk of AVR in older patients, the risk/benefit ratio of operation must be carefully assessed in the elderly. Improved methods of myocardial protection may reduce the risks for patients with AS and symptomatic 3-vessel CAD. Although age cannot be considered a contraindication to AVR, the estimated life expectancy, the quality of life, and the natural history of the disease must be balanced against the immediate and late postoperative risks of AVR in the elderly. Further improvement may be possible through modification of patient referral patterns, improvements in myocardial protection, and more critical assessment of the timing and indication for operation.

Intraaortic balloon pump counterpulsation during weaning from cardiopulmonary bypass or for circulatory support in the immediate postoperative period was analyzed in 2,498 patients undergoing AVR by Downing and associates[76] in Stanford, California. A total of 146 successful balloon insertions was performed in 155 attempts. Univariate analysis of individual factors delineated preoperative characteristics in patients having MVR and intraoperative factors in all patients that correlated with the use of the balloon pump. Multivariate analysis revealed a subset of male patients with mitral valve and CAD most likely to require counterpulsation. Overall survival rate was markedly reduced at 30 days (50 ± 5%) -vs- valve replacement only (96 ± 5%) and at 1 year, balloon 38%, valve replacement 89%. Patients requiring balloon pumping who had a preoperative diagnosis of AR had a lower 1-year survival than the total subgroup undergoing balloon counterpulsation. Similarly, patients treated by balloon counterpulsation who had postoperative renal failure had a significantly lower 1-year survival rate, 17% ± 5%, than those without renal failure, 66% ± 6%.

Anticoagulation in pregnancy

Lee et al[77] in Hong Kong used adjusted subcutaneous heparin and oral warfarin during 18 pregnancies in 16 women with artificial heart valves. Among these patients, oral warfarin was replaced by subcutaneous heparin as soon as pregnancy was confirmed. The heparin dosage was adjusted to maintain a partial thromboplastin time at 1.5 times the control values and treatment was administered during the first trimester and the last 3 weeks of gestation. Warfarin was used between the 13th and 37th weeks of pregnancy. In these patients, there were no maternal thromboembolic complications and none of the live-born babies demonstrated congenital malformations. Nevertheless, there were 9 spontaneous abortions, including 5 occurring in the first 12 weeks. The authors postulated that the early abortions may have been related to warfarin exposure at the beginning of pregnancy and recommend the preconception replacement of warfarin by heparin in patients with prosthetic heart valves requiring anticoagulation.

In an attempt to identify the best treatment for pregnant women with cardiac valve prostheses who are receiving oral anticoagulant therapy, Iturbe-Alessio and associates[78] from Mexico City, Mexico, studied 72 pregnancies prospectively. In 23 pregnancies (group I), the coumarin derivative acenocoumarol was discontinued and the patients received 5,000 U of subcutaneous heparin every 12 hours from the 6th to the 12th week of gestation. In 12 pregnancies (group II), heparin was not substituted for the coumarin derivative until after the 7th week, and in 37 pregnancies, detected after the first trimester (group III), the coumarin derivative was given throughout gestation. In most patients heparin was again substituted for the oral anticoagulant after the 38th week. Three mothers had thrombosis of a tilting-disk mitral prosthesis (2 cases were fatal) during heparin treatment. No differences were found in the rates of spontaneous abortion in the 3 groups. Coumarin embryopathy occurred in 25 and 29.6% of the pregnancies in groups II and III, respectively. The authors concluded that in the second and third trimesters of pregnancy, coumarin derivatives provide effective protection against thromboembolism while causing few fetopathic effects, but that these agents are contraindicated from the 6th to the 12th weeks of gestation.

Low-dose heparin does not protect against prosthetic-valve thrombosis, and the possibility that a larger dose might be more effective requires further exploration.

Prosthetic thrombosis

The main complication after implantation of a Björk-Shiley valve in the *tricuspid position* is late thrombotic obstruction. Boskovic and colleagues[79] studied 28 patients with tricuspid valve replacement at a mean follow-up of 5.2 years, 7 (25%) had thrombosis of the tricuspid prosthesis. There were 3 additional patients with a recurrent thrombotic malfunction for a total of 10 thromboses in 146 patient-years, yielding a rate of 6.8 per 100 patient-years. In all patients, the click of the prosthesis became inaudible and new diastolic or systolic murmurs occurred. Thrombolytic treatment with streptokinase was used. Two patients required 12 hours of therapy and 5 patients 24 hours of therapy. Thrombolysis was monitored by the thrombin time. Complete regression of thrombosis was seen in all 7 patients during the first 24 hours of therapy. There were no bleeding complications. One patient had signs of mild pulmonary emboli. Follow-up after successful treatment extended from 4–30 months (mean 16.5 months). Four patients had excellent long-term results. Three patients had rethrombosis at 4, 7, and 14 months. In each, repeat thrombolytic treatment was successful. This study and several others point out the usefulness of streptokinase for thrombosis of various disc and leaflet valves in all valve positions.

Ledain et al[80] in Pessac, France, evaluated 26 patients presenting with 28 instances of acute thrombotic occlusion of a prosthetic valve, including 16 mitral and 12 aortic valves. Patients were treated with fibrinolytic agents. In 15 cases, the patient presented with acute pulmonary edema and a low cardiac output, in 10 with CHF and embolism, and in 3 with peripheral embolism only. The diagnosis of thrombotic obstruction was made by echocardiography or cineradiography in patients in whom the disc of the prosthetic valve was immobile or barely moving. These patients were treated with fibrinolytic agents, including streptokinase (2,000,000 U for 10 hours, 14 cases), urokinase (4,500 U/kg/hour for 12 hours, 7 cases), or the 2 agents successively (7 cases). Fibrinolytic therapy was successful in 19 patients and 18 were alive and well without surgical intervention after a follow-up of 6–64 months. One patient had surgical revision after thrombolytic therapy. Fibrinolytic therapy was apparently successful in 2 patients, but recurrent obstruction developed at 4 and 19 months later, respectively, and the patients were again treated by fibrinolytic therapy. Fibrinolytic therapy failed in 2 patients leading to emergency surgery, and in 3 patients improvement was incomplete and death occurred shortly after treatment. There were 5 cases of systemic arterial embolism during the fibrinolytic therapy. No hemorrhagic complications occurred. Thus, fibrinolytic therapy is an alternative to surgical therapy in patients with thrombosed prosthetic valves, especially in patients who are critically ill and perhaps too unstable to undergo immediate surgery.

Morphologic studies

Sullivan and Roberts[81] from Bethesda, Maryland, described clinical and morphologic observations in 30 patients who underwent replacement *MVR for MS and either simultaneous replacement* (13 patients, group I) *or anuloplasty* (17 patients, group II) *of the tricuspid valve for pure TR.* Comparison of the 13 patients in group I with the 17 patients in group II disclosed similar mean ages (55 -vs- 58 years), similar average preoperative RV systolic pressures (64 -vs- 61 mmHg), similar average RA mean pressures (10 -vs- 9 mmHg), similar average LV systolic pressures (126 -vs- 120 mmHg), similar average PA wedge–LV mean diastolic pressures (16 -vs- 18 mmHg), similar mean heart weights (507 -vs- 535 g), and similar percents with grossly visible foci of LV necrosis (15 -vs- 12%) and fibrosis (23 -vs- 12%). Of the 13 patients in group I, 10 (77%) died early (≤60 days of tricuspid valve replacement) and 3 (23%) died late (29, 37, and 120 months); of the 17 patients in group II, 14 (82%) died early and 3 (18%) died late (4, 9, and 98 months). The causes of early death in the 2 groups were different: of the 10 patients in group I who died early, the cause was excessive bleeding in 5, low cardiac output of undetermined etiology in 3, dysfunction of both prostheses in 1, and cerebral insult in 1; of the 14 patients in group II who died early, none died from excessive bleeding, 4 from decreased cardiac output of uncertain cause, 5 from LV inflow obstruction (produced by a Starr-Edwards ball-valve prosthesis in 4 and from a Starr-Edwards disc prosthesis in 1), 1 from LV outflow obstruction (by a porcine bioprosthesis), 2 from technical mishaps (incision into LV free wall with rupture in 1 and litigation of the left circumflex coronary artery with resulting AMI in 1), and 2 died suddenly for reasons not determined. Of the 6 patients dying >60 days after operation, 4 died from CHF, 1 from a cerebral embolus, and 1 from prosthetic valve endocarditis.

Sullivan and Roberts[82] from Bethesda, Maryland, described clinical and morphologic observations in 12 patients who underwent *simultaneous replacement of the tricuspid, mitral, and aortic valves*. All 12 patients had MS, 10 AS, and 2 pure AR; 5 had tricuspid valve stenosis and 7 had pure TR. Of the 10 patients who died within 60 days of triple valve replacement, 7 had the low cardiac output syndrome, which in 4, and possibly 5, of the 7 was attributed to prosthetic aortic valve stenosis. In none of the 12 patients was the ascending aorta dilated, and in the 4 (possibly 5) patients with low cardiac output, the space between the surface of the caged poppet (4 patients) or margins of the tilting disc (1 patient) in the aortic valve position and the aortic endothelium appeared inadequate to allow unobstructed flow despite small-sized prostheses in all but 1 patient. Thus, aortic valve replacement in the setting of triple valve dysfunction is hazardous or potentially so. The relative small sizes of the hearts in these patients also make valve replacement more difficult (and hazardous) compared to hearts with larger ventricles and aortas.

Roberts and Sullivan[83] described necropsy findings in 6 patients who had MVR for MS combined with tricuspid valve replacement or commissurotomy for tricuspid valve stenosis.

Roberts and Sullivan[84] from Bethesda, Maryland, described clinical and necropsy findings in 54 patients, aged 25–83 years (mean 53), who died within 60 days of simultaneous replacements of both mitral and aortic valves (Table 6-11). The patients were separated into 4 groups on the basis of the presence of stenosis (with or without associated regurgitation) or pure regurgitation of each valve: 30 patients (56%) had combined MS and AS; 12 patients (22%) had MS and pure AR; 8 patients (15%) had pure regurgitation of both valves; and 4 patients (7%) had pure AR and MS. Necropsy examination in the 54 patients disclosed a high frequency (48%) of anatomic evidence of interference to poppet or disc movement in either the mitral or aortic valve position or both. Anatomic evidence of interference to movement of a poppet or disc in the aortic valve position was twice as common as anatomic evidence of interference to poppet or disc movement in the mitral position. Interference to poppet movement is attributable to the prosthesis's being too large for the ascending aorta or LV cavity in which it resided. The ascending

TABLE 6-11. *Pooled data in the 54 patients dying within 60 days after simultaneous replacement of both mitral and aortic valves*

		MS–AS	MS–AR	MR–AR	MR–AS	TOTAL
1	No. of patients	30 (56%)	12 (22%)	8 (15%)	4 (7%)	54
2	Age range (yr) (mean)	37–83 (57)	36–65 (50)	25–56 (43)	25–76 (56)	25–83 (53)
3	Men:women	14:16	3:9	6:2	4:0	27:27
4	Chronic atrial fibrillation	22/27 (81%)	12/12	3/8	2/3	39/50 (78%)
5	NYHA functional class					
	II:III:IV	2:19:9	0:9:3	0:7:1	0:4:0	2:39:13
6	Previous mitral					
	commissurotomy	7	3	0	0	10 (19%)
7	TR preoperatively	6	2	1	1	10 (19%)
8	TV anuloplasty	4	2	0	1	7
9	RV SP >30 mmHg (avg)	24/26 (92%) (57)	12/12 (66)	6/6 (46)	3/3 (102)	45/47 (96%) (60)
10	PA SP >30 mmHg (avg)	25/26 (96%) (55)	11/11 (65)	7/7 (53)	3/3 (102)	46/47 (98%) (60)
11	LV SP >140 mmHg (avg)	21/30 (71%) (169)	4/12 (136)	3/7 (141)	3/3 (154)	31/52 (60%) (157)
12	SA SP >140 mmHg (avg)	6/30 (20%) (125)	4/12 (138)	3/7 (149)	0/3 (123)	13/52 (25%) (131)
13	PAW-LV mdg (mmHg)	5–21 (13)	6–22 (12)	0	0	5–22 (13)
14	LV-SA psg (mmHg)	7–210 (43)	0	0	18–62 (32)	
15	CI <2.5 liters/min/m² (avg)	16/20 (80%) (2.2)	9/11 (2.0)	3/4 (2.1)	3/3 (1.9)	31/38 (82%) (2.1)
16	MR by LV cineangiogram	23/25 (92%)	10/12	7/7	4/4	44/48 (92%)
17	AR by AA cineangiogram	24/25 (96%)	12/12	7/7	3/3	46/47 (98%)
18	CA cineangiogram					
	(CA↓ >50% diameter)	14 (3)	2 (0)	1 (0)	3 (1)	20 (4) (20%)
19	Coronary bypass grafting	2	1	0	1	4 (7%)
20	Left Atrial thrombi-A only:					
	A + B	1:3	0:4	0:0	0:0	1:7
21	LA endocardial calcium	4	1	0	0	5
22	Death in operating room	7	5	1	2	15 (28%)
23	Excessive PO bleeding					
	without rupture	6	1	3	1	11 (20%)
24	Heart weight (g). range					
	(mean)					
	Men	450–900 (688)	575–710 (662)	570–1040 (815)	740–780 (763)	450–1040 (726)
	Women	370–740 (545)	310–620 (444)	515–530 (523)	—	310–740 (515)
25	Prosthetic dysfunction					
	(patients)	15	6	4	1	26 (48%)
	Mitral valve	4	3	1	1	9 (17%)
	Aortic valve	11	4	4	1	20 (37%)
26	Left-sided cardiac rupture	2	3	1	2	8 (15%)
	At PM stump	1	0	0	0	1
	Midway between PM &					
	anulus	0	2	1	1	4
	At mitral anulus	1	1	0	1	3
27	No. patients ≥1 CA					
	>75% ↓CSA	7	4	1	1	13 (24%)
28	No. LV fibrosis:necrosis					
	(hemorrhagic)	3:6 (4)	3:3 (3)	0:3 (0)	0:0 (0)	6 (11%):12 (22%) (7)
29	Dilated LV cavity @					
	necropsy	15	5	8	2	30 (56%)
30	Dilated LV cavity @					
	preoperative cine	5/25	3/12	7/7	2/4	17/48 (35%)
31	Prosthetic valve endocarditis	1	0	1	0	2 (4%)
32	Diffuse fibrosis, TV leaflets	5	5	0	0	10 (19%)

A = atrial appendage; AA = ascending aorta; AR = aortic regurgitation; B = body of left atrium; CA = coronary artery; CI = cardiac index; CSA = cross-sectional area; LA = left atrial; LV = left ventricular; mdg = mean diastolic gradient; MR = mitral regurgitation; NYHA = New York Heart Association; PA = pulmonary artery; PAW = pulmonary arterial wedge, PM = papillary muscle; PO = postoperative; psg = peak systolic gradient; RV = right ventricular; SA = systemic artery; SP = systolic pressure; TR = tricuspid regurgitation; TV = tricuspid valve.

aorta is infrequently enlarged in patients with combined mitral and aortic valve dysfunction irrespective of whether the aortic valve is stenotic or purely regurgitant. Likewise, the LV cavity is usually not dilated in patients with combined MS and AS, the most common indication for replacement of both left-sided cardiac valves. Of the 54 patients, 12 (22%) had 1 mechanical and 1 bioprosthesis inserted. It is recommended that both substitute valves should be mechanical prostheses or both should be bioprostheses.

References

1. HUTCHINS GM, MOORE GW, SKOOG DK: The association of floppy mitral valve with disjunction of the mitral anulus fibrosus. N Engl J Med 1986 (Feb 27); 314:535–40.
2. DEVEREUX RB, KRAMER-FOX R, BROWN WT, SHEAR K, HARTMAN N, KLIGFIELD P, LUTAS EM, SPITZER MC, LITWIN SD: Relation between clinical features of the mitral prolapse syndrome and echocardiographically documented mitral valve prolapse. J Am Coll Cardiol 1986 (Oct); 8:763–772.
3. RETCHIN SM, FLETCER RH, EARP J, LAMSON N, WAUGH RA: Mitral valve prolapse: disease or illness. Arch Intern Med 1986 (June); 146:1081–1084.
4. KOLIBASH AJ, KILMAN JW, BUSH CA, RYAN JM, FONTANA ME, WOOLEY CF: Evidence for progression from mild to severe mitral regurgitation in mitral valve prolapse. AM J Cardiol 1986 (Oct 1); 58:762–767.
5. PANIDIS IP, McALLISTER M, ROSS J, MINTZ GS: Prevalence and severity of mitral regurgitation in the mitral valve prolapse syndrome: a Doppler echocardiographic study of 80 patients. J Am Coll Cardiol 1986 (May); 7:975–981.
6. DEVEREUX RB, HAWKINS I, KRAMER-FOX R, LUTAS EM, HAMMOND IW, SPITZER MC, HOCHRETER C, ROBERTS RB, BELKIN RN, KLIGFIELD P, BROWN WT, NILES N, ALDERMAN MH, BORER JS, LARAGH JH: Complications of mitral valve prolapse: disproportionate occurrence in men and older patients. Am J Med 1986 (Nov); 81: 751–758.
7. NAGGAR CZ, PEARSON WN, SELJAN MP, MADDOCK LK, MASROF S, ELWOOD DJ: Frequency of complications of mitral valve prolapse in subjects aged 60 years and older. Am J Cardiol 1986 (Dec 1); 58:1209–1212.
8. MEYERS DG, STARKE H, PEARSON PH, WILKEN MK: Mitral valve prolapse in anorexia nervosa. Ann Intern Med 1986 (Sept); 105:382–383.
9. JOHNSON GL, HUMPHRIES LL, SHIRLEY PB, MAZZOLENI A, NOONAN JA: Mitral valve prolapse in patients with anorexia nervosa and bulimia. Arch Intern Med 1986 (Aug); 146:1525–1529.
10. PINES A, EHRENFELD M, FISMAN EZ, KAPLINSKY N, SAMRA Y, RONNEN M, KELLERMANN JJ: Mitral valve prolapse in psoriatic arthritis. Arch Intern Med 1986 (July); 146:1371–1373.
11. KREINDEL MS, SCHIAVONE WA, LEVER HM, COSGROVE D: Systolic anterior motion of the mitral valve after Carpentier ring valvuloplasty for mitral valve prolapse. Am J Cardiol 1986 (Feb 15); 57:408–412.
12. MIYATAKE K, IZUMI S, OKAMOTO M, KINOSHITA N, ASONUMA H, NAKAGAWA H, YAMAMOTO K, TAKAMIYA M, SAKAKIBARA H, NIMURA Y: Semiquantitative grading of severity of mitral regurgitation by real-time two-dimensional Doppler flow imaging technique. J Am Coll Cardiol 1986 (Jan); 7:82–88.
13. BLUMLEIN S, BOUCHARD A, SCHILLER NB, DAE M, BYRD BF, PORTS T, BOTVINICK EH: Quantitation of mitral regurgitation by Doppler echocardiogram. Circulation 1986 (Feb); 74:306–314.
14. HOCKREITER C, NILES N, DEVEREUX RB, KLIGFIELD P, BORER JS: Mitral regurgitation: relationship of noninvasive descriptors of right and left ventricular performance to clinical and hemodynamic findings and to prognosis in medically and surgically treated patients. Circulation 1986 (May); 73(5):900–912.
15. RAHKO PS, SALERNI R, REDDY PS, LEON DF: Extent of mitral calcific deposits determined by cineangiography in mitral stenosis and their effect on valve motion, hemodynamics and clinical signs. Am J Cardiol 1986 (July 1); 58:121–128.
16. NICOD P, HILLIS LD, WINIFORD MD, FIRTH BG: Importance of the "atrial kick" in determining the effective mitral valve orifice area in mitral stenosis. Am J Cardiol 1986 (Feb 15); 57:403–407.
17. BRYG RJ, WILLIAMS GA, LABOVITZ AJ, AKER U, KENNEDY HL: Effect of atrial fibrillation and mitral regurgitation on calculated mitral valve area in mitral stenosis. Am J Cardiol 1986 (Mar 1); 57:634–638.
18. SMITH M, HANDSHOE R, HANDSHOE S, KWAN OL, DeMARIA AN: Comparative accuracy of two-dimensional echocardiography and Doppler pressure half-time methods in assessing severity of mitral stenosis in patients with and without prior commissurotomy. Circulation 1986 (Jan); 73(1): 100–107.
19. KHANDHERIA BK, TAJIK AJ, REEDER GS, CALLAHAN MJ, NISHIMURA RA, MILLER FA, SEWARD JB: Doppler color flow imaging: a new technique for visualization and characterization of the blood flow jet in mitral stenosis. Mayo Clin Proc 1986 (Aug); 61:623–630.

20. BUTLER PM, LEGGETT SI, HOWE CM, FREYE CJ, HINDMAN NB, WAGNER GS: Identification of electrocardiographic criteria for diagnosis of right ventricular hypertrophy due to mitral stenosis. Am J cardiol 1986 (Mar 1); 57:639–643.

21. MATTINA CJ, GREEN SJ, TORTOLANI AJ, PADMANABHAN VT, ONG LY, HALL MH, PIZZARELLO RA: Frequency of angiographically significant coronary arterial narrowing in mitral stenosis. Am J Cardiol 1986 (Apr 1); 57:802–805.

22. REIS RN, ROBERTS WC: Amounts of coronary arterial narrowing by atherosclerotic plaques in clinically isolated mitral valve stenosis: analysis of 76 necropsy patients older than 30 years. Am J Cardiol 1986 (May 1); 57:1117–1123.

23. SATO S, KAWASHIMA Y, HIROSE H, NAKANO S, MATSUDA H, SHIRAKURA R: Long-term results of direct-current cardioversion after open commissurotomy for mitral stenosis. Am J Cardiol 1986 (Mar 1); 57:629–633.

24. ZAIBAG MA, KASAB SA, RIBEIRO PA, FAGTH MR: Percutaneous double-balloon mitral valvotomy for rheumatic mitral-valve stenosis. Lancet 1986 (Apr 5); 757–761.

25. BABIC UU, PEJCIC P, DJURISIC Z, VUCINIC M, GRUJICIC SM: Percutaneous transarterial balloon valvuloplasty for mitral valve stenosis. Am J Cardiol 1986 (May 1); 57:1101–1104.

26. HOAGLAND PM, COOK EF, WYNNE J, GOLDMAN L: Value of noninvasive testing in adults with suspected aortic stenosis. Am J Med 1986 (June); 80:1041–1050.

27. SMITH MD, DAWSON PL, ELION JL, WISENBAUGH T, KWAN OL, HANDSHOE S, DeMARIA AN: Systematic correlation of continuous-wave Doppler and hemodynamic measurements in patients with aortic stenosis. Am Heart J 1986 (Feb); 111:245–251.

28. ZOHGBI WA, FARMER KL, SOTO JG, NELSON JG, QUINONES MA: Accurate noninvasive quantification of stenotic aortic valve area by Doppler echocardiography. Circulation 1986; (Mar) 73(3):452–459.

29. OTTO CM, PEARLMAN AS, COMESS KA, REAMER RP, JANKO CL, HUNTSMAN LL: Determination of the stenotic aortic valve area in adults using Doppler echocardiography. J Am Coll Cardiol 1986 (Mar); 7:509–517.

30. OHLSSON J, WRANE B: Noninvasive assessment of valve area in patients with aortic stenosis. J Am Coll Cardiol 1986 (Mar); 7:501–508.

31. YEAGER M, YOCK PG, POPP RL: Comparison of Doppler-derived pressure gradient to that determined at cardiac catheterization in adults with aortic valve stenosis: implications from management. Am J Cardiol 1986 (Mar 1); 57:644–648.

32. PANIDIS IP, MINTZ GS, ROSS J: Value and limitations of Doppler ultrasound in the evaluation of aortic stenosis: a statistical analysis of 70 consecutive patients. Am Heart J 1986 (July); 112:150–158.

33. TEIRSTEIN P, YEAGER M, YOCK PG, POPP RL: Doppler echocardiographic measurement of aortic valve area in aortic stenosis: a noninvasive application of the Gorlin formula. J Am Coll Cardiol 1986 (Nov); 8:1059–1065.

34. MURAKAMI T, HESS OM, GAGE JE, GRIMM J, KRAYENBUEHL HP: Diastolic filling dynamics in patients with aortic stenosis. Circulation 1986 (June); 73(6):1162–1174.

35. FIFER MA, BOURDILLON PD, LORELL BH: Altered left ventricular diastolic properties during pacing-induced angina in patients with aortic stenosis. Circulation 1986 (Oct); 74:675–683.

36. McKAY RG, SAFIAN RD, LOCK JE, MANDELL VS, THURER RL, SCHNITT ST, GROSSMAN W: Balloon dilatation of calcific aortic stenosis in elderly patients: postmortem, intraoperative, and percutaneous valvuloplasty studies. Circulation 1986 (Jan); 74:119–125.

37. CRIBIER A, SAOUDI N, BERLAND J, SAVIN T, ROCHA P, LETAC B: Percutaneous transluminal valvuloplasty of acquired aortic stenosis in elderly patients: an alternative to valve replacement? Lancet 1986 (Jan 11) 63–67.

38. KING RM, GIULIANI ER, PIEHLER JM: Mechanical decalcification of the aortic valve. Ann Thorac Surg 1986 (Sept); 42:269–272.

39. GRAYBURN PA, SMITH MD, HANDSHOE R, FRIEDMAN BJ, DeMARIA AN: Detection of aortic insufficiency by standard echocardiography, pulsed Doppler echocardiograph, and auscultation: a comparison of accuracies. Ann Intern Med 1986 (May) 104:599–605.

40. PARAMESWARAN R, KOTLER MN, PARRY W, GOLDMAN AP: Echocardiographic analysis of left ventricular filling in isolated pure chronic aortic regurgitation. Am J Cardiol 1986 (Oct 1); 58:790–794.

41. TEAGUE SM, HEINSIMER JA, ANDERSON JL, SUBLETT K, OLSON EG, VOYLES WF, THADANI U: Quantification of aortic regurgitation utilizing continuous wave Doppler ultrasound. J Am Coll Cardiol 1986 (Sept); 8:592–599.

42. LABOVITZ AJ, FERRARA RP, KERN MJ, BRYG RJ, MROSEK DG, WILLIAMS GA: Quantitative evaluation

of aortic insufficiency by continuous wave Doppler echocardiography. J Am Coll Cardiol 1986 (Dec); 8:1341–1347.

43. KAWANISHI DT, MCKAY CR, CHANDRARATNA AN, NANNA M, REID CL, ELKAYAM U, SIEGEL M, RAHIM-TOOLA SH: Cardiovascular response to dynamic exercise in patients with chronic symptomatic mild-to-moderate and severe aortic regurgitation. Circulation 1986 (Jan); 73(2):62–72.

44. SHEN WF, FLETCHER PJ, ROUBIN GS, HARRIS PJ, KELLY DT: Relation between left ventricular functional reserve during exercise and resting systolic loading conditions in chronic aortic regurgitation. Am J Cardiol 1986 (Oct 1); 58:757–761.

45. HART G: Syphilis tests in diagnostic and therapeutic decision making. Ann Intern Med 1986 (Mar); 104:368–376.

46. THOMSEN NH, HORSLEV-PETERSEN K, BEYER JM: Ambulatory 24-hour continuous electrocardiographic monitoring in 54 patients with ankylosing spondylities. Eur Heart J 1986 (Mar); 7:240–246.

47. PATHAK R, PADMANABHAN VT, TORTOLANI AJ, ONG LY, HALL MH, PIZZARELLO RA: Angina pectoris and coronary artery disease in isolated, severe aortic regurgitation. Am J Cardiol 1986 (Mar 1); 57:649–651.

48. KLEAVELAND JP, REICHEK N, MCCARTHY DM, CHANDLER T, PRIEST C, MUHAMMED A, MAKLER PT, HIRSHFELD J: Effects of six-month afterload reduction therapy with hydralazine in chronic aortic regurgitation. Am J Cardiol 1986 (May 1); 57:1109–1116.

49. HOSHINO PK, GAASCH WH: When to intervene in chronic aortic regurgitation. Arch Intern Med 1986 (Feb); 146:349–352.

50. GOTT VL, PYERITZ RE, MAGOVERN GJ, CAMERON DE, MCKUSICK VA: Surgical treatment of aneurysms of the ascending aorta in the Marfan syndrome: results of composite-graft repair in 50 patients. N Engl J Med 1986 (Apr 24); 314:1070–1074.

51. KAYE D: Prophylaxis for infective endocarditis. Ann Intern Med 1986 (Mar); 104:419–423.

52. ROBBINS JM, FRATER RWM, SOEIRO R, FRISHMAN WH, STROM JA: Influence of vegetation size on clinical outcome of right-sided infective endocarditis. Am J Med 1986 (Feb); 80:165–171.

53. BUDA AJ, ZOTZ RJ, LEMIRE MS, BACH DS: Prognostic significance of vegetations detected by two-dimensional echocardiography in infective endocarditis. Am Heart J 1986 (Dec); 112:1291–1296.

54. DINUBILE MJ, CALDERWOOD SB, STEINHAUS DM, KARCHMER AW: Cardiac conduction abnormalities complicating native valve active infective endocarditis. Am J Cardiol 1986 (Dec 1); 58:1213–1217.

55. DOUGLAS A, MOORE-GILLON J, EYKYN S: Fever during treatment of infective endocarditis. Lancet (June 14); 1341, 1343.

56. SARELI P, KLEIN HO, SCHAMROTH CL, GOLDMAN AP, ANTUNES MJ, POCOCK WA, BARLOW JB: Contribution of echocardiography and immediate surgery to the management of severe aortic regurgitation from active infective endocarditis. Am J Cardiol 1986 (Feb 15); 57:413–418.

57. STERN HJ, SISTO DA, STROM JA, SOEIRO R, JONES SR, FRATER RWM: Immediate tricuspid valve replacement for endocarditis. Indications and results. J Thorac Cardiovasc Surg 1986 (Feb); 91:163–167.

58. CALDERWOOD SB, SWINSKI LA, KARCHMER AW, WATERNAUX CM, BUCKLEY MJ: Prosthetic valve endocarditis: an analysis of factors affecting outcome of therapy. J Thorac Cardiovasc Surg 1986 (Oct); 92:776–783.

59. KOSTUCKI W, VANDENBOSSCHE JL, FRIART A, ENGLERT M: Pulsed Doppler regurgitant flow patterns of normal valves. Am J Cardiol 1986 (Aug 1); 58:309–313.

60. SCHWARTZ ML, GOLDBERG SJ, WILSON N, ALLEN HD, MARX GR: Relation of Still's Murmur, small aortic diameter and high aortic velocity. Am J Cardiol 1986 (June); 57:1344–1348.

61. SUZUKI Y, KAMBARA H, KADOTA K, TAMAKI S, YAMAZATO A, NOHARA R, OSAKADA G, KAWAI C, KUBO S, KARAGUCHI T: Detection and evaluation of tricuspid regurgitation using a real-time, two-dimensional, color-coded, Doppler flow imaging system: comparison with contrast two-dimensional echocardiography and right ventriculography. Am J Cardiol 1986 (Apr 1); 57:811–815.

62. LEMBO NJ, DELL'ITALIA LJ, CRAWFORD MH, O'ROURKE RA: Diagnosis of left-sided regurgitant murmurs by transient arterial occlusion: a new maneuver using blood pressure cuffs. Ann Intern Med 1986 (Sept); 105:368–370.

63. HORTOP J, TSIPOURAS P, HANLEY J, MARON B, SHAPIRO JR: Cardiovascular involvement in osteogenesis imperfecta. Circulation 1986 (Jan); 73:54–61.

64. APONOW WS, SCHWARTZ KS, KOENIGSBERG M: Correlation of aortic cuspal and aortic root disease with aortic systolic ejection murmurs and with mitral anular calcium in persons older

than 62 years in a long-term health care facility. Am J Cardiol 1986 (Sept 15); 58:651–652.

65. RASHTIAN MY, STEVENSON DM, ALLEN DT, YOGANATHAN AP, HARRISON EC, EDMISTON WA, FAUGHAN P, RAHTMTOOLA SH: Flow characteristics of four commonly used mechanical heart valves. Am J Cardiol 1986 (Oct 1); 58:743–752.

66. PANIDIS IP, ROSS J, MINTZ GS: Normal and abnormal prosthetic valve function as assessed by Doppler echocardiography. J Am Coll Cardiol 1986 (Aug); 8:317–326.

67. RYAN T, ARMSTRONG WF, DILLON JC, FEIGENBAUM H: Doppler echocardiographic evaluation of patients with porcine mitral valves. Am Heart J 1986 (Feb); 111:237–244.

68. SAGAR K, WANN S, PAULSEN WHJ, ROMHILT DW: Doppler echocardiographic evaluation of Hancock and Björk-Shiley prosthetic valves. J Am Coll Cardiol 1986 (March); 7:681–687.

69. WILKINS GT, GILLAM LD, KRITZER GL, LEVINE RA, PALACIOS IF, WEYMAN AE: Validation of continuous-wave Doppler echocardiographic measurements of mitral and tricuspid prosthetic valve gradients: a simultaneous Doppler-catheter study. Circulation 1986 (Oct); 74:786–795.

70. MITCHELL RS, MILLER DC, STINSON EB, OYER PE, JAMIESON SW, BALDWIN JC, SHUMWAY NE: Significant patient-related determinants of prosthetic valve performance. J Thorac Cardiovasc Surg 1986 (June); 91:807–817.

71. BLOOMFIELD P, KITCHIN AH, WHEATLEY DJ, WALBAUM PR, LUTZ W, MILLER HC: A prospective evaluation of the Björk-Shiley, Hancock, and Carpentier-Edwards heart valve prostheses. Circulation 1986 (June); 73(6):1213–1222.

71A. DUNCAN JM, COOLEY DA, et al: Durability and low thrombogenicity of the St. Jude medical valve at 5 year follow-up. Ann Thorac Surg 1986 (Nov); 42:500–505.

72. LINDBLOM D, BJÖRK VO, SEMB BKH: Mechanical failure of the Björk-Shiley valve: incidence, clinical presentation, and management. J Thorac Cardiovasc Surg 1986 (Nov); 92:894–907.

73. GALLO I, NISTAL F, ARTINANO E: Six- to ten-year follow-up of patients with the Hancock cardiac bioprosthesis: incidence of primary tissue valve failure. J Thorac Cardiovasc Surg 1986 (July); 92:14–20.

74. FERRAZZI P, MCGIFFIN DC, KIRKLIN JW, BLACKSTONE EH, BOURGE RC: Have the results of mitral valve replacement improved? J Thorac Cardiovasc Surg 1986 (Aug); 92:186–197.

75. CHRISTAKIS GT, WEISEL RD, FREMES SE, TEOH KH, SKALENDA JP, TONG CP, AZUMA JY, SCHWARTZ L, MICKLEBOROUGH LL, SCULLY HE, GOLDMAN BS, BAIRD RJ: Can the results of contemporary aortic valve replacement be improved? J Thorac Cardiovasc Surg 1986 (July); 92:37–46.

76. DOWING RP, MILLER DC, STOFER R, SHUMWAY NE: Use of the intra-aortic balloon pump after valve replacement. J Thorac Cardiovasc Surg 1986 (Aug); 92:210–217.

77. LEE P-K, WANG RYC, CHOW JSF, CHEUNG KL, WONG VCW, CHAN T-K: Combined use of warfarin and adjusted subcutaneous heparin during pregnancy in patients wtih an artificial heart valve. J Am Coll Cardiol 1986 (July); 8:221–224.

78. ITURBE-ALESSIO I, FONSECA M, MUTCHINIK O, SANTOS MA, ZAJARIAS A, SALAZAR E: Risks of anticoagulant therapy in pregnant women with artificial heart valves. N Engl J Med 1986 (Nov 27); 315:1390–1393.

79. BOSKOVIC D, ELEZOVIC I, BOSKOVIC D, SIMIN N, ROLOVIC Z, JOSIPOVIC V: Late thrombosis of the Björk-Shiley tilting disc valve in the tricuspid position. Thrombolytic treatment with streptokinase. J Thorac Cardiovasc Surg 1986 (Jan); 91:1–8.

80. LEDAIN LD, OHAYON JP, COLLE JP, LORIENT-ROUDAUT FM, ROUDAUT RP, BESSE PM: Acute thrombotic obstruction with disc valve prostheses: diagnostic considerations and fibrinolytic treatment. J Am Coll Cardiol 1986 (Apr); 7:743–751.

81. SULLIVAN MF, ROBERTS WC: Mitral valve stenosis and pure tricuspid valve regurgitation: comparison of necropsy patients having simultaneous mitral and tricuspid valve replacements with necropsy patients having simultaneous mitral valve replacement and tricuspid valve anuloplasty. Am J Cardiol 1986 (Oct 1); 58:768–780.

82. SULLIVAN MF, ROBERTS WC: Clinical and morphologic observations after simultaneous replacement of the tricuspid, mitral and aortic valves. Am J Cardiol 1986 (Oct 1); 58:781–789.

83. ROBERTS WC, SULLIVAN MF: Combined mitral valve stenosis and tricuspid valve stenosis: morphologic observations after mitral and tricuspid valve replacements or mitral replacement and tricuspid valve commissurotomy. Am J Cardiol 1986 (Oct 1); 58:850–852.

84. ROBERTS WC, SULLIVAN MF: Clinical and necropsy observations early after simultaneous replacement of the mitral and aortic valves. Am J Cardiol 1986 (Nov 15) 58:1067–1084.

Myocardial Heart Disease

Morphologic studies

Unverferth and associates[1] from Columbus, Ohio, and Pittsburgh, Pennsylvania, studied the distribution of fibrosis and cellular hypertrophy in the hearts of 9 patients with idiopathic dilated cardiomyopathy (IDC). Transmural sections were removed from the LV and RV free walls and the ventricular septum of 9 patients with CHF and 6 control subjects. These sections were stained with hematoxylin-eosin (to determine cell size) and trichrome (to determine percent fibrosis). The sections were separated into equal areas from epicardium to endocardium in the RV and LV free walls and right to left across the ventricular septum. Percent fibrosis was greater in patients with IDC ($20 \pm 4\%$) than control subjects ($4 \pm 1\%$). A pattern of increasing fibrosis in the LV free wall from epicardium ($14 \pm 6\%$) to endocardium ($22 \pm 9\%$) was documented. Fibrosis was greater on the left ($21 \pm 12\%$) than the right ($15 \pm 6\%$) side of the septum. No pattern was evident in the RV free wall or in the control group. Myocardial cell diameter was greater in the CHF group ($22 \pm 5 \ \mu m$) than the control group ($17 \pm 2 \ \mu m$), but no pattern of hypertrophy across the walls was seen. The increased fibrosis, the pattern of fibrosis and the increased cell diameter in patients with IDC help to characterize IDC.

Immunologic studies

Gerli and associates[2] from Perugia, Italy, studied immune function, T-lymphocyte subsets, serum quantitative immunoglobulin levels, serum lysozyme levels, and circulating immune complex levels in patients with IDC. The percentage of helper/inducer T cells was higher and the percentage of suppressor/cytotoxic T cells was lower in IDC patients than in healthy controls and in patients with CAD. IDC patients, in addition, had higher 5/9+ T cells, a T-cell subset known to give maximal helper activity in B-cell differentiation assays. Peripheral blood mononuclear cells from IDC patients had a statistically greater ability to induce B-cell differentiation (helper T-cell function) into plasma cells and a hypofunctioning suppressor T-cell population in an *in vitro* pokeweed nitrogen-driven B-cell differentiation assay. Serum immunoglobulin IgM levels were higher in IDC patients, but serum lysozyme levels and serum immune complex levels in IDC patients were normal. These data verify that an immunoregulatory defect exists in IDC.

Peripartum

O'Connell et al[3] in Maywood, Illinois, studied 14 consecutive patients with peripartum cardiomyopathy attempting to define the clinical characteristics of this syndrome. Detailed histories and physical examinations, right-sided cardiac catheterizations, M-mode and 2-D echocardiograms, RNAs, and RV endomyocardial biopsies were obtained. These patients were then observed with sequential studies to determine prognostic indicators. Eight of these 14 patients were primiparous and an equal number first presented with CHF concomitant with or immediately before the onset of labor. These women were compared with 55 patients with IDC. Only mean age and onset of symptoms (29 ± 6 compared with 48 ± 14 years, respectively) and symptom duration (4 ± 8 compared with 19 ± 18 months) differed between the 2 groups. There were no differences in ventricular arrhythmias, LV chamber size, LVEF, or hemodynamics. Myocyte histologic findings were similar, but myocarditis was identified in 29% of patients with peripartum cardiomyopathy and in 9% of those with IDC. Seven patients with peripartum cardiomyopathy improved within 6 weeks of follow-up, and 6 died. Surviving patients had a higher LVEF (23 ± 12 compared with 11 ± 2%) and smaller LV cavity sizes. Thus, peripartum cardiomyopathy is clinically and hemodynamically indistinguishable from IDC, but is characterized by a relatively high frequency of histologic myocarditis and by either rapid, spontaneous improvement in CHF or progressive deterioration resulting in relatively rapid death.

Electrical stimulation

Stamato and associates[4] from Maywood and Hines, Illinois, assessed the response of patients with IDC to programmed electrical stimulation. Fifteen patients undergoing evaluation for CHF were studied. All patients underwent cardiac catheterization and coronary angiography and endomyocardial biopsy to exclude known causes of CHF. No patient had a history of syncope or sustained ventricular arrhythmias. All patients had severe LV dysfunction (mean EF 17%), and nonsustained VT on ambulatory monitoring or exercise testing. A protocol using up to 2 premature stimuli and burst pacing, from 2 RV sites, induced up to 4 repetitive ventricular responses but failed to induce a sustained ventricular arrhythmia in any patient. Patients with IDC, advanced ventricular arrhythmias, and depressed LV function respond differently to programmed electrical stimulation than do patients with CAD, advanced ventricular arrhythmias, and depressed LV function. Programmed electrical stimulation appears to have limited value in the evaluation of patients with IDC and nonsustained ventricular arrhythmias.

Poll and associates[5] from Philadelphia, Pennsylvania, determined the response to programmed electrical stimulation and the clinical outcome in 47 patients with IDC. Thirteen patients (group 1) presented with sustained uniform VT, 14 (group 2) presented with cardiac arrest and 20 (group 3) presented with nonsustained VT. The mean EF of the study population was $28 \pm 9\%$. The response to programmed stimulation was related to arrhythmia presentation. In all patients in group 1 sustained, uniform VT was induced, compared with 1 patient in group 2 and 2 patients in group 3. There were 14 sudden cardiac deaths and 1 cardiac arrest during a mean follow-up of 18 ± 14 months. The only 4 patients who presented with sustained VT or a cardiac arrest in whom sustained arrhythmia induction was suppressed with antiarrhythmic therapy remain alive. Nine of the 23 patients (4 in group 2 and 5 in group 3) in whom no sustained ventricular arrhythmia was induced died suddenly, with 5 of the 9 receiving empiric antiarrhythmic therapy. Three other patients, who had a slower and hemodynamically tolerated VT at the time of arrhythmia induction, died suddenly. Thus, in patients with IDC: 1) uniform, sustained VT is always and almost solely initiated in patients who present with this arrhythmia; 2) although few patients presenting with sustained VT or cardiac arrest have inducibility of the arrhythmias suppressed with therapy, if it is suppressed the patient appears to have a good prognosis; 3) a propensity for sudden cardiac death exists that is not predicted by the response to programmed stimulation (noninducibility during baseline stimulation or slowed arrhythmias on therapy) and is unrelated to arrhythmia presentation; and 4) empiric antiarrhythmic therapy does not improve outcome with respect to prevention of sudden cardiac death.

Das and associates[6] from Ann Arbor, Michigan, performed RV programmed stimulation with up to 3 extrastimuli in 24 patients (mean age 42 years) with IDC and no history of symptomatic ventricular arrhythmias. VT was induced in 8 patients and VF in 2. The VT was unimorphic in 2 and polymorphic in 6. No significant differences were noted between patients in whom arrhythmias were inducible and those in whom they were not with regard to age, symptomatic class, arrhythmia severity, or hemodynamic indexes. Over a mean follow-up of 12 months, 4 patients died, 3 suddenly and 1 with progressive CHF. Only 1 of the 3 who died suddenly had inducible VT. One other patient with induced sustained unimorphic VT later presented with spontaneous sustained VT similar in rate and configuration to induced VT. In conclusion, VT or VF may be induced in approximately 40% of patients with DC and no history of symptomatic VT or VF. Inducibility of polymorphic VT or VF does not correlate with clinical or hemodynamic variables or with the risk of sudden death. However, induction of unimorphic VT may predict later occurrence of spontaneous unimorphic VT.

Combined inotropic and vasodilator therapy

Much work has been reported regarding the mechanisms by which positive inotropic and vasodilator therapy effect systolic performance in CHF, but little is known about the effect of these agents on diastolic function. Carroll and co-investigators[7] in Chicago, Illinois recorded micromanometer LV and aortic pressure measurements simultaneously with 2-D targeted M mode echocardiography and thermodilution-determined cardiac output in 12 patients with IDC. Each patient received dopamine, dobutamine, and nitroprusside. Baseline hemodynamics were characterized by low cardiac index, high LV end-diastolic pressure, and increased end-diastolic and end-systolic dimensions (Fig. 7-1). All patients had abnormal LV pressure decay with a prolonged time constant and reduced peak diastolic lengthening rates. Dopamine and dobutamine decreased the time constant of relaxation and increased the peak lengthening rate. Dobutamine also reduced the minimum diastolic pressure from 14–10 mmHg; neither drug reduced the end-diastolic

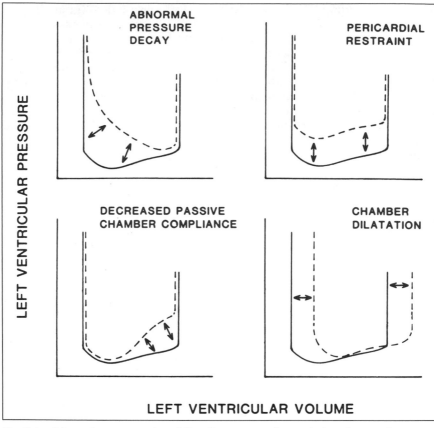

Fig. 7-1. Schematic representation of diastolic pressure-volume relations showing the types of changes involved in patients with dilated cardiomyopathy. For a given patient the pressure-volume relation may be modified with positive inotropic and vasodilator agents, which influence pressure decay, pericardial restraint, and chamber dilation. While abnormal myocardial properties may produce a decrease in passive chamber compliance in patients with congestive cardiomyopathy, no short-term effects on passive compliance occurred with these medications. Reproduced with permission from Carroll et al.[7]

pressure. Dopamine elevated end-diastolic pressures in 7 patients despite more rapid pressure decay. Diastolic pressure-dimension relations after dopamine and dobutamine administration showed a leftward shift with a reduced end-systolic chamber size, but no significant changes in passive chamber stiffness. Nitroprusside decreased LV minimum diastolic pressure and end-diastolic pressure; it did not consistently accelerate LV pressure decay at the doses tested. The decreased end-diastolic pressure with nitroprusside was due to a reduced end-diastolic dimension in 5 patients. In the other patients, all of whom had elevated RA pressures, diastolic pressure-dimension relations showed a parallel downward shift after administration of nitroprusside. Thus, positive inotropic therapy with beta$_1$-adrenoceptor agonists enhances early diastolic distensibility by accelerating relaxation, augmenting filling, and reducing end-systolic chamber size. Vasodilator therapy is much more effective in lowering diastolic pressures. In some patients this is due to a reduction in extrinsic restraint of the pericardium and/or RV interaction, whereas in others it simply reflects a decrease in chamber size without alterations in ventricular passive chamber properties.

HYPERTROPHIC CARDIOMYOPATHY

Postextrasystolic murmur

Kramer and associates[8] from Los Angeles and Torrance, California, performed phonocardiography during left-sided cardiac catheterization in 14 patients with HC, 40 with AS, and 4 with discreet subaortic stenosis, and they showed changes in the intensity of the murmur in response to increases in the postextrasystolic gradient. All patients showed increases in the gradient of the LV outflow tract during the postextrasystolic beat (Table 7-1). Of the 44 patients with AS and discreet subaortic stenosis, 42 (95%) had increases in murmur magnitude in contrast to 9 (64%) of the 14 patients with HC. Only 2 of the 7 patients with HC and resting gradients of >25 mmHg had murmur increases. This study shows, therefore, that the systolic murmur in HC, unlike the outflow tract murmur in AS or discreet subaortic stenosis, does not tract consistently with a magnitude of the outflow tract gradient.

Ventricular arrhythmias

Asymptomatic ventricular arrhythmias are common in patients with HC and are associated with sudden death. The variability of VPC and optimal duration of electrocardiographic monitoring necessary to exclude VT were assessed by Mulrow and associates[9] from London, UK, in 16 patients with HC in whom VT was detected during the first 48 hours of electrocardiographic monitoring. One hundred eight episodes of VT (range 0–10, mean 1.5/day) were recorded (52% incidence) during 48–168 hours of electrocardiographic monitoring (median 72) without cardiac medication within a 1-year period. The likelihood of excluding VT on electrocardiographic monitoring was determined. The probability of failing to detect VT in our selected group was 48% for 24 hours of electrocardiographic monitoring, 23% for 48 hours, and 11% for 72 hours. Daily VPC rates were 2 to 17,693 (median 187). Analysis of variance, applied to 10 patients with enough VPC for analysis, indicated that

TABLE 7-1. *Hemodynamic and phonocardiographic effects of the postextrasystolic beat in patients with hypertrophic cardiomyopathy and aortic or discrete subaortic stenosis. Reproduced with permission from Kramer et al.[8]*

| | REST GRADIENT* | POSTEXTRA-SYSTOLIC BEAT GRADIENT* | GRADIENT INCREASE* | PATIENTS WITH AORTIC PULSE PRESSURE | | PATIENTS WITH SYSTOLIC MURMUR INTENSITY | | |
				IN-CREASE	DE-CREASE	IN-CREASE	NO CHANGE	DE-CREASE
	←	mm Hg	→	←		*n*		→
Hypertrophic cardiomyopathy group 1	7.9 ± 10.4	103.6 ± 47.7	95.7 ± 42.8	0	7	7	0	0
Hypertrophic cardiomyopathy group 2	98.1 ± 34.3	166.4 ± 34.2	68.3 ± 30.6	0	7	2	3	2
Aortic or discrete subaortic stenosis	51.9 ± 29.1	84.7 ± 46.2	32.8 ± 20.0	37	7	42	2	0

* Values given as mean ±SD.

a 61% reduction of VPC in consecutive 24-hour periods was necessary to attribute an effect to the intervention rather than to spontaneous variability with 95% confidence. A sine wave curve fitted to the VPC counts revealed a circadian rhythm with a night frequency peak in 5 patients and an afternoon peak in 5. Thus, 48- to 72-hour electrocardiographic monitoring represents a pragmatic compromise in assessing drug intervention once VT is detected; longer periods (5–6 days) of electrocardiographic monitoring are required to exclude VT at initial evaluation, although the prognostic significance of VT detected after the first 72 hours is uncertain; and the frequency distribution of VPC shows substantial biologic variability and a circadian rhythm.

Doppler flow imaging

Nishimura and associates[10] from Rochester, Minnesota, evaluated 12 patients with HC by Doppler color flow imaging and continuous-wave Doppler echocardiography. Adequate color flow images were obtained in 10 of the 12 patients and MR was demonstrated in 6. An analysis of the color flow imaging revealed a temporal pattern in the LV outflow track that consisted of normal-velocity laminar flow during early systole followed by turbulent flow in midsystole. The maximal amount of MR on color flow imaging occurred late in systole after the appearance of turbulent flow in the LV outflow tract. The peak velocity detected in the LV outflow tract was positively correlated with the degree of systolic anterior motion of the anterior mitral leaflet. Patients with higher velocities in the LV outflow tract had prolonged ejection times. These findings support the concept of LV outflow obstruction in some patients with HC.

Yock et al[11] in Stanford, California, and Trondheim, Norway, evaluated the velocity characteristics of LV and aortic outflow in 25 patients with HC. Systematic pulsed and continuous-wave Doppler analysis combined with phonocardiography and M-mode echocardiography was used to establish the pattern and timing of outflow in the basal and provoked states. Examples of LV outflow jets recorded by continuous-wave Doppler or ultrasound in these patients are shown in Figure 7-2. Data obtained from these analyses sug-

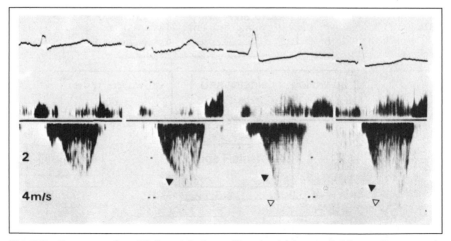

Fig. 7-2. Four examples of left ventricular outflow tract jets recorded by continuous wave Doppler ultrasound. Velocities range from 3.4 to 5.5 m/s. The increasing slope as the jets accelerate toward peak velocities (solid arrows) is typical for left ventricular outflow signals in hypertrophic cardiomyopathy. At the highest velocities, there is often some decrease in signal intensity or amplitude (open arrows). Reproduced with permission from Yock et al.[11]

gested that a) the high velocity LV outflow jet can be reliably discriminated from both aortic flow and the jet of MR using Doppler ultrasound; b) Doppler velocity contour responds in a characteristic fashion to provocative influences, including VPC and the Valsalva maneuver; c) the onset of MR occurs well before detectable systolic anterior motion of the mitral valve; d) LV flow velocities are elevated at the onset of systolic anterior motion of the mitral valve, suggesting a significant contribution of the Venturi effect in displacing the leaflets and chordae; e) the high velocities of the outflow jets are largely dissipated by the time flow reaches the aortic valve; and f) late systolic flow in the ascending aorta is nonuniform, with the formation of distinct eddies that may contribute to "preclosure" of the aortic valve.

Left ventricular filling

Gidding et al[12] in Ann Arbor, Michigan, analyzed LV filling patterns in 17 children and young adults with HC using M-mode echocardiographic and radionuclide techniques. Simultaneous Doppler ultrasound examination of the LV inflow, M-mode echocardiography, and phonocardiography were performed in the children and young adults: 10 had HC (ages 6–20 years) and 7 had a normal heart (ages 10–18 years). Measurements of various diastolic time intervals, peak flow velocity during rapid filling, and peak flow velocity during atrial contraction were obtained. From the M-mode studies, LV endocardia echocardiograms were digitized and peak rates of increase in LV dimension were determined and normalized for end-diastolic dimension. Diastolic time intervals, including isovolumic relaxation time were calculated from a phonocardiogram to determine end-systole. Isovolumic relaxation time was prolonged in patients with HC. Thus, altered patterns of LV filling are demonstrable by Doppler ultrasound techniques in young patients with HC. The prolongation of isovolumic relaxation times suggests a reduction in active LV relaxation in these patients.

Isovolumic relaxation

Betocchi et al[13] in Bethesda, Maryland, evaluated isovolumic relaxation in 90 patients with HC and 29 control subjects using RNA. The isovolumic relaxation period was determined automatically from LV time-activity curves as the interval between minimal volume and onset of rapid filling. In 17 patients, M-mode echocardiography performed simultaneously with RNA demonstrated that onset of MV opening correlated well with onset of rapid filling. In these patients, the isovolumic relaxation period was longer with HC than in control subjects (95 ± 44 compared with 50 ± 23 ms) and was longer in patients without an outflow tract gradient at rest than in patients with a gradient (109 ± 37 -vs- 86 ± 35 ms). In the patients without obstruction, there was a line or relation between the duration of the isovolumic period and peak filling rate. Filling was impaired in patients with HC as demonstrated by lower peak filling rate and prolonged time to peak filling rate compared with similar values in the normal volunteers. A prolonged isovolumic period was the main cause of the delay in time to peak filling rate. Oral verapamil (320–640 mg/day) was administered to 43 patients. Verapamil decreased the isovolumic relaxation time from 95 ± 42–80 ± 31 ms and improved filling as evidenced by an increase in peak filling rate and a decrease in the time to peak filling rate (Fig. 7-3). These data suggest that the delay in peak filling rate in patients with HC is related to a prolongation of the isovolumic period and that verapamil decreases isovolumic relaxation

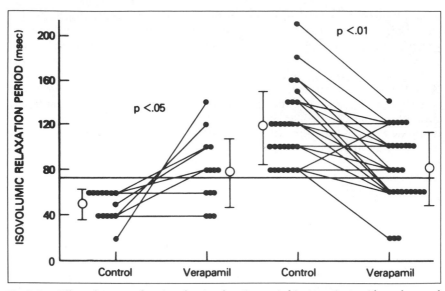

Fig. 7-3.   Effect of verapamil on isovolumic relaxation period in 14 patients with a subnormal or normal isovolumic period (left) and 29 patients with a prolonged isovolumic period (right). Horizontal line indicates mean normal value +1 SD. Open circles with vertical bars indicate mean values ±1 SD. Reproduced with permission from Belocchi et al.[13]

time and improves diastolic filling. Thus, impaired relaxation may be an important determinant of the decreased LV filling in patients with HC.

Intracavitary systolic pressure gradients

To correlate angiographic and hemodynamic events to HC, Grose and associates[14] from Bronx, New York, investigated 14 patients with HC using pressure recordings and caudocranial left anterior oblique contrast angiography. Patients were separated into 2 groups on the basis of the presence (group I) or absence (group II) of systolic anterior motion of the anterior mitral leaflet on caudocranial angiography. In group 1 (10 patients), the pressure gradient could be recorded with the LV catheter in the nonobliterated inflow region of the LV. Simultaneous micromanometer tracings and caudocranial angiography revealed that contact between the anterior mitral leaflet and the ventricular septum was an early systolic event (occurring 136 ± 33 ms after the R wave of the electrocardiogram) and was coincident with the onset of the pressure gradient. Cavitary obliteration was present in only 7 of 10 patients in group 1, and occurred late in systole well after the peak gradient (292 ± 28 ms after the R wave). In group II (4 patients), the pressure gradients could be recorded only from the obliterated portion of the ventricle distal to the level of the papillary muscles. Total LV cavitary obliteration was present in all group II patients. In 1 patient, simultaneous micromanometer pressure recording and caudocranial angiography revealed that cavitary obliteration preceded the peak gradient by 40 ms. Thus, in group I patients the onset of the pressure gradient is coincident with mitral leaflet–septal contact, while cavitary obliteration is an inconsistent late systolic event. In group II patients (no systolic anterior motion of the mitral valve) the pressure gradient could only be recorded in the LV apex, associated with total LV cavitary obliteration.

This study was followed by an editorial by Maron and Epstein.[15] They concluded that currently available data unequivocally support the concept that in patients with HC who have LV gradients measured at catheterization and who have associated marked SAM, a mechanical impediment to forward flow (and thus true obstruction to LV outflow) does exist. These authors also believe that the most important issue is not whether it is semantically appropriate to equate the presence of a gradient with the term "obstruction," but to appreciate that the gradient has important clinical implications by virtue of the markedly elevated intraventricular systolic pressures associated with it. These chronically elevated pressures are potentially detrimental to the left ventricle (a view held even by investigators opposed to the use of the term "obstruction" to describe the gradient in HC). Therefore, surgical obliteration of the gradient and normalization of these pressures remain an important and rational therapeutic objective in the severely symptomatic patients who have obstruction to LV outflow and who have failed to benefit from drug therapy.

Course of left ventricular thickening

Whether the magnitude and distribution of LV hypertrophy in patients with HC are established at birth or whether they evolve during the first years of life is unknown. Maron and associates[16] from Bethesda, Maryland, conducted serial echocardiographic studies in 39 children with a family history or morphologic evidence of HC. The patients were initially evaluated at 4–15 years of age (mean 11) and most recently at 9 to 20 years (mean 16). During a follow-up period of 2.5–6.8 years (mean 4), the magnitude and extent of preexisting LV hypertrophy markedly increased in 17 patients and the morphologic appearance of the heart evolved from normal to hypertrophic in 5 others. In these 22 patients the LV wall thickness increased strikingly (by 6–23 mm, a change of 101 ± 62%); these increases significantly exceeded those expected as a consequence of normal growth (13 ± 10%) and were not associated with symptomatic deterioration or related to subaortic obstruction. The authors concluded that LV hypertrophy may develop or progress spontaneously in patients with HC during childhood, when body growth is considerable. Since echocardiograms may be normal during childhood— before the morphologic features of hypertrophic cardiomyopathy develop—a single echocardiographic examination of young relatives of patients with HC may not exclude this disease.

Left ventricular dysfunction without severe hypertrophy

Spirito et al[17] in Bethesda, Maryland, studied 10 patients with nonobstructive HC and only mild localized LV hypertrophy with severe symptoms of CHF. During a mean follow-up period of 7 years, 6 of these 10 patients had a substantial increase in LV internal dimensions (6–15 mm, mean 10) as assessed with M-mode echocardiography, even though LV cavity size remained within normal limits in 5 of the 6 patients. Four patients had septal thinning (5–14 mm, mean 8). LV diastolic function assessed by RNA in 9 patients was impaired in 8 who demonstrated decreased peak filling rates and prolonged times to peak rate of filling (≥180 ms). In addition, LV systolic function, usually supernormal in patients with HC was depressed (LVEF ≤45%) in 6 patients. Therefore, in the subset of patients with nonobstructive HC and relatively mild and localized LV hypertrophy, symptoms of CHF developed. In most of these patients, both systolic and diastolic LV dysfunction was present and was associated with a progressive increase in LV internal dimension but without LV dilation.

Pulsus alternans

Pulsus alternans has been considered the sign of myocardial disease for >100 years. Cannon and co-investigators[18] in Bethesda, Maryland, noted LV pulsus alternans, a rhythmic beat-to-beat variation in LV systolic pressure and outflow gradient, in 35 of 200 patients with HC undergoing hemodynamic study (Fig. 7-4). LV pulsus alternans was not associated with significant systemic pulsus alternans, nor was RV pulsus alternans. All patients with LV pulsus alternans had severe outflow gradients at rest during provocation. Of 61 patients with severe basal outflow gradients >80 mmHg, 12 had LV pulsus alternans at rest. Eight of these patients underwent ventricular septal myotomy-myectomy; all had successful abolition of basal outflow gradient. Of the 7 of these 8 patients who underwent postoperative hemodynamic study and who were in sinus rhythm, none had LV pulsus alternans. Eleven of 60 patients with basal outflow gradients ranging from 10–70 mmHg had LV pulsus alternans during maneuvers provocative for outflow gradients. Two patients underwent ventricular septal myotomy-myectomy; neither had a gradient nor LV pulsus alternans during provocation postoperatively. Twelve additional patients with basal outflow gradients ranging from 0–115 mmHg had LV pulsus alternans after ectopic beats, generally occurring during maneuvers provocative for outflow gradients, associated with severe outflow gradients (mean gradient 130 ± 39 mmHg) during the

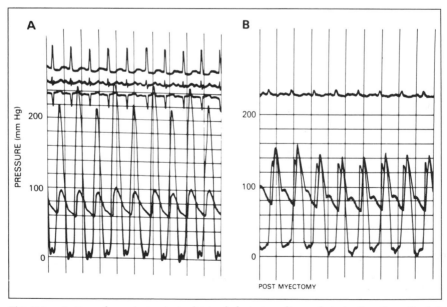

Fig. 7-4. A, Hemodynamic tracings obtained during cardiac catheterization from the left ventricle and brachial artery in a patient with severe left ventricular outflow obstruction at rest and sustained LVPA. Each horizontal division represents 20 mmHg; each vertical division is 0.5 sec. The prominent rhythmic alternation in left ventricular systolic pressure is associated with less prominent change in the arterial systolic pressure between strong and weak beats and the absence of rhythmic changes in left ventricular end-diastolic pressure. B, Hemodynamic tracings in the same patient 6 months after ventricular septal myotomy-myectomy demonstrating no basal gradient or LVPA. Reproduced with permission from Cannon et al.[18]

postextrasystolic beat. None of the 41 patients without an outflow gradient, basal or during provocation was found to have LV pulsus alternans. Thus, LV pulsus alternans is commonly seen in patients with HC and severe LV outflow gradients and may represent inadequate LV contractile function in the presence of high LV systolic pressures.

CARDIAC AMYLOIDOSIS

Echocardiographic assessment

Hongo and Ikeda[19] in Matsumoto, Japan, studied 28 patients with familial amyloid polyneuropathy by echocardiography to determine the evolution of amyloid heart disease. The incidence and degree of the abnormalities were correlated with neurologic disabilities, duration of the illness, and age in cross-sectional studies (Fig. 7-5). Studies were performed in 12 patients who were followed for a mean of 28 months. At the initial examination, LV diastolic function was reduced in 6 patients, while systolic function was preserved in 8. On follow-up there occurred significant increases in ventricular septal wall thickness and posterior LV wall thickness and reductions in the E-F slope of the mitral valve, percent fractional shortening, and LV internal diastolic dimension. At the final examination, marked LV hypertrophy was found in 3 patients, reduced LV diastolic function in all, impaired systolic function in 9, and decreased LV internal dimension in 3. Highly refractile myocardial echoes had appeared in 2 patients, pericardial effusion in 3, and valve thickening in 2. These investigators concluded that amyloid heart disease develops slowly but progressively.

Colchicine therapy

To determine whether colchicine prevents or ameliorates amyloidosis in patients with familial Mediterranean fever, Zemer and associates[20] from Tel-

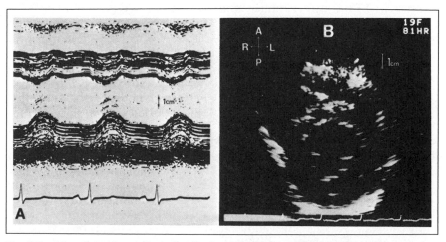

Fig. 7-5. M mode and two-dimensional echocardiograms obtained from a 54-year-old man (biopsy-proved cardiac amyloidosis) at the cross-sectional study. *A*, The interventricular septal wall and posterior wall are thickened. The maximal diastolic endocardial velocity of the posterior wall is markedly decreased, but %FS and mVcf are normal. *B*, Note a highly refractile appearance of the ventricular septum. L = left; R = right; A = anterior; P = posterior. Reproduced with permission from Hongo and Ikeda.[19]

Aviv, Israel, followed 1,070 patients with the latter disease for 4–11 years after they were advised to take colchicine to prevent febrile attacks. Overall, at the end of the study, the prevalence of nephropathy was one-third of that in a study conducted before colchicine was used to treat familial Mediterranean fever. Another group of patients had overt nephropathy when they started to take colchicine. Among 86 patients who had proteinuria but not the nephrotic syndrome, proteinuria resolved in 5 and stabilized in 68. Renal function deteriorated in 13 of the patients with proteinuria and in all of the 24 patients with the nephrotic syndrome or uremia. Thus, colchicine prevented amyloidosis in a high-risk population and it can prevent additional deterioration of renal function in patients with amyloidosis who have proteinuria but not the nephrotic syndrome. *These findings suggest that colchicine would also be useful in patients with cardiac amyloidosis.*

DOXORUBICIN CARDIOMYOPATHY

Palmeri and associates[21] from Bethesda, Maryland, prospectively assessed the role of rest and exercise RNA in predicting the cardiotoxic effects of doxorubicin in 48 patients who received a mean total doxorubicin dose of 522 mg/m^2 (range 480–600). Thirty-three patients also received cyclophosphamide (mean 5,220 mg/m^2). LVEF at rest progressively decreased from the baseline value of 55 ± 9–52 ± 8% after 338 mg/m^2–47 ± 8% after completion of doxorubicin therapy). In 42 patients (88%) EF at rest decreased after doxorubicin administration. Although no patient had known prior heart disease, the EF response to exercise was abnormal in 11 patients before doxorubicin. EF at rest after doxorubicin was significantly lower (41 ± 6 -vs- 49 ± 8%) in these 11 patients than in the 29 patients in whom the pretreatment EF response to exercise was normal, and in 4 of the 11 patients CHF developed. While age was an independent risk factor, cyclophosphamide did not appear to enhance the cardiotoxicity of doxorubicin. By multivariate analysis, age and EF at the midcourse of doxorubicin therapy were the most significant predictors of final EF after completion of doxorubicin therapy; neither rest nor exercise EF before doxorubicin appreciably improved the predictive value of age and EF at midcourse of therapy. Thus, some depression of LV function occurs in most patients receiving doxorubicin, and patients with abnormal baseline function appear to be at greater risk of clinical CHF after doxorubicin therapy. However, age and LVEF at the midcourse of doxorubicin treatment appear to be the most important determinants of subsequent LV function, and the clinical value of baseline testing before doxorubicin to predict LV function may be limited.

Strashun et al[22] in New York, New York, used serial gated blood pool scintigraphic monitoring of cardiac function with both the nonimaging scintillation probe and a conventional gamma camera-computer imaging system in 101 patients receiving doxorubicin hydrochloride (Adriamycin) chemotherapy. Comparison of probe- and camera-derived EF (n = 287) correlated significantly as did the interstudy (n = 183) change in EF. Significant discordance in probe- and camera-derived EF change occurred in 3 of 183 interstudy intervals. Average intrastudy variability of absolute probe-derived EF was 3%. Thirteen patients had clinical cardiotoxicity, including 4 at cumulative doxorubicin levels <450 mg/m^2. Mean absolute camera EF decline for these patients was 21% from baseline evaluation and mean absolute probe EF decline was 22%. The minimal absolute EF decline was 11% for patients with clinical CHF. Eight asymptomatic patients had therapy terminated before the development of cardiotoxicity after a mean decline in absolute camera EF of 19 ± 4% (SD) and in probe EF of 19 ± 9% into abnormal ranges. None of the 5 asymptomatic patients available for clinical follow-up at 6 months after termination of doxorubicin therapy subsequently had signs of ventricular dysfunction. Most patients (83%) studied at 450 mg/m^2-cumulative dose levels did not have a ≥15% decline from baseline into the abnormal EF range. These data suggest that a probe-derived EF measurement is similar to that derived from a conventional camera system and within acceptable limits for the characterization of cardiotoxicity resulting from doxorubicin.

ASSOCIATION WITH A CONDITION AFFECTING PRIMARILY A NONCARDIAC STRUCTURE(S)

Scleroderma

Raynaud's phenomenon and cardiac abnormalities are frequent in patients with systemic sclerosis. Ellis and associates[23] from Nashville, Tennessee, obtained radionuclide ventriculograms in 16 patients with Raynaud's phenomenon and systemic sclerosis or the related CREST syndrome and in 11 normal volunteers to evaluate changes in LV function that might be induced by exposure to cold. LV regional wall motion abnormalities developed in 9 of 16 patients during cooling compared with only 1 of 11 control subjects, despite a comparable increase in mean arterial pressure. The abnormalities occurred in 7 of 11 patients with systemic sclerosis, 1 of 4 with CREST syndrome, and 1 with Raynaud's disease. To test the potential protective effect of nifedipine, radionuclide ventriculograms were then obtained during cooling after sublingual nifedipine (20 mg). Only 5 of 13 patients had wall motion abnormalities, and the severity of the abnormalities was significantly less than during the first cooling period. Five of 8 patients who had cold-induced wall motion abnormalities during the first cooling period had none after nifedipine, whereas 2 other patients demonstrated small abnormalities only during the second cooling period after treatment with nifedipine. It is concluded that cold induces segmental myocardial dysfunction in patients with systemic sclerosis and that nifedipine may blunt the severity of this abnormal response.

Nitenberg and colleagues[24] from Limeil-Brevannes and Paris, France, compared the maximum coronary vasodilator capacity after intravenous dipyridamole (0.14 mg · kg^{-1} · min^{-1} × 4 minutes) in 7 patients with scleroderma myocardial disease with that of 7 control subjects. Hemodynamic data and LV angiographic data were not different in the 2 groups. The coronary flow reserve was evaluated by the dipyridamole/basal coronary sinus blood flow ratio and the coronary resistance reserve by the dipyridamole/basal coronary resistance ratio. Coronary reserve was greatly impaired in the group with scleroderma myocardial disease: dipyridamole/basal coronary sinus blood flow ratio was lower than in the control group (2.54 ± 1.37 -vs- 4.01 ± 0.56) and dipyridamole/basal coronary resistance ratio was higher than in the control group (0.47 ± 0.25 -vs- 0.23 ± 0.04). Such a decreased coronary flow and resistance reserve in patients with scleroderma myocardial disease was not explained by an alteration of LV function. Thus, reduced coronary flow and resistance reserve may be an important contributing factor in the pathogenesis of scleroderma myocardial disease.

Hyperthyroidism

Feldman et al[25] in Chicago, Illinois, evaluated 11 patients with hyperthyroidism to test the hypothesis that reduced afterload and increased preload and heart rate, rather than augmented contractility, are the major factors responsible for the increase in LV contractility in these patients. Ventricular hemodynamics were assessed by 2-D M-mode echocardiograms and callibrated carotid pulse tracings. Ventricular preload was estimated by end-diastolic dimension, whereas afterload was measured as end-systolic wall stress. LV performance was estimated by measuring the extent and velocity of ventricular wall shortening and myocardial work was assessed by measuring the ventricular systolic stress-length relations. After the initial studies, all patients were treated with propylthiouracil and this was followed by a subtotal thyroidectomy in 5 patients and treatment with iodine-131 in 2 patients. Results were compared with data obtained from 11 age-matched normal control subjects. With therapy, overall LV performance declined. This change was associated with no alteration in end-diastolic dimension or end-systolic wall stress, and a 24% reduction in heart rate. The end-systolic stress/rate–corrected shortening velocity relation decreased with the development of normal thyroid function (Fig. 7-6). In addition, there was a strong correlation between LV contractility and serum thyroid hormone levels. Ventricular minute work also declined with therapy. These data suggest that the altered

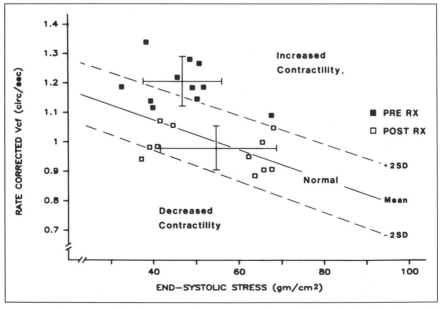

Fig. 7-6. Mean (solid line) and ± 2 SD confidence limits (dashed lines) for end-systolic stress/rate-corrected shortening velocity (Vcf) relation determined from a group of normal subjects (15). Vertical deviation from the mean regression line reflects a change in contractility for a given level of end-systolic wall stress independent of heart rate, preload and afterload. The end-systolic stress/rate-corrected shortening velocity relation for the 11 hyperthyroid subjects before (solid squares) and after (open squares) therapy is shown. Before treatment, values for all subjects were above the mean regression line, reflecting increased contractile state; 8 of the 11 points were above the ± 2 SD confidence limits. After treatment, all subjects showed a decline in the end-systolic stress/rate-corrected shortening velocity relation. One subject (value below the −2 SD confidence limit [lower left]) was hypothyroid. Reproduced with permission from Feldman et al.[25]

ventricular function of hyperthyroidism in humans is the result of augmented contractility rather than altered loading or chronotropic alterations.

Friedreich's ataxia

Child et al[26] in Los Angeles, California, evaluated 75 consecutive patients with Friedreich's ataxia to establish the prevalence and types of cardiac involvement in these patients. The patients included 39 males and 36 females, aged 10–66 years (mean 24). Electrocardiography was performed in all patients, echocardiography in 58 patients, and vectorcardiography in 34 patients. Among these patients, electrocardiographic and vectorcardiographic abnormalities occurred in 69 (92%). Electrocardiograms revealed ST-T-wave abnormalities in 79%, right-axis deviation in 40%, short PR intervals in 24%, and abnormal R waves in lead V_1 in 20%. In addition, abnormal inferolateral Q waves occurred in 14% of patients and LV hypertrophy was suggested on the electrocardiogram in 16%. Echocardiography revealed concentric LV hypertrophy in 11%, asymmetric septal hypertrophy in 9%, and globally decreased LV function in 7%. Two patients died, and postmortem examination revealed a dilated and atrophic left ventricle. These data indicate that most patients with Friedreich's ataxia have abnormal electrocardiograms and vectorcardiograms. Global LV dysfunction and concentric and asymmetric hypertrophy also occur in subsets of these patients.

Alboliras and associates[27] from Rochester, Minnesota, used combined 2-D and M-mode echocardiography to assess the cardiac status of 22 patients with Friedreich's ataxia and the findings were correlated with the clinical and electrocardiographic data. Mean age at onset of Friedreich's ataxia was 8 years (range 3–18); mean age at echocardiography was 18 years (range 8–39). Echocardiographic findings were abnormal in 19 patients (86%). The 3 patients with normal echocardiographic findings did not have cardiac symptoms, but 1 had electrocardiographic repolarization abnormalities. Concentric LV thickening, the most common echocardiographic finding, was found in 15 patients (68%) and in all 15 the papillary muscles were thickened. These 15 patients had electrocardiographic repolarization abnormalities and 5 had left-axis deviation; however, only 3 satisfied electrocardiographic criteria for LV or RV hypertrophy. Two of the 15 patients (9%) had symptoms of heart failure. Two patients had asymmetric septal thickening without clinical evidence of LV outflow tract obstruction; neither had cardiac symptoms, but both had electrocardiographic repolarization abnormalities. Two patients showed a dilated cardiomyopathy pattern; both had CHF and atrial flutter. One of these patients died, and necropsy revealed 4-chamber cardiac dilatation, RV and LV hypertrophy and histologic findings of diffuse interstitial fibrosis, myocellular hypertrophy, and necrosis. This study revealed a wide spectrum of cardiac abnormalities in patients with Friedreich's ataxia.

Myotonic dystrophy

In a family with myotonic dystrophy, 3 siblings showing electrocardiographic abnormalities were subjected to His bundle electrocardiographic studies by Hiromasa and associates[28] from Kanazawa, Japan. The duration of the disease ranged from 9 to 24 years. All 3 siblings had prolonged HV intervals (His-Purkinje conduction times) of 70–80 ms. The sister with the shortest duration of the disease had second-degree AV nodal block and left posterior fascicular block, the younger brother had left anterior fascicular block, and the elder brother with the longest history had first-degree AV block without bundle branch or fascicular block. With regard to associated arrhythmias, however, the elder brother had paroxysmal VT, apparently due to reentry involving the right bundle branch system, whereas the younger brother and sister had sinus bradycardia alone. This study reveals the prevalence of diffuse conduction disturbances of the specialized conducting system in a family with myotonic dystrophy.

References

1. UNVERFERTH DV, BAKER PB, SWIFT SE, CHAFFEE R, FETTERS JK, URETSKY BF, THOMPSON ME, LEIER CV: Extent of myocardial fibrosis and cellular hypertrophy in dilated cardiomyopathy. Am J Cardiol 1986 (Apr 1); 57:816–820.

2. GERLI R, RAMBOTTI P, SPINOZZI F, BERTOTTO A, CHIODINI V, SOLINAS P, GERNINI I, DAVIS S: Immunologic studies of peripheral blood from patients with idiopathic dilated cardiomyopathy. Am Heart J 1986 (Aug); 112:350–355.

3. O'CONNELL JB, COSTANZO-NORDIN MR, SUBRAMANIAN R, ROBINSON JA, WALLIS DE, SCANLON PJ, GUNNAR RM: Peripartum cardiomyopathy: clinical, hemodynamic, histologic and prognostic characteristics. J Am Coll Cardiol 1986 (July); 8:52–56.

4. STAMATO NJ, O'CONNELL JB, MURDOCK DK, MORAN JF, LOEB HS, SCANLON PJ: The response of patients with complex ventricular arrhythmias secondary to dilated cardiomyopathy to programmed electrical stimulation. Am Heart J 1986 (Sept); 112:505–508.

5. POLL DS, MARCHLINSKI FE, BUXTON AE, JOSEPHSON ME: Usefulness of programmed stimulation in idiopathic dilated cardiomyopathy. Am J Cardiol 1986 (Nov 1); 58:992–997.

6. DAS SK, MORADY F, DICARLO L, BAERMAN J, KROL R, DEBUITLEIR M, CREVEY B: Prognostic usefulness of programmed ventricular stimulation in idiopathic dilated cardiomyopathy without symptomatic ventricular arrhythmias. Am J Cardiol 1986 (Nov 1); 58:998–1000.

7. CARROLL JD, LANG RM, NEUMANN AL, BOROW KM, RAJFER SI: The differential effects of positive inotropic and vasodilator therapy on diastolic properties in patients with congestive cardiomyopathy. Circulation 1986 (Oct); 74:815–825.

8. KRAMER DS, FRENCH WJ, CRILEY JM: The postextrasystolic murmur response to gradient in hypertrophic cardiomyopathy. Ann Intern Med 1986 (May) 104:772–776.

9. MULROW JP, HEALY MJR, McKENNA WJ: Variability of ventricular arrhythmias in hypertrophic cardiomyopathy and implications for treatment. Am J Cardiol 1986 (Sept 15); 58:615–618.

10. NISHIMURA RA, TAJIK AJ, REEDER GS, SEWARD JB: Evaluation of hypertrophic cardiomyopathy by Doppler color flow imaging: initial observations. Mayo Clin Proc 1986 (Aug); 61:631–639.

11. YOCK PG, HATLE L, POPP RL: Patterns and timing of Doppler-detected intracavitary and aortic flow in hypertrophic cardiomyopathy. J Am Coll Cardiol 1986 (Nov); 8:1047–1058.

12. GIDDING SS, SNIDER R, ROCCHINI AP, PETERS J, FARNSWORTH R: Left ventricular diastolic filling in children with hypertrophic cardiomyopathy: assessment with pulsed Doppler echocardiography. J Am Coll Cardiol 1986 (Aug); 8:310–316.

13. BETOCCHI S, BONOW RO, BACHARACH SL, ROSING DR, MARON BJ, GREEN MV: Isovolumic relaxation period in hypertrophic cardiomyopathy: assessment by radionuclide angiography. J Am Coll Cardiol 1986 (Jan); 7:74–81.

14. GROSE R, STRAIN J, SPINDOLA-FRANCO H: Angiographic and hemodynamic correlations in hypertrophic cardiomyopathy with intracavitary systolic pressure gradients. Am J Cardiol 1986 (Nov 15); 58:1085–1092.

15. MARON BJ, EPSTEIN SE: Clinical significance and therapeutic implications of the left ventricular outflow tract pressure gradient in hypertrophic cardiomyopathy. Am J Cardiol 1986 (Nov 15); 1093–1096.

16. MARON BJ, SPIRITO P, WESLEY Y, ARCE J: Development and progression of left ventricular hypertrophy in children with hypertrophic cardiomyopathy. N Engl J Med 1986 (Sept 4); 315:610–614.

17. SPIRITO P, MARON BJ, BONOW RO, EPSTEIN SE: Severe functional limitation in patients with hypertrophic cardiomyopathy and only mild localized left ventricular hypertrophy. J Am Coll Cardiol 1986 (Sept); 8:537–544.

18. Cannon RO, Schenke WH, Bonow RO, Leon MB, Rosing DR: Left ventricular pulsus alternans in patients with hypertrophic cardiomyopathy and severe obstruction to left ventricular outflow. Circulation 1986 (Feb); 73(2):276–285.

19. Hongo M, Ikeda SI: Echocardiographic assessment of the evolution of amyloid heart disease: a study with familial amyloid neuropathy. Circulation 1986 (Feb); 73(2):249–256.

20. Zemer D, Pras M, Sohar E, Modan M, Cabill S, Gafni J: Colchicine in the prevention and treatment of the amyloidosis of familial Mediterranean fever. N Engl J Med 1986 (Apr 17); 314:1001–1005.

21. Palmeri ST, Bonow RO, Myers CE, Seipp C, Jenkins J, Green MV, Bacharach SL, Rosenberg SA: Prospective evaluation of doxorubicin cardiotoxicity by rest and exercise radionuclide angiography. Am J Cardiol 1986 (Sept 15); 58:607–613.

22. Strashun AM, Goldsmith SJ, Horowitz SF: Gated blood pool scintigraphic monitoring of doxorubicin cardiomyopathy: comparison of camera and computerized probe results in 101 patients. J Am Coll Cardiol 1986 (Nov); 8:1082–1087.

23. Ellis WW, Baer AN, Robertson RM, Pincus T, Kronenberg MW: Left ventricular dysfunction induced by cold exposure in patients with systemic sclerosis. Am J Med 1986 (Mar); 80:385–392.

24. Nitenberg A, Foult J-M, Kahan A, Perennec J, Devaux J-Y, Menkes C-J, Amor B: Reduced coronary flow and resistance reserve in primary scleroderma myocardial disease. Am Heart J 1986 (Aug); 112:309–315.

25. Feldman T, Borow KM, Sarne DH, Neumann A, Lang RM: Myocardial mechanics in hyperthyroidism: importance of left ventricular loading conditions, heart rate and contractile state. J Am Coll Cardiol 1986 (May); 7:967–974.

26. Child JS, Perloff JK, Bach PM, Wolfe AD, Perlman S, Kark RAP: Cardiac involvement in Friedreich's ataxia: a clinical study of 75 patients. J Am Coll Cardiol 1986 (June); 7:1370–1378.

27. Alboliras ET, Shub C, Gomez MR, Edwards WD, Hagler DJ, Reeder GS, Seward JB, Tajik AJ: Spectrum of cardiac involvement in Friedreich's ataxia: clinical, electrocardiographic and echocardiographic observations. Am J Cardiol 1986 (Sept 1); 58:518–524.

28. Hiromasa S, Ikeda T, Kubota K, Takata S, Hattori N, Nishimura M, Watanabe Y: A family with myotonic dystrophy associated with diffuse cardiac conduction disturbances as demonstrated by His bundle electrocardiography. Am Heart J 1986 (Jan); 111:85–91.

Congenital Heart Disease

In atrial septal aneurysm

Belkin and associates[1] from Durham, North Carolina, performed adequate contrast 2-D echocardiography in 13 of 16 patients with typical 2-D findings of atrial septal aneurysm. Five patients were referred for detection of intracardiac source of emboli after embolic stroke and 11 were evaluated for suspicion of valvular or other forms of heart disease. Contrary to findings of previous clinical studies, all 13 patients had 2-D evidence of right-to-left atrial level shunting. These findings represent the first clinical evidence of a high prevalence of atrial shunting in patients with atrial septal aneurysm.

ATRIOVENTRICULAR CANAL DEFECT

Operative treatment with associated right ventricular outflow obstruction

LeBlanc and colleagues[2] from Toronto, Canada, reviewed their results of total repair of atrioventricular septal defect (AVSD) in 29 children, 11 (group 1) with congenital RV outflow obstruction between 2 and 14 years of age, and 18 (group 2) operated between 0.2 and 12 years of age (mean × 6.0) who had previous PA banding 4.8 ± 3.6 years earlier. In group 1, a palliative infundibulectomy and pulmonary valvotomy had been previously performed in 1 child and 4 (36%) had a previous Blalock-Taussig shunt at a mean age of 2.8 years. A single patch technique of repair was used in 4 children and a double patch technique in the remaining 7. Five required a transanuluar patch to repair RV outflow obstruction. There were 2 deaths both from low cardiac output in patients aged 2 years at the time of repair. A third child died from dehiscence of the left AV valve 5 weeks later. Follow-up ranged from 13 months–15 years (mean × 5.5 years) and results were good in 5 patients, poor in 2 because of moderate to severe MR, and poor in 1 in whom complete heart block developed and who required a permanent pacemaker. Group 2 patients underwent complete repair between 0.2 and 12 years of age (mean × 6). Acquired infundibular obstruction was relieved in 4 directly and by patching a RV incision in 2. The remaining 14 were without infundibular stenosis and underwent repair and PA debanding. The PA band was removed in all; in 5 resection and direct end-to-end anastomosis was done and in 13 a pericardial patch was used to widen the band site. Although MR was present in 11, only 1 underwent MVR at the time of complete repair. There were 8 hospital deaths from low cardiac output in 7 and viral hepatitis in 1. There was no late mortality during the follow-up period ranging from 3.5–8.5 years (mean × 5.8). Results were good in 8 of 10 survivors who were asymptomatic and had normal exercise tolerance. One additional patient had residual RV outflow obstruction and a small residual VSD and another required pacemaker insertion for surgically acquired complete heart block. Analysis of multiple risk factors showed that overall death was more common when operations were performed in patients younger than 5 years of age and in those with preoperative moderate or severe MR. The authors recommended elective repair of AVSD with associated RV outflow obstruction when a child reaches a body weight of 15 kg, approximately 5 years of age. For those with AVSD alone, they recommended primary repair at any age and no longer advise initial PA banding. The latter is reserved for those with unbalanced forms or when concomitant disease precludes intracardiac repair.

Guo-wei et al[3] from Melbourne, Australia, reported their experience with the surgical management of 6 patients with complete AV canal, 4 with associated TF and 2 with double-outlet right-ventricle (DORV) and PS. Systemic-PA shunts were initially constructed in 4 patients ranging in age from 20 days–6 years. Four underwent complete repair using a transatrial approach and a comma-shaped Dacron® patch for VSD closure, a separate pericardial patch for atrial septation. Each survived and was followed between 6 and 43 months. Three of the 4 patients had a residual VSD that was later surgically closed in 2. The authors recommend corrective repair for these anomalies with selected initial use of systemic-PA shunting. There is a current tendency to perform modified Fontan-type operations in patients with more complex intracardiac defects such as those reported by Guo-wei. I (ADP) share the author's belief that a corrective repair is best for this group of malformations.

Vargas et al[4] from Boston, Massachusetts, reviewed their experience with 13 autopsy specimens and 13 patients who underwent repair of complete AV canal coexisting with TF between 1975 and 1985. A bridging left superior leaflet was present in 25 and the ostium primum component was either small or absent in 13. Anterior extension of the VSD with malalignment of the infundibular septum was present in each heart, but in 13, the VSD did not extend beneath the inferior leaflet. Leaflet tissue deficiency was present in 4, a single left papillary muscle in 3, an accessory valve orifice in 4, and ventricular dominance in 5 (LV in 4, RV in 1). Each had infundibular RV obstruction, 10 a hypoplastic pulmonary valve anulus, 1 pulmonary atresia, and 6 branch PA stenoses. At operation, the ostium primum was incised in 7 to aid in exposure, and the bridging left superior leaflet was divided obliquely and rightward so as to parallel the crest of the ventricular septum. This permitted the use of a single patch of pericardium sutured to close the VSD and minimize the risk of postrepair subaortic stenosis. The leaflets were then sutured to the pericardial patch which was then used to close the ostium primum defect. A transanular RV outflow patch was used in 10, an extracardiac RV-PA conduit in 1. The surgical group ranged from 16 months–16 years of age (mean 7 years) and 7 patients were <4 years of age. Preoperatively, AR was severe in 3 and mild to moderate in 4. There were no hospital deaths, 3 late deaths from AR in 2, and sepsis in 1. One patient with RV hypoplasia underwent a Fontan procedure within 24 hours of initial repair and 4 (31%) required left AVR which was early in 3 and late in 1. The authors indicate that improved preoperative diagnostic accuracy and a better understanding of the anatomic variables present in this combined condition have resulted in improved surgical results. They believe that the need for prosthetic valve replacement will continue to be required by some patients.

VENTRICULAR SEPTAL DEFECT

Spontaneous closure with ventricular septal aneurysm

Ramaciotti and associates[5] from San Francisco, California, reviewed 247 patients found to have an isolated perimembranous VSD on echocardiography. An aneurysm associated with a VSD was present in 77% and was found at the first echocardiographic examination in 94%. The median follow-up period was 27 months. In patients with aneurysm the VSD closed spontaneously in 11%, improved clinically in 33%, and required surgery in 11%. In patients without aneurysm the VSD closed spontaneously in only 2%, improved clinically in 16%, and required surgical closure in 47%. When considering only a larger VSD, 28% with aneurysm required surgery, whereas 84% without aneurysm required surgery. These authors found an important marker for perimembranous VSD in terms of tendency for closure. These data fit more with most clinicians' experience than the data by Bierman et al. (J Am Coll Cardiol, 1985; 5:118–123) as reported in *Cardiology 86*. This favorable prognosis was not found in patients with Down's syndrome because most of these patients did require surgical closure despite the presence of aneurysm. Thus, the formation of VSD aneurysm (or tricuspid valve pouch) is an important mechanism of VSD closure and its presence confers a more favorable prognosis in perimembranous VSD except in patients with Down's syndrome.

Color Doppler observations

Ludomirsky and associates[6] from Houston, Texas, compared color Doppler, standard echocardiography Doppler, and angiographic techniques in 51 patients age 3 months–25 years with VSD. Solitary VSD was present in 18, multiple VSD in 18, and intact ventricular septum in 15. At least 1 VSD was detected by color Doppler and standard echocardiography Doppler in all patients with angiographically proved VSD with no false positives. In the detection of multiple VSD, sensitivity of color Doppler was 72% and standard 2-D echocardiography Doppler was 38% with 100% specificity in both. Color Doppler failed to identify multiple VSDs in 5 patients: 2 weighed <4 kg; 3

had reduced pulmonary blood flow. These authors present important data that indicate the usefulness of color Doppler studies to detect multiple VSD. Further studies on large series of patients would be useful with this type of analysis to determine the diagnostic accuracy of this new technique for this application.

With associated aortic regurgitation

Craig and associates[7] from Toronto, Canada, studied 20 consecutive patients with VSD and aortic valve prolapse by cross-sectional echocardiography. Angiographic confirmation was available in all and surgical confirmation in 17. In 19, the right coronary cusp was involved and appeared to plug the defect in the precordial long- and short-axis cut. The cusp was deformed and appeared to pivot from the crest of the ventricular septum. In all 19, angiography demonstrated prolapse of the right cusp. Noncoronary cusp prolapse was observed in 2 by cross-sectional echocardiography and in 6 by angiocardiography. The VSD was perimembranous in 14 and doubly committed subarterial in 6 by echocardiography. Angiographically, the VSD was perimembranous in 15 and doubly committed in 5. AR was detected by Doppler interrogation in 7, all of whom underwent plication of the right coronary cusp. Angiographic evidence of AR was noted in 11, but 4 were mild and possibly related to catheter position. Five patients had associated muscular RV outflow tract obstruction and 3 had a subaortic ridge. Combined cross-sectional and pulsed Doppler echocardiography provided reliable assessment of right coronary cusp prolapse associated with VSD. Noncoronary cusp prolapse was more difficult to detect. This echocardiographic technique should help optimize the management of patients with VSD by providing a means of early detection of aortic valve prolapse before the development of AR.

PULMONIC VALVE STENOSIS

Doppler for measuring degree of stenosis

Although Doppler echocardiography has been demonstrated to accurately predict the pressure drop across the pulmonary valve in patients with PS, prior reports have stressed the need to correct for beam-flow intercept angles, to use simultaneous imaging, and to utilize the subcostal approach. Goldberg and associates[8] from Tucson, Arizona, determined the accuracy of estimating the pressure drop in PS patients by means of nonimaging Doppler applied without angle correction from precordial examination. Pressure drop estimated by Doppler was compared with that measured by strain-gauge manometry at catheterization. Data for 39 patients (21 simultaneous measurements; 18 nonsimultaneous) were evaluated. Results for the entire group showed a good correlation. The correlation for simultaneous measurement improved somewhat, but the difference was not significant. Comparison of the slope and intercept of data of this study to those of prior studies, which advocated more complex methodology, indicated that results were essentially similar and that use of the additional steps did not confer a significantly improved result. It was concluded that the simplified methodology utilized in this study provides accurate Doppler estimates of pressure gradient in patients with PS.

Percutaneous transluminal balloon valvuloplasty

Ali Khan and associates[9] from Riyadh, Saudi Arabia, performed percutaneous transluminal balloon pulmonary valvuloplasty 33 times in 32 patients. Patients ranged in age from 6 months–12 years (mean 4.5 years); average weight was 15 kg. Before dilatation, all patients had grade 4/6 late peaking systolic ejection murmurs, with right-axis deviation and RV hypertrophy. Moderate to severe PS (right ventricle-PA gradient 50 mmHg systolic) was confirmed both hemodynamically and angiographically. Balloon size was selected to be approximately 2 mm larger than the pulmonic valve anulus. Balloons were inflated to approximately 5 atm of pressure. Two patients required 2 simultaneous balloons as the pulmonary valve anulus was >25 mm. Predilatation peak systolic pressure gradients ranged from 50–245 mmHg (mean 99); postdilatation gradients ranged from 8–93 mmHg (mean 23). There were no deaths or complications. The systolic murmur with early systolic peak decreased in all but 3 patients. Systolic thrill disappeared in all but 3 patients. Follow-up at an average of 10 months revealed increasing exercise tolerance in two-thirds of patients. Fourteen patients underwent repeat catheterization >6 months after dilatation and showed persistent minimal gradient. Balloon valvuloplasty for PS is an effective, safe procedure.

Radtke and associates[10] from Boston, Massachusetts, reported percutaneous valvotomy for 27 patients, aged 6 days–19 years with unoperated typical PS using a balloon 7–60% (mean 30%) larger than the valve anulus. To achieve an oversized dilatation diameter in 3 patients, double balloons were inflated side by side. Reduction of transvalvular gradient occurred in all patients (mean $\pm$ SD 74 $\pm$ 15%) and average gradient decreased from 65 $\pm$ 19–16 $\pm$ 8 mmHg. A residual transvalvular gradient of <25 mmHg was achieved in 25 of 27 patients. No significant complications occurred. These authors presented the best results to date for reduction of gradient in PS although other previous results have been good. Oversized balloons are useful in achieving adequate reduction of gradient and can be used without added risk. These authors recommend balloons 20 to 40% larger than valve ring with the one caveat that a smaller balloon should be used initially in younger patients.

PULMONIC VALVE ATRESIA

Necropsy findings

Fyfe and associates[11] from Rochester, Minnesota, studied the necropsy findings in 17 hearts obtained from patients with pulmonary valve atresia and intact ventricular septum. Age at death ranged from 1 day–16 years (median 11 days). Coronary AV fistulas were found in 6 of 17 and 5 of 17 had coronary artery dysplasia. Evidence for myocardial ischemia was present in 10 of 17 hearts and correlated poorly with either RV coronary artery fistulas or coronary artery dysplasia. These authors demonstrated again the severity of myocardial ischemia that can occur in both right and left ventricles in patients with pulmonary atresia and intact ventricular septum. It has been postulated previously that coronary artery fistulas or coronary artery dysplasia might be the primary factors leading to ischemia. These data indicate that there are other determinants of ischemia. One might postulate that excessive myocardial oxygen demand of the hypertensive right ventricle and inadequate supply associated with cyanosis and possible systemic hypotension contributed significantly. This lesion continues to be a difficult one to treat and myocardial ischemia may well play a role in the high morbidity and mortality associated with this condition.

Right ventricular growth potential in neonates

In an effort to define RV growth potential in neonates with pulmonary atresia and intact ventricular septum, Lewis et al[12] from Los Angeles, California, reviewed their experience with 30 infants treated between 1970 and 1984. An index of RV cavity size was calculated by averaging the sum of the biplane dimensions of the tricuspid valve anulus, the RV inlet, and RV outlet at end diastole, normalized by the diameter of the descending aorta at the diaphragm. Fourteen group I patients received only a systemic-PA shunt. Eleven of these were treated before 1979 when a pulmonary valvotomy was not employed and an RV outflow tract was present in 9 (82%). Early and late mortality in group I was 50%. Preoperative RV index was 7 ± 3 and was unchanged at repeat cardiac catheterization studies performed in 3 of 7 surviving patients after an average interval of 4 years. Sixteen group II patients underwent pulmonary valvotomy and a concomitant shunt was made in 14. Overall mortality in group II was 19% and 11 patients underwent repeat studies at an average interval of 1.1 ± 0.9 years. RV size increased in all but 2 infants; RV index 8 preoperative -vs- 11 postoperative. The authors currently recommend initial use of prostaglandin E_1 for stabilization, cardiac catheterization with RV angiography to determine morphology and cavity size. Transventricular closed pulmonary valvotomy is performed in all infants in whom an RV outflow tract is angiographically identified and a Blalock-Taussig shunt performed in those whose RV index is <11. In the 10% of patients who have normal RV dimensions (RV index >11), a pulmonary valvotomy is the sole initial procedure and prostaglandin E_1 is continued for 3 to 5 days postoperatively. A subsequent shunt is recommended only if systemic arterial oxygen tension is <30 torr. Important residual RV outflow tract obstruction is present in 50% and more extensive secondary outflow tract reconstruction is required. This management program should result in a high percentage of patients suited to ultimate corrective repair.

Exercise response

Barber and associates[13] from Rochester, Minnesota, performed maximal exercise testing 35 times in 34 consecutive patients with pulmonary atresia and VSD. There were 14 studies in patients without repair, 11 studies in patients with RV to PA conduit without VSD closure, and 10 studies in patients with complete repair. Total work performed, maximal power achieved, exercise time, and maximal oxygen uptake were significantly greater in patients after partial or complete repair than in patients without repair. Patients in all 3 groups had a blunted heart rate response to exercise and the ventilatory equivalent for oxygen was increased both at rest and during exercise for patients without conduit repair and those with an RV to PA conduit without VSD closure. This study indicates that these patients have decreased exercise tolerance both before and after corrective surgery. Exercise tolerance does improve significantly after partial repair. No further improvement in exercise tolerance occurs after closure of the VSD although ventilatory function and systemic arterial blood saturation are improved.

These authors present another careful study in regard to exercise response in patients with pulmonary atresia plus VSD. These patients fared less well than those studied after repair of TF. In patients after repair of TF maximal oxygen consumption was 70% of predicted -vs- only 51% of predicted in the current study.

With juxtaductal left main pulmonary arterial obstruction

Momma and associates[14] from Tokyo, Japan, reviewed the morphology of the central PA by selective angiogram in 21 unoperated patients aged 11 days–21 years with pulmonary atresia plus VSD. Angiographic findings were confirmed at operation in 10 patients. There was juxtaductal stenosis of the left PA in 67% and complete left PA obstruction in 25% (Fig. 8-1). Six of 7 patients without juxtaductal obstruction had pulmonary valve atresia but all 9 patients with juxtaductal stenosis had complete atresia of the central pulmonary trunk. These authors presented an excellent demonstration of this unfortunately common problem in patients with pulmonary atresia plus VSD or TF. Data from a number of different observations suggest that this can be a progressive lesion possibly associated with the constriction of ductal tissue which extends into the left PA. These studies show that juxtaductal obstruction developed at both sides of the ductal junction with the PA but that it progressed more rapidly proximal to the junction. This is the first demonstration that juxtaductal obstruction appears to be an almost invariable finding in patients with atresia of the pulmonary trunk.

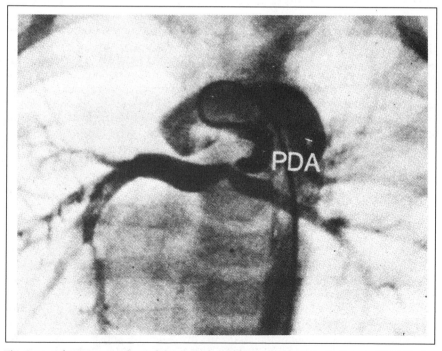

Fig. 8-1. Selective angiogram of the central pulmonary artery through the persistent ductus arteriosus (PDA) in case 11, showing cone-shaped stenotic ductus and juxtaductal stenosis of the left pulmonary artery. Stenosis of the ductus caused contrast material to be regurgitated into the aorta. Reproduced with permission from Momma et al.[14]

Operative repair

The use of prostaglandins and balloon atrial septostomy have significantly reduced the early mortality of patients with pulmonary atresia with intact ventricular septum. Opinions vary as to the optimal subsequent surgical management. Joshi et al[15] from Melbourne, Australia, reviewed their experience with 16 neonates (10 <1 day and 6 <6 days of age) initially treated by either a systemic-PA shunt, shunt with pulmonary valvotomy, and pulmonary valvotomy alone. Patients were categorized according to RV morphology by angiography. There was 1 death among 16 neonatal primary procedures, none among 4 secondary procedures and 1 among 5 delayed hemodynamic repairs. Patients with pulmonary valvotomy had significantly greater growth of the tricuspid valve than those who had shunt alone. There were 5 patients with major sinusoidal coronary artery communications and each was lacking an infundibular portion of the right ventricle. The authors current protocol that has evolved from this experience includes initial stabilization with ventilation, prostaglandin E_1 infusion and correction of acidosis. Echocardiographic evaluation and balloon septostomy under echocardiographic control is performed if the ASD is restrictive. Only selected patients are subjected to RV angiography. A 5-mm polytetrafluoroethylene shunt is placed from the left subclavian to the pulmonary trunk and closed pulmonary valvotomy is employed when all 3 portions of the right ventricle are present. A shunt without valvotomy is performed in selected patients with absent infundibulum or with major sinusoidal RV–coronary artery communications. Secondary valvotomy is done when good RV and tricuspid valve growth is observed. Hemodynamic repair is performed when adequate RV and tricuspid valve growth are present. Those with an adequate RV growth and/or persistent major sinusoidal communications are managed by a modified Fontan procedure. The authors believe that a systemic-PA shunt is the most important part of the neonatal palliative procedure, regardless of the morphology of the right ventricle.

Foker et al[16] from Minneapolis, Minnesota, reported their experience with pulmonary atresia with intact ventricular septum initially placing an RV outflow patch and continuation of PGE_1 infusion postoperatively until the need for a systemic-PA shunt can be determined. Each of the 15 neonates had suprasystemic RV pressure and preoperative stabilization with PGE_1. Initial RV outflow tract patching was accomplished in 13 and simultaneous PDA ligation in 2 in whom adequate postoperative RV function was confidently predicted. In 2 patients early in this experience, a shunt was performed as the initial procedure and an outflow patch planned at a second stage. In 9 patients, PGE_1 was infused postoperatively after outflow patching to provide pulmonary blood flow until RV function became adequate. There were 4 hospital deaths, 3 believed related to premature cessation of PGE_1 infusion. The fourth patient died from myocardial ischemia because of coronary artery stealing through RV sinusoids after an outflow patch and a shunt. There was 1 late death in 1 of the 2 patients in whom an initial shunt was performed. Each of the 10 hospital survivors subsequently underwent complete repair with no deaths. Five of the 10 had residual ASD with right-to-left shunting at the ages of 1–3 years, but balloon occlusion of the ASD during cardiac catheterization showed adequate RV function and subsequent closure was accomplished. The authors concluded that outflow patching can be performed as the initial procedure in the neonatal period with good results, maximizing the potential for RV growth. Pulmonary blood flow can be assured postoperatively with continued infusion of PGE_1. RV function often improves with time and the necessity for subsequent systemic-PA shunting can be assessed more properly, but seems to be needed only infrequently. Balloon occlusion of the ASD at late postoperative cardiac catheterization studies provides information regarding the advisability of surgical ASD closure. This is a unique experience in that all survivors of the initial hospital period have subsequently undergone definitive repair leaving the patient with a biventricular heart. The authors' current protocol of slowly tapering postoperative PGE$_1$ infusion and constructing a systemic-PA shunt only if pulmonary blood flow remains unsatisfactory after several days or longer (required in only 2 of 13 patients), is a most important part of their management program.

Metzdorff and colleagues[17] from Portland, Oregon, reviewed their experience between 1965 and 1982 with RV reconstruction after valvotomy for pulmonary atresia with intact ventricular septum. Twenty-five patients underwent initial valvotomy with or without concomitant shunt with 8 (32%) hospital deaths. Ten of the 17 hospital survivors subsequently underwent transannular RV outflow patching with no hospital deaths. RV systolic pressures were suprasystemic before reoperation and were near normal postoperatively. Nine of the 10 patients had tripartite RV morphology, but the right ventricle was hypoplastic in each. Tricuspid valve anular diameter was measured from the cineangiogram before the initial valvotomy and before RV reconstruction. Related to body length, anular diameter growth proceeded at a rate greater than normal as derived from autopsy data. The mean tricuspid valve anular diameter growth rate was also greater than that of patients with less favorable ventricular types treated with a systemic-PA shunt alone. The authors concluded that measurement of tricuspid anular diameter is a useful method of following RV growth and may aid in selecting patients for RV construction. They believe all patients should undergo recatheterization no later than 1 year after valvotomy, and if RV pressure remains elevated, outflow patch reconstruction should be advised.

Growth of hypoplastic PAs occurs in some patients after systemic-PA shunts or after establishing continuity between right ventricle and PA, leaving the VSD open. The latter procedure was employed by Millikan and associates[18] from Rochester, Minnesota, in 105 patients over an 8.5-year period. There were 12 (11%) hospital deaths and 11 (10%) late deaths before second stage repair. Twenty-five patients were awaiting late evaluation and the remaining 57 had follow-up studies, a mean of 33 months after initial palliation. In 31 (54%), final repair was deferred because of insufficient PA enlargement in 14, authorization abnormality in 9, or both in 8. The remaining 26 were advised to have second stage repair which was performed in 24. This included VSD closure in 24, RV outflow tract reconstruction in 18, relief of central PA stenosis in 14 and closure of systemic-PA collaterals in 10. There was 1 (4%) hospital death and 1 (4%) late death. Mean postrepair peak systolic RV–LV pressure ratio ranged between 0.32 and 1.0 (mean 0.67). Nineteen of 22 patients were followed and were in New York Heart Association class I or II. The authors believe this type of initial surgical treatment provides more rapid and complete PA growth and more efficient palliation than systemic-PA shunts. They indicate that the minimum acceptable size of PAs for permitting successful second stage repair is not precisely known. When the combined right and left PA *area* was ≥75% of normal, the postrepair RV–LV pressure ratio was <0.86 in all but 1 patient. Selection of patients for final repair includes those with adequate PA size as indicated above, distribution of unobstructed confluent PAs equivalent to at least 1 whole lung, and the presence of a predominant left-to-right shunt at the ventricular level in the absence of a restrictive RV–PA connection.

TETRALOGY OF FALLOT

Operative treatment

Vargas and colleagues[19] from Buenos Aires, Argentina, reported their experience with 77 patients who underwent surgical repair of TF with subarterial VSD. In this entity, the conal septum is absent or rudimentary and the VSD is committed to both the aortic and pulmonary valve rings. The initial 8 patients who underwent operation by these authors, did not have an enlarging patch placed either in the RV outflow tract or across the pulmonary valve anulus. There were 4 hospital deaths, each related to residual RV hypertension. It was thus recognized that closure of the subarterial VSD reduces the size of the infundibulum and results in postrepair RV outflow tract obstruction. A transanular patch was thought necessary for most and it was employed in 80% of the subsequent 49 patients with 2 hospital deaths (4%). In the most recent series of 20 patients, a transanular patch was employed in only 20% and a patch confined to the RV infundibulum in 75%. There was 1 hospital death (mortality 5%). The authors no longer recommend routine transanular patching in this entity but believe the pulmonary valve and its anulus can be preserved in most and residual RV hypertension avoided by the placement of an enlarging patch confined to the RV infundibulum.

A variety of surgical approaches have been used to manage the severely symptomatic neonate with TF and absent pulmonary valve. A uniform method of management has not yet been established and overall results have been mediocre. Ilbawi and associates[20] from Chicago, Illinois, reported their experience in 4 neonates treated during the first month of life with ligation of the main PA and insertion of a polytetrafluoroethylene systemic-PA shunt. The 2 survivors underwent operation at 2 and 3 days of age and achieved good palliation through 19 months of follow-up. The other 2 patients underwent operation at 3 and 4 weeks of age after unsuccessful medical treatment and ultimately died of sepsis and respiratory failure within 5 months of operation. The authors believe that this limited experience suggests that early palliation of this type will decrease the need for prolonged preoperative and postoperative ventilation and improve the outcome of these seriously ill neonates.

The high rate of premature calcification and degeneration of porcine heterograft valves placed in the aortic or mitral position or in extracardiac conduits has discredited their use in the pediatric population. Ilbawi et al[21] from Chicago, Illinois, reported their experience with 49 patients between 2 and 20 years of age who underwent *stent-mounted porcine valve insertion for control of pulmonary regurgitation after repair of TF*. In 9 the valve was placed at the initial repair and in 40 between 2 and 5 years postoperatively. Prosthetic valve stenosis or regurgitation occurred in 7 (14%) patients, 3–8 years after insertion, including 1 after bacterial endocarditis. The complication-free actuarial life of the bioprosthesis was 82% and the functional actuarial life was 84% at 10 years. Six of 17 (35%) valves with a diameter of ≤25 mm became dysfunctional, compared with only 1 of 32 (3%) of valves with a diameter of ≥27 mm. The actuarial functional life of smaller valves was <30% at 7 years compared with >95% at 10 years for the larger diameters. The degree of residual RV hypertension after valve replacement was also a factor determining late valve durability. Five of the 10 patients with a postrepair RV/LV pressure ratio of ≥50% had valve failure compared with only 2 (5%) among 39 whose pressure ratio was ≤50%. The actuarial functional life of the former group was 0% at 7 years compared with >90% at 10 years in the latter. The authors concluded that the porcine valve has satisfactory durability in the pulmonary position and that accelerated degeneration occurs with high RV pressure or small (<25 mm) anular size.

COMPLETE TRANSPOSITION OF THE GREAT ARTERIES

Arrhythmias after the Mustard operation

Hayes and associates[22] from New York, New York, presented follow-up data on 95 patients with TGA who underwent a Mustard intraatrial baffle operation. The patients were followed by scalar electrocardiography and 24-hour ambulatory monitoring. Twenty percent of patients had atrial arrhythmias at hospital discharge and new rhythm disturbances were recognized during each year of follow-up. By 6 years 75% had atrial rhythm disorders. Slow junctional rhythm was the most common abnormality found but complete heart block did not occur. SVT occurred late in 8 patients and was not documented before postoperative discharge. The incidence of sudden death was 3%. Six patients had pacemaker insertion with no deaths. These authors present very interesting data indicating the increasing incidence of atrial rhythm disturbances with long-term follow-up of the atrial baffle procedure. As with other studies, it appears that patients at risk for sudden death are those who had tachyarrhythmias that may or may not be associated with a bradycardia/tachycardia syndrome. Bradycardia in the range of 30–40 beats/minute during sleep was almost never associated with symptoms. Pacemakers were inserted for patients who had heart rates <30 beats/minute, patients with Stokes-Adams episodes, patients with a need for drug therapy other than digitalis for SVT, and patients with poor ventricular function with bradycardia, particularly those with documented ventricular ectopic activity.

Gillette and associates[23] from Charleston, South Carolina, and Houston, Texas, reported the use of pacemakers for 29 patients aged 3–19 years studied a mean of 5.5 years after the Mustard repair of TGA. Symptoms referrable to bradycardia were eliminated in each case and 4 patients who received an antitachycardia pacemaker no longer have symptomatic SVT. There have been 4 reoperations, 3 because of lead problems and 1 because of traumatic erosion of the pacemaker. Transvenous implantation was attempted in 18 patients and was successful in 16. These authors have had good results from the use of pacemakers and they have pioneered using the transvenous implant in younger pediatric patients. Their recommendations for use of a pacemaker include syncope or near syncope due to bradycardia, need for drugs other than digitalis, bradycardia <40 beats/minute while awake and/or ≤30 beats/minute while asleep.

Butto and associates[24] from Minneapolis, Minnesota, used transesophageal electrodes to study and treat 51 episodes of SVT in 13 patients with TGA who had undergone atrial baffle procedures. Tachycardia conversion was accomplished using 4 to 10 stimuli 9.9 ms in duration at 20–28 mA with an interstimulus interval of 50–100 ms < atrial cycle length. Esophageal stimulation converted 48 of 51 tachycardia episodes to sinus or junctional rhythm. Ten episodes in 6 patients were transiently converted to AF lasting 3 seconds–28 minutes. Acceleration of ventricular rate necessitated direct-current cardioversion in 1 episode. These authors have provided further data on the use of transesophageal treatment of SVT. A major problem with this technique has been patient acceptance. By shortening the number of stimuli, patient acceptance apparently has been increased significantly. Their protocol should be studied and tried by all physicians who have had difficulty in obtaining patient acceptance for this procedure.

Pulmonary venous obstruction after Mustard or Senning procedure

Smallhorn and associates[25] from Toronto, Canada, evaluated 63 patients after atrial repair of TGA using pulsed Doppler echocardiography. Using apical or subcostal 4-chamber orientation, satisfactory imaging and Doppler data were obtained in all patients. Obstruction produced a specific high velocity turbulent pattern either at midbaffle or at pulmonary venous atrium level. These authors have demonstrated the usefulness of Doppler recordings to diagnose pulmonary venous obstruction after atrial repair of transposition. Unfortunately, this complication can occur not only early but late after repair. The obstruction can become quite significant before symptoms occur. This modality should provide an easy and reliable method to demonstrate this problem early in its course.

The arterial switch operation

Quaegebeur and colleagues[26] from Leiden, Holland, presented a comprehensive analysis of 66 patients who underwent an arterial switch operation during an 8-year period. Twenty-three had TGA with intact ventricular septum, 33 TGA with large VSD and 10 with double-outlet right ventricle (DORV) with a subpulmonary VSD. There were 8 (12%) hospital deaths: 1 (4%) of 23 with TGA and intact septum; 6 (18%) of 33 with TGA, VSD; and 1 (10%) with DORV. Hospital mortality markedly decreased over the years so that between 1983 and 1985 it approached 0. The actuarial late survival (including hospital deaths) at 11 months was 81% for the 33 patients alive at that time. No additional deaths occurred among survivors alive at that time and followed for as long as 8 years. Low birth weight, TGA and VSD, DORV, PDA, earlier date of operation, and possibly a longer aortic cross-clamp time were incremental risk factors for death. Weight at operation, coronary artery anatomy and great artery position were not risk factors. Equations generated from this data predict a 1-year survival rate, including hospital mortality, after the arterial switch operation in 1985 at 100% for neonates with TGA and intact septum, and 100% for those with TGA and VSD, or DORV. Thus, the good late functional status, and the presence of sinus rhythm in 96% of the 55 surviving patients, indicates the superiority of this type of repair. This carefully analyzed superb surgical experience with the arterial switch operation will serve in the future as the basis for comparison for other series. It should be carefully studied by all interested in surgery for congenital heart disease.

The Jatene type of arterial switch operation is being applied with increased frequency to the various types of TGA. Since accurate transfer of the coronary arteries is essential to the success of this procedure, Kurosawa and associates[27] from Tokyo, Japan, reviewed the coronary anatomy present among 40 patients with varying types of TGA who underwent the Jatene operation. The overall perioperative mortality was 12.5%. There were 16 patients with TGA and intact septum, 11 of whom had undergone a previous PA banding and Blalock shunt. Coronary anatomy was normal (Shaher type 1) in 14 (88%) of this group. There were 12 patients with an aligned infundibular septum and a perimembranous VSD, 8 of whom had normal coronary anatomy. In contrast, this was present in only 4 of 12 patients with an anteriorly displaced infundibular septum and a malaligned VSD. The great arteries were anteroposteriorly related in 25 of the 40 patients and the coronary anatomy was normal in 22 (88%). In contrast, there were 3 patients with side-by-side great arteries and the coronary anatomy was normal in none, while among 12 patients with right obliquely related great arteries it was normal in 4. The authors beautifully detail the various types of coronary anatomy encountered and indicate the importance of understanding their variability. They believe that displacement of the infundibular septum not only determines the type of VSD and hemodynamics, but also often relates to the specific coronary anatomy. Hospital mortality was unrelated to coronary artery variations. They believe that displacement of the infundibular septum is important in determining the method of repair and recommend intraventricular rerouting when the great arteries are side-by-side and the VSD malaligned, and the Jatene type of arterial switch in the remaining type.

Left ventricular function before and after arterial repair

Arensman and associates[28] from Middlesex and London, UK, and Augusta, Georgia, studied LV function before and after arterial repair of TGA using computer-assisted analysis of 78 echocardiograms from 27 patients obtained 1 year before to 5 years after operation. Simple TGA was present in 16 of 27 patients and 11 of 27 had complex TGA with additional large VSD. Immediately after repair shortening fraction decreased from 46–33% with a corresponding drop in normalized peak shortening rate from 5.4–3.3 s^{-1}; normal septal motion was usually absent. Shortening fraction increased with time after repair and LV dimension increased appropriately for age. Septal motion was commonly absent after operation but improved subsequently. At 6 months after operation only 48% had absent septal motion and 20% had decreased septal motion. These data indicate the marked changes in LV contraction pattern which occurred after arterial repair of TGA. Despite obvious abnormalities in septal motion which are well known to occur after surgery, most of these patients have shown normal contractile function (Circulation 1983; 69:106–112). Further studies on assessment of contractile state and diastolic function would be quite useful in long-term assessment of the left ventricles in these patients.

Pulmonary trunk banding and arterial switching after the Mustard or Senning operation

Severe RV dysfunction occurs in 2–10% of patients within 10 years after venous switching by either the Mustard or Senning technique for TGA. Cardiac transplantation or a 2-stage operation consisting of initial preparation of the left ventricle by PA banding and later debanding, dismantling the atrial repair and arterial switching are potential surgical options. Thus, Mee[29] from Melbourne, Australia, reported his experience with anatomic repair in 2 patients. One had severe RV failure after undergoing VSD closure and a Senning procedure at 5 months of age. At age 2.5 years, a PA band was placed via a midline sternotomy incision and tightened to elevate the proximal PA systolic pressure to 60% of systemic. At catheter studies, 5 and 13 months later, this ratio was 0.58 and 1.0, respectively. Take-down of the Senning repair, debanding, and arterial switching were successfully accomplished with abolition of CHF, TR, and radionuclide demonstration of normal LV and RV function. A second patient underwent PA banding at the age of 10 years, after an initial Mustard operation at age 14 months and intervening severe RV failure. An LV/RV ratio of 0.52 was achieved and essentially persisted until age 14 years. Despite deteriorating LV function of uncertain etiology, the second stage procedure was performed successfully with a good result. This author recommends PA banding when decongestive therapy is needed for symptomatic RV dysfunction. An LV/RV pressure ratio of 0.55–0.65 should be achieved. The precise timing of debanding and arterial switching is not clear but may be guided by echocardiographic determination of LV wall thickness and catheter measurement of LV/RV pressures.

LEFT VENTRICULAR OUTFLOW OBSTRUCTION

Long-term results of open valvotomy for aortic valve stenosis

Hsieh and associates[30] from Boston, Massachusetts, reviewed the clinical course of 59 patients who underwent valvotomy for AS before 1968. All were >1 year of age at the time of operation and mean follow-up was 18 years. Actuarial analysis indicated that the probability of survival was 94% at 5 years and 77% at 22 years. Thirteen patients died, 7 suddenly. Among the latter, significant AS or AR was present in 4 of 7, 2 of 7 were symptomatic, and 2 of 7 had progression of a strain pattern on electrocardiography. Reoperation was carried out in 21 patients and 3 of 21 died. The probability of reoperation increased from 2% at 5 years to 44% at 22 years. Infective endocarditis occurred on 4 occasions in 3 patients with a frequency of 3.8 episodes/1,000 patient-years. Actuarial analysis of serious events defined as death, reoperation, and endocarditis indicated that the probability of being free of such an episode to be 92% at 5 years but decreased to 39% at 22 years.

Percutaneous transluminal balloon dilatation for discrete subaortic stenosis

Suarez de Lezo and associates[31] from Cordoba, Spain, reported percutaneous balloon dilatation of discrete subaortic stenosis in 7 patients aged 3–12 years. Peak LV pressure decreased from 181 ± 25–139 ± 11 mm Hg and peak systolic pressure gradient diminished from 65 ± 18–12 ± 9 mm Hg. Mild AR present in 6 patients before dilatation did not worsen. Four patients had reevaluation 7 ± 2 months later and had no significant increase in LV pressure or AR than that observed immediately after dilatation. These authors have presented a new indication for balloon dilatation.

Operative treatment of discrete and tunnel subaortic stenosis

Lavee and associates[32] from Tel Hashomer and Tel Aviv, Israel, reported a comparative experience among 42 patients who underwent surgical repair of discrete and tunnel type subaortic stenosis. Fifteen consecutive patients (group A) had "membranectomy" and myotomy, whereas 27 consecutive patients (group B) underwent "membranectomy" and myectomy. Two of group A and 9 of group B also had tunnel-type subaortic stenosis. There was no significant difference in the preoperative mean gradient across the LV outflow tract in each group. Postoperative cardiac catheterization studies at a mean follow-up period of 21 months showed a residual mean gradient of 29 ± 24 mmHg in group A and 10 ± 13 mmHg in group B, excluding those with tunnel-type obstruction. In the latter, mean postoperative gradients were 25 ± 7 and 30 ± 30 mmHg in groups A and B, respectively. The authors concluded that in the surgical management of discrete subaortic stenosis, deep myectomy in addition to membranectomy produces better relief of the LV outflow tract obstruction than does membranectomy and myotomy. In those with tunnel-type subaortic stenosis, myectomy is less effective than in the nontunnel type, but still produces acceptable results and may permit delay of more radical procedures.

AORTIC ISTHMIC COARCTATION

Echocardiographic studies in neonates

Morrow and associates[33] from Houston, Texas, performed quantitative analysis of the great vessels using 2-D echocardiography in 14 neonates with isolated coarctation and 14 normal control infants <1 month old. Coarctation patients showed transverse arch and isthmus diameters which were significantly smaller than in control subjects while the pulmonary valve and pulmonary trunk were significantly greater than in normal neonates. The descending aorta was not different between the 2 groups but the right innominate artery and the left carotid artery were significantly larger in the coarctation patients. These authors present interesting data regarding transverse arch hypoplasia and increased pulmonary valve and PA diameters in neonates with coarctation. These findings suggest decreased aortic arch flow and increased PA to PDA flow *in utero*. The data also indicate that postnatal constriction of the PDA is not the sole etiology for neonatal coarctation but that abnormalities are present before birth. Thus subtle abnormalities of the mitral or aortic valve might lead to decreased systemic flow early during fetal development with resultant decrease in isthmus size and progressive increase in LV afterload. These echocardiographic measurements can help considerably in making the echocardiographic diagnosis of coarctation in the young infant.

Doppler flow studies

Sanders and associates[34] from Boston, Massachusetts, studied 30 patients with unoperated coarctation, 9 patients with repaired coarctation, and 6 patients with interrupted arch or severe coarctation with large PDA using Doppler echocardiography to assess flow profile in the descending aorta. Control data were taken from 62 patients with various lesions without coarctation, including dilated cardiomyopathy and AS. The most useful discriminator was the peak systolic-to-peak diastolic frequency shift ratio that showed virtually no overlap with any of the other patient groups. Acceleration rate and time-to-peak velocity showed overlap both with cardiomyopathy and AS patients. Patients with coarctation or interrupted arch plus large PDA had normal Doppler profiles. These investigators have provided new data on attempting to make the diagnosis of coarctation in the infant or young child with coarctation. This is usually not a difficult diagnosis in patients with isolated coarctation and a constricted PDA. The authors also illustrated a well-known phenomenon in which a patient with a dilated PDA may show none of the typical signs of coarctation. In the era of early prostaglandin infusion, this finding limits the usefulness of Doppler data for coarctation diagnosis.

Magnetic resonance imaging

Boxer and associates[35] from Manhassett and Brooklyn, New York, studied 10 patients with coarctation of the aorta using magnetic resonance imaging. In all studies the sagittal and 60° left anterior oblique imaging planes adequately revealed the anatomy of the coarctation. Post-treatment imaging studies demonstrated effective relief in all patients. These authors present further data on the use of this new modality for coarctation imaging. This provides a new method for follow-up of coarctation patients particularly those in whom the question of aneurysm or recoarctation occurs. This should be particularly useful for studies of patients who have undergone balloon angioplasty.

Operative therapy

Kopf et al[36] from New Haven, Connecticut, reviewed their initial 5-year experience with repair of coarctation in 25 infants <3 months of age by subclavian flap angioplasty in 23, and pericardial patch aortoplasty in 2. There was 1 (4%) hospital death in a patient with an associated AV canal defect with RV dominance and a small LV cavity. Surviving patients were followed for an average of 61 months. There were 4 (17%) late deaths, each occurring in patients with additional severe intracardiac anomalies. Recurrent coarctation developed in 3 (13%) as defined by arm-to-leg gradients >15 mmHg. One underwent a patch aortoplasty at 18 months of age and the remaining 2 had balloon dilatation which was successful in 1. Overall, the actuarial freedom from recurrent coarctation was 88% at 96 months. However, among 14 patients who underwent repair at <2 weeks of age, there were 3 (21%) recurrences. The authors experience supports continued use of the subclavian flap angioplasty for infants with symptomatic coarctation. Their data also support avoiding concomitant PA banding for those with coexistent isolated VSD but recommend it for extremely small infants with VSD and additional complex cardiac disease.

Coarctation of the aorta, isolated or when associated with complex intracardiac defects, sometimes requires repair during the first month of life. Both the method of repair and the advisability of concomitant PA banding for certain subsets, remain controversial. Goldman and colleagues[37] from Denver, Colorado, reviewed their experience over a 7-year period with 64 neonates <30 days of age. Repair was performed by resection and end-to-end anastomosis in 6, patch aortoplasty using the subclavian flap in 48, the carotid artery in 2, and prosthetic material in 8. Preoperatively, patients were managed with prostaglandin E_1 infusion, correction of acidosis, and control of hypotension with dopamine. All patients were kept normothermic during the procedure. There were no early and 2 (7%) late deaths among 31 patients with isolated coarctation. Eighteen patients had a hemodynamically significant VSD and in addition to coarctation repair, PA banding was used in 7. There was 1 early and 2 late deaths. Fifteen patients had coarctation with large VSD as part of complex intracardiac defects. PA banding was used in 11 with 0 early and 2 late deaths, compared with 3 early and 1 late death among the 4 patients undergoing coarctation repair alone. Five (11%) patients who had subclavian flap aortoplasty required reoperation for recurrent coarctation. Residual ductal tissue may have played a role in this. This experience showed no significant difference in early or late mortality or duration of postoperative ventilator support, whether or not PA banding was added to coarctation repair in patients with associated isolated VSD. In contrast, a significantly lower mortality was present when PA banding was added to coarctation repair in those with a complex intracardiac lesion in addition to a large VSD. Therefore, the authors conclude that simultaneous PA banding should be used only for those with associated complex intracardiac defects. This experience helps to clarify the management of patients with coarctation associated with isolated VSD and with other complex defects. With regard to those with simple coarctation, considerable evidence is mounting to indicate that juxtacoarctation ductile tissue may be responsible for a disappointing incidence of recurrent coarctation after subclavian flap aortoplasty when performed during the first month of life. Excision of all ductal tissue coupled with repair by either end-to-end anastomosis or modified subclavian flap aortoplasty seems available.

Recognizing that recurrent coarctation occurs in some patients after subclavian flap aortoplasty, Sanchez et al[38] from Philadelphia, Pennsylvania, reviewed the records of 26 infants who underwent this procedure during the first 3 months of life. The coarctation was isolated in 12, associated with a significant VSD in 8, and with complex intracardiac anomalies in 6. There were 3 (12%) early deaths; over the follow-up period from 1.5 to 66 months (median 12), 5 (22%) survivors, each undergoing operation at <14 days of age, had severe recoarctation 1.5–6 months (median = 5) after repair. The obstruction appeared due to lumen obliteration by a shelf-like posterior wall tissue believed related to intrinsic abnormalities of the periductal aortic wall. Recoarctation correlated with younger age at aortoplasty but not with weight at operation. The authors concluded that other methods of repair should be considered in infants <3 weeks of age at operation but that the subclavian flap aortoplasty produces excellent results in older infants.

Division of the left subclavian artery is routinely employed in the classical subclavian flap aortoplasty for repair of coarctation of the aorta. Meier and associates[39] from Rio de Janeiro, Porto Allegre, and Aracaju, Brazil, reported their experience with 28 patients who underwent a new technique of coarctation repair. This method utilizes the left subclavian artery as an aortoplasty without distal division. The method consists of mobilization of the left subclavian artery, detaching it from its aortic origin, with an attached additional flap of the anterior wall of the aortic isthmus. A longitudinal incision is carried through the coarctate segment onto the distal aorta. The subclavian artery is incised posteriorly and translocated distally to be reimplanted on the aortic incision. This results in enlargement of the coarctate segment by the subclavian artery and also preserves blood flow to the left arm. Patients ranged in age from 2 months–25 years (mean 4 ± 5 years). There were no hospital deaths and the mean follow-up was 10 months. Postoperatively, femoral pulses were present in each patient and Doppler measurements showed normal pressures in the left arm and absent arm-leg pressure gradients. One late death occurred 7 months after coarctation repair, after an atrial switch operation for TGA. Four patients underwent recatheterization between 4 and 12 months postoperatively. Adequate correction was demonstrated and normal aortic growth at the coarctation site suggested. The authors believe this is the procedure of choice for most patients with coarctation of the aorta.

Hehrlein and colleagues[40] from Giessen and Bad Nauheim, Federal Republic of Germany, reported their experience with 317 patients who underwent repair of coarctation by either transverse closure of a longitudinal incision through the coarctate segment (group A), or enlargement of this longitudinal incision with a woven Dacron® or Teflon® patch (group B). Fifty-four patients were <12 months of age and 263 were >12 months of age at repair. The hospital mortality was 15% and 3%, respectively. During reinvestigation late postoperatively, an aneurysm at the site of repair was diagnosed in 18 of 285 group B patients and in none of 32 group A patients. Reoperation was performed in 15 of the 18 patients. Excision of the posterior ridge had been performed at the primary procedure in 12 of the 15 patients and the authors believe this is an essential predisposing factor for the development of late aneurysms. Microscopic examination of the aneurysmal wall revealed degeneration of the media in more than half of the patients. Aneurysms occurred whether silk suture or Prolene suture was used. The youngest patient in this group at the time of the primary procedure was 10 years of age and the mean age for the group with postoperative aneurysms was 20 years at the time of initial repair. The aneurysms occurred between 4 and 18 years after the initial surgical procedure. The authors concluded that in children >4 years of age, excision of the posterior fibrous ridge should be avoided. Synthetic patch graft repair of the coarctation should be viewed critically and used with limitation.

CONGENITALLY CORRECTED TRANSPOSITION

Ventricular function

Benson and associates[41] from Toronto, Canada, studied 8 asymptomatic patients with corrected transposition using equilibrium RNA at rest and during supine bicycle exercise. Ages ranged from 7–32 years and 5 patients had normal intracardiac hemodynamics, 2 had trivial AV valve regurgitation, and 1 had trivial PS. Average exercise duration was 11 ± 1 minute with limitation due only to fatigue. Normal increases in heart rate of 225% and systolic BP of 152% were found at peak exercise. Pulmonary ventricular EF at rest was 51% and did not change significantly at peak stress, 53%. Systemic ventricular EF was 48% at rest and increased to 64% at peak exercise. These authors presented further interesting data in patients with corrected transposition without significant associated intracardiac defects. Only 1 patient had a low value for systemic ventricular ejection at rest and all had a significant increase in exercise. In contrast, the pulmonary ventricle had low values in most patients at rest and a failure to increase the EF with exercise in all but 1 patient. The reason for the pulmonary ventricular dysfunction is unclear. The data on the systemic ventricle suggests that factors other than the RV functioning against systemic afterload contribute to the abnormal RVEF in patients with complete transposition who have undergone atrial repair.

Rhythm and conduction disturbances

Daliento and associates[42] from Padova, Italy, studied 17 patients with congenitally corrected transposition and no other complicating cardiac anomalies. Patient age ranged from 5–54 years and follow-up ranged from 5–37 years. Twenty-four-hour monitoring was performing in 15 of 17 and electrophysiologic studies, in 10 of 17 patients. There was 1 death: a 54-year-old woman died suddenly with complete AV block. Fifteen patients were without symptoms and 2 of 17 reported palpitations since childhood. First-degree AV block occurred in 2 of 17 and complete AV block in 5 of 17 patients. Electrophysiologic studies confirmed that AV block was supra-Hisian in 2 patients and proximal to the bifurcation in 1. Recurrent SVT was found in 2 patients and electrophysiologic study suggested a reentry mechanism, which in 1 patient was associated with a left lateral accessory pathway.

Holter monitoring showed significant ventricular arrhythmia in 8 and this finding was universal in the 4 patients studied with complete block. These investigators provide further data on conduction and rhythm disturbances in patients with corrected transposition. Complete AV block occurred at a mean age of 16 years with a range of from 4–30 years. Complete block was usually preceded by first and second-degree AV block. Unexpected ventricular arrhythmia and a sleeping heart rate <40 beats/minute were common in asymptomatic patients with complete heart block. The data indicate the need for careful follow-up and Holter monitoring in patients with corrected transposition who have complete heart block.

Systemic ventricular inflow and outflow obstruction

Marino and associates[43] from Boston, Massachusetts, studied 42 patients with congenitally corrected transposition using 2-D echocardiography. Obstruction of RV inflow and outflow was present and diagnosed by echocardiography in 5 of 42 patients. Diagnoses included supravalvular stenosing ring and subaortic obstruction due to infundibular hypertrophy in 3. In addition aortic coarctation was present in 4 of 42 patients and was diagnosed using suprasternal views. Systemic ventricular inflow and outflow obstruction was demonstrated in these studies in 12% of patients and thus is more common in this condition than previously recognized. Echocardiography is the ideal mode for diagnosing these important abnormalities.

Results of operative treatment

Lincoln and associates[44] from London, UK, studied 33 patients after anatomic correction of TGA or double-outlet right ventricle with subpulmonary VSD. There were no late deaths and clinical progress was excellent. Cardiac catheterization was performed in 17 patients 2 weeks–44 months after operation. Pressure gradients across RV outflow tract ranged from 5–72 mm Hg, being >40 mm Hg in 5 patients. No patient had important valvular regurgitation. LV function was assessed and was normal in most patients as was EF. Peak filling rate was increased above normal. Regional wall motion was abnormal in 7 of 11, showing anterior hypokinesia with delayed onset of inward wall motion. These authors presented interesting data showing a good functional result in TGA patients after arterial repair. These data, together with those from Harefield Hospital, also in London, UK, indicate excellent intermediate results for LV function in these patients. The wall motion abnormalities are of uncertain significance at this time and further long-term data are needed to evaluate the arterial repair.

MISCELLANEOUS TOPICS IN
PEDIATRIC CARDIOLOGY

Intracardiac blood flow studies in normal fetuses

Kenny and associates[45] from Boston, Massachusetts, used Doppler echocardiography to quantify changes in intracardiac flow velocities and RV and LV stroke volumes in 80 normal human fetuses from 19–41 weeks' gestation. Aortic and pulmonary diameters were measured at valve level and cross-sectional area calculated assuming a circular orifice. Diameters of PA and aorta increased linearly with gestational age, and PA diameter consistently exceeded aortic. In 44% of fetuses RV and LV stroke volumes were calculated with RV exceeding LV stroke volume by 28%. RV stroke volume increased exponentially from 0.7 ml at 20 weeks to 7.6 ml at 40 weeks and LV stroke volume from 0.7 ml at 20 weeks to 5.2 ml at 40 weeks. Flow velocity across tricuspid and mitral valves were consistently greater during atrial systole than during rapid ventricular filling. This is the latest attempt to determine whether or not RV dominance is present in the human fetus as it is in the lamb. These data suggest that there is a modest increase in RV -vs- LV output of approximately 25%, which is significantly less than the 50% greater RV output for the lamb. This difference is probably related to the much greater cerebral blood flow in the human -vs- the lamb fetus. These studies are useful in determining normal fetal cardiac development and thus may provide insight into changes in ventricular size and flow in fetuses with congenital anomalies.

Congenital heart disease in fetuses of mothers with a family history of congenital heart disease

Allan and associates[46] from London, UK, used fetal echocardiography to study recurrence rates in 1,021 mothers with a family history of congenital heart disease. The overall recurrence rate was 1 of 52 with a previously affected child and 1 of 10 with 2 previously affected children. Aortic valve atresia was associated with a recurrence rate of 1 of 28, coarctation of the aorta at a rate of 1 of 15, complex congenital heart disease at a rate of 1 of 11, and truncus arteriosus at 1 of 13. These findings indicate a much higher recurrence rate, particularly of complex defects, aortic valve atresia, and aortic coarctation than can be explained on the current polygenic theory. Fetal echocardiography may assume increasing importance, particularly for those mothers with a family history of defects that have a considerable increase in recurrence risk, than that previously considered.

Doppler echocardiography in patent ductus arteriosus

Swensson and associates[47] from San Diego, California, used Doppler color flow mapping to examine flow in the PA in 31 premature and term infants aged 4 hours–9 months with PDA as an isolated lesion or associated with other heart defects. The patterns were compared with 15 infants who did not have PDA with unconstricted PDA. Flow from aorta into PA was detected in late systole and early diastole along the superior leftward lateral wall of the main PA from the origin of the left PA back in a proximal direction toward the pulmonary valve. In constricted PDA and in associated with cyanotic heart disease, the position of the ductal shunt in the PA was more variable and often directed centrally or medially. Waveform spectral Doppler sampling could be performed in specific positions guided by the Doppler flow map to verify the phasic characteristics of the ductal shunt on spectral and audio outputs. Shunts through a small PDA were routinely detected in this group of infants and right-to-left ductal shunts could also be verified by the Doppler flow technique. These authors who have been in the forefront of evaluating Doppler color flow mapping have demonstrated the usefulness of this technique in detecting small PDA and right-to-left shunting. Although these diagnoses can usually be made with standard sector scanning and

Doppler techniques without color flow mapping, this technique shows promise for making such diagnoses more rapidly as well as providing a direct semiquantitative indication of shunt size.

Doppler echocardiography in total anomalous pulmonary venous connection

Smallhorn and Freedom[48] from Toronto, Canada, evaluated 38 patients with total anomalous pulmonary venous connection using pulsed Doppler echocardiography. There were no associated intracardiac anomalies in 29 of 38 patients, and 9 of 38 had complex intracardiac anatomy with low pulmonary flow. Multiple drainage sites were present in patients with venous obstruction. Flow in individual pulmonary veins and ascending or descending vein was nonphasic and varied only with respiration with obstruction. Flow in the absence of obstruction was phasic and varied with the cardiac cycle. Distal to the obstruction site the flow was nonlaminar and of high velocity irrespective of the amount of pulmonary blood flow (Fig. 8-2). These authors presented evidence for diagnosing obstruction or nonobstruction in this com-

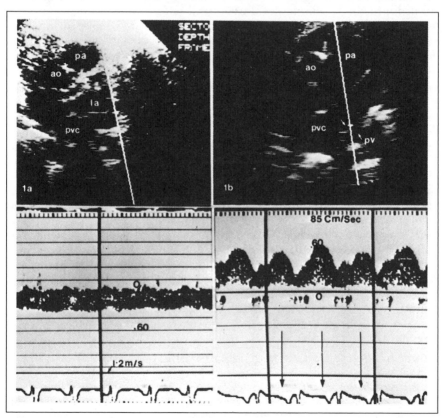

Fig. 8-2. a (left panels), Suprasternal frontal plane image with sample volume in a left upper lobe pulmonary vein (top). This patient had obstructed infracardiac drainage. Below is a Doppler spectral trace showing nonphasic flow. b (right panels), View with sample volume in a left pulmonary vein (pv) from a patient with unobstructed supracardiac total anomalous pulmonary venous connection. The spectral trace at bottom demonstrates phasic pulmonary venous flow. Biphasic and monophasic peaks are seen. ao = aorta; la = left atrium; pa = pulmonary artery; pvc = pulmonary venous confluence. Reproduced with permission from Smallhorn and Freedom.[48]

plex condition. The Doppler findings were quite useful regardless of whether there was associated complex intracardiac anatomy. These data are extremely helpful in evaluating preoperative patients with this condition.

Echocardiographic observations in the criss-crossed heart

Marino and associates[49] from Boston, Massachusetts, studied the echocardiographic anatomy of 14 patients aged 2 days–26 years with crisscrossed heart. Crossing of the AV valves could be seen in each case by scanning in a subxiphoid or apical 4-chamber view. Common anatomic features included normal viscera atrial situs and large VSD in all, TGA or double-outlet right ventricle in 13 of 14, subpulmonary stenosis with deficient subpulmonary infundibulum in 11 of 14, and subaortic infundibulum in 13 of 14 patients. Estimated RV sinus area was decreased in 7 patients with crisscrossed hearts in whom it could be measured and tricuspid valve diameter index was significantly smaller than age-matched controls. These authors present outstanding echocardiographic images of this complex anomaly. The article should be studied in detail by all physicians who deal with complex congenital heart disease. The particular combination of defects that are usually seen, which include large VSD, small right ventricle, and transposed great arteries or double-outlet right ventricle should alert physicians to this diagnosis.

Subaortic stenosis in the univentricular heart

Freedom and associates[50] from Toronto, Canada, examined 43 patients with univentricular hearts who underwent PA banding. Subaortic stenosis developed subsequent to banding in 31 of 43 patients (72%). The mean age at banding of those in whom AS developed was 0.21 years and stenosis was recognized at a mean age of 2.5 years. Stenosis usually resulted from progressive restriction of a wholly muscular interventricular communication. Banding of the PA may stimulate myocardial hypertrophy thus accelerating the potential for development of subaortic stenosis in these patients. These authors have presented further data on the development of subaortic stenosis in patients with univentricular hearts. This continues to be a problem that is difficult to treat and because of a tendency for recurrence after surgical enlargement of the interventricular communication. Experience with creation of a proximal PA-aortic window, transsection of the distal PA, and creation of a systemic-to-PA shunt indicates that this may be a preferred approach in the treatment of this unfortunate complication.

Home oxygen for Eisenmenger syndrome

Bowyer and associates[51] from London, UK, reported the use of long-term oxygen therapy at home for 9 children, ages 6 months–13 years with the Eisenmenger syndrome. Six additional children with similar findings were untreated. All had PA flow and pressures measured at cardiac catheterization and no significant change in PA pressure but a small change in pulmonary resistance with oxygen therapy. Long-term treatment consisted of home oxygen for a minimum of 12 hours/day for up to 5 years. Although a symptom score was devised and showed no difference between treated and untreated group, all 9 children receiving oxygen treatment survived while 5 of 6 not treated have died. This small study provides some new data on a difficult problem to study and to treat. It is suggestive that home oxygen may be beneficial in these patients and that a large-scale, carefully controlled trial might be useful in an attempt to improve the quality of life for this unfortunate group.

Changing trends in congenital heart disease in adults

Flanagan and associates[52] from Boston, Massachusetts, retrospectively analyzed 329 adults with congenital heart disease undergoing cardiac catheterization. All patients were >20 years of age. The diagnoses were divided into 5 groups: 1) simple left-to-right shunt lesions, including ASD, VSD, AV canal defect, and PDA; 2) simple valvular lesions, including PS, AS, subvalvular or supravalvular AS or PS, congenital AR, and isolated coarctation of the aorta; 3) multiple lesions, consisting of ≥2 distinct lesions such as coarctation with congenital MR or double-chambered right ventricle with VSD; 4) complex congenital heart disease including TF with or without pulmonary atresia, transposition complexes, single ventricle, tricuspid atresia, and Ebstein's malformation; and 5) hypertrophic cardiomyopathy. The patients also were divided into 2 groups, those undergoing cardiac catheterization from 1959–1964 and those having catheterization 1979–1984. The diagnoses in the patients having catheterization from 1979–1984 are summarized in Table 8-1. The frequency of ventricular dysfunction, dysrhythmia, and pulmonary vascular disease in the 202 patients seen from 1979–1984 are summarized in Table 8-2. Ventricular dysfunction was diagnosed by clinical features of CHF, LV end-diastolic pressure >12 mmHg or diminished systolic EF on angiography (<50%). Pulmonary vascular disease was deemed present when the pulmonary resistence was ≥5 Wood's units or 400 dynes s cm^{-5}. Dysrhythmias occurring within 5 years before or 1 year after cardiac catheterization were identified by review of the general medical records and electrocardiograms. Significant dysrhythmias were AF or flutter, SVT or VT, high-grade VPC, and second- and third-degree heart block. This retrospective analysis demonstrates that unlike 20 years ago, adults with congenital heart disease who now undergo cardiac catheterization often have more complex cardiovascular disease and have had prior surgery. Premature CAD is un-

TABLE 8-1. *Diagnostic distribution of complex CHD in 1979–1984. Reproduced with permission from Flanagan et al.*[52]

Ebstein's anomaly	5
Tricuspid atresia	6
Pulmonary atresia without VSD	0
Tetralogy of Fallot with pulmonary atresia	10
Tetralogy of Fallot	32
Simple d-transposition without VSD	0
Simple d-transposition with VSD	6
Complex d-transposition	1
l-Transposition	5
DORV	4
Single ventricle	9
Heterotaxy syndrome	3
TAPVC	2
Cor triatriatum	3
Truncus arteriosus	0
Other	1
Total	87

TABLE 8-2. *Acquired functional abnormalities (1979–1984, n = 202). Reproduced with permission from Flanagan et al.*[52]

	PERCENTAGE OF:		
	VENTRICULAR DYSFUNCTION	DYSRHYTHMIA	PULMONARY VASCULAR DISEASE
Simple shunt lesions	20/54(37)	22/54 (41)	12/54 (22)
<50 years age	5/38 (13)	6/38 (16)	8/38 (21)
>50 years age	15/16 (94)	16/16 (100)	4/16 (25)
Isolated valve lesions	12/44 (23)	4/44 (9)	1/44 (2)
Multiple lesions	7/16 (44)	3/16 (19)	5/16 (31)
Complex lesions	10/89 (11)	29/89 (33)	11/89 (12)
Hypertrophic cardiomyopathy	0/2 (0)	0/2 (0)	0/2 (0)
Surgery	13/117 (11)	31/117 (26)	9/117 (8)
Total	49/202 (24)	58/202 (29)	29/202 (14)
<50 years	29/179 (16)	41/179 (23)	25/179 (14)
>50 years	20/23 (87)	17/23 (74)	4/23 (17)

common. Ventricular dysfunction and dysrhythmias are common complications of congenital heart disease in adults.

Erythrocytosis in cyanotic congenital heart disease

Rosove and associates[53] from Los Angeles, California, studied 40 adults with cyanotic congenital heart disease and found 11 with especially pronounced erythrocytosis (mean hematocrit 66 ± 3%), repeatedly increasing hematocrit, recurring symptoms of hyperviscosity, and little or no shift of the hemoglobin/oxygen-dissociation curve. These patients were iron deficient as a result of many therapeutic phlebotomies; nevertheless their red-cell mass was comparable to that in iron-replete patients with similar, but stable, hematocrits. Iron repletion in the deficient patients resulted in rapidly increasing hematocrit and hyperviscosity. In 1 extreme case, erythropoiesis remained persistently iron deficient despite normal serum iron and ferritin levels. "Decompensated erythrocytosis" is an apt term for the excessive erythrocytic response and the associated phenomena.

Urate excretion in adults with cyanotic congenital heart disease

Ross and associates[54] from Los Angeles, California, studied renal function and urate metabolism in 10 adults ages 28–47 years with cyanotic congenital heart disease. Plasma uric acid was elevated in 9 of 10 patients but mean 24-hour excretion was normal while fractional excretion was low. Plasma creatinine concentration was normal; however, glomerular filtration rate was mildly reduced in all patients. Significant proteinuria was present in 3 of 10 patients and 1 patient was nephrotic. High plasma uric acid level was secondary to inappropriately low plasma uric acid excretion and not to urate overproduction. Elevated uric acid serves as a marker of abnormal intrarenal hemodynamics. These authors have made an important contribution to the understanding of the well-known clinical phenomenon, hyperuricemia, in older patients with cyanotic congenital heart disease. The patients in this study had an inability to normally excrete a water load, a finding which suggests hypoperfusion with increased reabsorption of fluid and urate from proximal tubules. These data provide important new information regarding this well-known complication of patients whose cyanosis is inadequately relieved by therapy for congenital defects.

Coronary arterial anomalies seen in adulthood

Roberts[55] from Bethesda, Maryland, reviewed major anomalies of coronary arterial origin seen in adulthood (Table 8-3) (Figs. 8-3, 8-4, 8-5, 8-6, 8-7 and 8-8).

Streptokinase for arterial and venous thrombus

LeBlanc and associates[56] from Vancouver, Canada, used low-dose streptokinase infusion in 8 children aged 6 days–11 years with aortic, aortico-PA or vena caval major thromboses. The thrombolytic agent was delivered to the area of thrombosis by percutaneously inserted catheters. The dose of streptokinase was 50–100 U/kg/hr. Therapy lasted for 2–11 days. Major bleeding occurred in 1 patient. Partial or complete lysis of clot occurred in 7 of 8 patients with major side effects of bleeding in only 1 patient. This therapy can be useful in selected infants and children with major thromboses. Careful patient follow-up in anticipation of possible bleeding problems are mandatory in this situation. Catheter-induced vascular thrombosis did not occur in this group.

Wessel and associates[57] from Boston, Massachusetts, reviewed 1,000 consecutive patients undergoing catheterization to determine the safety and efficacy of systemic fibrinolytic therapy for treatment of femoral thrombosis. Retrograde arterial catheterization was carried out in 771 patients, including 31 who had transarterial balloon dilatation procedures and all patients were given systemic heparin at the time of arterial cannulation. The overall incidence of femoral thrombosis was 28 of 771 (3.6%) including 12 of 31 (39%) patients undergoing balloon dilatation. Thrombosis occurred mainly in young patients with 27 of 28 weight <14 kg. After continuing heparin therapy for an average treatment period of 33 hours, 16 patients continued to have a pulseless extremity and were treated with streptokinase for an average duration of 13 hours. Normal pulses and systolic BP returned in 14 of 16 (88%) and were nearly normal in one other patient. The incidence of bleeding at the arterial puncture site in the streptokinase-treated patients was 25% and was highest in the patients who had a balloon dilation procedure. These authors present very detailed information regarding the risks of arterial thrombosis at cardiac catheterization in young patients. They have documented the increased morbidity associated with transarterial balloon dilatation procedures and have indicated that streptokinase therapy can be helpful in this situation. These data should be read carefully by all those who perform catheterizations in young children. It would appear that the risk of arterial thrombosis must be weighed before proceeding with transarterial balloon dilatation procedures in each individual patient.

Ventricular dimensions in tricuspid valve atresia after operative therapy

Graham and associates[58] from London, UK, compared echocardiographic measurements of LV wall stress and contractile function in 23 patients with tricuspid valve atresia after palliation only, in 19 patients after Fontan repair,

TABLE 8-3. *Anomalies of coronary arterial origin. Reproduced with permission from Roberts.*[55]

I. *Origin of 1 or more coronary arteries from the pulmonary trunk (PT) and 1 or more coronary arteries from the aorta*
  A. Left main (LM) from PT
  B. Right (R) from PT
  C. Left anterior descending (LAD) from PT
  D. Left circumflex (LC) from PT
  E. Accessory coronary artery from PT
II. Origin of 1 or 2 coronary arteries from the pulmonary trunk without origin of a coronary artery from the aorta
  A. R and LM from PT
  B. "Single coronary artery" from PT
III. *Anomalous origin of 1 or more coronary arteries from the aorta*
  A. LM and R from right aortic sinus
  B. LM and R from left aortic sinus
  C. LM and R from the posterior aortic sinus
  D. R and LC from right aortic sinus (or LC from R) and LAD from left sinus
  E. R and LAD from right aortic sinus (or LAD from R) and LC from left sinus
  F. R from posterior aortic sinus and LM from left sinus
  G. LM from posterior aortic sinus and R from right sinus
  H. LAD and LC from a separate ostium in the left aortic sinus and R from right aortic sinus
IV. *Origin of only 1 coronary artery from the aorta without origin of a coronary artery from the PT (single coronary ostium)*
  A. From the right aortic sinus
    1. R crosses crux and continues as the LC which continues as the LAD
    2. LM from R
      a. Coursing of LM posterior to aorta before dividing into LAD and LC
      b. Coursing of LM between aorta and PT before branching into LAD and LC
      c. Coursing of LM anterior to PT
      d. Coursing of LM in ventricular septum beneath right ventricular infundibulum
    3. LAD and LC from R with coursing of LC posterior to aorta and LAD anterior to right ventricle (RV)

4. LAD from R with coursing anterior to RV with R crossing crux to form LC
5. LAD from R with coursing between aorta and PT with R crossing crux to continue as LC
6. LAD from R with coursing between aorta and PT and LC from R with retroaortic course
7. LAD from R coursing anterior to RV, LC from R coursing between aorta and PT
8. LAD from R coursing retroaortic with R crossing crux to continue as LC
9. LAD from R with coursing to left side in ventricular septum beneath right ventricular outflow tract and LC from R with retroaortic course to left atrioventricular sulcus
  B. From left aortic sinus
    1. LAD and LC from single coronary artery with LC crossing crux to continue as R
    2. R, LAD, and LC from single coronary artery
      a. R posterior to aorta
      b. R between aorta and PT
      c. R anterior to RV
    3. R and LC from single coronary artery and LAD from R
      a. R between aorta and PT
      b. R posterior to aorta
    4. R and LAD from single coronary artery and of LC from LAD
      a. R between aorta and PT
      b. R posterior to PT
  C. From posterior aortic sinus
    1. Single coronary artery between aorta and PT with trifurcation into R, LAD, and LC
    2. Single coronary artery to left of PT with trifurcation into R, LAD, and LC
    3. Single coronary artery to right and when anterior to aorta giving rise to R and LM which subdivides into LAD and LC

and in 24 age-matched normal subjects. End-diastolic dimensions were increased above normal in both tricuspid atresia groups but palliation -vs- Fontan groups were similar. In addition, LV end-diastolic volume and wall mass were increased above normal in both patient groups, with both volume and mass showing greater values in palliated -vs- Fontan patients. Meridional end-systolic stress was increased in both patient groups. Contractile func-

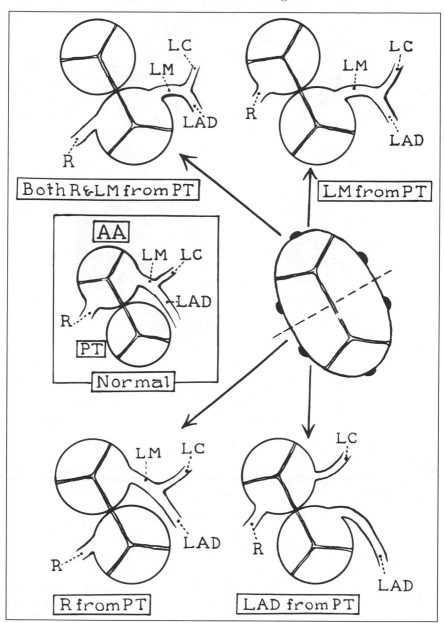

Fig. 8-3. Diagram illustrating the common arterial trunk arising from the heart in its early development with six potential coronary arterial ostia and the possible coronary anomalies resulting when inappropriate ostia do not regress. *AA* = ascending aorta; *LAD* = left anterior descending coronary artery; *LC* = left circumflex coronary artery; *LM* = left main coronary artery; *PT* = pulmonary trunk; *R* = right coronary artery. Reproduced with permission from Roberts.[55]

tion estimated by rate-corrected circumferential fiber shortening velocity as a function of end-systolic stress was abnormal in 9 of 23 (39%) palliated patients and in 5 of 23 (26%) Fontan patients. Contractile function was depressed in 1 of 11 palliated patients younger than 5 years of age and in 8 of 12 older than 5.3 years. These studies reveal that despite Fontan repair in tricuspid valve atresia LV volume overload and hypertrophy remain and abnormal contractile function persists in a significant number of patients. Ab-

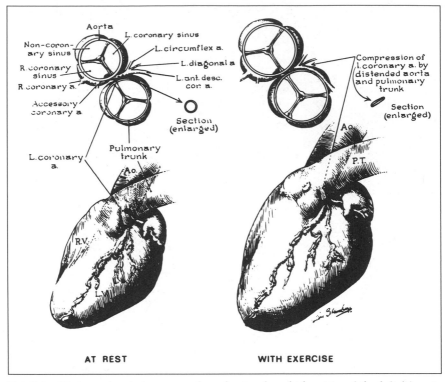

Fig. 8-4. Diagram showing a proposed mechanism by which origin of the left (L) main coronary artery (a) from the right sinus of Valsalva causes nonfatal or fatal cardiac dysfunction. Reproduced with permission from Roberts.[55]

normal contractile function is prevalent in patients >5 years of age with palliation only and suggests that earlier Fontan repair could result in improved late contractile function.

Exercise tolerance after the Fontan operation

Driscoll and associates[59] from Rochester, Minnesota, compared the results for graded exercise response of 81 patients with tricuspid valve atresia or functional single ventricle studied preoperatively with those of 29 patients studied postoperatively. Postoperative patients ranged in age from 4–36 years at the time of Fontan operation and from 6–36 years at the time of exercise testing. Total work performed was 25% of predicted preoperatively and increased to 37% postoperatively. Duration of exercise was 42% preoperatively and increased to 58% postoperatively. Maximal oxygen uptake averaged 43% preoperatively and increased to 50% postoperatively. A negative correlation was found between the age at exercise and exercise tolerance both preoperatively and postoperatively. Patients with a direct RA-PA connection had greater exercise tolerance than those with RA-RV connection. ST-T segment abnormalities occurred in 27% of preoperative patients and 38% of postoperative patients. Cardiac arrhythmia was noted at rest in 14% of preoperative and 21% of postoperative patients. Arrhythmia during exercise was present in 28% at rest and in 38% during exercise. These authors demonstrated improvement in exercise response after Fontan operation. The response to exercise, however, remains abnormal in most patients even after successful repair. The negative correlation between age and exercise tolerance postoperatively provides further suggestive evidence that there is deterioration of ventricular pump function that results from chronic volume overload and cyanosis in the functional single ventricle.

MISCELLANEOUS TOPICS IN PEDIATRIC CARDIAC SURGERY

Operative treatment of absent pulmonic valve syndrome

Karl and colleagues[60] from London, UK, reviewed their experience with 19 children aged 5 days–11 years who received various forms of surgical treatment over a 7-year period. There were 9 infants <1 year of age with intractable respiratory symptoms and CHF, 5 of whom required preoperative ventilation. All patients had patch closure of the VSD and reconstruction of the RV outflow tract using a patch alone in 2, orthotopic xenograft valve insertion in 2, homograft monocusp patch in 5, Dacron® xenograft conduit in 1, or aortic homograft valved conduit in 8. Each of the older children survived operation, but among the 9 infants, there were 5 hospital deaths. The mean age at operation for the infant group was 17 weeks (SD = 10 weeks). The 4 survivors in the infant group each had insertion of an aortic homograft valved conduit and resection of the main PA and the anterior portion of the right and left branches. The authors recommended complete intracardiac

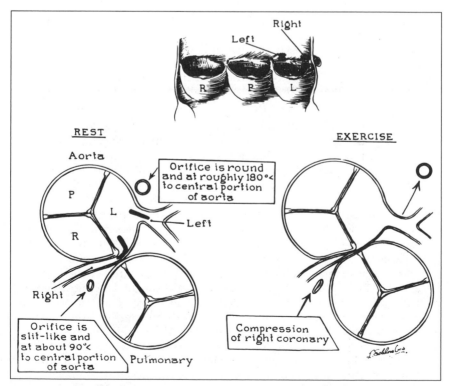

Fig. 8-5. Diagram showing mechanism by which origin of the right coronary artery arising from the left sinus of Valsalva might cause fatal or nonfatal cardiac dysfunction. (From Roberts WC, et al: Am J Cardiol 49:863, 1982. Reproduced by permission.)

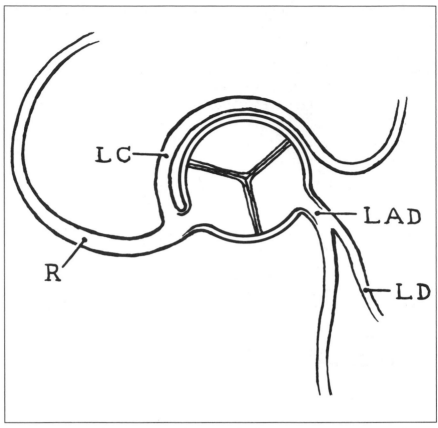

Fig. 8-6.   Diagram showing origin of left circumflex *(LC)* coronary artery arising as the first branch of the right *(R)* coronary artery and then coursing posterior to the aorta before reaching the left atrioventricular sulcus. The left anterior descending *(LAD)* coronary artery arises from the left sinus of Valsalva. *LD* = left diagonal. Reproduced with permission from Roberts.[55]

repair with VSD closure, interposition of a homograft valved conduit and PA resection for these patients. It is clear that some patients with this malformation escape problems during infancy and present for elective repair at an older age. In this group, PA resection is generally not needed, the use of an orthotopic homograft valve is probably advisable, although overall results are good despite the reparative methods employed. The group of patients who present in infancy with severe respiratory problems represent a continued surgical challenge. Rabinovitch and colleagues (Rabinovitch M, Grady S, David I, Van Praagh R, Sauer U, Buhlmeyer K, Castaneda AR, Reid L, Silva DK: Compression of intrapulmonary bronchi by abnormally branching pulmonary arteries associated with absent pulmonary valves. Am J Cardiol 50:804–813, 1982.) thoroughly studied the arterial and bronchial trees of 3 infants with absent pulmonary valve syndrome at necropsy. They found diffuse bronchovascular changes which would not be completely relieved by eliminating compression at the main bronchus level. These findings may prevent a high rate of surgical success despite the management program employed. The articles by Ilbawi and colleages and Karl and colleagues present different surgical recommendations with similar degrees of failure. It is intriguing to consider the possibility that surgical treatment during the first few days of life may provide the best chance of success by eliminating additional tracheobronchial injury which seems likely to occur from PA dilatation and the large

RV stroke volume. Whether this should be by complete repair with homo-graft valve replacement as recommended by Karl or by PA ligation and sys-temic-PA shunting as recommended by Ilbawi remains for future delinea-tion.

Park et al[61] from San Antonio, Texas, utilized initial PA banding and an aorto-PA shunt as the initial surgical management of a 9-day-old infant with TF and absent PV syndrome and hyperinflation of the right lower lung field. The patient was dismissed on the tenth postoperative day, and subsequent intracardiac repair employing transannular patching was successfully done at 28 months of age. The authors reasoned that a PA band decreases the diameter, pressure, and pulsatility of the PA and the shunt maintains ade-quate pulmonary blood flow. They believe this is preferable to complete ligation of the PA because it avoids subsequent prosthetic conduit replace-ment of the PA and the inherent risks involved in a totally shunt-dependent circulation. They recommended that neonates with this syndrome be fol-lowed closely and if evidence of respiratory distress or pulmonary hyperinfla-

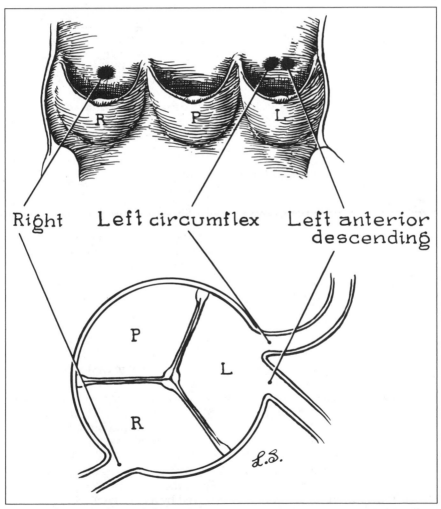

Fig. 8-7. Drawing of aorta showing origin of each of the left circumflex and left anterior descending coronary arteries from a separate ostium in the left *(L)* sinus of Valsalva. *R* = right and *P* = posterior sinus of Valsalva or cusp. Reproduced with permission from Roberts.[55]

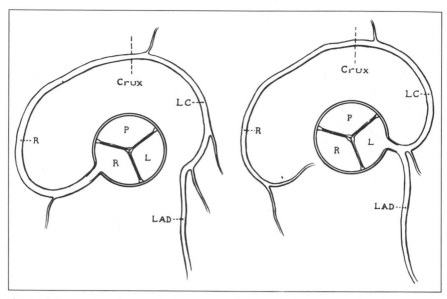

Fig. 8-8. Drawings of the two most common varieties of single coronary ostium. In one (*left*), the single ostium arises in the right aortic sinus and in the other (*right*), the single ostium arises in the left (*L*) aortic sinus. When the single coronary artery arises from the right aortic ostium, the right (*R*) coronary artery crosses the crux to continue as the left circumflex (*LC*), which in turn continues as the left anterior descending (*LAD*). When the single ostium is located in the left aortic sinus, the left main gives rise to the LAD and the LC, and LC crosses the crux to continue as the right coronary artery. Reproduced with permission from Roberts.[55]

tion develop, PA banding with or without a shunt should be done before progressive air trapping and tracheobronchial malacia occur.

Operative treatment of double-outlet right ventricle

Kirklin and associates[62] from Birmingham, Alabama, reported a rigorous analysis of their experience with 127 patients undergoing repair of double-outlet right ventricle (DORV) over an 18-year period. The overall actuarial survival at 12 years was 38%. Statistical analysis indicated that the current 2-week survival rate after the intraventricular tunnel repair for DORV with subaortic VSD in 6-month-old infants is 99% and the 10-year survival rate, 97%. Reoperation after tunnel repair in this entity was required in only 1 of 56 patients and the late functional results were excellent. Similar results were present in patients with DORV and a doubly committed VSD, except that 2 of 10 patients had discrete localized subaortic stenosis late postoperatively. In this experience, early and late results in patients with DORV and subpulmonary VSD were poor when an atrial switch operation was part of the repair. When an intraventricular tunnel repair connecting the LV with the aorta was combined with a RV-PA conduit, no early deaths occurred but late mortality was high. For this type of DORV, the authors currently recommended either an intraventricular tunnel connecting the VSD with the PA and an arterial switch operation, or an intraventricular tunnel connecting the LV with the aorta without obstructing the pathway from the RV to the PA. Patients with DORV with noncommitted VSD were repaired by a variety of methods. They had only a 22% overall 10-year survival rate and results were particularly poor when an intraventricular tunnel was employed. In this subset there were 12 deaths among 16 patients who underwent an LV-aortic tunnel repair, compared with only 1 among 7 in whom an atrial switch repair was performed. When PS was present in this subset, the authors believe the surgical choices should be between a Fontan-type operation, or an atrial switch repair with closure of the VSD, closure of PA, and a valved extracardiac conduit from LV to PA. There is uncertainty as to which of these operations is best. When PS is absent, either of these 2 types of repair may be considered after initial PA banding in infancy. Additionally, the possibility of enlarging the VSD superiorly and creating a tunnel connecting it to the PA can also be done.

A number of surgical options exist for repair of DORV with subpulmonary VSD. Doty[63] from Salt Lake City, Utah, presented an original operation for intraventricular repair of this defect when the aorta is directly anterior to the PA. He used a tubular Dacron® prosthesis that was sutured to the VSD and ventricular septum on 1 end, and coursed anteriorly along the free RV wall to insert onto the subaortic conus. The tube graft itself was used to widen the ventriculotomy incision so as not to compromise residual RV volume. Although this operation has the disadvantage of leaving a long tubular conduit pathway which may not grow, it does leave the left ventricle as the systemic ventricle and offers additional flexibility among the surgical options used to repair this complex and variable cardiac defect. This is an interesting and unique addition to the surgical options available to repair of DORV. Its future use will probably be somewhat limited, but should remain in the surgeon's armamentarium. The primary operations currently employed are the Jatene type of arterial switch, and the intraventricular repair described by Patrick and McGoon. The latter is somewhat similar to what Doty describes and although it is probably more complex to perform, it leaves autologous cardiac structures forming most of the intraventricular tunnel. The use of the Damus-Stansel-Kaye procedure and an intraventricular tunnel connecting VSD to PA, coupled with venous switching, have taken a smaller place among the surgical options available. When the great arteries are side by side, the tunnel repair connecting the VSD with the aorta as described by Kawashima is the simplest available procedure and when applicable, should be used in this particular anatomic arrangement.

Seven patients with DORV and subpulmonary VSD (the Taussig-Bing anomaly) underwent repair between 1.5 and 33 months (mean 14) of age. Four had previous PA banding, 2 previous coarctation repair, and 1 a previous surgical septectomy. The great arteries had a side-by-side relation in 5 and were anteroposterior in 2. The VSD was patched to direct the LV outflow to the original pulmonary trunk. This was done transatrially in 5 and through a right ventriculotomy in 2. A Jatene-type of arterial switch with coronary artery transfer was performed in each. Continuity between the RV and distal PA was accomplished directly in 3, with interposition of a Dacron® tube in 1 and using the LeCompte maneuver in 3. There was 1 (14%) hospital death occurring in a patient with side-by-side great arteries in whom the LeCompte maneuver was initially employed and subsequently dismantled and a tube of bovine pericardium interposed between the proximal and distal PA. There were no late deaths in 6 survivors followed between 6 and 31 months (mean 15). Reoperation was required in 1 patient to close a large residual VSD and to relieve residual RV outflow tract obstruction. This patient has persistent respiratory symptoms, but the remaining 5 survivors are asymptomatic. Postoperative cardiac catheterization was performed in 5. A large residual VSD was identified in the patient mentioned above. An additional patient had a small unimportant residual VSD but no patient had AR or a pressure gradient measured from LV to aorta. Three patients had residual subvalvar RV outflow tract obstruction which was repaired in 1. The authors recommended anatomic correction at the arterial level for patients with DORV.

Damus-Stansel-Kaye procedure for complete transposition of the great arteries or for double-outlet right ventricle

The operation described by Damus, Stansel, and Kaye is applicable to patients with TGA and similar types of cardiac malformations. It consists of division of the pulmonary trunk with anastomosis of its proximal portion to the side of the ascending aorta, closure of the VSD, and placement of an extracardiac conduit from right ventricle to distal main PA. Closure of the aortic valve leaflets or subvalvar area by patching has been a controversial detail. DeLeon and associates[65] from Chicago, Illinois, presented their experience with 2 patients, 1 with TGA and another with the DORV, in whom significant AR developed after the Damus-Stansel-Kaye procedure. One required late closure of the aortic valve and the other is awaiting this procedure. In contrast, AR did not develop among 7 patients with a univentricular heart and subaortic stenosis who underwent creation of an aortopulmonary window followed postoperatively up to 7 years (mean 43 months). Postoperative angiograms suggested that the development of AR after the Damus-Stansel-Kaye procedure may have been caused by aortic valve prolapse. The authors concluded that the aortic valve or subaortic region should be closed at the initial repair in patients with low pulmonary vascular resistance who are undergoing the Damus-Stansel-Kaye procedure to minimize the need of reoperation for AR.

Complications after the Fontan operation

Mayer et al[66] from Boston, Massachusetts, reviewed their experience from 1973 through 1985 with 167 consecutive patients who underwent a modified Fontan-type operation. Of these, 109 (65%) failed to meet $\geq$1 of the original 10 selection criteria proposed by Fontan's group in the areas of age, anomalies of systemic and/or pulmonary venous connection, PA deformity, and pulmonary vascular hemodynamics. Sixteen (62%) of 26 patients who had a mean PA pressure >15 mmHg survived. Sixteen (84%) of 19 patients who had anomalies of systemic and/or pulmonary venous connection survived. There were 26 (59%) survivors among 44 patients <4 years of age at operation and 23 (92%) among 25 patients >15 years. PA distortion resulting from prior palliative operations was present in 34 patients and 17 (50%) survived the modified Fontan operation. Pulmonary arteriolar resistance was >2 units · m^2 in 26 and 14 (54%) survived, while 81 (87%) of 93 with a resistance <2 units · m^2 survived. Pulmonary arteriolar resistance and PA distortion were identified by multivariate analysis as significant incremental risk factors for death within 30 days of operation. Age and anomalies of systemic and/or pulmonary venous connection and PA pressure were not independent predictors of outcome. Elevated pulmonary arteriolar resistance and PA distortion from prior palliative operations increased the risk of this operation. Higher PA pressure alone should not contraindicate a Fontan operation if pulmonary arteriolar resistance is low.

Coronary venous return via the coronary sinus is often subjected to higher than normal pressure after the classic Fontan operation. Thus, Ilbawi and colleagues[67] from Chicago, Illinois, performed experimental and clinical studies to determine if elevated coronary sinus pressure affected LV function. In 13 canine studies, coronary sinus pressure was increased in stepwise fashion from 5–25 torr. When the pressure reached 15 torr, there was a significant decrease in cardiac index (3.60 ± 0.5–2.70 ± 0.6 liters/min/m^2), coronary blood flow (14 ± 3–7 ± 2 ml/min), rate of rise of LV pressure, and an increase in coronary arteriovenous saturation. Postoperative cardiac catheterization studies were performed in 24 patients 1–4 years after the Fontan operation for tricuspid atresia or other types of single ventricle. Patients with a mean RA pressure <15 torr had LV EF of $93 \pm 6\%$ of predicted, whereas those with a RA pressure ≥ 15 torr had an LV EF of $75 \pm 13\%$ of predicted. The authors believe these data demonstrate that elevated coronary sinus pressure has deleterious effects on ventricular function after the Fontan procedure. They recommend modifications of the procedure such as using the rudimentary right ventricle when feasible or diverting coronary sinus flow to the pulmonary venous atrium, to decrease postrepair coronary sinus hypertension and improve ventricular function.

Complete closure of defects in the atrial septum is an essential part of the Fontan procedure as residual defects will result in persistent cyanosis from right-to-left shunting. Rumisek and colleagues[68] from Philadelphia, Pennsylvania, called attention to the presence of coronary sinus septal defects, which were found in 2 of 10 patients with tricuspid valve atresia who underwent a modified Fontan procedure over a 12-month period. The defects in these 2 patients were not recognized preoperatively or intraoperatively and the postrepair arterial oxygen tension was 45 and 52 mmHg in each. Postoperative selective angiography the day after operation in 1 and contrast echocardiography on the day of surgery in the other demonstrated an isolated coronary sinus septal defect which was subsequently closed by a second procedure. Arterial oxygen tension increased to 167 and 370 mmHg after repair. A review of 150 postmortem specimens of tricuspid valve atresia demonstrated a coronary sinus septal defect in 2, one with normally related and 1 with transposed great arteries. Two additional specimens showed multiple punctate fenestrations in the sinus septum connecting the coronary sinus with the left atrium. Although the incidence of coronary sinus septal defects in patients with tricuspid atresia is probably <5%, leaving them untreated results in severe postoperative cyanosis. The authors believe that intraoperative diagnosis is possible but cannot be reliably predicted by inspection of RA anatomy alone. Although the coronary sinus orifice may be closed within the atrium, the authors suggested that routine baffling of the coronary sinus orifice into the left atrium would obviate this problem and also possibly reduce the potential for myocardial edema by diverting the coronary venous return into the lower pressure left atrium after repair.

DeLeon and colleagues[69] from Chicago, Illinois, reviewed their experience with 4 of 44 patients who had undergone a Fontan operation who subsequently underwent early takedown of the procedure because of severe low cardiac output. The patients ranged from 4–7 years of age, 3 with tricuspid valve atresia and 1 with double-inlet left ventricle. Three of the 4 had undergone previous PA banding and had had subaortic stenosis with gradients ranging from 35–80 mmHg. At the time of the Fontan procedure, a simultaneous Glenn shunt was performed in 2 patients. Early postoperatively, each of the 4 had profound low cardiac output associated with mean RA pressures ranging from 21–31 mmHg. Takedown with construction of systemic-PA shunts was accomplished in each patient between 6 and 65 hours postoperatively. A simultaneous Glenn shunt was performed in 1. There were 2 hospital survivors who remained well at 5 months and 4 years postoperatively and

2 early deaths from persistent low cardiac output. The authors believe that patients who have profound low cardiac output after the Fontan operation should be considered for takedown of the orthoterminal connection, recognizing its significant risk.

Kirklin et al[70] from Birmingham, Alabama, reviewed their experience with 102 patients, 0.7–38 years of age, who underwent a Fontan-type operation for a wide variety of cardiac malformations. Complete follow-up information was obtained over the 10-year study period with a median follow-up time of 33 months. Actuarial survival at 9.4 years was 81% for those with tricuspid valve atresia compared with 63% for the overall group. High postrepair RA pressure correlated with the probability of early death, and the risk increased rapidly when the pressure was >14 mmHg. Hypertrophy of the ventricular main chamber was a significant risk factor for early and late death, which in part explained the lesser risk of the Fontan procedure in patients with tricuspid atresia. Although younger age was a risk factor for early postoperative death, it was neutralized by recent date of operation. The authors believe the Fontan operation should be done electively between the ages of 2 and 4 years to avoid increasing ventricular hypertrophy. Older age, per se, is not a contraindication to the procedure.

A variety of surgical techniques have evolved since the original descriptions of the RV exclusion operation by Fontan and Kreutzer. Lee and colleagues[71] from Rochester, Minnesota, compared the clinical results of a direct valveless atriopulmonary connection (n = 60) -vs- an AV connection using the native pulmonary valve (n = 24) and the subpulmonary ventricular chamber among 84 patients with tricuspid valve atresia and ventriculoarterial concordance. Preoperative characteristics of the 2 groups were similar except for a greater frequency of Waterston shunts (38 -vs- 17%) and a higher mean pulmonary arteriolar resistance (1.9 ± 0.7 units $\cdot$ m^2 -vs- 1.1 ± 0.8 units $\cdot$ m^2) in the atriopulmonary group compared with the AV group. The latter had a higher frequency of Glenn shunts (46 -vs- 15%). Operative mortality was 5% for the atriopulmonary group and 4% for the AV group and at 3.5 years postoperatively, the overall survival rate was $89 \pm 4\%$ -vs- $88 \pm 7\%$, respectively. The atriopulmonary group had an early postoperative mean RA pressure of 18 ± 3 mmHg compared with 16 ± 3 mmHg for the AV group. This difference was not reflected in early or late results. The authors concluded that there is no important difference in the clinical outcome of patients undergoing modified Fontan/Kreutzer repair for tricuspid atresia with AV concordance with either method. They believe the choice of the connection should be dictated by the anatomy, such as presence of pulmonary valve or arterial stenoses, size of outlet chamber, and the presence of coronary artery anomalies.

Late follow-up after operative therapy of aortico-left ventricular tunnel

Meldrum-Hanna and colleagues[72] from London, UK, reported their experience with 6 patients undergoing repair of aortico-LV tunnel since 1970. At operation they were between 5 and 34 years of age and tunnel closure was accomplished working through the aorta by direct suture in 5 and patch closure in 1. Coexisting valve pathology included AS in 2, AR in 3, cuspal defects in 2, and healed infective endocarditis in 1. There were no hospital deaths and at early postoperative examination, 67% had mild AR. Three patients (50%) underwent subsequent AVR for progressive AR at a mean of 10 years postoperatively. The authors' experience and review of published reports lead them to believe that early operation is advisable not only to prevent CHF, but also to prevent progression of aortic valve damage and progressive AR. Careful postoperative follow-up is necessary since 50% of their patients ultimately required AVR.

Operative therapy of total anomalous pulmonary venous connection

Oelert and colleagues[73] from Hanover, West Germany, reviewed their experience with 53 infants who underwent corrective repair of total anomalous pulmonary venous connection (TAPVC) between 1973 and 1984. It was supercardiac in 41%, cardiac in 17%, infracardiac in 36%, and mixed in 6%. Hospital mortality was highest at 42% in the infracardiac group and 23% overall. Over the years of the study, overall hospital mortality decreased to 11%. Factors related to hospital mortality were the anatomic type of lesion, the degree of pulmonary venous obstruction, the severity of pulmonary hypertension, younger age of the patient, and earlier date of operation. The authors currently recommended prompt surgical repair for highly symptomatic patients with TAPVC.

The site of venous drainage in most patients with TAPVC lies within the conventional classification of supracardiac, cardiac, infracardiac, and mixed types. Arciprete et al[74] from Liverpool and Near Manchester, UK, reported 3 infants whose pulmonary veins entered a confluence which then emptied by 2 separate connections, 1 to the coronary sinus and a second via the left vertical vein to the left innominate vein. These 3 were among 98 patients who underwent operation for TAPVC between 1970 and 1984. Preoperatively, the diagnosis of double connection was not made in 2 patients, each thought to have a mixed type of TAPVC with drainage of the left upper lobe to the left innominate vein and drainage of the remaining veins to a confluence emptying into the coronary sinus. Initial repair consisted of incision of the common coronary sinus–left atrial wall and closure of the coronary sinus orifice and ASD. Both required reoperation for closure of the left vertical vein 3 years later. The diagnosis in the third patient was made by passing the cardiac catheter down the vertical vein into the confluence and injecting contrast medium that showed the second communication between the confluence and the coronary sinus. Primary complete repair was successfully performed. The authors emphasized the necessity for complete and accurate preoperative diagnosis by cardiac catheterization methods to permit primary complete surgical repair. They also indicated the incompleteness of the currently used Darling classification and recommended describing this entity as a left cardinal type of TAPVC with double connection to an ascending vein and coronary sinus. The risk of operation for repair of TAPVC has progressively declined and is now quite low. Although there is a tendency to advise operation based on preoperative echocardiographic diagnosis, we support the authors' contention that complete and accurate diagnosis is best obtained by cardiac catheterization methods and provides useful information for the planning of proper and complete surgical repair. The uncommon pathology described by the authors can be nicely delineated preoperatively by contrast media injection into the pulmonary confluence via the left vertical vein.

Operative treatment of interrupted aortic arch

A variety of surgical methods have been used to repair neonates with interrupted aortic arch (IAA). Creation of a large anastomosis between the 2 aortic segments after complete excision of ductal tissue seems preferable to the interposition of prosthetic tubes. Since the ascending aorta is often small, the placement of a partial occlusion clamp to facilitate construction of the anastomosis risks complete occlusion of the ascending aorta and has been 1 factor leading some surgeons to the use of cardiopulmonary bypass with profound hypothermia and circulatory arrest. Galla and colleagues[75] from Brooklyn, New York, reported primary aortic arch reconstruction in 3 neonates with IAA and VSD. Patients were surface-cooled to 32°C and the operation performed through a left thoracotomy. A partial occlusion clamp was placed on the ascending aorta and carotid arteries, purposely resulting in complete obstruction of the ascending aorta. This permitted a large aortotomy that extended onto the left carotid artery so that a wide anastomosis to the descending aorta could be easily constructed. Aortic occlusion time varied between 12 and 21 minutes. Each patient survived the initial hospital period without neurologic deficit; 1 died 3 months postoperatively from sepsis. Femoral pulses were normal in each. The authors indicated that this technique is of value only if a functional VSD is present to allow LV decompression during the period of aortic crossclamping. A PA band is not utilized when the intracardiac defect is an isolated VSD, but is employed when complex associated defects are present.

The management of patients with IAA and associated intracardiac defects remains controversial. Complete primary repair -vs- arch repair and palliation of the intracardiac defects are the surgical options. Hammon and colleagues[76] from Nashville, Tennessee, reviewed their 10-year experience with 16 infants, 9 with IAA between the left carotid and subclavian arteries (type B) and 7 just distal to the left subclavian artery (type A). The associated intracardiac defects were VSD in 7, aortopulmonary window in 4, truncus arteriosus type I in 2, TGA and VSD in 1, and single ventricle in 2. Eight of the 16 patients (including 3 with VSD) underwent palliation with 6 hospital and 2 late deaths. Since 1980, 8 patients (4 with VSD and 4 with aortopulmonary window) underwent complete repair with no hospital and 1 late death. The authors concluded that primary complete repair of IAA is clearly advisable for patients with associated VSD or aortopulmonary window. The poor results obtained by palliating those with more complicated associated lesions support future attempts for primary repair in this group as well.

Operative treatment of supravalvular mitral stenosis

Sullivan and associates[77] from London, UK, reviewed the clinical data, echocardiographic findings, and operative anatomy in 14 patients who underwent surgery for membranous supravalvular MS between 1978 and 1985. Patients ages ranged from 6 weeks–13 years and associated lesions included mitral valve abnormalities (8), VSD (7), coarctation (5), left superior vena cava (6), subaortic stenosis (3), and ASD (1). Successful removal of a supravalvular membrane, which was usually adherent to the valve, was possible in 12 of 14 and 2 of 14 patients who underwent MVR. There were no operative deaths. Eleven patients had follow-up in excess of 1 year with 1 late death. Of the remaining patients, 8 of 10 are asymptomatic and 7 of 10 have no clinical evidence of residual MS.

Valve replacement in children

The timing of operation, type of valve substitute, and need for long-term anticoagulation remain controversial aspects of cardiac valve replacement in children. Milano et al[78] from Paris, France, reviewed their experience with

166 children ≤15 years of age who underwent AVR (53) or MVR (90), or both (23). Eighty-four received a bioprosthesis, (71) a mechanical prosthesis, and 11 a mitral bioprosthesis and an aortic mechanical prosthesis. Hospital mortality was 9%. All but 8 patients (95%) were followed for a mean interval of 4.1 years for the bioprosthesis group, 3.3 years for the mechanical prosthesis group, and 3.5 years for the mitral bioprosthesis group. Actuarial survival at 7 years was 63 ± 6% for the bioprosthesis group and 70 ± 7% for the mechanical prosthesis group. There were no significant differences between the 2 groups for valve related mortality, thromboembolism (greater after MVR), or endocarditis. Wafarin anticoagulation was advised indefinitely for those in the mechanical prosthesis group and for only 3 months after operation for those in the bioprosthesis group. The linearized rates of reoperation were 10 ± 2% per patient-year in the bioprosthesis group and 2 ± 1% per patient-year in the mechanical prosthesis group. Primary tissue failure was the main cause of reoperation and the overall mortality at the secondary procedure was 12%. The incidence of reoperation for tissue failure was 8 ± 2% per patient-year for those with a porcine bioprosthesis and 20 ± 6% per patient-year for those with a pericardial bioprosthesis. The authors concluded that satisfactory early and late results can be achieved when the aortic valve is replaced with a mechanical prosthesis. They suggest the use of antiplatelet therapy in addition to Wafarin for this subset. Porcine or pericardial valve substitutes should be avoided in children. In the mitral position, early and late results are less than satisfactory with either type of substitute primarily because of early degeneration of the bioprosthesis and a higher risk of thromboembolism (4% per patient-year) with an mechanical prosthesis. They believe every effort should be made to repair the diseased mitral valve in children and if valve replacement is absolutely necessary that a mechanical prosthesis be used with indefinite long-term anticoagulation.

Spevak and associates[79] from Boston, Massachusetts, reported results of 70 valve replacements in 63 children <5 years of age between 1966 and 1984. There were 49 mitral, 6 aortic, 11 tricuspid, and 1 multiple valve replacement performed. Tissue valves were used in 20%, but since 1980 only Björk-Shiley and St. Jude's valves have been used. The most common indication for valve replacement was MR after repair of AV canal (34%). Mortality decreased considerably over time and was 22% since 1982. More than 67% of the fatalities were operative deaths, usually within 3 days of surgery. Survival curves since 1980 predict 1-and 5-year survival of 73 and 51%, respectively. For the 46 operative survivors, 1- and 5-year valve survival was 97 and 70%, respectively. All but 1 patient with nontissue valve received anticoagulant therapy and thromboembolism rate was 1.6/100 patient-years and hemorrhage 0.8/100 patient-years. These patients represent a heterogenous group with significant congenital abnormalities of the mitral valve and systemic AV valve regurgitation in patients with TGA. For this complex group the present results are good but problems remain in terms of thromboembolism, valve dysfunction, and septic complications.

Verrier et al[80] from San Francisco, California, reviewed their experience with 51 children aged 1–23 years (mean 13) who received aspirin (n = 45) or aspirin with dipyridamole (n = 6) for anticoagulation after mechanical AVR. All but 2 patients were followed between 3 and 100 months (mean 37). A Björk-Shiley standard tilting disc was used in 50 patients and a St. Jude Medical in 1. There were no postoperative thrombotic or thromboembolic events. Four patients (6%) had minor hemorrhagic complications, 3 having nosebleeds and 1 an upper gastrointestinal hemorrhage. Five patients were altered to warfarin anticoagulation because of physician preference. There were 4 late deaths, 2 from prosthetic valve endocarditis and 2 from other medical problems. There were no mechanical valve failures but 1 reoperation was performed 9 months later for paravalvular leakage. Each patient was in sinus rhythm or a paced rhythm, none in AF. The authors concluded that aspirin (or aspirin and dipyridamole) may be the anticoagulant of choice in children with mechanical aortic valves.

Fate of right ventricular to pulmonary arterial conduit after Rastelli operation

Palik and associates[81] from Nashville, Tennessee, studied 18 patients with partially obstructed RV to PA conduits 1–9 years after a Rastelli operation. Age at the initial conduit procedure was 1–8 months in 7 patients (group I) and 2–9 years in the remaining 11 patients (group II). All but 7 patients were free of symptoms at the time of the postoperative study. Neither peak RV pressure nor RV to PA gradients were different between groups. RVEF was decreased in group II but was normal in the infant group. There was a significant inverse relation between RVEF and age at repair. RV end-diastolic volume was normal or increased in all patients and did not differ between the groups. LVEF also was decreased in the older but normal in the infant group. There was a decrease in RV and/or LVEF from pre- to postoperative studies in only 1 of 6 group I patients compared with 4 of 5 group II patients. RNA with exercise was performed in 8 patients and RVEF responses were abnormal in all of them, whereas LVEF responses were abnormal in 7 of 8. A decrease of RVEF with exercise of >5 EF units was associated with a resting gradient from RV to PA of >60 mmHg. These data indicate that RVEF is usually abnormal in patients with obstructed RV to PA conduits who undergo operation after infancy. The progressive decrease in RVEF with age indicates the inadequacy of hypertrophy to normalize RV pump function with time. The additional data of abnormal LVEF in these patients indicate that inadequate myocardial protection at the time of surgery may have been present in the older patient group.

Operative treatment of left ventricular diverticulum

Congenital diverticulum of the ventricle is a rare malformation with fewer than 80 cases reported. When accompanied by malrotation of the heart, intracardiac anomalies, defects of the lower sternum, pericardium, diaphragm and abdominal wall, it has been known as Cantrell's syndrome. Okereke and colleagues[82] from Houston, Texas, reported their experience with 10 patients surgically treated over a 20-year period. They ranged in age from 3 months–37 years. A LV diverticulum was present in each, being apical in location in 7, in the LV outflow tract in 2, and at the AV junction and LV free wall in 1. The LV diverticulum was the only intracardiac abnormality in 2, whereas the remaining patients had varying intracardiac defects. Symptoms were related mainly to associated malformations including intracardiac, midline thoracic, diaphragmatic, and abdominal wall defects. Nine patients underwent operation solely to correct the ventricular diverticulum in 3 and also to correct associated cardiac diaphragmatic or midline abnormalities in 6. Resection of the ventricular diverticulum without cardiopulmonary bypass was used in 3 cases because of the narrow necks connecting the diverticulum to the true ventricle. In the remaining 6, cardiopulmonary bypass was used in 3 because of associated intracardiac anomalies and in 3 because it was not feasible to apply a clamp to the neck of the diverticulum. There were no hospital deaths, 1 patient died 1 month after dismissal from hemopericardium, and another 5 years later of prosthetic valve related etiology. The remaining 7 patients are alive and well. The authors recommended surgical treatment for all patients with a congenital ventricular diverticulum to avoid the complications of spontaneous rupture or CHF.

Bovine parietal pericardium for operative repair

Crawford and colleagues[83] from Charleston, South Carolina, used preserved bovine pericardium in the repair of a wide variety of congenital heart defects in 105 patients. It was not a contributing factor in the 12 hospital and 6 late deaths. The material was found to be flexible and easy to use, and in follow-up ranging from 6–60 months (mean 30), no patient had patch calcium. The authors recommended the use of glutaraldehyde-preserved bovine pericardium in this group of patients but indicate that longer follow-up will be necessary to determine if calcium and patch distortion will occur. An alternative and less expensive approach is the use of autologous parietal pericardium that has been rinsed in glutaraldehyde to improve its tensile strength and handling characteristics.

References

1. BELKIN RN, WAUGH RA, KISSLO J: Interatrial shunting in atrial septal aneurysm. Am J Cardiol 1986 (Feb 1); 57:310–312.

2. LeBLANC JG, WILLIAMS WG, FREEDOM RM, TRUSLER GA: Results of total correction in complete atrioventricular septal defects with congenital or surgically induced right ventricular outflow tract obstruction. Ann Thorac Surg 1986 (Apr); 41:387–391.

3. GUO-WEI H, MEE RBB: Complete atrioventricular canal associated with tetralogy of Fallot or double-outlet right ventricle and right ventricular outflow tract obstruction: a report of successful surgical treatment. Ann Thorac Surg 1986 (June); 41:612–615.

4. VARGAS FJ, OTERO COTO E, MAYER JE JR, JONAS RA, CASTANEDA AR: Complete atrioventricular canal and tetralogy of Fallot: surgical considerations. Ann Thorac Surg 1986 (Sept); 42:258–263.

5. RAMACIOTTI C, KEREN A, SILVERMAN NH: Importance of (perimembranous) ventricular septal aneurysm in the natural history of isolated perimembranous ventricular septal defect. Am J Cardiol 1986 (Feb); 57:268–272.

6. LUDOMIRSKY A, HUHTA JC, VICK W, MURPHY DJ, DANFORD DA, MORROW WR: Color Doppler detection of multiple ventricular septal defects. Circulation 1986 (Dec) 74:1317–1322.

7. CRAIG BG, SMALLHORN JF, BURROWS P, TRUSLER GA, ROWE RD: Cross-sectional echocardiography in the evaluation of aortic valve prolapse associated with ventricular septal defect. Am Heart J 1986 (Oct); 112:800–807.

8. GOLDBERG SJ, VASKO SD, ALLEN HD, MARX GR: Can the technique for Doppler estimate of pulmonary stenosis gradient be simplified? Am Heart J 1986 (Apr); 111:709–713.

9. ALI KHAN MA, AL YOUSEF S, MULLINS CE: Percutaneous transluminal balloon pulmonary valvuloplasty for the relief of pulmonary valve stenosis with special reference to double-balloon technique. Am Heart J 1986 (July); 112:158–166.

10. RADTKE W, KEANE JF, FELLOWS KE, LANG P, LOCK JE: Percutaneous balloon valvotomy of congenital pulmonary stenosis using oversized balloons. J Am Coll Cardiol 1986 (Oct); 8:909–15.

11. FYFE DA, EDWARDS WD, DRISCOLL DJ: Myocardial ischemia in patients with pulmonary atresia and intact ventricular septum. J Am Coll Cardiol 1986 (Aug); 8:402–6.

12. LEWIS AB, WELLS W, LINDESMITH GG: Right ventricular growth potential in neonates with pulmonary atresia and intact ventricular septum. J Thorac Cardiovasc Surg 1986 (June); 91:835–840.

13. BARBER G, DANIELSON GK, PUGA FJ, HEISE CG, DRISCOLL DJ: Pulmonary atresia with ventricular septal defect: preoperative and postoperative responses to exercise. J Am Coll Cardiol 1986 (Mar); 7:630–638.

14. Momma K, Takao A, Ando M, Nakazawa M, Satomi G, Imai Y, Takanashi T, Kurosawa H: Juxtaductal left pulmonary artery obstruction in pulmonary atresia. Br Heart J 1986 (Jan); 55:39–44.

15. Joshi SV, Brawn WJ, Mee RBB: Pulmonary atresia with intact ventricular septum. J Thorac Cardiovasc Surg 1986 (Feb); 91:192–199.

16. Foker JE, Braunlin EA, St Cyr JA, Hunter D, Molina JE, Moller JH, Ring WS: Management of pulmonary atresia with intact ventricular septum. J Thorac Cardiovasc Surg 1986 (Oct); 92:706–715.

17. Metzdorff MT, Pinson CW, Grunkemeier GL, Cobanoglu A, Starr A: Late right ventricular reconstruction following valvotomy in pulmonary atresia with intact ventricular septum. Ann Thorac Surg 1986 (July); 42:45–51.

18. Millikan JS, Puga FJ, Danielson GK, Schaff HV, Julsrud PR, Mair DD: Staged surgical repair of pulmonary atresia, ventricular septal defect, and hypoplastic, confluent pulmonary arteries. J Thorac Cardiovasc Surg 1986 (June); 91:818–825.

19. Vargas FJ, Kreutzer GO, Pedrini M, Capelli H, Coronel AR: Tetralogy of Fallot with subarterial ventricular septal defect. Diagnostic and surgical considerations. J Thorac Cardiovasc Surg 1986 (Nov); 92:908–912.

20. Ilbawi MN, Fedorchik J, Muster AJ, Idriss FS, DeLeon SY, Gidding SS, Paul MH: Surgical approach to severely symptomatic newborn infants with tetralogy of Fallot and absent pulmonary valve. J Thorac Cardiovasc Surg 1986 (Apr); 91:584–589.

21. Ilbawi MN, Idriss FS, DeLeon SY, Muster AJ, Berry TE, Paul MH: Long-term results of porcine valve insertion for pulmonary regurgitation following repair of tetralogy of Fallot. Ann Thorac Surg 1986 (May); 41:478–482.

22. Hayes CJ, Gersony WM: Arrhythmias after the Mustard Operation for transposition of the great arteries: a long-term study. J Am Coll Cardiol 1986 (Jan); 7:133–137.

23. Gillette PC, Wampler DG, Shannon C, Ott D: Use of cardiac pacing after the mustard operation for transposition of the great arteries. J Am Coll Cardiol 1986 (Jan); 7:138–141.

24. Butto F, Dunnigan A, Overholt ED, Benditt DG, Benson DW: Transesophageal study of recurrent atrial tachycardia after atrial baffle procedures for complete transposition of the great arteries. Am J Cardiol 1986 (June); 57:1356–1362.

25. Smallhorn JF, Gow R, Freedom RM, Trusler GA, Olley P, Pacquet M, Gibbons J, Vlad P: Pulsed Doppler echocardiographic assessment of the pulmonary venous pathway after the mustard or senning procedure for transposition of the great arteries. Circulation 1986 (April); 73:765–774.

26. Quaegebeur JM, Rohmer J, Ottenkamp J, Buis T, Kirklin JW, Blackstone EH, Brom AG: The arterial switch operation. An eight-year experience. J Thorac Cardiovasc Surg 1986 (Sept); 92:361–384.

27. Kurosawa H, Imai Y, Takanashi Y, Hoshino S, Sawatari K, Kawada M, Takao A: Infundibular septum and coronary anatomy in Jatene operation. J Thoracic Cardiovasc Surg 1986 (Apr); 91:572–583.

28. Arensman FW, Radley-Smith R, Grieve L, Gibson DG, Yacoub MH: Computer assisted echocardiographic assessment of left ventricular function before and after anatomical correction of transposition of the great arteries. Br Heart J 1986 (Feb); 55:162–167.

29. Mee RBB: Severe right ventricular failure after Mustard or Senning operation. Two-stage repair: pulmonary artery banding and switch. J Thorac Cardiovasc Surg 1986 (Sept); 92:385–390.

30. Hsieh K-S, Keane JF, Nadas AS, Bernhard WF, Castaneda AR: Long-term follow-up of valvotomy before 1986 for congenital aortic stenosis. Am J Cardiol 1986 (Aug) 58:338–341.

31. Suarez de Lezo J, Pan M, Sancho M, Herrera N, Arizon J, Franco M, Concha M, Valles F, Romanos A: Percutaneous transluminal balloon dilatation for discrete subaortic stenosis. Am J Cardiol 1986 (Sept) 58:619–621.

32. Lavee J, Porat L, Smolinsky A, Hegesh J, Neufeld HN, Goor DA: Myectomy versus myotomy as an adjunct to membranectomy in the surgical repair of discrete and tunnel subaortic stenosis. J Thorac Cardiovasc Surg 1986 (Nov); 92:944–949.

33. Morrow WR, Huhta JC, Murphy DJ, McNamara DG: Quantitative morphology of the aortic arch in neonatal coarctation. J Am Coll Cardiol 1986 (Sept); 8:616–20.

34. Sanders SP, MacPherson D, Yeager SB: Temporal flow velocity profile in the descending aorta in coarctation. J Am Coll Cardiol 1986 (Mar); 7:603–609.

35. Boxer RA, LaCorte MA, Singh S, Cooper R, Fishman MC, Goldman M, Stein HL: Nuclear magnetic resonance imaging in evaluation and follow-up of children treated for coarctation of the aorta. J Am Coll Cardiol 1986 (May); 7:1095–1098.

36. Kopf GS, Hellenbrand W, Kleinman C, Lister G, Talner N, Laks H: Repair of aortic coarctation in the first three months of life: immediate and long-term results. Ann Thorac Surg 1986 (Apr); 41:425–430.

37. Goldman S, Hernandez J, Pappas G: Results of surgical treatment of coarctation of the aorta in the critically ill neonate. Including the influence of pulmonary artery banding. J Thorac Cardiovasc Surg 1986 (May); 91:732–737.

38. Sanchez GR, Balsara RK, Dunn JM, Mehta AV, O'Riordan AC: Recurrent obstruction after subclavian flap repair of coarctation of the aorta in infants. Can it be predicted or prevented? J Thorac Cardiovasc Surg 1986 (May); 91:738–746.

39. Meier MA, Lucchese FA, Jazbik W, Nesralla IA, Mendonca JT: A new technique for repair of aortic coarctation. Subclavian flap aortoplasty with preservation of arterial blood flow to the left arm. J Thorac Cardiovasc Surg 1986 (Dec); 92:1005–1012.

40. Hehrlein FW, Mulch J, Rautenburg HW, Schlepper M, Scheld HH: Incidence and pathogenesis of late aneurysms after patch graft aortoplasty for coarctation. J Thorac Cardiovasc Surg 1986 (Aug); 92:226–230.

41. Benson LN, Burns R, Schwaiger M, Schelbert HR, Lewis AB, Freedom RM, Olley PM, McLaughlin P, Rowe RD: Radionuclide angiographic evaluation of ventricular function in isolated congenitally corrected transposition of the great arteries. Am J Cardiol 1986 (Aug); 58: 319–324.

42. Daliento L, Corrado D, Buja G, John N, Nava A, Thiene G: Rhythm and conduction disturbances in isolated, congenitally corrected transposition of the great arteries. Am J Cardiol 1986 (Aug); 58:314–318.

43. Marino B, Sanders SP, Parness IA, Colan SD: Obstruction of right ventricular inflow and outflow in corrected transposition of the great arteries (S,L,L): two-dimensional echocardiographic diagnosis. J Am Coll Cardiol 1986 (Aug); 8:407–411.

44. Lincoln C, Redington AN, Li K, Mattos S, Shinebourne EA, Rigby ML: Anatomical correction for complete transposition and double outlet right ventricle: intermediate assessment of functional results. Br Heart J 1986 (Nov); 56:259–266.

45. Kenny JF, Plappert T, Doubilet P, Saltzman DH, Cartier M, Zollers L, Leatherman GF, St. John Sutton M: Changes in intracardiac blood flow velocities and right and left ventricular stroke volumes with gestational age in the normal human fetus: a prospective Doppler echocardiographic study. Circulation 1986 (Dec); 74:1208–1216.

46. Allan LD, Crawford DC, Chita SK, Anderson RH, Tynan MJ: Familial recurrence of congenital heart disease in a prospective series of mothers referred for fetal echocardiography. Am J Cardiol 1986 (Aug); 58:334–337.

47. Swensson RE, Valdes-Cruz, LM, Sahn DJ, Sherman FS, Chung KJ, Scagnelli S, Hagen-Ansert S: Real-time Doppler color flow mapping for detection of patent ductus arteriosus. J Am Coll Cardiol 1986 (Nov); 8:1105–1112.

48. Smallhorn JE, Freedom RM: Pulsed Doppler echocardiography in the preoperative evaluation of total anomalous pulmonary venous connection. J Am Coll Cardiol 1986 (Dec); 8:1413–1420.

49. Marino B, Sanders SP, Pasquini L, Giannico S, Parness IA, Colan SD: Two-dimensional echocardiographic anatomy in crisscross heart. Am J Cardiol 1986 (Aug); 58:325–333.

50. Freedom RM, Benson LN, Smallhorn JF, Williams WG, Trusler GA, Rowe RD: Subaortic stenosis, the univentricular heart, and banding of the pulmonary artery: an analysis of the courses of 43 patients with univentricular heart palliated by pulmonary artery banding. Circulation 1986 (April); 73:758–764.

51. Bowyer JJ, Busst CM, Denison DM, Shinebourne EA: Effect of long-term oxygen treatment at home in children with pulmonary vascular disease. Br Heart J 1986 (April); 55:385–390.

52. Flanagan MF, Leatherman GF, Caris A, Keane JF, Selwyn AP, Lock JE: Changing trends of congenital heart disease in adults; a catheterization laboratory perspective. Cathet Cardiovasc Diagn 1986 (Nov); 12:215–218.

53. Rosove MH, Hocking WG, Canobbio MM, Perloff JK, Child JS, Skorton DJ: Chronic hypoxemia and decompensated erythrocytosis in cyanotic congenital heart disease. Lancet 1986 (Aug 9); 313–314.

54. Ross EA, Perloff JK, Danovitch GM, Child JS, Canobbio MM: Renal function and urate metabolism in late survivors with cyanotic congenital heart disease. Circulation 1986 (March); 73:396–400.

55. Roberts WC: Major anomalies of coronary arterial origin seen in adulthood. Am Heart J 1986 (May); 5:941–963.

56. LeBlanc JG, Culham JAG, Chan KW, Patterson MW, Tipple M, Sandor GG: Treatment of grafts

and major vessel thrombosis with low-dose streptokinase in children. Ann Thorac Surg 1986 (June); 41:630–635.

57. WESSEL DL, KEANE JF, FELLOWS KE, ROBICHAUD H, LOCK JE: Fibrinolytic therapy for femoral arterial thrombosis after cardiac catheterization in infants and children. Am J Cardiol 1986 (Aug); 58:347–351.

58. GRAHAM TP, FRANKLIN RCG, WYSE RKH, GOOCH V, DEANFIELD JE: Left ventricular wall stress and contractile function in childhood: normal values and comparison of Fontan repair versus palliation only in patients with tricuspid atresia. Circulation 1986 (Sept); 74 Suppl I:I-61–I-69.

59. DRISCOLL DJ, DANIELSON GK, PUGA FJ, SCHAFF HV, HEISE CT, STAAT BA: Exercise tolerance and cardiorespiratory response to exercise after the Fontan operation for tricuspid atresia or functional single ventricle. J Am Coll Cardiol 1986 (May); 7:1087–1094.

60. KARL TR, MUSUMECI F, DE LEVAL M, PINCOTT JR, TAYLOR JFN, STARK J: Surgical treatment of absent pulmonary valve syndrome. J Thorac Cardiovasc Surg 1986 (April); 91:590–597.

61. PARK MK, TRINKLE JK: Absent pulmonary valve syndrome: a two-stage operation. Ann Thorac Surg 1986 (June); 41:669–671.

62. KIRKLIN JW, PACIFICO AD, BLACKSTONE EH, KIRKLIN JK, BARGERON LM JR: Current risks and protocols for operations for double-outlet right ventricle. Derivation from and 18 year experience. J Thorac Cardiovasc Surg 1986 (Nov); 92:913–930.

63. DOTY DB: Correction of Taussig-Bing malformation by intraventricular conduit. J Thorac Cardiovasc Surg 1986 (Jan); 91:133–138.

64. KANTER K, ANDERSON R, LINCOLN C, FIRMIN R, RIGBY M: Anatomic correction of double-outlet right ventricle with subpulmonary ventricular septal defect (the "Taussig-Bing" anomaly). Ann Thorac Surg 1986 (March); 41:287–292.

65. DELEON SY, IDRISS FS, ILBAWI MN, MUSTER AJ, PAUL MH, BERRY TE, DUFFY CE, QUINONES J: The Damus-Stansel-Kaye procedure. Should the aortic valve or subaortic valve region be closed? J Thorac Cardiovasc Surg 1986 (May); 91:747–753.

66. MAYER JE, HELGASON H, JONAS RA, LANG P, VARGAS FJ, COOK N, CASTANEDA AR: Extending the limits for modified Fontan procedures. J Thorac Cardiovasc Surg 1986 (Dec); 92:1021–1028.

67. ILBAWI MN, IDRISS FS, MUSTER AJ, DELEON SY, BERRY TE, DUFFY CE, PAUL MH: Effects of elevated coronary sinus pressure on left ventricular function after Fontan operation. An experimental and clinical correlation. J Thorac Cardiovasc Surg 1986 (Aug); 92:231–237.

68. RUMISEK JD, PIGOTT JD, WEINBERG PM, NORWOOD WI: Coronary sinus septal defect associated with tricuspid atresia. J Thorac Cardiovasc Surg 1986 (July); 92:142–145.

69. DELEON SY, ILBAWI MN, IDRISS FS, MUSTER AJ, GIDDING SS, BERRY TE, PAUL MH: Persistent low cardiac output after the Fontan operation. Should takedown be considered? J Thorac Cardiovasc Surg 1986 (Sept); 92:402–405.

70. KIRKLIN JK, BLACKSTONE EH, KIRKLIN JW, PACIFICO AD, BARGERON LM JR: The Fontan operation. Ventricular hypertrophy, age, and date of operation as risk factors. J Thorac Cardiovasc Surg 1986 (Dec); 92:1049–1064.

71. LEE CN, SCHAFF HV, DANIELSON GK, PUGA FJ, DRISCOLL DJ: Comparison of atriopulmonary versus atrioventricular connections for modified Fontan/Kreutzer repair of tricuspid valve atresia. J Thorac Cardiovasc Surg 1986 (Dec); 92:1038–1048.

72. MELDRUM-HANNA W, SCHROFF R, ROSS DN: Aortico-left ventricular tunnel: late follow-up. Ann Thorac Surg 1986 (Sept); 42:304–306.

73. OELERT H, SCHAFERS H, STEGMANN T, KALLFELZ H, BORST HG: Complete correction of total anomalous pulmonary venous drainage: experience with 53 patients. Ann Thorac Surg 1986 (April); 41:392–394.

74. ARCIPRETE P, McKAY R, WATSON GH, HAMILTON DI, WILKINSON JL, ARNOLD RM: Double connections in total anomalous pulmonary venous connection. J Thorac Cardiovasc Surg 1986 (July); 92:146–152.

75. GALLA JD, LANSMAN SL, LOWERY RC, ERGIN MA, GRIEPP RB: Primary reconstruction of interrupted aortic arch by total aortic outflow obstruction. J Thorac Cardiovasc Surg 1986 (Feb); 91:200–204.

76. HAMMON JW JR, MERRILL WH, PRAGER RL, GRAHAM TP JR, BENDER HW JR: Repair of interrupted aortic arch and associated malformations in infancy: indications for complete or partial repair. Ann Thorac Surg 1986 (July); 42:17–21.

77. SULLIVAN ID, ROBINSON PJ, DELEVAL M, GRAHAM TP JR: Membranous supravalvular mitral stenosis: a treatment form of congenital heart disease. J Am Coll Cardiol 1986 (July); 8:159–164.

78. Milano A, Vouhe PR, Baillot-Vernant F, Donzeau-Gouge P, Trinquet F, Roux PM, Leca F, Neveux JY: Late results after left-sided cardiac valve replacement in children. J Thorac Cardiovasc Surg 1986 (Aug); 92:218–225.

79. Spevak TJ, Freed MD, Castaneda AR, Norwood WI, Pollack KT: Valve replacement in children less than 5 Years of Age. J Am Coll Cardiol 1986 (Oct); 8:901–908.

80. Verrier ED, Tranbaugh RF, Soifer SJ, Yee ES, Turley K, Ebert PA: Aspirin anticoagulation in children with mechanical aortic valves. J Thorac Cadiovasc Surg 1986 (Dec); 92:1013–1020.

81. Palik I, Graham TP Jr., Burger J: Ventricular pump performance in patients with obstructed right ventricular-pulmonary artery conduits. Am Heart J 1986 (Dec); 112:1271–1276.

82. Okereke OU, Cooley DA, Frazier OH: Congenital diverticulum of the ventricle. J Thorac Cardiovasc Surg 1986 (Feb); 91:208–214.

83. Crawford FA, Sade RM, Spinale F: Bovine pericardium for correction of congenital heart defect. Ann Thorac Surg 1986 (June); 41:602–605.

Congestive Heart Failure

Effects of eating on cardiac performance

To determine whether significant spontaneous hemodynamic changes occurred without therapeutic intervention, Cornyn and associates[1] from San Francisco, California, and Columbus, Ohio, studied 15 patients with stable CHF without active treatment during an 8-hour period. Significant changes that mimic those seen during treatment with vasodilating medications were found. Increases were seen in heart rate (minimum 82 ± 19 beats/min, maximum 88 ± 18 beats/min) and cardiac index (minimum 2.14 ± 0.45 liters/min/m^2, maximum 2.42 ± 0.79 liter/min/m^2). Decreases were observed in PA wedge pressure (maximum 24 ± 7 mm Hg, minimum 21 ± 7 mm Hg) and systemic vascular resistance (maximum 1,600 ± 280 dynes s cm^5, minimum 1,390 ± 310 dynes s cm^{-5}). Except for the decrease in PA wedge pressure, all hemodynamic changes appeared to be related to eating. In addition, a statistically significant postprandial decrease in mean BP (before meal 85 ± 12 mm Hg, after meal 78 ± 11 mm Hg) was seen. These data reinforce the need for caution in interpreting small hemodynamic changes, even if statistically significant, and they indicate the desirability of including placebo groups or phases in drug studies and of performing hemodynamic measurements in the postabsorptive state.

Siemienczuk and associates[2] from Portland, Oregon, assessed the effects of ingestion of a meal on cardiac performance in patients with chronic severe CHF. A group of 32 patients underwent right-sided cardiac catheterization on the day before the study. The patients then fasted for 12 hours overnight. In the morning baseline hemodynamic measurements were obtained; then, 11 patients (group I) consumed a liquid meal of 317 kcal, and 21 patients (group II) received a placebo medication and continued fasting. Hemodynamic measurements were then obtained at intervals over 2 hours. Significant changes were seen in group I only. Cardiac index increased 22%, stroke work index increased 14%, PA wedge pressure decreased 20%, and systemic vascular resistance decreased 22% in group I. This study demonstrates an important effect on ingestion of a meal on cardiac performance in patients with CHF. To avoid overestimating the beneficial effects of therapy, eating must be carefully controlled when assessing the effects of various therapies in these patients.

Serum sodium concentration

Thirty to 50% of patients with advanced LV dysfunction who remain symptomatic taking digitalis and diuretic drugs will die within 1 year, and 60% to 80% will die within 2 years. Although past reports have identified a variety of prognostic factors in patients with severe chronic CHF, previous studies have not evaluated the interaction of prognostic variables and drug treatment. Lee and Packer[3] in New York, New York, analyzed the association of 30 clinical, hemodynamic, and biochemical variables with survival in 203 consecutive patients with severe CHF; all variables were assessed just before initiation of treatment with a variety of vasodilator drugs, and all patients were subsequently followed for 6 to 94 months. By regression analysis, pretreatment serum sodium concentration was the most powerful predictor of cardiovascular mortality, with hyponatremic patients having a substantially shorter median survival than did patients with a normal serum sodium concentration (164 -vs- 373 days). The unfavorable prognosis for hyponatremic patients appeared to be related to the marked elevation of plasma renin activity that the investigators noted in these patients, since hyponatremic patients fared significantly better when treated with angiotensin converting-enzyme inhibitors than when treated with vasodilator drugs that did not interfere with angiotensin II biosynthesis. In contrast, there was no selective benefit of the converting-enzyme inhibition on the survival of patients with a normal serum sodium concentration, in whom plasma renin activity was low. This interaction between serum sodium concentration, drug treatment, and long-term outcome suggests that the renin-angiotensin system may exert a deleterious effect on the survival of some patients with chronic heart failure, which can be antagonized by converting-enzyme inhibition, and provides a clinical counterpart for the similar prognostic role that has been postulated for angiotensin II in experimental preparations of CHF.

Atrial natriuretic peptide

To define the relation between atrial pressures and the release of atrial natriuretic peptide (ANP), Raine and associates[4] from Basel, Switzerland, measured plasma concentrations of the peptide in 26 patients with cardiac disease—11 with normal atrial pressures and 15 with elevated atrial pressures. Mean peptide levels in the peripheral venous blood were increased in 11 patients with cardiac disease and normal atrial pressures compared with 60 healthy controls (48 ± 14 -vs- 17 ± 2 pmol/liter). In the patients with elevated AP, peptide concentrations were increased twofold in peripheral venous, RA, PA, and systemic arterial plasma, compared with the concentrations in the patients with normal AP. A step-up in peptide concentration was seen between the venous and RA plasma and between the pulmonary and systemic arterial plasma, suggesting release of the peptide from the atria. A linear relation was found between RA pressure and RA peptide concentration and between PA wedge pressure and the systemic arterial peptide concentration. RA pressure and the peptide concentration both increased with exercise testing in the 9 patients evaluated. The authors concluded that the release of ANP is at least partly regulated by RA and LA pressures.

Noninvasive evaluation of left ventricular function

The M-mode echocardiogram is widely used to follow patients with CHF, but the value of M-mode echocardiography for this purpose is unclear. In 49 patients with symptomatic CHF, Baker and colleagues[5] from Little Rock, Arkansas, obtained M-mode echocardiograms during baseline evaluation to determine the value of M-mode echocardiography for predicting 1-year survival or maximal oxygen uptake during exercise. The cause of CHF was CAD in 12 patients and idiopathic dilated cardiomyopathy in 37 patients. Overall mortality at 1 year was 10 of 49 (20%), but was higher in patients with CAD (42%) compared with those with idiopathic dilated cardiomyopathy (14%). M-mode echocardiographic indexes of LV contractility were greater in survivors in whom shortening fraction averaged 16 ± 8 -vs- $10 \pm 4\%$ in nonsurvivors. Velocity of circumferential fiber shortening averaged 0.53 ± 0.25 Hz in survivors -vs- 0.35 ± 0.15 Hz in nonsurvivors. No LV dimensions, including systolic and diastolic diameters, volume, wall thickness, and mass differed significantly between survivors and nonsurvivors. No M-mode echocardiographic measure of LV dimensions or contractility correlated significantly with maximal oxygen uptake during exercise. Thus, M-mode echocardiography may be useful in predicting survival but not functional capacity in patients with CHF.

Rahko and associates[6] from Pittsburgh, Pennsylvania, determined the usefulness of systolic time intervals, diastolic time intervals, and echocardiography in evaluating LV function in 69 patients with severe CHF. All systolic time intervals were markedly abnormal (preejection period/LV ejection time 0.59 ± 0.18 -vs- 0.30 ± 0.04, preejection period index 170 ± 37 -vs- 117 ± 11, LV ejection time index 372 ± 26 -vs- 410 ± 17; patients -vs- control subjects). Diastolic time intervals in patients were not different from those in control subjects. Echocardiographic measurements were all markedly abnormal (LV end-diastolic dimension 6.9 ± 1.0 -vs- 4.8 ± 0.4 cm, patients -vs-control subjects). No pattern of abnormalities distinguished ischemic cardiomyopathy from idiopathic dilated cardiomyopathy. The presence of LV conduction delay did not substantially alter results, except that exclusion of patients with LV conduction delay normalized the total time of systole (QA2) index (from 542 ± 40 to 531 ± 31 ms) and reduced but did not normalize prolongation in the preejection period index (from 170 ± 37 to 162 ± 29 ms). No systolic or diastolic interval strongly correlated with any hemodynamic or other independent measure of LV performance. Twenty-four patients were given inotropic or unloading agents, which significantly improved hemodynamic values. Systolic and diastolic intervals were measured at baseline and at maximal hemodynamic effect. The correlation of changes in hemodynamics with changes in systolic and diastolic intervals was only modest. Thus, although systolic time intervals and associated echocardiographic measurements can detect abnormal LV function, they cannot reliably detect a change in LV function or distinguish gradations of abnormality. Diastolic intervals correlate only modestly with changes in hemodynamic values.

Lipkin and associates[7] from London, UK, studied 26 patients, aged 36–68 years, with stable chronic CHF (New York Heart Association functional class II and III) and 10 normal subjects of similar age range. Exercise capacity was assessed by determining oxygen consumption reached during a maximal treadmill exercise test and by measuring the distance each patient walked in 6 minutes. There were significant differences in the distance walked in 6 minutes among normal subjects, patients with class II CHF, and those with class III CHF (683 m, 558 m, and 402 m, respectively). The relation between maximal oxygen consumption and the distance walked in 6 minutes was curvilinear (Fig 9-1); thus, the distance walked varied considerably in those with a low maximal oxygen consumption, but varied little in patients and normal subjects with a high maximal oxygen consumption. All subjects preferred performing the 6-minute walking test to the treadmill exercise test, considering it to be more closely related to their daily physical activity. The 6-minute test is a simple objective guide to disability in patients with CHF and could be of particular value in assessing patients with severe CHF but less useful in assessing patients with mild CHF.

Catecholamines

The importance of sympathetic nervous overactivity in the pathophysiology of CHF is partly based on observations that the sympathetic neurotransmitter norepinephrine is present in increased concentrations in the plasma. Plasma concentration of norepinephrine is determined by the rates of both release of norepinephrine to the plasma and removal of norepinephrine from plasma. Hasking and co-workers[8] in Melbourne, Australia, used the analysis of plasma kinetics of the sympathetic neurotransmitter, norepinephrine, to estimate sympathetic nervous activity (integrated nerve-firing rate) for the

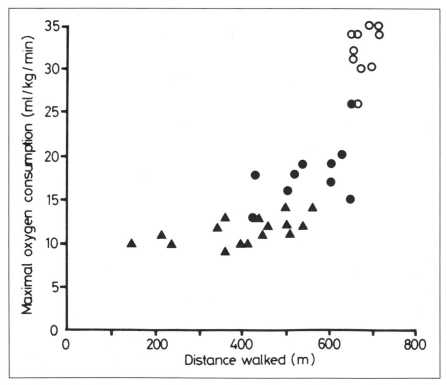

Fig. 9-1. Relation between maximal oxygen consumption and distance walked during six minute test. Normal subjects (O); patients with New York Heart Association class II heart failure (●); patients with New York Heart Association class III heart failure (▲). Reproduced with permission from Lipkin et al.[7]

body as a whole and for individual organs. In 12 patients with CHF (LVEF 10–39%), the mean arterial plasma norepinephrine concentration was 557 pg/ml compared with 211 pg/ml in 15 subjects without CHF. The difference was due to both increased release of norepinephrine to plasma (indicating increased "total" sympathetic activity) and reduced clearance of norepinephrine from plasma. The increase in sympathetic activity did not involve all organs equally. Cardiac and renal norepinephrine spillover were increased by 540% and 206%, respectively, but norepinephrine spillover from the lungs was normal. Adrenomedullary activity was also increased in the patients with CHF, whose mean arterial plasma epinephrine concentration was 181 pg/ml compared with 71 pg/ml in control subjects. There is marked regional variation, inapparent from measurements of plasma norepinephrine concentration, in sympathetic nerve activity in patients with CHF. Thus, the findings of increased cardiorenal norepinephrine spillover has important pathophysiologic and therapeutic implications.

High peripheral vascular resistance is a hallmark of advanced CHF and several neurohumoral factors may contribute, which include increased activity of the renin-angiotensin system, elevated levels of arginine vasopressin, and increased activity of the sympathetic nervous system. The high levels of circulating norepinephrine could reflect increased sympathetic neural activity or result from altered synthesis, release, or metabolism of norepinephrine. Leimbach and co-investigators[9] in Iowa City, Iowa, used microneurography (peroneal nerve) to directly record sympathetic nerve activity to muscle (mSNA) and also measured plasma norepinephrine levels in patients with CHF and in normal control subjects. The goal was to determine whether sympathetic nerve activity is increased in patients with CHF and whether plasma norepinephrine levels correlate with levels of mSNA in CHF. Resting muscle sympathetic nerve activity in 16 patients with moderate-to-severe CHF (54 bursts/minute) was significantly higher than the levels of activity in either 9 age-matched control subjects (25 bursts/minute) or 19 "young" normal control subjects (24 bursts/minute). The investigators found a significant correlation between plasma norepinephrine levels and mSNA. Neither mSNA nor plasma norepinephrine levels correlated with total systemic vascular resistance, cardiac index, LVEF, or heart rate. However, both mSNA and plasma norepinephrine levels showed significant positive correlations with LV filling pressures and mean RA pressure. The results of the study provide the first direct evidence of increased central sympathetic nerve outflow in patients with CHF and the first direct evidence that plasma norepinephrine levels show a reasonable correlation with sympathetic nerve activity to muscle in these patients. Furthermore, the data suggest that preload is an important determinant of SNA in these patients.

Beta-adrenergic receptors

Fowler and co-investigators[10] in Salt Lake City, Utah, developed methods for identifying beta-adrenergic receptors in human RV endomyocardial biopsy tissue with the radioligand $(-)$ $[^{125}I]$ iodocyanopindolol (ICYP). Specific ICYP binding in a crude, high-yield membrane preparation derived from endomyocardial biopsy tissue was high (specificity greater than 90%), of high affinity (K_D around 20 pM), saturable and stereospecific for the $(-)$ -vs- the $(+)$ isomer of isoproterenol. Subjects with mild-moderate and severe biventricular dysfunction had respective decreases in beta-adrenergic receptor density of 38% and 58% when normalization methods were averaged, with no significant differences in ICYP dissociation constant. The patients were divided into 2 groups according to their LVEF at rest. Group A consisted of 7 patients with no or mild CHF and LVEF >0.40; subgroup B consisted of 11 patients with moderate to severe CHF and LVEF <0.30. Graded sequential infusions of dobutamine and calcium gluconate were administered. Those with severe cardiac dysfunction had marked impairment of the dobutamine dP/dt and stroke index response, whereas those responses to calcium did not differ in the 2 groups. These data indicate that in the intact human heart 1) endomyocardial biopsy may be used for direct analysis of beta-adrenergic receptors, 2) CHF associated myocardial beta-adrenergic down-regulation begins with mild-moderate ventricular dysfunction, 3) reduction in myocardial beta-receptor density is related to degree of CHF, and 4) beta-receptor down-regulation is associated with pharmacologically specific impairment of the beta-agonist-mediated contractile response.

Arginine vasopressin

Ten patients with advanced CHF were treated with an arginine vasopressin antagonist during hemodynamic monitoring to determine the contribution of vasopressin to systemic vasoconstriction by Creager et al[11] in Boston, Massachusetts. In these studies, the vasopressin antagonist caused a decrease in systemic vascular resistance in 3 patients whose plasma vasopressin was >4.0 pg/ml; the average plasma vasopressin level was 2.4 ± 0.6 pg/ml for the entire group. Plasma vasopressin concentration correlated with the percent decrease of systemic vascular resistance, serum sodium, and serum creatinine values (Fig. 9-2). The relative roles of vasopressin and the renin-angiotensin and sympathetic nervous systems in causing systemic arterial vasocon-

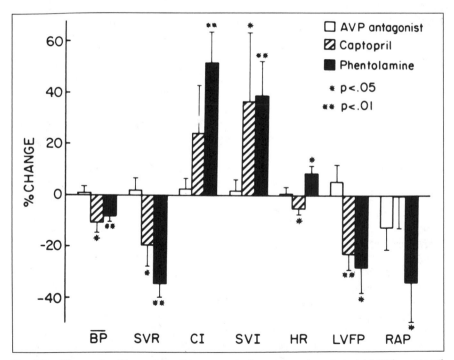

Fig. 9-2.   The maximal hemodynamic response to the vasopressin antagonist (AVP), captopril and phentolamine. Hemodynamic variables are indicated as percent change (mean ± SEM) from pretreatment values. $\overline{BP}$ = mean blood pressure; CI = cardiac index; HR = heart rate; LVFP = left ventricular filling pressure; RAP = right atrial pressure; SVI = stroke volume index; SVR = systemic vascular resistance. Reproduced with permission from Creager et al.[11]

striction were compared by administering captopril and phentolamine to these patients. Captopril decreased systemic vascular resistance by 20%, primarily in patients with high plasma renin activities. Levels of plasma renin activity ranged between 1 and 46 ng/ml/hour and correlated with serum sodium, serum creatinine, and RA pressures Phentolamine decreased systemic vascular resistance in all patients by an average of 34%, but the decrease did not correlate with the pretreatment norepinephrine serum concentrations. Norepinephrine levels were elevated in all patients with a mean of 694 ± 110 pg/ml and correlated with baseline stroke volume indexes and plasma renin activities. Thus, vasopressin and the renin-angiotensin system each contribute to systemic vasoconstriction in some patients with CHF, but the sympathetic nervous system consistently contributes to vasoconstriction in these patients.

Goldsmith et al[12] in Minneapolis, Minnesota, and Milwaukee, Wisconsin, evaluated the effects of exogenously administered arginine vasopressin in 11 patients with chronic CHF. Infusion rates of 0.1 to 0.8 pmol/kg/min increased plasma arginine vasopressin from 6.5 ± 2.7 (SD) pg/ml initially to 63 ± 39 pg/ml at the highest infusion rate of arginine vasopressin. In association with the administration of arginine, there were progressive decreases in cardiac output and stroke volume and increases in systemic vascular resistance and PA wedge pressure. Only minor changes occurred in heart rate and BP with the administration of arginine. Changes in cardiac output, stroke volume, and systemic vascular resistance were evident from the first infusion rate (Fig. 9-3). Therefore, relatively small changes in arginine vasopressin level cause modest but significant adverse circulatory effects in patients with CHF. These data are consistent with the possibility that circulating arginine vasopressin in physiologic concentrations may influence hemodynamics in patients with CHF.

TREATMENT

Captopril

To evaluate the influence of renal function on the efficacy of the converting-enzyme inhibitor, captopril, Packer and associates[13] from New York, New York, measured the long-term hemodynamic and clinical responses to captopril in 101 consecutive patients with chronic severe CHF grouped according to pretreatment serum creatinine concentration (group I, <1.4 mg/dl; group II, 1.4–2.8 mg/dl; and group III, >2.8 mg/dl). After 1 to 3 months of treatment, patients with preserved renal function (group I) had greater increases in stroke volume index and greater decreases in LV filling pressure and systemic vascular resistance than did patients with renal impairment (groups II and III). Clinical improvement paralleled these hemodynamic benefits; only 2 of 12 patients with severe renal insufficiency (group III) improved clinically compared with 29 of 40 patients with preserved renal function (group I) and 29 of 49 patients with mild-to-moderate renal impairment (group II). Therapy-limiting rash and dysgeusia occurred most frequently in patients with renal impairment. The findings support an important role for the kidneys in mediating the beneficial actions of captopril in patients with severe CHF.

The effects of captopril as long-term treatment in 20 patients with CHF was studied in a double-blind trial conducted by Cleland and associates[14] from Glasgow, Scotland. Captopril caused a significant increase in serum

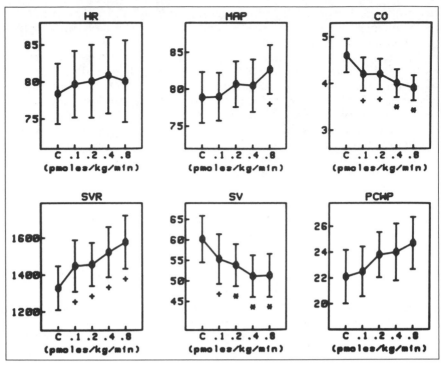

Fig. 9-3. Overall hemodynamic responses to arginine vasopressin infusions. Data are shown as mean ± SD for each infusion rate. See text for the arginine vasopressin levels corresponding to the infusion rate. ^+p <0.05; $^*p$ <0.01. CO = cardiac output (liters/min); HR = heart rate (beats/min); MAP = mean arterial pressure (mm Hg); PCWP = pulmonary capillary wedge pressure (mm Hg); SV = stroke volume (ml); SVR = systemic vascular resistance (dynes·s·cm^{-5}). Reproduced with permission from Goldsmith et al.[12]

digoxin levels. No patients had evidence of digoxin toxicity. Serum and total body potassium increased and the frequency of ventricular arrhythmias showed a modest decline. Creatinine clearance and radioisotopically measured glomerular filtration rate decreased, but there was a poor relation between these and the increase in serum digoxin. In a further open study on 12 patients, creatinine, urea, and digoxin clearance were significantly reduced by captopril. However, digoxin clearance declined more than creatinine clearance (89 ± 25–69 ± 22 μmol/liter and 81 ± 14–72 ± 19 μmol/liter, respectively). Fractional excretion of urea and digoxin filtered at the glomerulus declined, indicating greater tubular reabsorption or reduced tubular secretion of these compounds. Captopril causes an increase in serum digoxin by reducing renal clearance of the drug.

Enalapril

Kromer and associates[15] from Wurzburg, Federal Republic of Germany, investigated the effectiveness of converting enzyme inhibition on cardiac performance of patients with CHF (New York Heart Association functional class II). Twelve outpatients were treated with enalapril, 5–10 mg twice daily, in addition to stable doses of digitalis and diuretic drugs. Before and after 4 and 12 weeks of treatment, a treadmill exercise test and echocardiography were performed. Maximal oxygen uptake and exercise tolerance increased significantly and mean arterial pressure at rest and on exertion decreased significantly. Heart rate did not change. LV end-diastolic diameter decreased significantly. Serum angiotensin-converting enzyme activity was reduced to nearly 0; plasma renin concentration, which was already elevated, increased further. Plasma norepinephrine levels did not change significantly. Treatment was tolerated well by all patients. Enalapril decreased preload and afterload, suggesting that they might have had an inappropriately elevated arteriolar and venous tone owing to a moderately stimulated renin angiotensin system and sympathetic nervous system. These conditions may lead to further deterioration of cardiac performance.

Captopril -vs- enalapril

To evaluate the concept that long duration of action is an advantageous property of angiotensin-converting enzyme inhibitors in the treatment of severe CHF, Packer and associates[16] from New York, New York, randomly assigned 42 patients to therapy with either a short-acting inhibitor (captopril 150 mg/day) or a long-acting inhibitor (enalapril, 40 mg/day) for 1–3 months while concomitant therapy with digoxin and diuretic drugs was kept constant. The treatment groups had similar hemodynamic and clinical characteristics at baseline evaluation and similar initial responses to converting-enzyme inhibition. During long-term therapy, captopril and enalapril produced similar decreases in systemic BP, but the hypotensive effects of enalapril were more prolonged and persistent than those of captopril. Consequently, although the patients in both groups improved hemodynamically and clinically during the study, serious symptomatic hypotension (syncope and near syncope) was seen primarily among those treated with enalapril. Sustained hypotension also probably accounted for the decline in creatinine clearance and the notable retention of potassium observed in the patients treated with enalapril but not in those treated with captropril. The authors concluded that when large, fixed doses of converting-enzyme inhibitors are used in the treatment of patients with severe CHF, long-acting agents may produce prolonged hypotensive effects that may compromise cerebral and renal function, and thus they may have disadvantages in such cases, compared with short-acting agents.

Prazosin

Packer et al[17] in New York, New York, used right-sided cardiac catheterization before and during long-term therapy with prazosin in 27 patients with severe CHF to determine a) the efficacy of prazosin and b) whether the renin-angiotensin system plays a role in the development of hemodynamic tolerance to long-term prazosin administration. During 3–12 weeks of treatment with prazosin, doses of digoxin and furosemide remained constant. Eleven of 27 patients were assigned to concomitant therapy with spironolactone, whereas the remaining 16 patients did not receive the aldosterone antagonist. The initial doses of prazosin resulted in marked increases in cardiac index and decreases in mean arterial pressure, LV filling pressure, and systemic vascular resistance in all of the patients studied, but these effects were rapidly attenuated in both groups after 48 hours and remained reduced during long-term therapy (Fig. 9-4). Three to 12 weeks of therapy was associated with cardiac index returning to pretreatment levels and a failure of it to decrease when the drug was withdrawn. Mean arterial pressure, LV filling pressure, and systemic vascular resistance remained decreased although attenuated after 3–12 weeks of therapy and increased to pretreatment values when the drug was withdrawn. Spironolactone therapy did not alter the

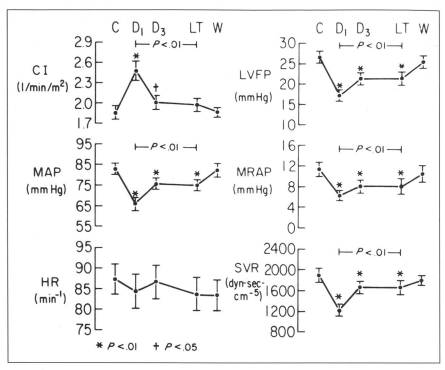

Fig. 9-4. Values for cardiac index (CI), mean arterial pressure (MAP), heart rate (HR), left ventricular filling pressure (LVFP), mean right atrial pressure (MRAP) and systemic vascular resistance (SVR) before prazosin (C), after the first dose of the drug (D_1), after 48 hours of therapy (D_3), during long-term treatment (3 to 12 weeks, LT) and 48 hours after drug withdrawal (W). Symbols indicate significance of differences from control values: p values at the top of each panel indicate significance of differences between D_1 and LT. Data are shown as mean ± SEM. Reproduced with permission from Packer et al.[17]

magnitude and time course of these responses. Fourteen of the 24 patients (58%) demonstrated loss of hemodynamic efficacy to prazosin during long-term hemodynamic study without changes in plasma renin activity or body weight. These data suggest that prazosin produces long-term hemodynamic and clinical benefit in only 30–40% of patients with severe CHF, and they do not support a role for the renin-angiotensin system in the development of tolerance to alpha$_1$-adrenergic blockade.

Captopril -vs- prazosin

Mettauer and co-investigators[18] in Quebec, Canada, infused 15 ml/kg body weight waterload to 50 patients with CHF and measured systemic hemodynamic, renal function, and neurohumoral parameters before 2 days and 1 month after randomly allocating patients to prazosin or captopril therapy. Both prazosin and captopril caused similar and persistent hemodynamic changes, but important differences existed between their renal and neurohumoral effects. After 1 month of continuous therapy, captopril increased creatinine clearance from 71–84 ml/min/1.73^2, increased the waterload excreted in 5 hours from 50–71%, and increased 5-hour sodium excreted from 6.8–14/7 mEq. Captopril also caused a decrease in plasma norepinephrine from 568–448 pg/ml, in plasma epinephrine from 94–73 pg/ml, and in plasma aldosterone from 57–28 ng/dl, without changing plasma vasopressin.

These beneficial effects were greater after 1 month of therapy than after 2 days. The only beneficial effect of prazosin was to increase water excretion from 49–59%. The long-term response to captopril was similar in patients with higher and lower renin levels. In patients with lower renin levels, prazosin decreased PA wedge pressure (25–22 mmHg), decreased plasma arginine vasopressin (1.16–0.75 pg/ml), increased water excretion (62–85%), and decreased plasma epinephrine (81–46 pg/ml), whereas in patients with higher renin levels none of these beneficial effects were noted. The investigators concluded 1) that captopril produces long-term beneficial renal and neurohumoral effects that prazosin does not despite similar hemodynamic changes with the 2 drugs, 2) that these effects are at least partially dependent on the initial neurohumoral and hemodynamic status of the patient, and 3) that through hemodynamic improvements vasodilators may chronically interrupt vasopressin overstimulation.

Packer and associates[19] from New York, New York, compared short- and long-term hemodynamic and clinical responses to sequential therapy with prazosin (15 mg/day for 3–12 weeks) and captopril (75–300 mg/day for 2–15 weeks) in 22 patients with severe chronic CHF. First doses of prazosin produced marked increases in cardiac index and stroke volume index, but these effects were lost during long-term treatment. First doses of captopril produced only modest increases in both variables, but these persisted without attenuation during prolonged therapy. Both drugs produced immediate decreases in LV filling pressure, mean arterial pressure, mean right atrial pressure and systemic vascular resistance; these changes became significantly attenuated with prazosin but not with captopril. At the end of treatment, stroke volume index was significantly higher and RV and LV filling pressures were significantly lower with captopril than with prazosin. Only 8 of the 22 patients (36%) treated with prazosin benefited clinically, whereas 14 of 19 patients (74%) treated with captopril believed they had improved. These differences could not have been predicted by comparing responses to first doses of the 2 drugs. These findings indicate that the choice of 1 vasodilator drug over another in patients with CHF should be based on studies that compare long-term rather than short-term hemodynamic and clinical effects.

Prazosin -vs- hydralazine + isosorbide dinitrate

To evaluate the effects of vasodilator therapy on mortality among patients with chronic CHF, Cohn and associates[20] of the Veterans Administration Cooperative Study randomly assigned 642 men with impaired cardiac function and reduced exercise tolerance who were taking digoxin and a diuretic drug to receive additional double-blind treatment with placebo, prazosin (20 mg/day), or the combination of hydralazine (300 mg/day) and isosorbide dinitrate (160 mg/day). Follow-up averaged 2.3 years (range 6 months–5.7 years). Mortality over the entire follow-up period was lower in the group that received hydralazine and isosorbide dinitrate than in the placebo group (Fig. 9-5). This difference was of borderline statistical significance. For mortality by 2 years, a major endpoint specified in the protocol, the risk reduction among patients treated with both hydralazine and isosorbide dinitrate was 34%. The cumulative mortality rates at 2 years were 26% in the hydralazine–isosorbide dinitrate group and 34% in the placebo group; at 3 years, the mortality rate was 36% -vs- 47%. The mortality-risk reduction in the group treated with hydralazine and isosorbide dinitrate was 36% by 3 years. The mortality in the prazosin group was similar to that in the placebo group. LVEF (measured sequentially) increased significantly at 8 weeks and at 1

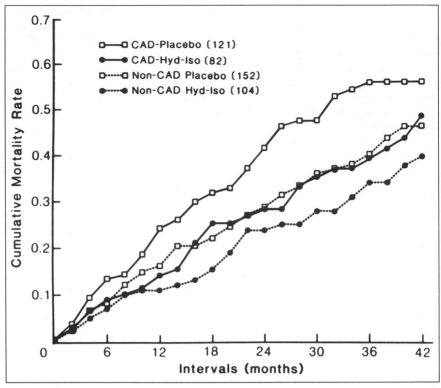

Fig. 9-5. Cumulative mortality among patients with (n = 203) and without (n = 256) coronary artery disease (CAD) treated with placebo or hydralazine–isosorbide dinitrate (Hyd–Iso). Reproduced with permission from Cohn et al.[20]

year in the group treated with hydralazine and isosorbide dinitrate but not in the placebo or prazosin groups. The data suggest that the addition of hydralazine and isosorbide dinitrate to the therapeutic regimen of digoxin and diuretic drugs in patients with chronic CHF can have a favorable effect on LV function and mortality.

Milrinone

Cody and colleagues[21] in New York, New York, developed an isolated limb preparation to evaluate the direct vasoactive properties of cardioactive drugs on the forearm vasculature in patients with CHF. Using this model, the investigators infused milrinone in subsystemic doses (1, 10, and 20 μg/minute per 100 ml forearm volume) into the brachial artery of 13 patients with moderate-to-severe CHF. Forearm and systemic hemodynamics were monitored and milrinone plasma concentrations from both the forearm venous effluent and PA were measured. Compared with the baseline forearm blood flow, the 3 doses of milrinone resulted in increases in forearm blood flow; this was associated with a reduction of forearm vascular resistance from the baseline values. Forearm vasodilatation occurred without change in systemic hemodynamics or therapeutic milrinone plasma concentrations in the PA. In 5 patients the response to intraarterial milrinone was compared to that of nitroprusside. Response to nitroprusside was greater than that to milrinone. Milrinone was administered by a systemic intravenous route, the magnitude of forearm vasodilatation was not as great as that with intraarterial milrinone, suggesting different sensitivities of vasodilatation in alternate vascular beds or the influence of baroreceptor autoregulation. This study identified direct vasodilator properties of milrinone that are independent of the drug's inotropic activity.

The cardiac bipyridines, including milrinone, reduce cardiac filling pressures and systemic vascular resistance and increase cardiac output in patients with CHF. To determine the relative contributions of milrinone's positive inotropic and vasodilator actions in patients with severe CHF, Ludmer and co-investigators[22] in Boston, Massachusetts, administered the drugs by constant infusion directly into the LM coronary artery of 11 patients with New York Heart Association functional class III or IV CHF. Intracoronary infusion of milrinone at rates up to 50 μg/minute had no effect on mean arterial pressure or systemic vascular resistance but resulted in dose-related increases in peak positive dP/dt (+21%), stroke volume index (+18%), and stroke work index (+21%), and decreases in heart rate (−3%), mean RA pressure (−25%), and LV end-diastolic pressure (−17%). In 8 patients, intravenous administration (75 μg/kg) after the intracoronary infusion resulted in significant decreases in mean arterial pressure (−14%) and systemic vascular resistance (−40%), further increase in stroke volume index compared with intracoronary administration, and further decreases in mean RA and LV end-diastolic pressures compared with intracoronary administration. These data indicate that milrinone exerts both positive inotropic and vasodilator actions that contribute significantly to the drug's overall hemodynamic effect.

Baim et al[23] in Boston, Massachusetts, evaluated the long-term efficacy and safety of oral milrinone therapy during a 2.5-year period in 100 patients with severe CHF despite their receiving conventional medical therapy. Oral milrinone therapy (27 ± 8 mg/day initial dose) was well tolerated. Drug-associated side effects occurred in only 11% of patients and resulted in the withdrawal of milrinone in only 4% of patients. Among 94 patients evaluated after 1 month of therapy, 51% had improved by at least 1 New York Association functional class. Nevertheless, despite clinical improvement, mortality rates for patients treated with milrinone did not appear to be reduced; 39% of these patients died by 6 months and 63% at 1 year (Fig. 9-6). The clinical variables that predicted death within 6 months included a) advanced functional class, b) impaired renal function, c) reduced RVEF, d) presence of nonsustained VT on 24-hour ambulatory electrocardiography, e) more impaired baseline hemodynamic function, and f) absence of clinical improvement after 1 month on milrinone therapy. Multivariate analysis identified lower baseline cardiac index and aortic systolic pressure as the most important variables in predicting death during a short-term follow-up. Patients who died of progressive CHF had less frequent use of antiarrhythmic drugs and greater increases in diuretic and milrinone doses than did those who died suddenly. Therefore, although milrinone is well tolerated and produces early symptomatic benefit in approximately half of the patients with CHF not adequately responsive to conventional therapy, there is no evidence that it reduces the high mortality risk for patients with this problem.

Milrinone is a promising new inotrope, but its arrhythmogenic potential has not been defined. Anderson and associates[24] from Salt Lake City, Utah, monitored ventricular arrhythmias during a 24-hour baseline and 48-hour milrinone infusion period in 12 patients with chronic CHF. Patients were characterized by mean age of 58 years and LVEF of 21%. Nine (75%) were men, 9 had primary idiopathic dilated cardiomyopathy, and 3 had CAD. None had a history of cardiac arrest or sustained VT. Milrinone was given as a loading dose (mean 53 μg/kg/10 minutes; range 37.5–75) followed by a

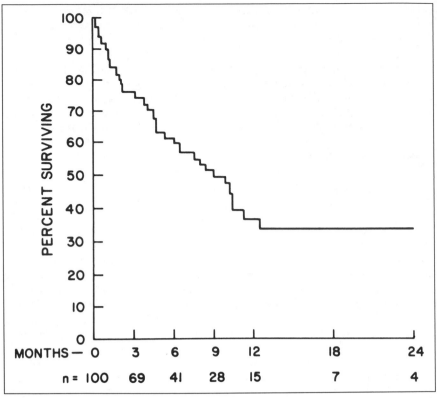

Fig. 9-6. Survival curve for the 100 patients receiving chronic oral milrinone therapy. The figures at the bottom refer to the number of patients at risk at the indicated times. Reproduced with permission from Baim et al.[23]

48-hour maintenance infusion (mean 0.53 μg/kg/min; range 0.25–0.75). Acutely, cardiac index increased by 27% and PA wedge pressure decreased by 30% during milrinone administration; changes were maintained during continued therapy. Ventricular arrhythmia response was variable, with no significant overall difference. However, a trend toward increased ectopic activity was noted. No sustained tachyarrhythmias occurred. Mean frequency of VPC was 87 ± 48 VPC/hour during baseline monitoring and 141 ± 69/hour after infusion of the drug. Mean frequency of couplets was 6.0 ± 4.9/hour before drug infusion and 14.3 ± 11.0/hour during infusion. Mean frequency of runs was 0.9 ± 0.8/hour before and 2.7 ± 2.4/hour during drug infusion. Two patients met criteria for proarrhythmia (increased VPC of >4× and/or repetitive forms of >10×). However, neither proarrhythmia patient required reduction in the dosage of milrinone or additional antiarrhythmic therapy. Milrinone may be safely administered for prolonged periods (2 days) with excellent clinical tolerance and low arrhythmogenic potential, and it produces significant and beneficial hemodynamic effects in patients with advanced CHF. However, to exclude arrhythmogenic effects, continuous electrocardiography is advised, as for other intravenous inotropes.

Grose et al[25] in Bronx, New York, studied the effects of dobutamine and milrinone given intravenously on systemic hemodynamics, coronary blood flow, and selected aspects of myocardial metabolism in 11 patients with severe CHF. In this study, milrinone and dobutamine increased cardiac index similarly from 1.9 ± 0.4–2.5 ± 0.4 liters/min/m² and from 1.9 ± 0.4–2.8 ± 0.8 liters/min/m², respectively. Milrinone also decreased LV end-diastolic

pressure to a greater extent than dobutamine (Fig. 9-7). Milrinone also reduced mean systemic arterial and RA pressure, whereas dobutamine did not.
Dobutamine increased the first derivative of LV pressure (dP/dt) but milrinone did not. Blood flow and myocardial oxygen consumption were increased by dobutamine but were unchanged by milrinone. Both dobutamine
and milrinone significantly decreased coronary vascular resistance and myocardial oxygen extraction but did not change myocardial lactate extraction.
Therefore, dobutamine and milrinone produce similar improvements in cardiac index, but dobutamine produces more direct increase in cardiac contractility and milrinone more substantial vasodilating effect.

Administration of the positive inotropic vasodilator milrinone results in
immediate improvement in the maximal and submaximal metabolic responses to exercise. To determine whether these effects persist during long-
term therapy, Ribeiro and associates[26] from Boston, Massachusetts, evaluated 9 patients with severe CHF by upright maximal exercise testing before
therapy (baseline), after 10 ± 1 weeks of oral therapy, and during double-
blind, placebo-controlled readministration of intravenous milrinone after
withdrawal of oral drug for 24 hours. During long-term oral therapy, maximal oxygen uptake was unchanged (baseline 792 ± 72 ml/minute, oral therapy 820 ± 83 ml/minute), whereas the anaerobic threshold was increased
significantly from 570 ± 53 ml/minute–681 ± 61 ml/minute. After withdrawal of milrinone, maximal oxygen uptake and anaerobic threshold decreased significantly; subsequent intravenous administration caused significant increases in maximal oxygen uptake and anaerobic threshold, back to
the values measured during oral therapy. After oral milrinone withdrawal,
maximal oxygen uptake decreased below baseline values, suggesting progression of the underlying disease. The anaerobic threshold expressed as a percent of maximal oxygen uptake was significantly increased during oral therapy (baseline 73 ± 2%, oral therapy 84 ± 2%) and remained significantly

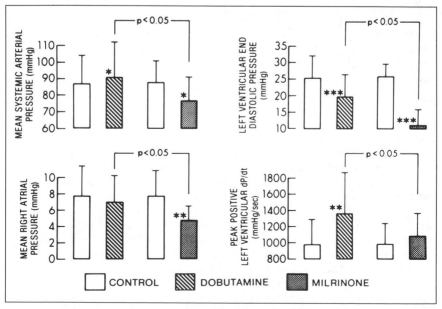

Fig. 9.7 Comparative effects of dobutamine and intravenous milrinone on systemic
hemodynamic variables. Horizontal bars indicate ±SD. * p <0.05; ** p <0.01: *** p <0.001
versus control. Reproduced with permission from Grose et al.[25]

increased after drug withdrawal, suggesting a peripheral circulatory effect. These results indicate that in selected patients with severe CHF, milrinone exerts persistent effects on the metabolic responses to both maximal and submaximal exercise. Because of progressive deterioration in exercise capacity during long-term oral therapy, the effects of milrinone may not be apparent unless it is withdrawn. The relation of milrinone therapy to disease progression is not known.

Dobutamine -vs- amrinone

Gage and co-workers[27] in Bronx, New York, evaluated the effects of amrinone, dobutamine, and a combination of the 2 drugs on peak positive LV dP/dt and LV performance in 11 patients with chronic CHF. When administered alone, dobutamine (10.9 μg/kg/min) and intravenous amrinone (1.9 mg/kg/min) significantly increased left ventricular dP/dt and performance. When compared with dobutamine alone, the addition of amrinone resulted in further increases in LV dP/dt and cardiac index. The combination also induced a further reduction in LV end-diastolic pressure (from 18–15 mmHg) when compared with amrinone alone. The combination of dobutamine and amrinone increased heart rate slightly when compared with either drug alone. It did not further reduce systemic arterial pressure when compared with amrinone alone. The dose-response curve of LV dP/dt and performance during titration of dobutamine with and without the addition of intravenous amrinone was evaluated in 7 patients. The addition of amrinone to any dose of dobutamine produced higher cardiac index and lower systemic vascular resistance than dobutamine or amrinone alone. Thus, when compared with dobutamine alone in patients with chronic CHF, the addition of intravenous amrinone to dobutamine results in an additive improvement in LV performance through the dose range.

Enoximone (MDL 17,043)

Weber and associates[28] from Chicago, Illinois, examined the efficacy and safety of enoximone for chronic clinically stable CHF secondary to ischemic or myopathic heart disease. Thirty-one patients were enrolled into an early phase II trial. The hemodynamic response to intravenous and oral enoximone was assessed and compared with the response to dobutamine therapy (5–10 μg/kg/min). Maximal O_2 uptake, an objective measure of effort tolerance, was serially monitored. Intravenous (1–2 mg/kg) and oral (1–2 mg/kg) enoximone improved cardiac index, while reducing right atrial and wedge pressures to a greater extent than dobutamine. The salutary hemodynamic response to oral enoximone was sustained for 6–8 hours and was not associated with subacute drug tolerance. Maximal O_2 uptake was increased at 2, 4, 8, 12, 24, and 52 weeks of oral enoximone therapy (1.4 ± 0.5 mg/kg every 8 hours), whereas radionuclide EF at 65 weeks increased from baseline (39 ± 16 -vs- 30 ± 9%). Nine patients, 8 of whom were in functional class III or IV on enrollment, died after a mean of 18 weeks: 4 from cardiac failure and 5 suddenly. Two patients had adverse gastrointestinal effects. Oral enoximone (1–2 mg/kg every 8 hours) appears to be useful in the short- and long-term management of clinically stable, chronic CHF.

Dobutamine -vs- enoximone

Likoff and associates[29] from Philadelphia, Pennsylvania, compared the acute hemodynamic response to intravenous dobutamine with intravenous

MDL 17,043 in 8 patients with severe chronic CHF. Simultaneous RNA was performed with gated equilibrium blood pool imaging to derive LV volumes and EF during serial hemodynamic measurements. Six patients had an optimal dobutamine dose of 10 $\mu g/kg/min$; 2 others were compared at a dose of 7.5 $\mu g/kg/min$; comparisons with MDL 17,043 were obtained after a 1.5-mg/kg bolus dose in all 8 patients. Dobutamine and MDL 17,043 caused significant and similar increases in cardiac index and stroke volume index. Dobutamine significantly increased heart rate and MDL 17,043 did not. MDL 17,043 significantly decreased PA wedge, mean PA, and RA pressures; dobutamine did not. Dobutamine increased end-diastolic volume in 4 patients, with little concomitant decrease in wedge pressure; MDL 17,043 caused no change or a decrease in LV end-diastolic volume in 5 patients, but consistently decreased wedge pressure in all. Thus, the LV pressure-volume curve was displaced downward to a more favorable position after MDL 17,043 but not after dobutamine. In patients with chronic CHF, acute myocardial performance was more optimally influenced by MDL 17,043 than dobutamine administration.

Uretsky and associates[30] from Pittsburgh, Pennsylvania, compared the peak hemodynamic effect and hormonal response of the phosphodiesterase inhibitor enoximone (MDL 17,043) with those of dobutamine in 10 patients with severe CHF. Both agents significantly increased cardiac index, stroke volume index, and heart rate. Enoximone tended to decrease mean systemic arterial and PA wedge pressures, whereas dobutamine did not. Both agents decreased systemic vascular resistance. The increase in heart rate was greater with dobutamine than with enoximone. Plasma renin activity increased significantly with dobutamine (from 11 ± 14–18 ± 15 ng/ml/hour) and with enoximone (from 14 ± 18–17 ± 19 ng/ml/hour). Dobutamine suppressed plasma norepinephrine level and enoximone did not. Neither agent affected the plasma vasopressin level. These data demonstrate a similar acute hemodynamic and hormonal profile for both enoximone and dobutamine. Further, dobutamine, like other β agonists, provokes renin secretion and may do so to a greater extent than enoximone.

Ibopamine

N-Methyldopamine (epinine), one of the few modifications of the dopamine (DA) molecule that retains agonists activity at the DA_1 receptor, was administered orally by Rajfer and co-investigators[31] in Chicago, Illinois, as a diisobutyric ester, ibopamine (100, 200, and 300 mg), to 15 patients with CHF. An increase in cardiac index and decline in systemic vascular resistance was observed with each dose, and these hemodynamic effects persisted for 3–6 hour (Table 9-1). Small transient increments in RA and PA wedge pressures occurred 0.5 hour after ingestion of 200 and 300 mg of ibopamine, but these pressures returned to baseline of lower levels within 30 minutes. Heart rate and mean arterial pressure were unchanged. Plasma concentrations of epinine peaked 0.5 hour after administration of the drug and then declined to minimal levels at 3 hours. Ten patients enrolled in a trial to evaluate the efficacy of long-term therapy with ibopamine; after 8 weeks of treatment, the initial hemodynamic responses to the drug were attenuated and no significant improvement in oxygen uptake at peak exercise was observed. A decline in plasma norepinephrine concentrations, which could be attributed to activation of alpha$_2$-adrenoceptors and/or DA_2 receptors on sympathetic nerves, was observed after initial administration of ibopamine and persisted after long-term drug ingestion; no long-term hemodynamic benefit could be ascribed to the reduction in sympathetic activity.

TABLE 9-1. *Hemodynamic responses to short- and long-term administration of ibopamine in nine patients with congestive heart failure. Reproduced with permission from Rajfer et al.[31]*

	INITIAL STUDY		LONG-TERM STUDY	
	BASELINE	AFTER TREATMENT	BASELINE	AFTER TREATMENT
Cardiac index (liters/min/m²)	1.90 ± 0.10	2.30 ± 0.17[C]	1.88 ± 0.13	2.04 ± 0.14
Stroke volume index (ml/beat/m²)	23.8 ± 1.5	28.0 ± 2.5[C]	24.7 ± 2.4	26.1 ± 2.7
Mean arterial pressure (mm Hg)	82 ± 4	84 ± 4	85 ± 4	87 ± 4
Systemic vascular resistance (dyne · sec · cm⁻⁵)	1727 ± 149	1494 ± 133[C]	1775 ± 151	1701 ± 153
Mean pulmonary capillary wedge pressure (mm Hg)	21 ± 2	22 ± 2	24 ± 2[B]	27 ± 2[A]
Mean right atrial pressure (mm Hg)	8 ± 2	9 ± 3	10 ± 2	12 ± 2
Heart rate (beats/min)	80 ± 2	84 ± 3	78 ± 3	81 ± 4

Values are mean ±SEM.
[A]$p < .05$ for the difference from the baseline value for the long-term study; [B]$p < .05$ for the difference between baseline values for the initial and long-term studies; [C]$p < .01$ for the difference from the baseline value for the initial study.

Viprostol -vs- nitroprusside

Prostaglandins have been shown to stimulate renin release through a direct effect on the juxtaglomerular cells and on the macula densa. The responsiveness of the renin-angiotensin system to hemodynamic changes in patients with CHF is reduced and this could be due to a defect of the juxtaglomerular apparatus. To test this hypothesis, Olivari and co-workers[32] in Minneapolis, Minnesota, compared the responses to viprostol, an analog of prostaglandin E_2 (PGE_2) that is known to stimulate both the macula densa and the juxtaglomerular cells, to nitroprusside in patients with CHF. An average reduction in mean arterial pressure of 6 mmHg with viprostol was associated with a 5-fold increase in plasma renin activity. In contrast plasma renin activity did not change with nitroprusside despite a significant decrease in preload and an average decrease in mean arterial pressure of 16 mmHg. These data demonstrate that 1) the renin-angiotensin system could be activated by PGE_2 in patients with CHF, 2) this activation is not related to the global hemodynamic changes induced by PGE_2, and 3) previously reported unresponsiveness of the renin-angiotensin system in patients with CHF cannot be attributed to a defective response of the juxtaglomerular apparatus.

Nitroglycerin

Jordon and associates[33] from Little Rock, Arkansas, and Summit, New Jersey, administered *transdermal* nitroglycerin, 60 mg/24 hours, to 8 patients or placebo to 7 patients in a double-blind fashion, and monitored PA wedge pressure and nitroglycerin plasma levels for 24 hours. After placebo administration, nitroglycerin plasma levels and PA wedge pressure remained unchanged. During transdermal nitroglycerin administration, the plasma nitroglycerin level increased from 0.04 ± 0.12 ng/ml at baseline to near peak levels at 2 hours (7.43 ± 7.21 ng/ml). Between 2 and 24 hours, levels fluctuated at a steady state. PA wedge pressure decreased from 22 ± 7 mmHg at control to a nadir of 14 ± 5 mmHg at 4 hours. Despite persistently high plasma nitroglycerin levels, by 18 hours PA wedge pressure was no longer significantly reduced (20 ± 9 mmHg). These results indicate that rapid development of tolerance is the cause of attenuated hemodynamic efficacy of transdermal nitroglycerin.

To clarify the continuing controversy concerning the use of transdermal nitroglycerin, Packer and associates[34] from New York, New York, evaluated the short-term hemodynamic responses to sublingual, oral, and transcutaneous nitrates in 22 patients with severe chronic CHF. Sixteen patients had favorable hemodynamic effects with transdermal nitroglycerin, but the doses needed to achieve this response varied greatly: 10 mg/24 hours in 6 patients, 20 mg/24 hours in 5 patients, 40 mg/24 hours in 3 patients, and 60 mg/24 hours in 2 patients. Of the 6 remaining patients, 3 did not respond to high-dose transdermal nitroglycerin even though they had marked effects after

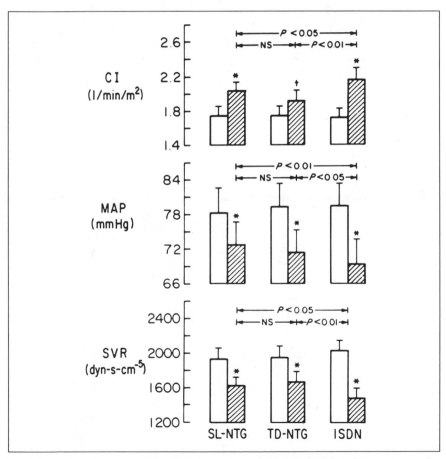

Fig. 9-8. Values for cardiac index (C1), mean arterial pressure (MAP) and systemic vascular resistance (SVR) before (*open bars*) and after (*shaded bars*) administration of sublingual nitroglycerin (SL-NTG, 5 to 15 minutes), transdermal nitroglycerin (TD-NTG, 1 hour) and oral isosorbide dinitrate (ISDN, 15 to 45 minutes). Significance of difference between pre- and posttreatment values for each drug: *p <0.01, †p <0.05. The p values above the bars designate significance of differences among the 3 drugs. NS = not significant.

sublingual and oral nitrate administration; 3 others did not respond to any nitrate formulation by any route. Transdermal nitroglycerin produced immediate increases in cardiac index and decreases in RV and LV filling pressure, mean arterial pressure and systemic vascular resistance (Figs 9-8 and 9-9). These effects, however, became rapidly attenuated within 3–6 hours; after 18–24 hours, only modest decreases in RV and LV filling pressures were observed. After removal of transdermal nitroglycerin treatment, rebound decreases in cardiac index and rebound increases in mean arterial pressure and systemic vascular resistance occurred, but RV and LV filling pressures returned to pretreatment values without rebound changes. Isosorbide dinitrate, 40 mg orally, produced hemodynamic effects that were greater in magnitude than effects seen after administration of transdermal nitroglycerin,

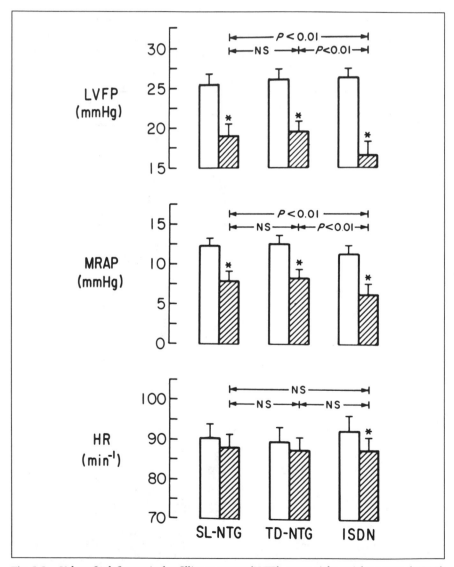

Fig. 9-9. Values for left ventricular filling pressure (LVFP), mean right atrial pressure (MRAP) and heart rate (HR) before (*open bars*) and after (*shaded bars*) administration of sublingual nitroglycerin, transdermal nitroglycerin and oral isosorbide dinitrate. Format, abbreviations and symbols as in Figure 3.

but 4 patients in whom tolerance to transdermal nitroglycerin developed showed reversible cross tolerance to oral isosorbide dinitrate. In conclusion, the use of transdermal nitroglycerin in patients with severe chronic CHF is limited by the large doses of the drug that are needed in some patients, by the rapid attenuation of its beneficial effects during prolonged therapy, by the potential for cross tolerance to other nitrates, and by the occurrence of rebound phenomena after drug withdrawal.

Nicardipine

Ryman and associates[35] from New York, New York, studied the hemodynamic response to vasodilation induced by a new calcium channel antagonist, nicardipine, in 10 patients with severe, chronic CHF. Rest and exercise hemodynamics were evaluated in the baseline state and after 1 week of oral nicardipine therapy (30 mg 3 times daily). In addition, respiratory gas exchange and arteriovenous oxygen difference were measured to assess changes in oxygen utilization. The responses of the sympathetic nervous system were evaluated by measuring plasma norepinephrine concentrations at rest and during maximal exercise. At rest, nicardipine administration was associated with significant reductions in mean systemic arterial pressure, systemic vascular resistance, PA wedge pressure and PA pressure, and significant increases in cardiac index and stroke volume index. These effects were maintained during exercise. In contrast to findings with other calcium antagonists, no negative inotropic effect of nicardipine was identified. Nicardipine administration was associated with reduction of arteriovenous oxygen difference. Nicardipine had no effect on plasma norepinephrine concentrations, suggesting absence of reflex sympathetic nervous activation. Thus, nicardipine-mediated vasodilation leads to significant improvements in both rest and exercise cardiac performance.

Nortriptyline

Roose and associates[36] from New York, New York, measured the effect of nortriptyline on LVEF and BP in 21 depressed patients with LV impairment. EF was unchanged by nortriptyline treatment and orthostatic hypotension developed in only 1 of the 21 patients. Nortriptyline, therefore, emerges as a relatively safe treatment for depression in patients with LV impairment.

References

1. CORNYN JW, MASSIE BM, UNIVERFERTH DV, LEIER CV: Hemodynamic changes after meals and placebo treatment in chronic congestive heart failure. Am J Cardiol 1986 (Feb 1); 57:238–241.
2. SIEMIENCZUK D, GREENBERG B, BROUDY DR: Effects of eating on cardiac performance in congestive heart failure. Chest 1986 (Aug); 193–197.
3. LEE WH, PACKER M: Prognostic importance of serum sodium concentration and its modification by converting-enzyme inhibition in patients with severe chronic heart failure. Circulation 1986 (Feb); 257–267.
4. RAINE AEG, ERNE P, BURGISSER E, MULLER FB, BOLLI P, BURKART F, BUHLER FR: Atrial natriuretic peptide and atrial pressure in patients with congestive heart failure. N Engl J Med 1986 (Aug 24); 315:533–537.
5. BAKER BJ, LEDDY C, GALIÈ N, CASEBOLT P, FRANCIOSA JA: Predictive value of M-mode echocardiography in patients with congestive heart failure. Am Heart J 1986 (Apr); 111:697–701.

6. RAHKO PS, SHAVER JA, SALERNI R, URETSKY BF, MATESIC C: Noninvasive evaluation of systolic and diastolic function in severe congestive heart failure secondary to coronary artery disease or idiopathic dilated cardiomyopathy. Am J Cardiol 1986 (June 1); 57:1315–1322.

7. LIPKIN DP, SCRIVEN AJ, CRAKE T, POOLE-WILSON PA: Six minute walking test for assessing exercise capacity in chronic heart failure. Br Med J 1986 (Mar); 292:653–655.

8. HASKING GJ, ESLER MD, JENNINGS GL, BURTON D, JOHNS JA, KORNER PI: Norepinephrine spillover to plasma in patients with congestive heart failure: evidence of increased overall and cardiorenal sympathetic nervous activity. Circulation 1986 (Apr); 73(4):615–621.

9. LEIMBACH WN, WALLIN G, VICTOR RG, AYLWARD PE, SUNDLOF G, MARK AL: Direct evidence from intraneural recordings for increased central sympathetic outflow in patients with heart failure. Circulation 1986 (May); 73(5):913–919.

10. FOWLER MB, LASER JA, HOPKINS GL, MINOBE W, BRISTOW MR: Assessment of the β-adrenergic receptor pathway in the intact failing human heart: progressive receptor down-regulation and subsensitivity to agonist response. Circulation 1986 (Dec); 74:1290–1302.

11. CREAGER MA, FAXON DP, CUTLER SS, KOHLMANN O, RYAN TJ, GAVRAS H: Contribution of vasopressin to vasoconstriction in patients with congestive heart failure: comparison with the renin-angiotensin system and the sympathetic nervous system. J Am Coll Cardiol 1986 (Apr); 7:758–765.

12. GOLDSMITH SR, FRANCIS GS, COWLEY AW JR, GOLDENBERG IF, COHN JN: Hemodynamic effects of infused arginine vasopressin in congestive heart failure. J Am Coll Cardiol 1986 (Oct); 8:779–783.

13. PACKER M, LEE WH, MEDINA N, YUSHAK M: Influence of renal function on the hemodynamic and clinical responses to long-term captopril therapy in severe chronic heart failure. Ann Intern Med 1984 (Feb); 104:147–154.

14. CLELAND JGF, DARGIE HJ, PETTIGREW A, GILLEN G, ROBERTSON NIS: The effects of captopril on serum digoxin and urinary urea and digoxin clearances in patients with congestive heart failure. Am Heart J 1986 (July); 112:130–135.

15. KROMER EP, RIEGGER GAJ, LIEBAU G, KOCHSIEK K: Effectiveness of converting enzyme inhibition (enalapril) for mild congestive heart failure. Am J Cardiol 1986 (Feb 15); 57:459–462.

16. PACKER M, LEE WH, YUSHAK M, MEDINA N: Comparison of captopril and enalapril in patients with severe chronic heart failure. N Engl J Med 1986 (Oct 2); 315:847–853.

17. PACKER M, MEDINA N, YUSHAK M: Role of the renin-angiotensin system in the development of hemodynamic and clinical tolerance to long-term prazosin therapy in patients with severe chronic heart failure. J Am Coll Cardiol 1986 (Mar); 7:671–680.

18. METTAUER B, ROULEAU J, BICHET D, KORTAS C, MANZINI C, TREMBLAY G, CHATTERJEE K: Differential long-term intrarenal and neurohormonal effects of captopril and prazosin in patients with chronic congestive heart failure: importance of initial plasma renin activity. Circulation 1986 (Mar); 73(3):492–502.

19. PACKER M, MEDINA N, YUSHAK M: Comparative hemodynamic and clinical effects of long-term treatment with prazosin and captopril for severe chronic congestive heart failure secondary to coronary artery disease or idiopathic dilated cardiomyopathy. Am J Cardiol 1986 (June 1); 57:1323–1327.

20. COHN JN, ARCHIBALD DG, PHIL M, ZIESCHE S, FRANCIOSA JA, HARSTON WE, TRISTANI FE, DUNKMAN WB, JACOBS W, FRANCIS GS, FLOHR KH, GOLDMAN S, COBB FR, SHAH PM, SAUNDERS R, FLETCHER RD, LOEB HS, HUGHES VC, BAKER B: Effect of vasodilator therapy on mortality in chronic congestive heart failure: results of a Veterans Administration cooperative study. N Engl J Med 1986 (June 12); 314:1547–1552.

21. CODY RJ, MULLER FB, KUBO SH, RUTMAN H, LEONARD D: Identification of the direct vasodilator effect of milrinone with an isolated limb preparation in patients with chronic congestive heart failure. Circulation 1986 (Jan); 73(1):124–129.

22. LUDMER PL, WRIGHT RF, ARNOLD MO, GANZ P, BRAUNWALD E, COLUCCI W: Separation of the direct myocardial and vasodilator actions of milrinone administered by an intracoronary infusion technique. Circulation 1986 (Jan); 73(1):130–137.

23. BAIM DS, COLUCCI WS, MONRAD ES, SMITH HS, WRIGHT RF, LANOUE A, GAUTHIER DF, RANSIL BJ, GROSSMAN W, BRAUNWALD E: Survival of patients with severe congestive heart failure treatment with oral milrinone. J Am Coll Cardiol 1986 (Mar); 7:661–670.

24. ANDERSON JL, ASKINS JC, GILBERT EM, MENLOVE RL, LUTZ JR: Occurrence of ventricular arrhythmias in patients receiving acute and chronic infusions of milrinone. Am Heart J 1986 (Mar); 111:466–474.

25. GROSE R, STRAIN J, GREENBERG M, LeJEMTEL TH: Systemic and coronary effects of intravenous milrinone and dobutamine in congestive heart failure. J Am Coll Cardiol 1986 (May); 7:1107–1113.

26. RIBEIRO JP, WHITE HD, ARNOLD JMO, HARTLEY LH, COLUCCI WS: Exercise responses before and after long-term treatment with oral milrinone in patients with severe heart failure. Am J Med 1986 (Nov); 81:759–764.

27. GAGE J, RUTMAN H, LUCIDO D, LeJEMTEL TH: Additive effects of dobutamine and amrinone on myocardial contractility and ventricular performance in patients with severe heart failure. Circulation 1986 (Feb); 74:367–373.

28. WEBER KT, JANICKI JS, JAIN MC: Enoximone (MDL 17,043) for stable, chronic heart failure secondary to ischemic or idiopathic cardiomyopathy. Am J Cardiol 1986 (Sept 15); 58:589–595.

29. LIKOFF MJ, ULRICH S, HAKKI A, ISKANDRIAN AS: Comparison of acute hemodynamic response to dobutamine and intravenous MDL 17,043 (enoximone) in severe congestive heart failure secondary to ischemic cardiomyopathy or idiopathic dilated cardiomyopathy. Am J Cardiol 1986 (June 1); 57:1328–1334.

30. URETSKY BF, GENERALOVICH T, VERBALIS JG, VALDES AM, REDDY PS: Comparative hemodynamic and hormonal response of enoximone and dobutamine in severe congestive heart failure. Am J Cardiol 1986 (July 1); 58:110–116.

31. RAJFER SI, ROSSEN JD, DOUGLAS FL, GOLDBERG LI, KARRISON T: Effects of long-term therapy with oral ibopamine on resting hemodynamics and exercise capacity in patients with heart failure: relationship to the generation of N-methyldopamine and to plasma norepinephrine levels. Circulation 1986 (Apr); 73(4):740–748.

32. OLIVARI MT, DEVINE TB, COHN JN: Evidence for a direct renal stimulating effect of prostaglandin E_2 on renin release in patients with congestive heart failure. Circulation 1986 (Dec); 74:1203–1207.

33. JORDAN RA, SETH L, CASEBOLT P, HAYES MJ, WILEN MM, FRANCIOSA J: Rapidly developing tolerance to transdermal nitroglycerin in congestive heart failure. Ann Intern Med 1986 (Mar); 104:295–298.

34. PACKER M, MEDINA N, YUSHAK M, LEE WH: Hemodynamic factors limiting the response to transdermal nitroglycerin in severe chronic congestive heart failure. Am J Cardiol 1986 (Feb 1); 57:260–267.

35. RYMAN KS, KUBO SH, LYSTASH J, STONE G, CODY RJ: Effect of nicardipine on rest and exercise hemodynamics in chronic congestive heart failure. Am J Cardiol 1986 (Sept 15); 58:583–588.

36. ROOSE SP, GLASSMAN AH, GIARDINA EGV, JOHNSON LL, WALSH BT, WOODRING S, BIGGER JT: Nortriptyline in depressed patients with left ventricular impairment. JAMA 1986 (Dec); 256:3253–3257.

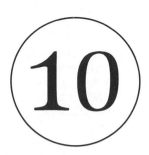

Miscellaneous Topics

Total 12-lead QRS voltage in autopsied men

Use of the total 12-lead QRS electrocardiographic voltage as a criterion for LV hypertrophy has been of recent interest. Although upper and lower limits of QRS voltage for individual electrocardiographic leads have been reported in clinically healthy men and women, the upper limit of total 12-lead QRS voltage has not been established in adults free of cardiopulmonary disease by clinical and necropsy criteria. Therefore, Odom and associates[1] from Little Rock, Arkansas, and Bethesda, Maryland, determined total QRS voltage from all 12 electrocardiographic leads in 30 autopsied men known to be free of cardiopulmonary disease by clinical assessment and by a special cardiac examination using postmortem coronary angiography and chamber partition determination of LV weight. Gross heart weight, LV weight, and total QRS voltage are reported. Comparisons were made between disease-free patients and previously reported patients with AS, AR, and cardiac amyloidosis with respect to total 12-lead QRS voltage and gross heart weight. Total QRS voltage and gross heart weight were significantly greater in patients with severe AS (mean 245 mm) and severe AR (mean 274 mm) than in the patients without cardiopulmonary disease (mean 127 mm). Total QRS voltage was significantly less, whereas gross heart weight was significantly greater in patients with cardiac amyloidosis (mean 101 mm) than in normal subjects (mean 127 mm). These data provide a basis for evaluating the total 12-lead QRS voltage as a criterion for LV hypertrophy.

Left ventricular filling

Gardin and associates[2] from Orange and Long Beach, California, evaluated the usefulness of pulsed Doppler flow velocity measurements for evaluating LV diastolic filling. In normal persons these measurements are affected by age and respiration, but not by gender, body surface area, or normal BP. Additional factors that may influence these measurements include the imaging view and sample volume location. In this study, the effects of imaging view and sample volume location were evaluated in 52 normal subjects, aged 21 to 78 years. Pulsed Doppler recordings were obtained from the apical 4-chamber and apical 2-chamber views with the sample volume located both in the left atrium and at the level of the mitral valve leaflet tips. Doppler measurements were slightly, but not significantly, higher (4% on average) for recordings obtained from the apical 4-chamber than from the 2-chamber view for peak flow velocity in both early and late diastole. However, apical 4-chamber recordings from a sample volume in the left atrium resulted in measurements significantly lower for both early and late diastolic mitral peak flow velocity than those obtained near the mitral leaflet tips (peak flow velocity in early diastole = 43 ± 12 -vs- 57 ± 12 cm/s and peak flow velocity in late diastole = 36 ± 7 -vs- 46 ± 11 cm/s, respectively). The higher mitral peak flow velocity values recorded in early and late diastole near the mitral leaflet tips may be related to the smaller flow area at the mitral valve orifice compared with the left atrium. Neither imaging view nor sample volume location resulted in significant differences in the ratio of late-to-early diastolic peak flow velocity. Pulsed Doppler mitral flow velocity measurements must be standardized for sample volume location when evaluating ventricular diastolic filling.

Aortic flow velocity in exercise

Although Doppler echocardiography is useful in the assessment of LV function at rest, little information is available on the application of this technique during exercise. Gardin and associates[3] from Orange, California, performed Doppler aortic flow studies in 17 young normal subjects during and after supine bicycle exercise to determine the feasibility of recording Doppler aortic flow velocity with a suprasternal notch transducer during exercise and to assess the changes in normal aortic flow velocity during exercise and early recovery (Fig. 10-1). Each subject exercised until fatigue; mean duration of exercise was 10 minutes. Heart rate increased from a mean of 69 beats/minute at control to 159 beats/minute during peak exercise. On average, aortic peak flow velocity increased by 45% from control, reaching its maximum at 2 minutes after exercise. Ejection time decreased by 34% during exercise, being shortest at peak exercise. Heart rate, peak flow velocity, and ejection time had not returned to normal by 10 minutes after exercise. Aortic flow velocity integral (a relative measure of stroke volume) decreased by 10% at peak exercise compared with control, but had returned to control at 2 minutes after exercise. Despite mild aliasing and increased respiratory rate during maximal exercise, aortic flow velocity measurements could be recorded using the suprasternal technique. These baseline Doppler exercise data should be useful in further studies of exercise hemodynamic changes in patients with heart disease.

Relation of intensity of exercise training to functional capacity

Gossard and associates[4] from Stanford, California, evaluated the effects of 12 weeks of home-based exercise training on peak exercise oxygen consumption (VO₂ max) in healthy sedentary middle-aged men, mean age 49 ± 6 years. Twenty-one men trained at low intensity, 23 trained at high inten-

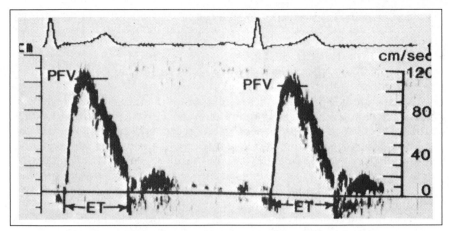

Fig. 10-1. Spectral display of a normal aortic flow velocity recording demonstrating method for making measurements of peak flow velocity (PFV, cm/s) and ejection time (ET, ms).

sity, and 20 were control subjects. Individually prescribed low- and high-intensity training was performed 5 times per week within a range of 42–60% and 63–81% of baseline VO_2 max, corresponding to average heart rates of 102–122 and 128–148 beats/minute, respectively. Caloric expenditure per training session approximated 350 kcal in both groups; adherence was at least 90% in both groups. VO_2 max increased 8% in patients who trained at low intensity, 17% in those who trained at high intensity, and not at all in control subjects. Low-intensity exercise training at home significantly augments functional capacity in healthy sedentary middle-aged men.

Postexercise hypotension

Although a decrease in systolic BP occurring during treadmill exercise is often a sign of severe LV dysfunction, the prevalence and significance of postexertional hypotension is unclear. Fleg and Lakatta[5] from Baltimore, Maryland, analyzed the postexercise systolic BP response to maximum treadmill exercise in 781 asymptomatic volunteers, aged 21–96 years (mean 51), from the Baltimore Longitudinal Study on Aging. Fifteen subjects (2%) had a postexercise decrease in systolic BP of ≥20 mmHg from preexercise sitting values, to a level of ≤90 mmHg. The prevalence of postexercise hypotension was 3% (14 of 449) in subjects <55 years of age but only 0.3% (1 of 332) in those >55 years of age. Before exercise the 15 subjects had a slight orthostatic decrease in systolic BP of −1.7 ± 4.8 mmHg compared with an increase of 5.3 ± 5.1 mmHg in age-matched control subjects. The lowest systolic BP averaged 78 ± 9 mmHg (range 62–90) and occurred between 4 and 9 minutes after exercise in 80% of cases. All but 3 episodes were symptomatic, with dizziness dominant. In only 2 subjects was the hypotension associated with vagal symptoms and bradycardia. Compared with control subjects, subjects with postexercise hypotension had higher maximal heart rates (184 ± 15 -vs- 173 ± 11 beats/minute), but showed no difference in exercise tolerance or systolic BP at submaximal or maximal effort. Postexercise ST-segment abnormalities suggesting ischemia occurred in one-third of the hypotensive subjects but in none of the control subjects. No subject with hypotension had cardiovascular morbidity or mortality over a follow-up period averaging 4 years. Thus, in a general population, hypotension after treadmill exercise occurs primarily in younger persons with high maximal heart rates. It may be a cause for an ischemic electrocardiographic response but appears to have a benign prognosis.

Changes in aerobic work performance with age

To determine the physiologic mechanisms of the decline in aerobic work performance with age, Higginbotham and associates[6] from Durham, North Carolina, performed a cross-sectional study involving 24 sedentary male volunteers, aged 20 to 50 years, and they underwent right-sided cardiac catheterization, arterial cannulation, RNA, and expired gas analysis for detailed evaluation of central and peripheral cardiovascular function during submaximal and maximal exercise. Habitual physical activity level varied but was well matched across the age range. Over the 3-decade age range studied, there was no detectable change in cardiovascular function at rest. When peak exercise variables were examined, an age-related 25% decrease in O_2 consumption was noted; this was associated with a 25% decrease in peak cardiac index and a 20% decrease in peak heart rate. In addition, there was an age-related increase in calculated systemic and pulmonary vascular resistances and an increase in LV ejection time. No age relation was seen for exercise stroke volume index, end-diastolic volume index, end-systolic volume index, pulmonary artery wedge pressure, EF, or arteriovenous O_2 difference. These results indicate that the age-related decline in aerobic work performance among men aged 20–50 years results primarily from a reduced exercise heart rate in older subjects rather than from a reduction in stroke volume or peripheral O_2 utilization.

Effect of exercise on platelet aggregability

Platelet function along with lipoprotein and the arterial vessel wall has been postulated to be centrally involved in the development of atherosclerosis. There are currently no definitive data on the long-term effects of regular physical exercise on platelet function in humans. Rauramaa and co-workers[7] in Kuopio, Finland, assessed the influence of regular moderate-intensity physical exercise (brisk walking to slow jogging) on platelet aggregation in a population-based sample of middle-aged, overweight, mildly hypertensive men in eastern Finland. In this controlled study, the investigators evaluated the net effect of exercise on platelet aggregation by studying changes in optical density and ATP release in platelet-rich plasma. A significant inhibition of secondary platelet aggregation from 27–36% was observed in the men taking regular exercise. These findings give new insight into the possible protective effects of exercise against the risk of ischemic heart disease.

Effects of beta-adrenergic blockade on exercising

Exercise training improves function of the heart, peripheral circulation, and skeletal muscle that results in enhanced physical work capacity. Since the specific influence of beta-adrenergic stimulation on these various adaptations has not been clear, Wolfel and co-workers[8] in Denver, Colorado, studied the effect of beta$_1$-selective and nonselective beta-adrenergic blockade on the exercise conditioning response of 24 healthy, sedentary men after an intensive 6-week aerobic training program. Subjects randomly assigned to receive placebo, 50 mg twice daily of *atenolol* (selective), or 40 mg twice daily of *nadolol* (nonselective) were tested before and after training both with and without drugs. Comparable reductions in maximal exercise heart rate occurred with atenolol and nadolol, indicating equivalent $beta_1$-adrenergic blockade. Vascular $beta_2$-adrenergic selectivity was maintained with atenolol as determined by calf plethysmography during intravenous infusion of epinephrine. At maximal exercise, subjects receiving placebo increased their exercise duration and oxygen pulse significantly greater than those receiving atenolol or nadolol. During submaximal exercise there were reductions in heart rate and heart rate–blood pressure product in all 3 groups, but these reductions were greater with placebo than with either drug. Leg blood flow during submaximal exercise decreased 24% in the placebo group but was unchanged in the atenolol and nadolol groups. Lactates in arterialized blood during submaximal exercise were reduced equivalently in all 3 groups after training. Capillary/fiber ratio in vastus lateralis muscle biopsy specimens increased 31% in the placebo group and 21% in the atenolol group and tended to increase in the nadolol group. Succinic dehydrogenase and cytochrome oxidase activities in muscle biopsy specimens increased equivalently in all 3 groups after training. Thus, although exercise conditioning developed to some extent in both drug groups, especially during submaximal exercise, these changes were less marked than that with placebo. While beta-adrenergic blockade attenuated the exercise conditioning response, skeletal muscle adaptations including increases in oxidative enzymes, capillary supply, and decreases in exercise blood lactates were unaffected. Cardiac and peripheral vascular adaptations do appear to be affected by beta-adrenergic blockade during training, but cardioselectivity does not seem to be important in modifying these effects.

Left ventricular mechanics in distance runners

Mickelson and associates[9] from San Francisco, California, assessed heart size and mechanics at rest in highly trained distance runners. They compared 62 runners (>40 miles/week) and 84 nonrunners by 2-dimensional echocardiography. LV end-diastolic volume index and mass index were larger in runners than in nonrunners and in men than in women. However, LV end-diastolic and end-systolic volume/mass ratios were similar for runners and nonrunners. Noninvasive estimates of end-systolic and peak-systolic meridional and circumferential wall stresses were lower in runners than in nonrunners. Lower wall stress resulted from lower myocardial area/cavity area ratios, and thus average radius/thickness ratios (measured from the parasternal short-axis view), in runners than in nonrunners. These investigators detected a subtle change in ventricular shape among the distance runners; basilar hypertrophy accounted for increased myocardial thickness with normal cavity size in the parasternal short-axis view, as might be expected in hearts working under sustained pressure elevations during prolonged training periods. However, cavity length and therefore ventricular volume were increased in the apical views, leading to a normal overall volume/mass ratio. These hearts have thus adjusted to periods of volume, and to pressure overload. Race performance is determined by a complex interaction between the heart, vascular, and skeletal muscle systems. In this study no parameter of myocardial size or function predicted 10 km or marathon race times, just as no physical characteristic or training record predicted LV mass, end-diastolic or end-systolic volume. Myocardial adaptation and performance are unique characteristics of these persons.

Electrocardiography during parachute jumping

Using 2-channel 24-hour ambulatory electrocardiographic recording, Tak and associates[10] from Amsterdam, The Netherlands, studied 7 healthy young

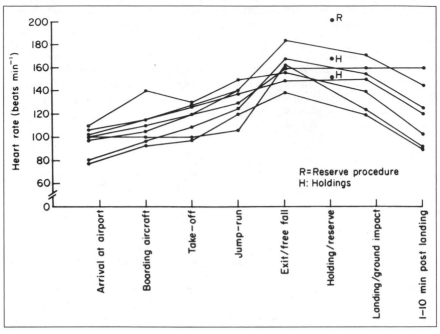

Fig. 10-2. Heart rates during various stages of competitive parachute jumping (day 1) in 7 healthy volunteers 20–30 years of age. For subjects who performed more than one jump, the average heart is depicted. Reproduced with permission from Tak et al.[10]

men during 1 day of parachute jumping competition (day 1), compared with 1 control day (day 2). A symptom-limited exercise test was also performed on day 2. Maximal heart rates attained during exercise testing were of the same order as during parachute jumping (Fig. 10-2). In the phases just before "exit," short periods of striking sinus arrhythmia with slow atrial rhythm were present in 3 subjects. Only 1 of these had slow atrial rhythm during the control day. Atrial and ventricular premature complexes, when present, disappeared with higher heart rates under all circumstances. No AV conduction disturbances were found.

Effect of digoxin on electrocardiogram during exercise

Sundqvist and associates[11] from Stockholm, Sweden, studied the effect of digoxin on the electrocardiogram at rest and during and after exercise in 11 healthy subjects. Exercise was performed on a heart rate–controlled bicycle ergometer with stepwise increased loads up to a heart rate of 170 beats/ minute. The subjects were studied after peroral intake of digoxin at 2 dose levels and after withdrawal of digoxin. Administration of digoxin induced significant ST-T depression at rest and during exercise even at the small dose (2.4 ± 0.8 μg/kg body weight, mean ± standard deviation). The ST-T changes were numerically small and dose-dependent. The most pronounced ST and T depression occurred at a heart rate of 110–130 beats/minute. At higher heart rates the ST depression was less pronounced but still statistically significant. During the first minutes after exercise no significant digitalis-induced ST-T depression was seen. This reaction is not of the type usually seen in myocardial ischemia. Fourteen days after withdrawal of the drug there were no significant digitalis-induced ST-T changes at rest or during or after exercise.

Mechanism of loss of physiologic S_3 with age

A third heart sound is frequently audible in normal children and adolescents, but its presence in persons >40 years of age is usually associated with underlying heart disease such as LV failure of various origins or excessive flow through the mitral valve in early diastole. To study the mechanism of disappearance of the physiologic third heart sound (S_3) with advancing age, Van de Werf and co-investigators[12] in Leuven, Belgium, quantitatively analyzed combined phonoechocardiographic and phonomechanocardiographic recordings from 165 subjects between 6 and 62 years old. Nearly all subjects <40 years old had a recordable S_3. Although recordable in 39% of the 44 subjects >40 years old, the physiologic S_3 found in the older adults was less intense and occurred later in ventricular diastole compared with that in children and adolescents. Marked changes in LV filling hemodynamics were observed with aging, including an increase in LV wall thickness and mass, a prolongation of the LV isovolumetric relaxation period, a decrease in LV early diastolic filling and wall thinning rates, and a reduction in the height and steepness of the rapid filling wave measured on the calibrated left apexcardiogram. Although less pronounced, these changes were very similar to the diastolic abnormalities found in patients with pressure overload LV hypertrophy. Therefore, the higher pressure load imposed on the LV wall due to the well-known gradual increase in BP that occurs during normal growth and adulthood appears to be the most likely explanation for the observed changes in diastolic filling. It was concluded that the later occurrence, the diminishing amplitude, and the eventual complete disappearance of the physiologic S_3 with age results from a decrease in early diastolic LV filling and subsequent deceleration of inflow caused by the development of relative LV hypertrophy in adulthood as compared with childhood.

PERICARDIAL HEART DISEASE

Recurrent acute pericarditis

Fowler et al[13] in Cincinnati, Ohio, evaluated 31 patients with recurrent pericarditis observed for periods of 2–19 years. Twenty-four had idiopathic pericarditis, 4 had postoperative or posttraumatic pericarditis, 2 had postinfarction pericarditis, and 1 had recurrent pericarditis after anticoagulant-induced intrapericardial bleeding. Among 24 patients (group I), recurrent pericarditis was documented by a) electrocardiographic changes; b) electrocardiographic evidence of pericardial fluid; and c) a pericardial friction rub and chest pain typical of pericarditis. In 7 patients (group II), recurrent pericarditis was documented only by increased white blood cell count, erythrocyte sedimentation rate, or fever in addition to chest pain. The duration of the active or recurrent process was ≥5 years in 19 patients and ≥8 years in 7 patients. Three patients had cardiac tamponade with the initial episode of pericarditis, but no patient had tamponade during recurrent pericarditis. In addition, no patient had CHF, constrictive pericarditis, or life-threatening cardiac arrhythmias with recurrent pericarditis. Most patients required adrenal steroid therapy to obtain pain relief, and withdrawal of steroids subsequently was usually difficult. Nine patients underwent pericardiectomy, but in only 2 was this followed by definite pain relief. Thus, these data suggest that recurrent attacks of chest pain are the major disabling features of recurrent pericarditis.

Percutaneous pericardial catheter drainage

Kopecky and associates[14] from Rochester, Minnesota, analyzed results of 42 consecutive patients having pericardial effusion treated with percutaneous pericardial drainage. Intermittent (79%) or continuous (21%) drainage through a 60-cm pigtail catheter (No. 6Fr–8Fr) was used. Clinical indications were urgent or semiurgent treatment of large (38%), life-threatening (24%), recurrent (21%), or acute (traumatic) (17%) pericardial effusion. Sixteen patients had a malignant cause for the effusion. Mean duration of use of the indwelling pericardial catheter was 3.5 days (range <1–19 days). Two of the 9 catheters in patients on continuous drainage but only 1 of 33 catheters in patients on intermittent drainage became occluded. There was only 1 possible infective complication. Six patients had subsequent elective surgical intervention. Placement of an indwelling pericardial catheter guided by 2-D echocardiography is safe and effective for initial treatment of selected pericardial effusions.

ATRIAL NATRIURETIC FACTOR

In CARDIOLOGY 1986 considerable space was given to the atrial natriuretic peptide (ANP). Needleman and Greenwald[15] reviewed recent findings on ANP, a peptide hormone that is intimately involved in the regulation of renal and cardiovascular homeostasis. This peptide, which is stored in the atrial cardiocyte, is capable of exerting potent, selective, and transient effects on fluid and electrolyte balance and on BP. Hundreds of publications have appeared since the announcement of the discovery of this structure in 1984. The present article is an interpretive review to provide a framework for understanding current and future findings about ANP and their implications. The schematic overview of Figure 10-3 shows how ANP links the heart, kidneys, adrenal glands, blood vessels, and brain in a complex hormonal system involved in volume and pressure homeostasis. Basal levels of ANP exist in the circulation, suggesting that it is released continuously at low levels. Increases in the plasma level of ANP can be elicited by atrial stretch caused by volume expansion, constrictor agents that elevate atrial pressure, immersion in water, atrial tachycardia, and high salt diets. Although the peptide is stored as the high-molecular-weight prohormone, the primary form that is isolated from the plasma is the low-molecular weight carboxy-terminal fragment atrial peptin-28. Thus, a very selective enzymatic cleavage of the largely inactive peptide occurs during the release process. Once in the circulation, the peptide exerts a number of effects through specific extracellular receptors, to produce a multiplicity of actions involved in renal and cardiovascular functions. The combined effects that alter salt and water metabolism arise from direct renal effects, which produce an increase in glomerular filtration and pronounced natriuresis and diuresis; inhibition of aldosterone secretion by the cells in the adrenal zona glomerulosa, regardless of the stimulus; suppression of vasopressin release that is elevated by dehydration or hemorrhage; and inhibition of the angiotensin-induced drinking response. The influence of ANP on BP has been observed in its capacity to suppress elevated

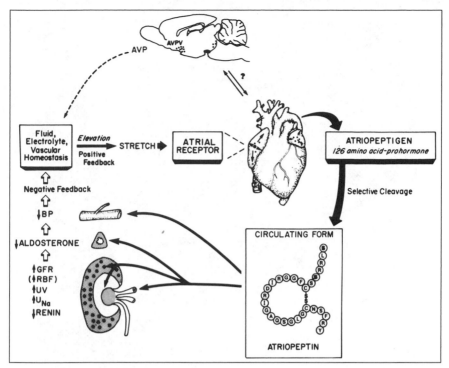

Fig. 10-3. Schematic diagram of the atriopeptin hormonal system. Reproduced with permission from Needleman and Greenwald.[15]

plasma levels of renin and to relax blood vessels directly, thereby reducing vascular resistance. The discovery and characterization of ANP heralds a unique opportunity for the development of new pharmacologic agents for the therapeutic manipulation of circulatory, volume, and salt homeostasis.

To evaluate the relation between plasma levels and immunoreactive ANP and different hemodynamic parameters, Bates and co-workers[16] in Ann Arbor, Michigan, studied 34 patients undergoing right sided cardiac catheterization. Plasma levels of ANP in blood samples withdrawn from the femoral vein, right ventricle, and left ventricle were determined by radioimmunoassay. RA pressure, PA wedge pressure, heart rate, and mean arterial pressure were found to be independent and significant predictors of ANP plasma levels. The closest correlations were between RA pressure and either RV ANP or femoral vein ANP levels. Five patients with isolated LV failure had elevated ANP levels out of proportion to that of RA pressure levels. PA wedge pressure also correlated with RV ANP levels and with femoral vein ANP levels. However, ventricular levels were twice femoral vein levels and were closely correlated, and RV and LV levels were almost identical. Patients with volume overload states had elevated ANP levels. The investigators concluded that distention of either atrium may act as a potent stimulus for ANP release, although circulating levels may be clinically ineffective in producing diuresis and natriuresis.

Rodeheffer et al[17] in Nashville, Tennessee, studied the regulation of intravascular volume through measurements of the ANP. Intracardiac pressures and plasma ANP concentrations in the central circulation were measured in 34 patients with different cardiovascular disorders. In these studies, plasma ANP concentration increased from the inferior vena cava to the right atrium (76 ± 24–162 ± 37 pg/ml) and from the vena cava to the aorta (76 ± 24–177 ± 46 pg/ml). Mean RA pressure was correlated positively with ANP con-

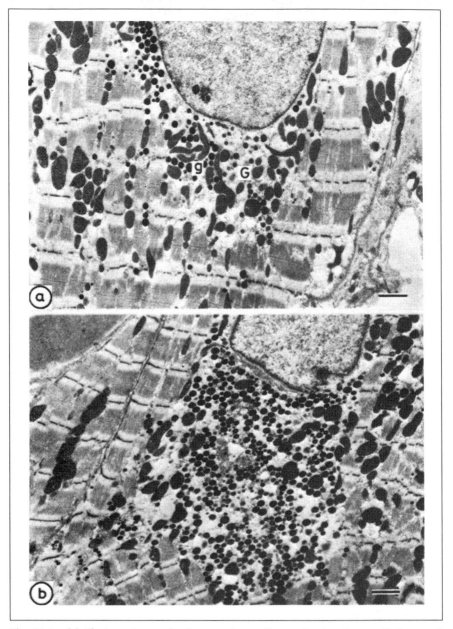

Fig. 10-4. (a) Electronmicrograph of a granular cardiocyte showing the myofibrils, a well developed Golgi apparatus (G), and the granules (g). (b) Electronmicrograph of an atrial cardiocyte of a rat on a sodium free diet for 30 days showing a great increase in granularity. Reproduced with permission from Genest.[18]

centration in the PA, and mean PA wedge pressure was correlated positively with ANP concentration in the aorta. In 6 patients, increased atrial pressure was associated with increased ANP concentration in the PA and aorta. These data suggest that ANP exists in human atrial myocardium and that it is released in response to increased atrial pressure.

Genest[18] from Montreal, Canada, updated the information on the ANP which was discovered initially only 3 years ago (Fig. 10-4). This article and a preceding editorial by Linden and Knapp[19] provide a good review of this fascinating cardiac hormone.

CARDIAC NEOPLASMS

Electrocardiographic markers of metastases

Cardiac metastases are often clinically inapparent but have important prognostic significance. Cates and colleagues[20] from Nashville, Tennessee, studied 1,046 consecutive autopsies performed between 1981 and 1983, and 210 patients with both premortem and autopsy diagnoses of cancer were found, in whom a recent (<3 months before death) electrocardiogram was available. Of these patients, 47 had cardiac metastases (group I) and 163 did not (group II). In group I, 19 patients had new electrocardiographic changes suggestive of myocardial ischemia or injury, including either diffuse T wave inversion (10%), segmental (electrocardiographic pattern suggestive of a specific coronary distribution) T-wave inversion (80%), or ST elevation (10%). No patient had symptoms suggestive of myocardial ischemia. In group II, 6 patients had electrocardiographic changes suggestive of myocardial ischemia or injury: 4 patients with preterminal sepsis, 1 with AMI, and 1 with Aspergillus nodules within the myocardium. New atrial arrhythmias (7 patients) and low voltage (10 patients) were found with greater frequency in group I patients. Patients with normal electrocardiograms were unlikely to have cardiac metastases; however, the finding of nonspecific ST-T wave changes was not helpful in differentiating the 2 groups. In clinically stable patients with cancer and no cardiac symptoms suggestive of ischemia, any new electrocardiographic change should raise the suspicion of cardiac metastases. The electrocardiographic finding of myocardial ischemia or injury has high specificity (96%) for cardiac metastases.

Multiple recurrent cardiac myxomas

McCarthy and associates[21] from Rochester, Minnesota, reviewed the records of 56 patients who underwent operation for cardiac myxoma and 29 cases in which cardiac myxoma was found at autopsy. Five patients had a "complex" of unusual findings including multiple pigmented skin lesions, myxoid fibroadenomas of the breast, skin myxomas, and primary pigmented nodular adrenocortical disease. Four of these 5 patients had multiple cardiac myxomas. Three of the 4 patients who underwent surgical excision had recurrent myxomas and these were the only recurrences in the series. Thus, the occurrence of multiple and recurrent myxomas in patients with the "myxoma complex" was significantly higher than in the rest of the patients with sporadic myxomas. The authors recommended a thorough search for multiple tumors at operation, close postoperative follow-up, and careful screening of family members when these cardiac lesions are associated with the complex noncardiac conditions.

OBESITY

Electrocardiogram

Frank et al[22] in Springfield, Illinois, evaluated the electrocardiograms in 1,029 obese subjects and correlated them with the severity of obesity and with age, sex of the patient, and BP. With increasing obesity, the heart rate,

PR interval, QRS duration, QTc interval and voltage increased, and the QRS vector shifted to the left. These changes were independent of age, sex of the patient, and BP. Bradycardia was found in 19% of the obese patients and ST- and T-wave abnormalities in 11%. Low voltage was present in only 4% of the patients and QTc prolongation occurred in 28%. These data suggest that the heart rate of QRS voltage increase with increasing obesity, conduction is slowed, and the QRS vector shifts toward the left. These changes should be considered when evaluating electrocardiograms in obese patients.

Twin study

Stunkard and associates[23] from Philadelphia, Pennsylvania, and Washington, D.C., assessed height, weight, and body mass index in 1,974 monozygotic and in 2,097 dizygotic male twin pairs. Concordance rates for different degrees of overweight were twice as high for monozygotic twins as for dizygotic twins. Classic twin methods estimated a high heritability for height, weight, and body mass index, both at age 20 years (0.80, 0.78, and 0.77, respectively) and at a 25-year follow-up (0.80, 0.81, and 0.84, respectively). Height, weight, and body mass index were highly correlated across time, and a path analysis suggested that the major part of that covariation was genetic. These results were similar to those of other twin studies of these measures and suggest that human fatness is under substantial genetic control.

Adoption study

Stunkard and associates[24] from Philadelphia, Pennsylvania, Copenhagen, Denmark, and Houston, Texas, examined the contributions of genetic factors in the family environment to human fatness in a sample of 540 adult Danish adoptees who were selected from a population of 3,580 and divided into 4 weight classes: thin, medium weight, overweight, and obese. There was a strong relation between the weight class of the adoptees and the body-mass index of their biologic parents. There was no relation between the weight class of the adoptees and the body-mass index of their adoptive parents. Cumulative distributions of the body-mass index of parents showed similar results; there was a strong relation between the body-mass index of biologic parents and adoptee weight class and no relation between the index of adoptive parents and adoptee weight class. Furthermore, the relation between biologic parents and adoptees was not confined to the obesity weight class, but was present across the whole range of body fatness—from very thin to very fat. The authors concluded that genetic influences have an important role in determining human fatness in adults, whereas the family environment alone has no apparent effect. This article was followed by an editorial entitled "Bad News and Good News About Obesity" by Theodore B. Van Itallie[25].

PULMONARY HYPERTENSION

New histologic classification

Roberts[26] from Bethesda, Maryland, proposed a simple histologic classification of PA hypertension and it consisted of only 3 grades based on histo-

TYPES AND GRADING OF MORPHOLOGIC PULMONARY ARTERIAL CHANGES

CHANGE (S)	GRADE	MORPHOLOGY
Normal or Thin-Walled	0	
Medial Thickening (MT)	I	
MT + Intimal Thickening (IT)	II	
MT + IT + Plexiform Lesion	III	

Reproduced with permission from Roberts.[26]

logic alterations irrespective of the etiology of, or the time of appearance of, the PA hypertension. The major changes in the pulmonary arteries include: 1) medial thickening (MT), 2) intimal thickening (IT), and 3) plexiform lesions (PL). Grade 1 includes MT only; grade 2, MT plus IT; and grade 3, MT plus IT plus PL (Fig. 10-5).

Doppler studies

Isobe and associates[27] from Tokyo, Japan, used Doppler echocardiography to estimate PA pressure in 45 adult patients with various kinds of heart disease and the patterns were compared with those of 32 normal control subjects. Doppler signals obtained in the RV outflow tract just proximal to the pulmonary valve and electrocardiogram were recorded simultaneously. Doppler velocity time intervals were measured as follows: RV preejection period, accelerated time from the onset of the RV ejection flow velocity to the peak, and RV ejection time. Thirty patients had PA hypertension and 16 patients had a low cardiac index. The best correlation with PA pressure was achieved by the RV preejection period/acceleration time index. Sensitivity and specificity for predicting PA hypertension were 93% and 97%, respectively. Acceleration time correlated best with the logarithm of PA mean pressure. Patients were separated into 2 groups according to cardiac index. In those patients with a cardiac index of <2.5 liters/min/m^2, both RV preejection period/acceleration time and acceleration time were significantly correlated with PA mean pressure and log (PA mean pressure), respectively. However, the slope of the regression line for acceleration time and log (PA mean pressure) was significantly steeper than that for patients with a cardiac index of ≥2.5 liters/min/m^2, whereas the relation between RV preejection period/ acceleration time and PA mean pressure in the 2 groups could not be differentiated statistically from each other. Other intervals and ratios were less quantitative because of late systolic turbulent flow and individual variability. Thus, RV preejection period/acceleration time is a new, highly quantitative and convenient predictor of PA pressure even in the presence of a low cardiac output state.

Martin-Duran and associates[28] from Santander, Spain, assessed the use of pulsed Doppler echocardiography to measure PA pressure. PA flow at the RV outflow tract was analyzed in 51 patients. Attention was focused on PA flow morphologic pattern, RV systolic intervals, time to peak flow and acceleration time index. Correlation was made with PA pressure and total pulmonary resistance. Three morphologic patterns of PA flow were found: type I indicates normal PA pressure (sensitivity 85%, specificity 100%) and types II and III indicate PA hypertension (sensitivity 100%, specificity 85%). The RV preejection/RV ejection ratio, time to peak flow and acceleration time index show a good correlation coefficient improved when a logarithmic function was applied. The best correlation was achieved with time to peak flow and especially with acceleration time index. Analysis of pulmonary flow is a reliable new tool for evaluating PA pressure and is even better for evaluating total pulmonary resistance. Acceleration time index is the parameter that correlates best with these 2 variables.

Masuyama and co-workers[29] in Osaka, Japan, used continuous-wave Doppler echocardiography to estimate PA pressures by measuring pulmonary regurgitant flow velocity in 21 patients with pulmonary hypertension (mean PA pressure >20 mmHg) and 24 patients without pulmonary hypertension. The pulmonary regurgitant flow velocity patterns, characterized by a rapid increase in flow velocity immediately after closure of the pulmonary valve and a gradual deceleration until the next pulmonary valve opening, were successfully obtained in 18 of the 21 patients with pulmonary hypertension and in 13 of the 24 patients without pulmonary hypertension. As PA pressure increased, pulmonary regurgitant flow velocity became higher; the RV pressure gradient in diastole (PG) was estimated from the pulmonary regurgitant flow velocity (v) by means of the simplified Bernoulli equation ($PG = 4V^2$). The Doppler-determined pressure gradient at end-diastole correlated well with the catheter measurement of the pressure gradient at end-diastole and with PA end-diastolic pressure. The peak of Doppler-determined pressure gradient during diastole correlated well with mean PA pressure. These investigators concluded that continuous-wave Doppler echocardiography was useful in measuring pulmonary regurgitant flow velocity for the noninvasive estimation of PA pressures.

PULMONARY EMBOLISM

Echocardiographic findings

Kasper and colleagues[30] from Freiburg and Mainz, West Germany, performed echocardiographic studies in 105 patients with acute and recurrent pulmonary emboli. Pulmonary embolism was confirmed by pulmonary angiography (n = 48), necropsy (n = 6), and lung perfusion scintigraphy (n = 51). Seventy of 93 patients (75%) displayed a dilated right ventricle, 38 of 91 patients (42%) had reduced LV cavity dimension, 41 of 82 patients (50%) had decreased EF slope of the mitral valve, and 78 of 101 patients (77%) had dilated right PAs. The motion of the ventricular septum was abnormal in 41 of 93 patients (44%). Right-sided thrombi were seen in 13 patients within the right PA (n = 11) and in the right ventricle (n = 3); in 1 patient they were found in the superior vena cava, in the innominate vein, and the right atrium. Two patients had right-sided endocarditis. Thus, echocardiographic changes were frequently found in patients with proved pulmonary emboli. The echocardiographic findings of right-sided cardiac and PA abnormalities indicate hemodynamically active pulmonary emboli.

Tissue-type plasminogen activator therapy

Goldhaber and associates[31] from Boston and West Roxbury, Massachusetts, gave recombinant human tissue-type plasminogen activator (TPA) via a peripheral vein to 36 patients with angiographically documented pulmonary embolism. The regimen was 50 mg/2 hours followed by repeat angiography and, if necessary, an additional 40 mg/4 hours. By 6 hours, 34 of 36 patients had angiographic evidence of clot lysis, slight in 4, moderate in 6, and marked in 24. The quantitative score improved 21% by 2 hours and 49% by 6 hours. Fibrinogen decreased 30% from baseline at 2 hours and 38% from baseline at 6 hours. Two patients had major complications; in 1, bleeding from a pelvic tumor required surgery; in the other, who had had CABG 8 days earlier, pericardial tamponade developed. These initial results in selected patients make a case for expanded investigational use of peripheral intravenous TPA in pulmonary embolism.

Embolectomy

Pulmonary embolism is a common emergency, yet nearly 80 years after Trendelenberg's first pioneering operation, there is no clear consensus on the role of surgical therapy. Clarke and Abrams[32] from Birmingham, UK, report 55 pulmonary emboletomy procedures. They report the use of inflow occlusion without cardiopulmonary bypass. A total of 65 patients underwent operation with a diagnosis of massive pulmonary embolism, most of them in shock and half of them having had VF or asystole before operation. In 7 patients, the diagnosis was in error. Fifty-five patients ultimately had pulmonary emboli removed during the operation. The time from embolism to operation ranged from 20 minutes–24 hours (mean 5 hours). The overall surgical mortality was 44%. In the view of the authors, normothermic venous inflow occlusion is ideal for pulmonary embolectomy, particularly in small hospitals without standby cardiopulmonary bypass. The investigators suggest that profound circulatory disturbances caused by pulmonary emboli are attended by a poor prognosis. They suggest that observation is not acceptable, nor is thrombolytic enzyme therapy. In properly selected patients, the procedure may be lifesaving. Whether cardiopulmonary bypass is necessary may not be the question; rather, one should consider if the procedure should be performed and with what frequency.

ANTITHROMBOTIC THERAPY

In 1984, the American College of Chest Physicians in conjunction with the National Heart, Lung, and Blood Institute, appointed a special working group to evaluate the indications for anticoagulant and antiplatelet agents. The special working group was charged to critically review the current literature and accumulated experience and to use the information to make recommendations on indications for antithrombotic therapy, selection of the most appropriate entithrombotic agent, optimal dosage regimens, and the optimal duration of therapy. The group was divided into 8 task forces to examine the use of antithrombotic therapy in the following conditions: CAD, valvular heart disease, prosthetic heart valves, CABG, AF, venus thrombosis and pulmonary embolism, peripheral vascular disease, and cerebral vascular disease. After each task force reached a consensus within their area, their recommendations were presented to the entire working group. After further discussions and revision, the working group prepared the final recommendation. The recommendations were published in 11 articles, each of which was usually no more than a page in length.[33-44] The following recommendations were included in some of the articles from this group: 1) It was strongly recommended that long-term warfarin therapy sufficient to prolong the prothrombin time to 1.5–2.0 times control using rabbit brain thromboplastin (standardized INR = 3.0–4.5) be used in patients with rheumatic mitral valve disease who have documented systemic embolism. (I [WCR] presume this means only patients with MS and not those with pure MR.) It was recommended that if recurrent systemic embolism occurred despite adequate warfarin therapy, dipyridamole (400 mg/day) should be added. It was recommended that long-term warfarin therapy sufficient to prolong the prothrombin time to 1.2–1.5 times control be used in all patients with rheumatic mitral valve disease with associated chronic or paroxysmal AF. 2) It was recommended that patients with MVP who had documented but unexplained transient ischemic attacks should be treated with long-term aspirin therapy. The dose currently recommended is 1 gm/day. Also, if transient ischemic attacks recur in a patient with MVP despite aspirin therapy, long-term warfarin therapy (1.2–1.5 times control) should be used. It was also strongly recommended that patients with MVP who had documented systemic embolism be treated with long-term warfarin therapy (1.5–2.0 times control). It was also recommended that patients with MVP complicated by chronic or paroxysmal AF should be treated with long-term warfarin therapy to prolong prothrombin time to 1.2–1.5 times control. 3) Patients with mitral anular calcium complicated by systemic thromboembolism should be treated with long-term warfarin therapy to prolong prothrombin time to 1.5–2.0 times control. It was recommended that patients with mitral anular calcium with associated AF should be treated with long-term warfarin therapy to prolong prothrombin time to 1.2–1.5 times control. (I [WCR] very much disagree with this recommendation.) 4) It was strongly recommended that all patients with mechanical prosthetic heart valves be treated with long-term warfarin at a dose sufficient to prolong the prothrombin time to 1.5–2.0 times control using rabbit brain thromboplastin. It was also recommended that patients with mechanical prosthetic heart valves who had systemic emboli despite adequate therapy with warfarin be treated with dipyridamole (400 mg/day) in addition to warfarin. It was recommended that when a major episode of bleeding occurred in a patient with a mechanical prosthetic valve who is being treated with long-term warfarin, lower doses of warfarin (prothrombin time 1.2–1.5 times control) may be used. 5) It was recommended that all patients with bioprosthetic valves in the mitral position be treated for the first 3 months after bioprosthetic insertion with less intense warfarin (prothrombin time 1.2–1.5 above control). It was also recommended that patients with bioprosthetic valves who had a history of systemic embolism or had evidence of LA thrombus at surgery or who had AF be treated with long-term warfarin therapy. (In my view [WCR] these patients should never receive a bioprothesis; they should be given a mechanical valve.) 6) It was recommended that aspirin in combination with dipyridamole be used in patients undergoing CABG although the evidence for that recommendation was unconfirmed. The clearest evidence is for aspirin 1 g/day in combination with dipyridamole, 225 mg/day. Aspirin should be administered the day of surgery. Dipyridamole should begin 2 days before surgery at a larger dose (400 mg/day). Aspirin 100 mg/day alone, beginning the day of surgery, may also be considered. 7) It was strongly recommended that all patients with AMI receive a minimum of low-dose heparin, 5,000 IV/SC every 12 hours until fully ambulatory to prevent venous thromboembolism. It was also recommended that patients with AMI at increased risk of systemic emboli because of transmural anterior wall AMI receive heparin therapy followed by warfarin therapy to prolong prothrombin time to an INR of 2.0–3.0 for 1–3 months (1.2–1.5 times control using rabbit brain thromboplastin). It was strongly recommended that patients with AMI at increased risk of systemic emboli because of AF, history of previous systemic or pulmonary emboli, or CHF receive heparin therapy followed by warfarin therapy to prolong prothrombin time to an INR of 2.0–3.0 (1.2–1.5 times control using rabbit brain thromboplastin) for at least 3 months. 8) It was strongly recommended that patients with unstable angina pectoris be treated with aspirin for 2 years at 3–5 mg/day. The routine use of anticoagulant therapy was not recommended in patients with unstable angina. 9) It was strongly recommended that long-term warfarin therapy (INR of 3.0–4.5; prothrombin time 1.5–2.0 times control using rabbit brain thromboplastin) be used in patients with AF who had documented systemic embolism.

MISCELLANEOUS CARDIOLOGIC TOPICS

Asymptomatic neck bruits

Chambers and Norris[45] from Toronto, Canada, followed 500 asymptomatic patients with cervical bruits prospectively by clinical and Doppler examination for up to 4 years (mean 23 months) to identify the variables predicting outcome. Thirty-six patients had strokes or transient ischemic attacks, 51 had cardiac ischemic events, and 45 died. At 1 year the incidence of cerebral ischemic events (transient ischemic attacks and strokes) was 6%, that of cardiac ischemic events was 7%, and that of death was 4%. The overall incidence of stroke at 1 year was 2% (1% in patients without previous transient ischemic attacks), but the incidence was 5.5% in patients with severe carotid-artery stenosis (>75%). Cerebral ischemic events were most frequent in patients with severe carotid-artery stenosis, progressing carotid-artery stenosis or heart disease and in men. The degree of carotid-artery stenosis on initial presentation was a powerful predictor of neurologic sequelae. Patients with asymptomatic cervical bruits have a higher risk of a cardiac ischemic event than of a stroke. Although the risk of cerebral ischemic events is highest in patients with severe carotid-artery stenosis, in most instances even these patients do not have strokes without some warning.

Use of "routine" chest radiographs

Tape and Mushlin[46] from Rochester, New York, evaluated the usefulness of admission and preoperative chest radiographs in enhancing patient care. Calculations based on estimates of the accuracy of chest radiographs and the likelihood of disease suggest that routine chest radiography may result in more misleading than helpful results. Patients in whom chest radiographs are likely to improve outcome are best identified by a careful history and physical examination. The authors recommend that the practice of performing routine chest radiographs on admission and preoperatively be stopped and that the procedure be reserved for patients with clinical evidence of chest disease and patients having intrathoracic surgery.

Medical standards for civilian airmen

Engelberg and associates[47] from Chicago, Illinois, and Salt Lake City, Utah, summarized the report of a comprehensive review by the American Medical Association of the medical standards for civilian airmen. The present standards were promulgated by the Federal Aviation Administration in 1959 and the alcoholism and cardiovascular standards were revised in 1982. Included in this article are recommended standards for the cardiovascular system. An applicant shall have no established medical history or clinical diagnosis of: 1) AMI, 2) angina pectoris, 3) CAD that has required treatment or, if untreated, is or has been symptomatic or clinically significant, 4) any form of heart or arterial surgery, including PTCA or permanent pacemaker insertion, 5) any form of congenital heart disease, 6) any significant precordial murmur or valvular heart disease, 7) any evidence of pericarditis or cardiomyopathy, 8) any significant disturbance of heart rhythm or conduction, 9) a sitting BP ≥150/95 mmHg or a systolic BP >160 mmHg, or a history of any hypertensive medication within the last year, or any history of surgery or angioplasty for the treatment of systemic hypertension, and 10) any evidence of significant peripheral arterial-vascular obstructive disease or aneurysm or a history of surgery for these conditions.

For airmen who fly in a single-crew cockpit operation, at age 50 years, the applicant must have a total serum cholesterol level <300 mg/dl. On initial certification, and at age 35 years, 40 years, and annually after age 40 years, the applicant must demonstrate an absence of any significant electrocardiographic abnormality, including myocardial infarction. An electrocardiogram recorded according to acceptable standards and techniques ≤30 days before an examination for a first-class certificate is accepted at the time of the physical examination.

Echocardiographic-morphologic correlation of left ventricular hypertrophy

To determine the accuracy of echocardiographic dimensions and mass measurements for detection and quantification of LV hypertrophy, Devereux and associates[48] from New York, New York, and Philadelphia, Pennsylvania, blindly read antemortem echocardiograms and compared LV mass measurements in them to LV mass measurements made at necropsy in 55 patients. LV mass was calculated using M-mode LV measurements by Penn and the American Society of Echocardiography (ASE) conventions and cube function and volume correction formulas in 52 patients. Penn-cube LV mass correlated closely with necropsy LV mass and overestimated it by only 6%; sensitivity in 18 patients with LV hypertrophy (necropsy LV mass >215 g) was 100% (18 of 18 patients) and specificity was 86% (29 of 34 patients). ASE-cube LV mass correlated similarly to necropsy LV mass, but systematically overestimated it (by a mean of 25%); the overestimation could be corrected by the equation: LV mass = 0.80 (ASE-cube LV mass) + 0.6 g. Use of ASE measurements in the volume correction formula systematically underestimated necropsy LV mass (by a mean of 30%). In a subset of 9 patients, 3 of whom had technically inadequate M-mode echocardiograms, 2-D echocardiographic LV mass by 2 methods was also significantly related to necropsy LV mass. Among other indexes of LV anatomy, only measurement of myocardial cross-sectional area was acceptably accurate for quantitation of LV mass or diagnosis of LV hypertrophy (sensitivity = 72%, specificity = 94%). In conclusion, M-mode echocardiographic LV mass by the Penn-cube method accurately diagnoses and quantitates LV hypertrophy, as does LV mass by the ASE-cube method after correction by a simple regression equation; 2-D echocardiography may increase the proportion of patients in whom LV mass can be measured; and measurements of LV cross-sectional area detect and quantify LV hypertrophy with moderate accuracy, whereas other echocardiographic measurements are less useful for this purpose.

Electrocardiogram -vs- echocardiogram for diagnosing "left atrial enlargement"

Van Dam and associates[49] from Utrecht, The Netherlands, in 100 unselected consecutive adult patients with a variety of cardiac diseases studied the agreement between elecrocardiogram and echocardiogram for diagnosing "LA enlargement." In only 4 patients did both methods agree with respect to this diagnosis. Mainly as a result of supraventricular arrhythmia, the P wave of the electrocardiogram could not be analyzed in 19 patients. In 13 of the 19, the electrocardiogram showed enlargement of the left atrium. Four of the remaining 81 patients had positive electrocardiographic criteria for LA enlargement and 20 patients had LA enlargement on their electrocardiogram. Thus, there is no agreement between the electrocardiographic diagnosis of LA enlargement and the LA cavity size as measured from the echocardiogram. The echocardiogram is the reference method for assessing LA size (Fig. 10-6).

Cardiovascular findings in quadriplegia and paraplegia

Kessler and associates[50] from Miami, Florida, determined various cardiac variables in 7 normal, 7 paraplegic and 7 quadriplegic patients. Quadriplegic patients had a 26% lower LV mass index (75 ± 13 g/m^2) compared with normal volunteers (102 ± 16 g/m^2) or paraplegic patients (110 ± 26 g/m^2). Six quadriplegic and 3 paraplegic patients had an unusual pattern of LV posterior wall asynergy, which was associated with a significant rightward shift of the frontal-plane QRS axis (92 ± 22° -vs- 42 ± 41°) and smaller LA

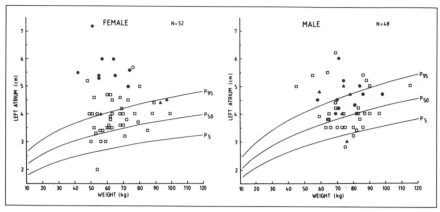

Fig. 10-6. Nomograms of the 5th, 50th and 95th percentile curves of the left atrial dimension of a healthy population, plotted against weight and sex. The following represent the individual echocardiographic measurements: ○, subjects without analyzable P wave on the ECG; △, subjects with electrocardiographic left atrial enlargement; □, subjects without left atrial enlargement on the ECG. Reproduced with permission from Van Dam et al.[49]

dimensions (2.4 ± 0.4 -vs- 3.0 ± 0.2 cm). The quadriplegic group had a significantly reduced mean BP (67 ± 7 -vs- 88 ± 8 mmHG in normal subjects), high normal peripheral resistances (22 ± 5 -vs- 17 ± 5 U in normal subjects), and a markedly reduced calculated cardiac output (3.2 ± 0.6 -vs- 5.4 ± 1.4 liters/minute in normal subjects). Hemodynamic data for the paraplegic patients were similar to those in the normal group. A decrease in LV wall stress, mediated primarily by a decrease in venous return, appeared to result in the "adaptive" cardiac atrophy seen in these quadriplegic patients. LV asynergy was common and also may be related to a decrease in cardiac filling.

Myocardial contusion from blunt chest trauma

One of the many potential complications of nonpenetrating chest injury is myocardial contusion. Sutherland and associates[51] from London, Canada, examined the immediate hemodynamic sequelae of blunt chest trauma complicated by acute myocardial contusion in multiple traumatized patients. Focal defects of ventricular wall motion defined by gated cardiac scintigraphy identified acute myocardial contusion in 28 of 43 patients, involving the RV wall alone in 18 (group 1A), the LV wall in 4 (group 1B), and both RV and LV walls in 6 (group 1C). Qualitatively normal ventricular wall motion was found in the 15 patients (group 2). Although there was no difference between groups 1A and 2 in mean systemic oxygen transport (620 ±189 -vs- 627 ± 105 ml/min/m²), LVEF (52 ± 14 -vs- 60 ± 9%) or calculated LV end-diastolic and end systolic volumes, mean RVEF was significantly lower in group 1A (29 ± 9%) than in group 2 (47 ± 7%). Concomitantly, evidence of RV systolic dysfunction was apparent in group 1A (RV end-systolic volume 104 ± 56 ml/m²). RV stroke work was similar between the groups, and RV pump function was identical by virtue of a larger RV preload n group 1A (RV end-diastolic volume 143 ± 63 ml/m²) than in group 2 (RV end-diastolic volume 93 ± 26 ml/m²). Thus, use of the RV Frank-Starling mechanism in patients with traumatic RV contusion maintains RV pump function at a level similar to that in traumatized patients without acute myocardial contusion.

McBride and associates[52] from St. Paul and Minneapolis, Minnesota, retrospectively studied 36 victims of high-voltage electrical contact injuries to determine the incidence and possible source of elevated creatine kinase (CK)-MB enzyme in their serum. Only 2 sustained AMI (1 late) according to history, electrocardiography, and clinical course. Serum lactate dehydrogenase isoenzyme levels were abnormal but revealed no AMI patterns. CK total activity, however, reached 1.5–1,140 times normal in 92% and the CK-MB level was abnormal in 50% despite the low incidence of AMI damage. Skeletal muscle CK and CK-MB levels in 4 nonelectrically injured patients were comparable to those in normal muscle, whereas CK and CK-MB activity were elevated in 6 such electrical injuries. There was a gradient in CK-MB activity, with greatest CK-MB activity in "normal" muscle near the injury site, lesser amounts in border tissue, and least in the worst-injured site. The authors concluded that 1) AMI injury is uncommon in high-voltage electrical injury, and 2) skeletal muscle injured by high electrical voltage is stimulated to produce and to release CK-MB.

Cigarette smoking decreases energy

Hofstetter and associates[53] from Lausanne, Switzerland, studied the effect of cigarette smoking on energy expenditure in 8 healthy cigarette smokers who spent 24 hours in a metabolic chamber on 2 occasions, once without smoking and once while smoking 24 cigarettes per day. Diet and physical exercise (30 minutes of treadmill walking) were standardized on both occasions. Physical activity in the chamber was measured by use of a radar system. Smoking caused an increase in total 24-hour energy expenditure (from a mean value [± standard error of the mean] of 2,230 ± 115–2,445 ± 120 kcal/24 hours), although no changes were observed in physical activity or mean basal metabolic rate (1,545 ± 80 -vs- 1,570 ± 70 kcal/24 hours). During the smoking period, the mean diurnal urinary excretion of norepinephrine increased from 1.25 ± 0.14–1.82 ± 0.28 µg/hour, and mean nocturnal excretion increased from 0.73 ± 0.07–0.91 ± 0.08 µg/hour. These short-term observations demonstrate that cigarette smoking increases 24-hour energy expenditure by approximately 10%, and that this effect may be mediated in part by the sympathetic nervous system. The findings also indicate that energy expenditure can be expected to decrease when people stop smoking, thereby favoring the gain in body weight that often accompanies the cessation of smoking.

Echocardiographic findings in pheochromocytoma

Shub and associates[54] from Rochester, Minnesota, used M-mode and 2-D echocardiography to study 26 consecutive, unselected patients with pheochromocytoma. Only 1 patient had CHF. More than half had no cardiac symptoms or abnormalities. The most common (80% of patients) echocardiographic pattern was normal LV mass with normal or even increased systolic performance. When LV mass was increased, LV systolic function was either normal or only borderline depressed in most of the patients. Patients with echocardiographic LV hypertrophy had symmetric thickening of ventricular walls; no case of asymmetric septal hypertrophy was found. There was no correlation between 24-hour urinary norepinephrine excretion and any of the echocardiographic variables studied. In some patients, increased LV wall thicknesses did not correlate with increased LV mass as calculated by the Woythaler echocardiographic method. LA enlargement was not seen in any patient, including those with increased LV mass. The electrocardiogram and echocardiogram may be discordant: electrocardiographic LV hypertrophy was seen in 6 patients, of whom 5 had normal echocardiographic LV mass.

In patients with pheochromocytoma who have no cardiac symptoms or other clinical evidence of cardiac involvement, echocardiographic findings are usually normal.

Somatostatin analogue for the carcinoid syndrome

The carcinoid syndrome has excited interest and posed a therapeutic challenge since it was first described >30 years ago. The disorder usually, of course, is associated with carcinoid tumors of the small bowel that are metastatic to the liver. Clinically, the syndrome is manifested by episodic flushing and diarrhea and in about half the patients by a specific type of valvular and mural endocardial heart disease. The precise chemical mechanisms of the syndrome have not been clearly defined although an increase of serotonin production is almost always observed. An increase in urinary excretion of the serotonin metabolite 5-hydroxyindoleacetic acid (5-HIAA) is the most reliable laboratory finding for diagnosis of this syndrome. Effective treatment has been lacking. Kvols and associates[55] from Rochester, Minnesota, studied the effects of a long-acting analogue of somatostatin (SMS 201-995, Sandoz) in 25 patients with histologically proved metastatic carcinoid tumors and the carcinoid syndrome. This drug was self-administered by subcutaneous injection at a dose of 150 μg 3 times daily. Flushing and diarrhea associated with the syndrome were promptly relieved in 22 patients. All 25 patients had an elevated 24-hour urinary excretion of 5-HIAA (mean 265 mg/24 hours; range 14–1,079), which served as an objective indicator of disease activity. Eighteen of the 25 patients (72%) had a decrease ≥50% in their urinary 5-HIAA levels compared with the pretreatment values. The median duration of this biochemical response was >12 months (range 1–18). Since no serious toxicity was observed, the authors concluded that SMS 201-995 may be appropriate for use as early therapy in patients with symptoms due to the carcinoid syndrome who have not responded to simpler measures. This article was followed by an editorial by John Oates[56].

Complications of central venous catheterization

Sznajder and associates[57] from Haifa, Israel, prospectively studied the results of 714 attempts at central vein catheterization during an 8-month period in their intensive care department. They compared the rates of failure of catheterization and early complications among 3 percutaneous approaches: subclavian, anterior jugular, and posterior jugular veins. The procedures were performed by experienced staff or resident physicians and inexperienced interns and residents under teaching supervision. Overall rates of failure and complication were similar for each percutaneous approach within each group of physicians. Overall failure rate was 10% for the experienced group and 19% for the inexperienced. The complication was 5% for experienced and 11% for inexperienced. Among inexperienced physicians, the success rate was 87% and the complication rate 8% in unconscious patients, whereas in conscious patients these rates were 79 and 14%, respectively. The inexperienced physicians caused fewer complications in mechanically ventilated than in spontaneously breathing patients. The authors suggest that inexperienced physicians should first attempt central vein catheterizations in unconscious and mechanically ventilated patients.

Years of life lost from cardiovascular disease

Cardiovascular diseases (CVD) (ICD 390-398, 402, 404-429) remain the leading cause of death in the USA, despite a persistent decline in the mortality rate of about 2%/year since 1968[58]. CVD ranks third in years of potential life lost (YPLL) before age 65, a measure that generally highlights death in the early years. This ranking reflects the large number of people who die prematurely from CAD (ICD 410-414). Other categories of CVD accounting for YPLL are acute rheumatic fever (ICD 410-414), chronic rheumatic heart disease (ICD 393-398), hypertensive disease (ICD 401-405), diseases of pulmonary circulation (ICD 415-417), and other forms of heart disease (ICD 420-429). Total YPLL, as well as YPLL for men and women, has continued to decline since 1968 (Fig. 10-7). In 1983, the most recent year for which complete age-, sex-, race-, and cause-specific mortality data are available, CVD accounted for 1,620,219 YPLL before age 65; this respresents 16% of YPLL for all causes of death in 1983. CAD accounted for 1,001,875 YPLL (62% of all CVD). Thus, CAD alone would rank as the fourth highest cause of YPLL behind unintentional injuries, malignant neoplasms, and suicide. In 1983, white males continued to account for most (67%) of YPLL from CAD, followed by white females (18%), black males (9%), black females (5%), and all others (1%). However, the crude rates of YPLL indicate similar risks for CAD mortality among white and black males (691 and 651 YPLL/100,000, respectively). The rate for black females was 1.75 times higher than that for white females (315 -vs- 180 YPLL/100,000). Rates for males and females of other races were substantially lower than those for their white counterparts.

CARDIAC TRANSPLANTATION

Heart transplantation has now achieved a therapeutic status similar to that of cadaveric renal transplantation. Depending on patient selection criteria, it is estimated that as many as 15,000 people per year could conceivably benefit from a heart transplant, but the actual number of persons who will benefit is severely constrained by donor supply. Evans and associates[59] from Millwood, Virginia, estimated the availability of heart donors in the USA per year as only 400 to 1,100 viable donor hearts. A donor supply is the most critical determinant of the future of heart transplantation because it will dictate the number of transplants performed, the survival of transplant recipients, the total program expenditures associated with heart transplantation, the nature of the legal and ethical issues involved, the number of cardiac transplant programs required to make optimal use of the available donor hearts, and the future role of mechanical circulatory support systems.

Characteristics of the donor heart may affect short- and long-term survival of cardiac transplant patients. Emery and associates[60] from Tucson, Arizona, describe their experience with 223 cardiac donor referrals: 62 were accepted for transplantation (15 local, 23 regional [<370 km], and 24 distant [370–1,556 km]). Although there was no difference in initial myocardial function, median survival with follow-up through June 30, 1985, of patients receiving locally, regionally, and distantly procured organs, was 59, 18, and 21 months, respectively (Fig. 10-8). Cumulative proportion 1-year survival was 93%, 56%, and 61%, respectively. The 2-year survival was 85% for patients given locally procured hearts, 43% for those with regionally procured hearts, and 38% for those with a heart from a distant donor. There were no

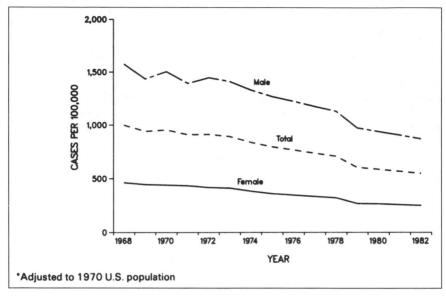

Fig. 10-7. Rate* of years of potential life lost (YPLL) from ischemic heart disease (IHD), by year—United States, 1968–1982. Reproduced with permission from MMWR.[58]

differences in the time from injury to the declaration of brain death or the time from declaration of brain death to cardiectomy among the local, regional, or distant groups. There were no differences in early cardiac function in donor hearts, whether obtained locally, regionally, or distantly. Thus, although late survival varied with donor procurement location, early survival did not. Other variables of the donor that did not influence long-term survival included age, hypotensive event before transplantation, cardiac arrest requiring closed-chest massage before cardiectomy, inotropic support at any time before cardiectomy, and donor ischemic time. There was a striking difference in long-term survival (but not short-term) in distantly procured hearts in the University of Arizona experience. The use of catecholamines pretransplant in the donor, donor ischemic time, and, presumably, number of rejection episodes did not predict the less satisfactory survival of patients undergoing transplantation with regionally or distantly procured hearts. This is surprising and is not the experience among other transplant centers. The data cannot be ignored, however, and may urge regionalization of donor procurement.

Levine and associates[61] from Minneapolis, Minnesota, studied abnormal sympathetic nervous system activity in severe CHF in 14 patients before and 3–6 months after orthotopic heart transplantation. Before transplantation plasma norepinephrine levels at rest were elevated (909 ± 429 pg/ml, compared with normal, 185 ± 60 pg/ml). No reflex activation of the sympathetic nervous system was seen with infusion of sodium nitroprusside despite a significant decrease in arterial pressure. The response to orthostatic tilt also was blunted in the patients before transplantation. Exercise capacity was reduced in these patients and plasma norepinephrine increased promptly at low exercise loads. After cardiac transplanation plasma norepinephrine levels returned to normal (319 ± 188 pg/ml) and the sympathetic response to the stresses of orthostatic tilt (320 ± 196–419 ± 197) and nitroprusside infusion (255 ± 94–555 ± 130) normalized within 6 months after transplantation. Exercise capacity increased and the increase in plasma norepinephrine levels at various exercise loads was reduced for any given workload. Therefore, abnormal adrenergic activity in patients with severe CHF results mostly from the reduction in LV pump function and is reversible if adequate pump function is restored.

Hardesty and associates[62] from Pittsburgh, Pennsylvania, described their experience in cardiac transplantation in a group of terminally ill patients. Cardiac transplantation started in 1980 at their center and all of the initial recipients were in New York Heart Association functional class IV, but many were ambulant. There were, however, a group of patients who were more clearly terminally ill. They were characterized by systolic arterial pressure of <80/mmHg, a cardiac index of <2 liters/min/m², evidence of reduced blood flow as indicated by urine output of <20 ml/hour, impaired mental function, and signs of decreased peripheral perfusion. In 1985, 40% of patients who had transplants at Pittsburgh met those criteria for terminal illness. Thus, the authors report the results of 33 patients who either required intravenous inotropic support or diastolic augmentation to sustain life until a donor heart became available. During the same period, 44 patients who were in class IV but did not meet these criteria also received transplants. In the 33 terminally ill patients, 18 had a creatinine level >1.5 mg/dl, and the maximal creatinine level was 2.5 ml/dl. Immunosuppression included large initial doses of corticosteroids and cyclosporine with rat antithymocyte globulin as rescue therapy for acute rejection. Actuarial survival at 30 months for the group of terminally ill patients was 75% compared with 67% for the less critically ill group. Actuarial survival at 30 months for the combined group of 77 patients was 67%. The authors commented that the average waiting period for a donor heart for the critically ill patients was 11 days and for those less ill, 42 days. The pretransplantation interval was managed without central venous pulmonary arterial or systemic arterial monitoring to minimize the possibility from sepsis due to catheters. A right-sided cardiac catheterization was performed to assess the pulmonary vascular resistance in each instance but a left-sided cardiac catheterization and ventriculogram were avoided. The postoperative care was more complex and the hospitalization more prolonged. However, the long-term survival was equally good in these terminally

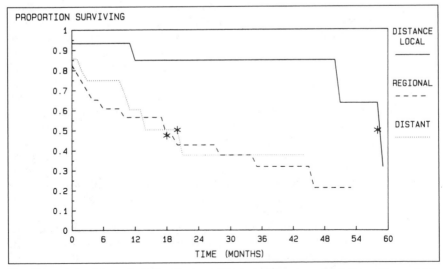

Fig. 10-8. Actuarial survival of patients undergoing cardiac transplantation with respect to distance of donor organ procurement. Survival is significantly better in those patients with locally procured hearts (p <0.05). The end point for the data shown was June 30, 1985. (* = median survival.) Reproduced with permission from Emery et al.[60]

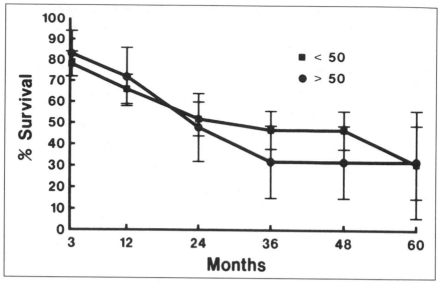

Fig. 10-9.   Actuarial survival of 62 transplant patients. One year survival was 66 ± 7% for those patients under 50 and 72 ± 14% for those over 50 years old. Reproduced with permission from Carrier et al.[63]

ill patients, the oldest of whom was 58 years old. This large and successful transplant center has had excellent results in patients termed critically ill. Most other centers are seeing similar patients and expanding their criteria to include older and younger patients and those with creatinine levels >2.0 mg/dl.

Carrier et al[63] in Tuscon, Arizona, evaluated 62 patients undergoing cardiac transplantation at the University of Arizona from March 1979 to March 1985. Thirteen patients, including 11 men and 2 women were >50 years of age at the time of transplantation and 49 were <50 years old. The mean age of the patients >50 was 53 ± 1 years. Eight patients were treated with conventional immunosuppressive therapy, including azathioprine, prednisone, and rabbit antithymocyte globulin, and 5, beginning in January 1983 were treated with cyclosporine, prednisone, and rabbit antithymocyte globulin. Among these patients, early mortality was 16% in the group >50 years -vs- 18% for those <50 years of age (Fig. 10-9). The late mortality (>90 days) were 36 and 33%, respectively. In both groups, rejection and infection were the main causes of death. The incidence of infection was 1.9 ± 0.5 episodes per patient in those >50 years and 1.9 ± 1.4 in those <50 years of age. The frequency of rejection was 1.3 episodes per patient-year in those >50 years and 1.7 episodes per patient-year in those <50 years of age. Actuarial survival at 1 year was 72 ± 14% in the group >50 and 66 ± 7% in the group <50 years of age. These data indicate that the results of cardiac transplantation for patients >50 years do not differ significantly from those patients aged <50 years. Thus, each potential transplant recipient must be evaluated in terms of individual risk and benefit from the procedure.

Heart and heart-lung transplant recipients at Stanford, California, are routinely prescribed long-term calcium carbonate antacid therapy to aid in the prevention of peptic ulcer and osteoporosis associated with glucocorticold immunosuppressive therapy. Patients consumed 4–>10 g/day of elemental calcium. Since calcium carbonate also provides the essential ingredients for the development of the milk-alkali syndrome, Kapsner and associates[64] from Stanford, California, reviewed the laboratory flow sheets of

297 heart and heart-lung transplant recipients to determine the frequency of hypercalcemia: 65 patients had significant hypercalcemia after transplantation; 31 were alkalotic at the time of hypercalcemia; and 37 had impairment in renal function. It is likely that most of these patients became eucalcemic by discontinuing calcium carbonate therapy; intravenous hydration and forced diuresis were used to treat severe cases. It is possible that the incidence of the milk-alkali syndrome will increase with the current popularity of prescribing calcium carbonate for the prevention and treatment of osteoporosis.

Singer and associates[65] from London, UK, measured plasma atrial natriuretic peptide (ANP) by radioimmunoassay 6–77 weeks after operation in 8 cardiac transplant recipients with no appreciable evidence of cardiac failure or rejection and in 8 control subjects matched for age, sex, race, and BP. Plasma ANP concentrations were significantly higher in the cardiac transplant recipients (mean 19.4 ng/liter) than in the controls (7.3 ng/liter). The mechanisms underlying these raised values were not clear. These findings suggest that the transplanted atria may secrete atrial peptides and that innervation is not obligatory for secretion of ANP to occur. Before this can be confirmed, however, what the relative contribution of donor and recipient atrial tissue is to the secretion of these peptides remains to be established.

Aortic valve atresia is the worst heart disease known to man and womankind. It is the most common cause of death from heart disease in the first week of life. Surgical correction of this anomaly is fruitless. Heart replacement by allotransplantation is a potentially definitive form of treatment for this condition. Bailey and associates[66] from Loma Linda, California, described their experience with orthotopic cardiac transplantation in 3 newborns with aortic valve atresia. These same investigators performed a cardiac xenotransplantation in a newborn with aortic valve atresia in October 1984. Subsequently these investigators were referred 21 newborns for cardiac transplantation, and 20 had hypoplastic left-heart syndrome (aortic valve atresia), and 1 had idiopathic cardiomyopathy. Seven of these 21 infants accepted for transplantation died before any surgery could be performed while they were awaiting allografts. Only 3 of the 21 received cardiac transplants, and they were the basis of the present report. All 3 are alive and apparently well. These workers indicated that following infants with cardiac allografts has been relatively uncomplicated. They suggested that serial endomyocardial biopsies were undesireable in this age group. This article was followed by an editorial by Shroeder and Hunt[67].

Burke and associates[68] from Stanford, California, reviewed their results in 27 patients who underwent 28 heart-lung transplant operations between March 1981 and August 1985: 8 patients died in the perioperative period and adhesions related to previous thoracic surgery proved to be a major risk factor for postoperative hemorrhage. Obliterative bronchiolitis developed in half of the 20 long-term survivors, a mean of 11 months (range 2–35) after surgery: 4 of these patients died, 3 are functionally limited, 2 were successfully treated with corticosteroids, and the remaining patient underwent successful retransplantation. The other 10 long-term survivors returned to a normal life with essentially normal pulmonary function measured at a mean of 22.6 months (range 4–42) after transplantation. All the surviving patients have evidence of renal impairment related to cyclosporin nephrotoxicity. The results indicate that, although heart-lung transplantation is compatible with essentially normal long-term pulmonary function, the procedure should not yet be regarded as a routine clinical intervention.

Little published information is available about the temporary use of a *univentricular or biventricular prosthetic heart* to provide time to procure a

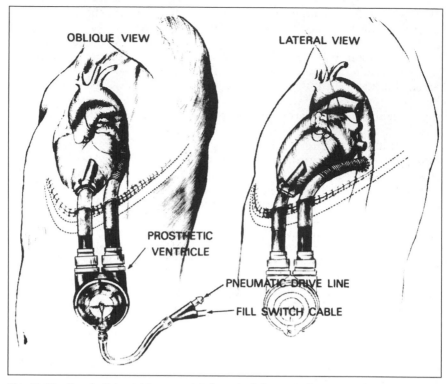

Fig. 10-10.   Prosthetic ventricle connected from the left ventricular apex and returning blood flow to the descending aorta. Reproduced with permission from Hill et al.[69]

donor heart. Hill and associates[69] from San Francisco, California, reported the successful use of a prosthetic left ventricle as a bridge to transplantation in a 47-year-old man in cardiogenic shock after massive AMI. At 1 year the patient is well and works part-time (Fig. 10-10). This study was followed by an editorial entitled, "Artificial Hearts—Permanent and Temporary," by Arnold Relman.[70] Relman advocated, as have several experts, that further use of the Jarvik-7 artificial heart for permanent implantation should cease. Relman was not against further research in developing an artificial heart, but since 3 of the 5 recipients of the Jarvik-7 artificial heart were dead and the other 2 are seriously disabled, and none had enjoyed even a few months of life outside the hospital, it was time to cease using this device.

OTHER CARDIOVASCULAR SURGICAL TOPICS

Use of "routine" electrocardiogram before noncardiac surgery

Goldberger and O'Konski[71] from Boston, Massachusetts, and San Diego, California, analyzed available data regarding the necessity for obtaining a baseline or screening electrocardiogram in all adult patients before surgery involving general or regional anesthesia or on hospital admission for other indications (Fig. 10-11). To reduce costs related to unnecessary tests and false-positive results, routine use of the electrocardiogram is warranted only

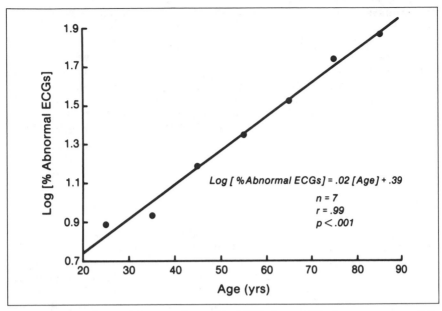

Fig. 10-11. Prevalence of electrocardiographic (ECG) abnormalities increases exponentially with age. The mean frequency of abnormal ECG findings in seven age groups, weighted by the total number of patients in each population in four studies (2, 9, 12, 13), is plotted. Reproduced with permission from Goldberger and O'Konski.[71]

in selected subsets of hospitalized patients, including those with cardiac signs or symptoms and those at risk for occult heart disease, particularly older patients.

Complications of intraaortic balloon pumping

Kantrowitz and associates[72] from Detroit, Michigan, analyzed findings in 872 attempts at intraaortic balloon pumping (IABP) in 733 patients in which the balloon was inserted between June 1967 and December 1982. Nearly 75% of the patients were men; the proportion of women increased in recent years. The principal indication for IABP support initially was cardiogenic shock, but over the years, preoperative support, weaning from cardiopulmonary bypass, and unstable angina have become the primary indications. Complications of IABP were classified and distributed by severity (minor: I [15%] and II [26%]; major: III [3%] and IV [1%]) and type (vascular [22%], infectious [22%], and bleeding [7%]). Vascular complication rates were higher in women (32 -vs- 18%), in diabetic patients (32 -vs- 20%), and in hypertensive patients (27 -vs- 20%). These did not vary with the duration of IABP support (range of duration 0–76 days). The rate of infectious complications was related to location of IABP (coronary care unit 26%, operating room 12%). The rate of fever and bacteremia increased significantly with duration of IABP support, but the rate of local wound infection did not. In conclusion, most IABP complications are minor, resolve after balloon removal, are related to vascular status of the patient and, with the exception of bacteremia, are independent of IABP duration.

Intraoperative epicardial echocardiography

Van Herwerden and associates[73] from Rotterdam, The Netherlands, evaluated the usefulness of intraoperative epicardial 2-D echocardiography using a commercially available 5-MHz mechanical sector scanner in 200 patients.

The scanhead was inserted into a gas-sterilized plastic bag and placed on the exposed heart. Unsuspected new diagnoses were made in 7 patients. In 68 patients additional morphologic information was obtained. This information influenced surgical maangement in 32 patients. Intraoperative echocardiographic analysis of the surgical correction revealed the expected results in 184 patients. In 16 patients the investigation provided important information in the decision of immediate reoperation. The authors concluded that epicardial 2-D echocardiography performed by the surgeon familiar with the interpretation of echocardiographic cross sections yields important information for surgical management. The technique has become an important adjunct in their cardiac surgery department for immediate decision making and leads to optimal results.

Late warm-blood cardioplegia

The controversy continues surrounding the best delivery mode for cardioplegia (clear or blood), the best solution for cardioplegia (simply potassium, oxygenated, or substrate-enhanced), and the appropriate reperfusion vehicle. Teoh and associates[74] from Toronto, Canada, offer information supporting the use of terminal warm cardioplegic infusion after cold-blood cardioplegia. They performed a prospective, randomized trial in 20 patients undergoing elective CABG. Eleven patients received cold-blood cardioplegia and 9 patients received cold-blood cardioplegia followed by warm-blood cardioplegia before crossclamp removal (hot shot). The hot shot provided oxygen and removed excess lactate from the arrested heart. After the hot shot, lactate was extracted by the heart and tissue ATP, and glycogen concentrations were preserved. Atrial pacing and volume loading 3 and 4 hours postoperatively resulted in decreased myocardial lactate extraction after cold-blood cardioplegia but increased lactate extraction after the hot shot. LA pressures were higher at similar end-diastolic volumes (by nuclear ventriculography), which suggested decreased diastolic compliance after cold-blood cardioplegia. These investigators concluded that terminal warm-blood cardioplegia caused accelerated myocardial metabolic recovery, preserved high-energy phosphates, improved the metabolic response to postoperative hemodynamic stress, and reduced LA pressures. The infusion of potassium-rich warm blood or substrate-enhanced blood before terminating the ischemic cardioplegic period may enhance myocardial recovery and improve hemodynamic function. Such a procedure did so in this group of patients. However, as in many other studies of cardioplegia, the subjects had relatively good ventricular function. What is needed is a study similar to the Toronto study done in high risk patients, so that clear improvement in outcome can be demonstrated.

Protamine after cardiopulmonary bypass

The administration of protamine sulfate for reversing the anticoagulant effect of heparin during cardiopulmonary bypass is occasionally associated with severe hemodynamic alterations. The mechanisms responsible for these phenomena have not been elucidated. Complement activation during cardiopulmonary bypass and the level of C3a 3 hours after cardiopulmonary bypass and protamine administration has been shown to be a risk factor for postoperative morbidity. Kirklin and associates[75] from Birmingham, Alabama, studied 19 patients prospectively before and after administration of protamine sulfate after cardiopulmonary bypass. After protamine administration, C3a, C4a, and C4d were elevated. The peak levels of C3a and C4a were in samples taken 10 minutes after protamine administration. Only C3a was elevated after cardopulmonary bypass and before protamine administration. *In vitro*, only the combination of protamine sulfate and heparin, and neither alone, resulted in increased C3a and C4a. Administration of protamine was associated with small and transient decreases in total white cells, granulocytes, and platelets, and with small and transient reductions in systemic and PA and LA and RA pressures. Systemic vascular resistance decreased and pulmonary vascular resistance increased but the change could be the result of chance. These data and those reported by others support the inference that complement activation occurs during cardiopulmonary bypass by the alternative pathway and again during protamine administration by the classic pathway. The authors suggested that this accompanies a whole body inflammatory reaction with blood cell and hemodynamic changes which, when extreme, could result in severe hemodynamic derangement.

Desmopressin after cardiac surgery

Bleeding after cardiopulmonary bypass necessitates reexploration of the chest in approximately 3% of patients who have had operations on the heart. Salzman and associates[76] from Boston, Massachusetts, examined the possibility that this problem might be alleviated by desmopressin acetate (DDAVP), which increases the plasma level of von Willebrand factor and improves hemostasis in mild hemophilia and other conditions associated with defective platelet function. In a double-blind, prospective, randomized trial, the authors studied the effect of intraoperative desmopressin acetate in 70 patients undergoing various cardiac operations requiring cardiopulmonary bypass. Patients undergoing uncomplicated primary CABG were excluded. The drug significantly reduced mean operative and early postoperative blood loss (1,317 ± 486 ml in the treated group -vs- 2,210 ± 1,415 ml in the placebo group); of the 14 patients whose 24-hour blood loss exceeded 2,000 ml, 11 had received the placebo. Plasma levels of von Willebrand factor were higher after desmopressin acetate than after placebo. Patients with the most bleeding had relatively low levels of von Willebrand factor before operation, suggesting a role for this factor in the hemorrhagic tendency induced by extracorporeal circulation. There were no untoward side effects of desmopressin acetate. The authors concluded that the administration of desmopressin acetate can be recommended to reduce blood loss in patients undergoing complex cardiac operations. The beneficial effect of the drug on hemostasis after cardiopulmonary bypass may be related to its effect on von Willebrand factor.

This study was followed by an editorial entitled "Bleeding After Cardiopulmonary Bypass," by Lawrence Harker[77] from La Jolla, California. This author pointed out that if the results of this trial are found to apply to other types of cardiac operations (there are >200,000 such operations each year in the USA), therapy with desmopressin acetate could produce a substantial savings in blood supplies. Additional benefits would include a reduced risk of transfusion-transmitted diseases and the obvious advantage of a reduced rate of reoperation. It would be important, however, to determine in patients undergoing CABG whether preoperative desmopressin increases the possibility of graft occlusion. Since the overall statistical benefit reported in these studies probably depends on protecting a relatively small proportion of vulnerable patients, it remains to be determined in future trials whether these patients can be identified either preoperatively, on the basis of lower-range circulating levels of von Willebrand factor, or postoperatively on the basis of persistent prolongation of the bleeding time. If either of these strategies is valid, desmopressin could then be given to patients who are at particular risk of bleeding, rather than to all patients undergoing cardiopulmonary bypass.

Cerebral consequences of cardiopulmonary bypass

Smith and associates[78] from London, UK, investigated preoperatively and 8 days and 8 weeks postoperatively 55 patients undergoing CABG and compared findings with those of 20 patients having thoracic or major vascular surgery for changes in neuropsychologic status, psychiatric state, cerebral blood flow, and neurologic signs, this last being assessed also at 24 hours. Major persisting neurologic changes were rare, but minor abnormalities were significantly more common after CABG than after thoracic or vascular surgery. Neuropsychologic deficits were common at 8 days in both CABG and comparison groups and persisted at 8 weeks in about one-third of all patients. Cerebral blood flow was reduced at 8 days in some CABG patients, but this was not significant for the group. Preexisting cerebral vascular disease was not predictive, but low profusion pressure and long bypass time were associated with postoperative deficits.

PUBLISHED SYMPOSIA ON
CARDIOVASCULAR DISEASE IN 1986

In Table 10-1 are listed the symposia published in THE AMERICAN JOURNAL OF CARDIOLOGY IN 1986[79], and in Table 10-2 are listed the symposia on cardiovascular disease published in THE AMERICAN JOURNAL OF MEDICINE in 1986.

TABLE 10-1. *SYMPOSIA in the AJC in 1986*

NO.	PUBLICATION DATE	SUBJECT	GUEST EDITOR	NO. ARTICLES	NO. PAGES	SPONSOR
A	January 24	Diuretics	Andrew Whelton	9	56	Hoffman-LaRoche
B	January 31	Ventricular arrhythmias in congestive heart failure	J. Thomas Bigger Jr	8	48	Mead Johnson
C	February 12	Lipids and hypertension	Walter M Kirkendall Paul Samuel	12	72	Sandoz
D	February 26	Calcium antagonists in hypertension	John H Laragh	21	112	Knoll AG
E	March 28	*Guanfacine* for hypertension	Donald G Vidt Peter A Van Zweiten	13	73	A H Robins
F	April 25	Non-selective beta blockers	Stephen E Epstein Robert J Lefkowitz	10	56	Merck, Sharp & Dohme
G	May 30	Hyperlipidemia	Antonio M Gotto Jr	8	48	Warner-Lambert
H	June 27	*Probucol* for hypercholesterolemia	Howard A Eder	9	56	Merrell Dow
A	July 31	Diuretics	James C Melby	5	24	Merck, Sharp & Dohme
B	August 15	Silent myocardial ischemia	Bramah N Singh	10	64	Key
C	August 29	Encainide	Donald C Harrison Joel Morganroth	18	120	Mead Johnson
D	September 30	Calcium antagonists in hypertension	William W Parmley Henry A Solomon	11	46	Miles
E	November 26	*Bevantolol*	Stanley H Taylor	9	48	Warner-Lambert
13				143	823	

TABLE 10-2.   *Cardiovascular Symposia in The American Journal of Medicine in 1986*

SYMPOSIUM NUMBER	SUBJECT OF SYMPOSIUM	GUEST EDITOR(S)	NO. ARTICLES	NO. PAGES	SPONSORING COMPANY
2A (February 14)	Prazosin, lipids and hypertension	Robert I. Levy Paul Leren	20	136	Pfizer
2B (February 28)	Congestive heart failure	Mark M. Applefeld	13	88	Eli Lilly
4A (April 25)	Potassium, magnesium cardio-vascular death and triam-terene/hydrochlorothiazide	Norman K. Hollenberg	6	40	Lederle
4C (April 30)	Myocardial ischemia	Myron L. Weisfeldt	8	64	Pfizer
5A (May 16)	Diabetes mellitus in the elderly	Loren G. Lipson	8	72	Pfizer (Roerig)
5B (May 23)	Terazosin and hypertension	Marvin Moser	17	112	Abbott
4A (October 20)	Myocardial ischemia and nifedipine	Peter F. Cohn	6	40	Pfizer
4C (October 31)	Enalapril for hypertension and congestive heart failure	Aram V. Chobanian James V. Warren	10	56	Merck Sharp & Dohme
6A (December 15)	Nifedipine for systemic hypertension	Aram V. Chobanian	8	48	Pfizer
6C (December 31)	Hydrochlorothiazide and systemic hypertension	William B. Stason Mark V. Pauly	9	56	Smith Kline & French
10			105	712	

SOME GOOD CARDIOLOGIC BOOKS
PUBLISHED IN 1986

This piece briefly mentions some of the better books that have crossed my desk in 1986.[80]

1. Cheng TO, editor. *The International Textbook of Cardiology*. New York: Pergamon Press, 1986:1299, $125.00.

The intent of this fine book is to give "serious students of international cardiology a source of reference in one single textbook." Cheng assembled 136 contributors, two-thirds of whom are from the USA, to produce 83 chapters occupying 1,272 pages. This book is about 35% smaller and it costs about 20% more than either the Braunwald or Hurst cardiologic textbooks.

2. Kaplan NM. *Clinical Hypertension*. 4th ed. Baltimore: Williams & Wilkins, 1986:492, $54.95.

This book, in my view, is the best of the clinical books on systemic hypertension. Although the book covers all forms of systemic hypertension, the most common forms receive the most attention. This is a very practical book by one of the best teachers in medicine.

3. Antman EM, Rutherford JD. *Coronary Care Medicine. A Practical Approach*. Boston: Martinus Nijhoff, 1986:384, $69.95.

This book covers virtually all aspects of management of patients with coronary problems necessitating hospitalization in a coronary care unit.

4. Conti CR, editor. *Coronary Artery Spasm. Pathophysiology, Diagnosis, and Treatment*. New York: Marcel Dekker, 1986:347, $59.75.

This book is the best one on this subject. It records what is known and pertinent about coronary artery spasm.

5. Grossman W, editor. *Cardiac Catheterization and Angiography*. 3rd ed. Philadelphia: Lea & Febiger, 1986:562, $49.50.

This book is a classic and a must possession of physicians who spend time in a cardiac catheterization laboratory.

6. Vlietstra RE, Holmes DR, Jr., editors. *PTCA Percutaneous Transluminal Coronary Angioplasty*. Philadelphia: FA Davis, 1986:268, $49.00.

A timely book.

7. Iskandrian AS. *Nuclear Cardiac Imaging: Principles and Applications*. Philadelphia: FA Davis, 1986:527, $75.00.

This fine book by a single author provides an in-depth analysis of the usefulness of the most commonly available cardiac imaging modalities: thallium-201 scintigraphy, myocardial infarct avid imaging, and radionuclide ventriculography. The emphasis is on the implications of these diagnostic procedures on patient management rather than on detailed technical considerations.

8. McArdle WD, Katch FI, Katch VL. *Exercise Physiology. Energy, Nutrition, and Human Performance*. 2nd ed. Philadelphia: Lea & Febiger, 1986:696, $32.50.

This is an excellent book combining information on nutrition, energy and exercise performance. The price is right.

9. Schneeweiss A. *Drug Therapy in Cardiovascular Diseases*. Philadelphia: Lea & Febiger, 1986:835, $84.50.

This is a drug-oriented scholarly book. The drugs are classified by their pharmacologic properties and each chapter deals with 1 drug. Three-fourths of the book is devoted to 4 major drug classes: beta blockers, calcium-channel blockers, converting-enzyme inhibitors and antiarrhythmic agents. The remainder of the book is devoted to 32 other drugs. The purpose of this book is not to suggest which drug to use but to supply information about available drugs.

10. Schneeweiss A. *Drug Therapy in Infants and Children with Cardiovascular Diseases*. Philadelphia: Lea & Febiger, 1986:398, $45.00.

This book is organized similarly to the one above by the same author, and it should be of great value to physicians who care for children with cardiovascular disease. A section on diuretics is not included in either book by Schneeweiss.

11. Opie LH, editor; Chatterjee K, Gersh BJ, Harrison DC, Kaplan NM, Marcus FI, Singh BN, Sonnenblick EH, Thadani U, collaborators. *Drugs for the Heart*. 2nd ed. Orlando, FL: Grune & Stratton, 1987:238, $18.95.

This pocket-sized compendium provides information on 10 kinds of cardiovascular drugs—beta blockers; nitrates; calcium antagonists; digitalis, sympathomimetics, and inotropic-dilators; diuretics; vasodilators; angiotensin-converting-enzyme inhibitors; antithrombotic agents; and lipid-lowering agents—their uses, doses and side effects. This is a wonderfully useful book.

12. Barlow JB. *Perspectives on the Mitral Valve*. Philadelphia: FA Davis, 1987:381, $49.00.

John Barlow's name, of course, is synonymous with mitral valve prolapse. This well-done book summarizes his 30-year experience with the Barlow syndrome and with the many other conditions that affect the mitral valve.

13. Furman S, Hayes DL, Holmes DR Jr. *A Practice of Cardiac Pacing*. Mount Kisco, NY: Futura, 1986:480, $59.50.

A book on pacing co-authored by Seymour Furman is one to take note of. This text discusses and illustrates how pacemakers work and what telemetric, radiologic and electrocardiographic findings are associated with normal and abnormal function. The book provides a personal approach from 2 large cardiac pacing practices, the Montefiore Medical Center and the Mayo Clinic.

14. Benditt DG, Benson DW Jr., editors. *Cardiac Preexcitation Syndromes. Origins, Evaluation, and Treatment*. Boston: Martinus Nijhoff, 1986:556, $105.00.

I suspect that this book will be the gospel on preexcitation for some time to come.

15. Huhta JC. *Pediatric Imaging/Doppler Ultrasound of the Chest: Extra-cardiac Diagnosis.* Philadelphia: Lea & Febiger, 1986:225, $42.50.

16. Swischuk LE, Sapire DW. *Basic Imaging in Congenital Heart Disease.* 3rd ed. Baltimore: Williams & Wilkins, 1986:312, $58.95.

17. Williams RG, Bierman FZ, Sanders SP. *Echocardiographic Diagnosis of Cardiac Malformations.* Boston: Little, Brown, 1986:237, $48.50.

I think No. 14 is the best of the 3.

18. Perloff JK. *The Clinical Recognition of Congenital Heart Disease.* 3rd ed. Philadelphia: WB Saunders, 1987:705, $95.00.

This book, an update and expansion of the second edition appearing in 1978, focuses entirely on the clinical diagnosis of congenital heart disease. The 32 chapters contain 733 figures, 54 (7%) of which are echocardiograms (all cross-sectional except for 1 Doppler) and 3,539 references. This book by a master clinician has been a classic since its beginning.

19. Roberts WC, editor. *Adult Congenital Heart Disease.* Philadelphia: FA Davis, 1987:752, $75.00.

When an editor reviews his own handiwork the reader is at least clearly forewarned that the impartial judgments will be from the author's point of view. This book is an outgrowth of *Congenital Heart Disease in Adults* which FA Davis published in 1979 as part of their Cardiovascular Clinics Series. The 1979 book was the first ever published on congenital heart disease in adults. During these past 7 years, much new information on this subject has been accumulated, and although the present book is an outgrowth of the 1979 book, the new one is different. Five chapters have been added, 20 of the remaining 22 have been expanded, and several have additional or new authors. The publisher is to be complimented for the attractiveness of the book.

20. Roberts WC, editor: Mason DT, Rackley CE, Willerson JT, Graham TP Jr., Pacifico AD, Karp RB, contributors. *Cardiology 1986.* New York: Yorke Medical Books, 1986:444, $55.00.

21. Harvey WP, Kirkendall WM, Laks H, Resnekov L, Rosenthal A, Sonnenblick EH, editors. *1986 Yearbook of Cardiology.* Chicago: Year Book Medical Publishers, 1986:364, $44.95.

The 2 books are quite different. The Yorke book (no. 20), which appeared in June 1986, contains summaries of 771 articles, all published in 1985, plus 112 figures, 31 tables and 444 pages. The Yearbook (no. 21), published in August 1986, contains summaries of 309 articles, 42 (14%) of which were published in 1984 and only 21 (7%) of which were published in October–December 1985, plus 49 figures, 17 tables and 364 pages. All summaries in the Yorke book (no. 20) were selected by and written by the physician authors; all summaries in the Yearbook (no. 21) were selected by the physician editors who wrote brief comments, but the articles themselves were summarized by the publisher. Separation of the editors' comments from the summaries themselves is the unique feature of the Yearbook. The Yorke book costs 18% more than the Yearbook, but it contains 18% more pages, it summarizes 60% more articles, and it provides 56% more figures and 45% more tables.

22. Paul O. *Take Heart. The Life and Prescription For Living of Dr. Paul Dudley White.* Boston: Harvard University Press, 1986:315, $18.95.

23. Meijler FL, Burchell HB, editors. *Professor Dirk Durrer. 35 Years of Cardiology in Amsterdam. A Selection of Papers and Full Bibliography.* Amsterdam: North-Holland, 1986:678, $101.75.

24. Cournand AF with the collaboration of Meyer M. *From Roots to Late*

Budding. The Intellectual Adventures of a Medical Scientist. New York: Gardner Press, 1986:232, $18.95.

Three good books for the cardiologic historian.

CARDIOLOGIC HISTORIC NOTES

Howell[81] from Ann Arbor, Michigan, reviewed some of the enormous changes that have occurred in cardiology during the present century. These changes included the cardiology societies, the cardiology journals, how cardiology subdivisions have operated in departments of pediatrics, medicine and surgery, and how cardiology subdivisions have operated in hospitals themselves. This is a fine article.

The year 1985 saw the deaths of 3 prominent innovators in the cardiac catheterization laboratory—Andreas R. Gruentzig, Melvin Judkins and F. Mason Sones, Jr[82]. The year 1986 saw the loss of 2 great pediatric cardiologists, Helen Brooke Taussig and William J. Rashkind, and a leader and producer in adult cardiology for 50 years, George Edward Burch[83].

References

1. Odom H, Davis JL, Dinh H, Baker BJ, Roberts WC, Murphy ML: QRS voltage measurements in autopsied men free of cardiopulmonary disease: a basis for evaluating total QRS voltage as an index of left ventricular hypertrophy. Am J Cardiol 1986 (Oct 1); 58:801–804.
2. Gardin JM, Dabestani A, Takenaka K, Rohan MK, Knoll M, Russell D, Henry WL: Effect of imaging view and sample volume location on evaluation of mitral flow velocity by pulsed Doppler echocardiography. Am J Cardiol 1986 (June 1); 57:1335–1339.
3. Gardin JM, Kozlowski J, Dabestani A, Murphy M, Kusnick C, Allfie A, Russell D, Henry WL: Studies of Doppler aortic flow velocity during supine bicycle exercise. Am J Cardiol 1986 (Feb 1); 57:327–332.
4. Gossard D, Haskell WL, Taylor CB, Mueller JK, Rogers F, Chandler M, Ahn DK, Miller NH, Debusk RF: Effects of low- and high-intensity home-based exercise training on functional capacity in healthy middle-aged men. Am J Cardiol 1986 (Feb 15); 57:446–449.
5. Fleg JL, Lakatta EG: Prevalence and significance of postexercise hypotension in apparently healthy subjects. Am J Cardiol 1986 (June 1); 57:1380–1384.
6. Higginbotham MB, Morris KG, Williams RS, Coleman RE, Cobb FR: Physiologic basis for the age-related decline in aerobic work capacity. Am J Cardiol 1986 (June 1); 57:1374–1379.
7. Rauramaa R, Salonen JR, Seppanen K, Salonen R, Venalanen JM, Ihanainen M: Inhibition of platelet aggregability by moderate intensity physical exercise: a randomized clinical trial in overweight men. Circulation 1986 (Nov); 74:939–944.
8. Wolfel EE, Hiatt WR, Brammell HL, Carry MR, Ringel SP, Travis V, Horwitz LD: Effects of selective and nonselective B-adrenergic blockade on mechanisms of exercise conditioning. Circulation 1986 (Oct); 74:664–674.
9. Mickelson JK, Byrd BF III, Bouchard A, Botvinick EH, Schiller NB: Left ventricular dimensions and mechanics in distance runners. Am Heart J 1986 (Dec); 112:1251–1256.
10. Tak T, Cats VM, Dunning AJ: Ambulatory ECG recording during competitive parachute jumping in apparently healthy young men: more evidence for intermittent vagal dominance during enhanced sympathetic activity. Eur Heart J 1986 (Feb); 7:110–114.
11. Sundqvist K, Atterhog J, Jogestrand T: Effect of digoxin on the electrocardiogram at rest and during exercise in healthy subjects. Am J Cardiol 1986 (Mar 1); 57:661–665.
12. Van de Werf F, Geboers J, Kesteloot H, De Geest H, Barrios L: The mechanism of disappearance of the physiologic third heart sound with age. Circulation 1986 (May); 73(5):877–884.

13. Fowler NO, Harbin AD: Recurrent acute pericarditis: Follow-up study of 31 patients. J Am Coll Cardiol 1986 (Feb); 7:300–305.

14. Kopecky SL, Callahan JA, Tajik K, Seward JB: Percutaneous pericardial catheter drainage: report of 42 consecutive cases. Am J Cardiol 1986 (Sept 15); 58:633–635.

15. Needleman P, Greenwald JE: Atriopeptin: cardiac hormone intimately involved in fluid, electrolyte, and blood-pressure homeostasis. N Engl J Med 1986 (Mar 27); 314:828–834.

16. Bates ER, Shenker Y, Grekin RJ: The relationship between plasma levels of immunoreactive atrial natriuretic hormone and hemodynamic function in man. Circulation (June); 73(6):1155–1161.

17. Rodeheffer RJ, Tanaka I, Imada T, Hollister AS, Robertson D, Inagami T: Atrial pressure and secretion of atrial natriuretic factor into the human central circulation. J Am Coll Cardiol 1986 (July); 8:18–26.

18. Genest J: The atrial natriuretic factor. Br Heart J 1986 (Oct); 56:302–316.

19. Linden RJ, Knapp MF: Is atrial natriuretic peptide really a hormone? Br Heart J 1986 (Oct); 56:299–301.

20. Cates CU, Virmani R, Vaughn WK, Robertson RM: Electrocardiographic markers of cardiac metastasis. Am Heart J 1986 (Dec); 112:1297–1303.

21. McCarthy PM, Piehler JM, Schaff HV, Pluth JR, Orszulak TA, Vidaillet HJ, Carney JA: The significance of multiple, recurrent, and "complex" cardiac myxomas. J Thorac Cardiovasc Surg 1986 (Mar); 91:389–396.

22. Frank S, Colliver JA, Frank A: The electrocardiogram in obesity: Statistical analysis of 1,029 patients. J Am Coll Cardiol 1986 (Feb); 7:295–299.

23. Stunkard AJ, Foch TT, Hrubec Z: A twin study of human obesity. JAMA 1986 (July 4); 256:51–54.

24. Stunkard AJ, Sorensen TIA, Hanis C, Treasdale TW, Chakraborty R, Schull WJ, Schulsinger F: An adoption study of human obesity. N Engl J Med 1986 (Jan 23); 314:193–198.

25. Van Itallie TB: Bad news and good news about obesity. N Engl J Med 1986 (Jan 23); 314:239–240.

26. Roberts WC: A simple histologic classification of pulmonary arterial hypertension. Am J Cardiol 1986 (Aug 1); 58:385–386.

27. Isobe M, Yazak Y, Takaku F, Koizumi K, Hara K, Tsuneyoshi H, Yamaguchi T, Machii K: Prediction of pulmonary arterial pressure in adults by pulsed Doppler echocardiography. Am J Cardiol 1986 (Feb 1); 57:316–321.

28. Martin-Duran R, Larman M, Trugeda A, Vazquez De Prada JA, Ruano J, Torres A, Figueroa A, Pajaron A, Nistal F: Comparison of Doppler-determined elevated pulmonary arterial pressure with pressure measured at Cardiac catheterization. Am J Cardiol 1986 (Apr 1); 57:859–863.

29. Masuyama T, Kodama K, Kitabatake A, Sato H, Shinsuke N, Inoue M: Continuous-wave Doppler echocardiographic detection of pulmonary regurgitation and its application to noninvasive estimation of pulmonary artery pressure. Circulation 1986 (Mar); 74:484–492.

30. Kasper W, Meinertz T, Henkel B, Eissner D, Hahn K, Hofmann T, Zeiher A, Just H: Echocardiographic findings in patients with proved pulmonary embolism. Am Heart J 1986 (Dec); 112:1284–1290.

31. Goldhaber SZ, Markis JE, Meyerovitz MF, Kim DS, Dawley DL, Sasahara A, Vaughan DE, Selwyn AP, Loscalzo J, Kessler CM, Sharma GVRK, Grossbard EB, Braunwald E: Acute pulmonary embolism treated with tissue plasminogen activator. Lancet 1986 (Oct 18); 886–888.

32. Clarke DB, Abrams LD: Pulmonary embolectomy: a 25 year experience. J Thorac Cardiovasc Surg 1986 (Sept); 92:442–445.

33. Dalen JE, Hirsh J: American College of Chest Physicians and the National Heart, Lung, and Blood Institute National Conference on Antithrombotic Therapy. Arch Intern Med 1986 (Mar); 146:462–463.

34. Sherman DG, Dyken ML, Harrison MJG: Cerebral embolism. Arch Intern Med 1986 (Mar); 146:471–472.

35. Genton E, Clagett GP, Salzman EW: Antithrombotic therapy in peripheral vascular disease. Arch Intern Med (Mar); 146:470–471.

36. Dunn M, Alexander J, De Silva R, Hildner F: Antithrombotic therapy in atrial fibrillation. Arch Intern Med (Mar); 146:470.

37. Resnekov L, Chediak J, Hirsh J, Lewis D: Antithrombotic agents in coronary artery disease. Arch Intern Med (Mar); 146:469.

38. STEIN PD, COLLINS JJ, KANTROWITZ A: Antithrombotic therapy in mechanical and biological prosthetic heart valves and saphenous vein bypass grafts. Arch Intern Med (Mar); 146:468–469.

39. LEVINE HJ, PAUKER SG, SALZMAN EW: Antithrombotic therapy in valvular heart disease. Arch Intern Med 1986 (Mar); 146:467–468.

40. HYERS TM, HULL RD, WEG JG: Antithrombotic therapy for venous thromboembolic disease. Arch Intern Med 1986 (Mar); 146:467.

41. LEVINE MN, RASKOB G, HIRSH J: Hemorrhagic complications of long-term anticoagulant therapy. Arch Intern Med 1986 (Mar); 146:466.

42. HIRSCH J, DEYKIN D, POLLER L: Therapeutic range for oral anticoagulant therapy. Arch Intern Med 1986 (Mar); 146:466.

43. HIRSH J, FUSTER V, SALZMAN E: Dose antiplatelet agents: The relationship among side effects and antithrombotic effectiveness. Arch Intern Med 1986 (Mar); 146:465–466.

44. SACKETT DL: Rules of evidence and clinical recommendations on the use of antithrombotic agents. Arch Intern Med 1986 (Mar); 146:464–465.

45. CHAMBERS BR, NORRIS JW: Outcome in patients with asymptomatic neck bruits. N Engl J Med 1986 (Oct 2); 315:860–865.

46. TAPE TG, MUSHLIN AI: The utility of routine chest radiographs. Ann Intern Med 1986 (May); 104:663–670.

47. ENGLEBERG AL, GIBBONS HL, DOEGE TC: A review of the medical standards for civilian airmen: synopsis of a two-year study. JAMA 1986 (Mar 28); 255:1589–1599.

48. DEVEREUX RB, ALONSO DR, LUTAS EM, GOTTLIEB GJ, CAMPO E, SACHS I, REICHEK N: Echocardiographic assessment of left ventricular hypertrophy: comparison to necropsy findings. Am J Cardiol 1986 (Feb 15); 57:450–458.

49. VAN DAM I, ROELANDT J, DE MEDINA OR: Left atrial enlargement: an electrocardiographic misnomer? An electrocardiographic–echocardiographic study. Eur Heart J 1986 (Feb); 7:115–117.

50. KESSLER KM, PINA I, GREEN B, BURNETT B, LAIGHOLD M, BILSKER M, PALOMO AR, MYERBURG RJ: Cardiovascular findings in quadriplegic and paraplegic patients and in normal subjects. Am J Cardiol 1986 (Sept 1); 58:525–530.

51. SUTHERLAND GR, CHEUNG HW, HOLLIDAY RL, DRIEDGER AA, SIBBALD WJ: Hemodynamic adaptation to acute myocardial contusion complicating blunt chest injury. Am J Cardiol 1986 (Feb 1); 57:291–297.

52. McBRIDE JW, LABROSSE KR, McCOY HG, AHRENHOLZ DH, SOLEM LD, GOLDENBERG IF: Is serum creatine kinase-MB in electrically injured patients predictive of myocardial injury? JAMA 1986 (Feb 14); 255:764–768.

53. HOFSTETTER A, SCHUTZ Y, JEQUIER E, WAHREN J: Increased 24-hour energy expenditure in cigarette smokers. N Engl J Med 1986 (Jan 9); 314:79–82.

54. SHUB C, CUETO-GARCIA L, SHEPS SG, ILSTRUP DM, TAJIK J: Echocardiographic findings in pheochromocytoma. Am J Cardiol 1986 (Apr 15); 57:971–975.

55. KVOLS LK, MOERTEL CG, O'CONNELL MJ, SCHUTT AJ, RUBIN J, HAHN RG: Treatment of the malignant carcinoid syndrome: evaluation of a long-acting somatostatin analogue. N Engl J Med 1986 (Sept 11); 315:663–666.

56. OATES J: The carcinoid syndrome. N Engl J Med 1986 (Sept 11); 315:702–704.

57. SZNAJDER JI, ZVEIBIL FR, BITTERMAN H, WEINER P, BURSZTEIN S: Central vein catheterization: Failure and complication rates by three percutaneous approaches. Arch Intern Med 1986 (Feb); 146:259–261.

58. Years of life lost from cardiovascular disease. MMWR 1986 (Oct 24); 35:653–655.

59. EVANS RW, MANNINEN DL, GARRISON LP, MAIER AM: Donor availability as the primary determinant of the future of heart transplantation. JAMA 1986 (Apr 11); 255:1892–1898.

60. EMERY RW, CORK RC, LEVINSON MM, RILEY JE, COPELAND J, McALEER MJ, COPELAND JG: The cardiac donor: a six-year experience. Ann Thorac Surg 1986 (Apr); 41:356–362.

61. LEVINE TB, OLIVARI MT, COHN JN: Effects of orthotopic heart transplantation on sympathetic control mechanisms in congestive heart failure. Am J Cardiol 1986 (Nov 1); 58:1035–1040.

62. HARDESTY RL, GRIFFITH BP, TRENTO A, THOMPSON ME, FERSON PF, BAHNSON HT: Mortally ill patients and excellent survival following cardiac transplantation. Ann Thorac Surg 1986 (Feb); 41:126–129.

63. CARRIER M, EMERY RW, RILEY JE, LEVINSON MM, COPELAND JG: Cardiac transplantation in patients over 50 years of age. J Am Coll Cardiol 1986 (Aug); 8:285–288.

64. KAPSNER P, LANGSDORF L, MARCUS R, KRAEMER FB, HOFFMAN AR: Mil-alkali syndrome in patients treated with calcium carbonate after cardiac transplantation. Arch Intern Med 1986 (Oct); 146:1965–1968.

65. SINGER DRJ, BUCKLEY MG, MACGREGOR GA, KHAGHANI A, BANNER NR, YACOUB MH: Raised concentrations of plasma atrial natriuretic peptides in cardiac transplant recipients. Br Med J 1986 (Nov 19); 293:1391–1392.

66. BAILEY LL, NEHLSEN-CANNARELLA SL, DOROSHOW RW, JACOBSON JG, MARTIN RD, ALLARD MW, HYDE MR, BUI RHD, PETRY EL: Cardiac allotransplantation in newborns as therapy for hypoplastic left heart syndrome. N Engl J Med 1986 (Oct 9); 315:949–951.

67. SHROEDER JS, HUNT SA: Cardiac transplantation: Where are we? N Engl J Med 1986 (Oct 9); 315:961–963.

68. BURKE CM, BALDWIN JC, MORRIS AJ, SHUMWAY NE, THEODORE J, TAZELAAR HD, MCGREGOR C, ROBIN ED, JAMIESON SW: Twenty-eight cases of human heart-lung transplantation. Lancet 1986 (Mar 8); 517–519.

69. HILL JD, FARRAR DJ, HERSHON JJ, COMPTON PG, AVERY GJ, LEVIN BS, BRENT BN: Use of a prosthetic ventricle as a bridge to cardiac transplantation for postinfarction cardiogenic shock. N Engl J Med 1986 (Mar 6); 314:626–628.

70. RELMAN, A: Artificial hearts—permanent and temporary. N Engl J Med 1986 (Mar 6); 314:644–645.

71. GOLDBERGER AL, O'KONSKI M: Utility of the routine electrocardiogram before surgery and on general hospital admission. Ann Intern Med 1986 (Oct); 105:552–557.

72. KANTROWITZ A, WASFIE T, FREED PS, RUBENFIRE M, WAJSZCZUK W, SCHORK MA: Intraaortic balloon pumping 1967 through 1982: Analysis of complications in 733 patients. Am J Cardiol 1986 (Apr 15); 57:976–983.

73. VAN HERWERDEN LA, GUSSENHOVEN WJ, ROELANDT J, BOS E, LIGTVOET CM, HAALEBOS MM, MOCHTAR B, LEICHER F, WITSENBURG M: Intraoperative epicardial two-dimensional echocardiography. Eur Heart J 1986 (May); 7:386–395.

74. TEOH KH, CHRISTAKIS GT, WEISEL RD, FREMES SE, MICKLE DAG, ROMASCHIN AD, HARDING RS, IVANOV J, MADONIK M, ROSS IM, MCLAUGHLIN PR, BAIRD RJ: Accelerated myocardial metabolic recovery with terminal warm blood cardioplegia. J Thorac Cardiovasc Surg 1986 (June); 91:888–895.

75. KIRKLIN JK, CHENOWETH DE, NAFTEL DC, BLACKSTONE EH, KIRKLIN JW, BITRAN DD, CURD JG, REVES JG, SAMUELSON PN: Effects of protamine administration after cardiopulmonary bypass on complement, blood elements, and the hemodynamic state. Ann Thorac Surg 1986 (Feb); 41:193–199.

76. SALZMAN EW, WEINSTEIN MJ, WEINTRAUB RM, WARE JA, THURER RL, ROBERTSON L, DONOVAN A, GAFFNEY T, BERTELE V, TROLL J, SMITH M, CHUTE LE: Treatment with desmopressin acetate to reduce blood loss after cardiac surgery: A double-blind randomized trial. N Engl J Med 1986 (May 29); 213:1402–1406.

77. HARKER LA: Bleeding after cardiopulmonary bypass. N Engl J Med 1986 (May 29); 213:1446–1447.

78. SMITH PL, NEWMAN SP, ELL PJ, TREASURE T, JOSEPH P, SCHNEIDAU A, HARRISON MJG: Cerebral consequences of cardiopulmonary bypass. Lancet (Apr 12); 823–825.

79. ROBERTS WC: The AJC in 1986. Am J Cardiol 1987 (Feb 1); 59:391–392.

80. ROBERTS WC: Some good cardiologic books published in 1986. Am J Cardiol 1986 (Dec); 58:1271–1272.

81. HOWELL JD: The changing face of twentieth-century American cardiology. Ann Intern Med 1986 (Nov); 105:772–782.

82. PROUDFIT WL: F. Mason Sones, Jr., M.D., (1918–1985): the man and his work. Cleve Clin Q 1986 (summer); 53:121–124.

83. ROBERTS WC: George Edward Burch, MD, 1910–1986. Am J Cardiol 1986 (July 1); 58:162–167.

Author Index

Subject Index

in atrial flutter, 217–18
Atrial septal defect, 373
Atrioventricular block, 147–48,
254–55
Atrioventricular canal defect,
373–75

Balloon dilation during PTCA, 386
Bepridil
in angina pectoris, 90
in ventricular arrhythmias,
240–41
Beta-adrenergic receptors, 423–24
Beta blockers
in AMI, 177–81
in angina pectoris, 84, 87–91
effect on exercise, 446–47
in hypertension, 286–91
in ventricular arrhythmias,
234–35
Betaxolol, 84
Bioprostheses, 339–50, 410–12
Blacks, acute myocardial infarction
in, 130–31
Blood pressure
and insulin levels, 264
measurement, 265
monitoring, 265–66
Bruits, in neck, 459–60
Bundle branch block (BBB), 253–
54

Calcium
channel blockers
in AMI, 177–81
deficiency hypothesis, 273–74
deposits, 49–50
echographic detection of, 338–
39
supplementation, 284
in valvular heart disease, 338–39
Cancer, 453
Captopril
in congestive heart failure, 425–
26
-vs- enalapril, 427
-vs- prazosin, 428–29
in hypertension, 294
-vs- propranolol -vs- methyldopa, 289–91
Carcinoid syndrome, somatostatin
for, 464
Cardiac amyloidosis, 365–66
colchicine therapy, 365–66
echocardiographic assessment,
365
Cardiac arrest, 243–52

in Air Force recruits, 244
cardiopulmonary resuscitation,
246–48
definitions and causes, 243
effect of therapy, 249–52
in infants, 244
risk factors, 243
in Southeast Asian refugees,
244–46
survivors after resuscitation,
248–49
symptoms preceding, 244
Cardiac neoplasms, 453
markers of metastases, 453
multiple recurrent myxomas,
453
Cardiac surgery, 470–74
cardioplegia, 472
desmopressin after, 473
intraaortic balloon pumping
complications, 471
intraoperative echocardiography,
471–72
protamine after, 472–73
Cardiac transplantation, 465–70
Cardiac valve replacement,
Cardiodefibrillator, automatic, 242
Cardiologic books in 1986, 475–78
Cardiomyopathies
doxorubicin, 366–67
hypertrophic, 359–65
Doppler flow study, 360–61
intracavitary systolic pressure
gradient, 362–63
isovolumic relaxation, 361–62
left ventricular disfunction
without hypertrophy, 363–
64
left ventricular filling, 361
left ventricular thickening, 363
postextrasystolic murmur, 359
pulsus alternans, 364–65
idiopathic dilated, 355–58
immunologic studies, 355–56
peripartum, 356
programmed electrical stimulation, 356–57
therapy for, 357–58
inducing, for tachycardia, 219–
20
ischemia, in acute myocardial
infarction, 157–59
Cardioplegia, 472
Cardiopulmonary bypass, 472–74
Cardiopulmonary resuscitation
acid-base state, 247
1986 guidelines, 246–47
in rural areas, 247–48
survivors after, 248–49

Still's murmur, origin of, 336–37
Streptokinase
  in acute myocardial infarction,
    187–96, 197–201
  in congenital heart disease, 397
Sudden death. *See* Cardiac arrest
Supraventricular tachycardia
  in acute myocardial infarction,
    148
  atrial natriuretic factor, 221
  catheter ablation, 223
  after coronary artery bypass
    grafting, 114
  esmolol, 222
  flecainide in, 221
  flestolol in, 222–23
  inducing cardiomyopathy, 219–
    20
  initiating atrial fibrillation, 219
  pindolol + verapamil, 223
  propafenone in, 221–22
  symptom frequency, 218–19
Surgery
  transplantation, cardiac, 465–70
  See also Cardiac surgery; Cardio-
    vascular surgery; Coronary
    artery bypass grafting; Con-
    genital heart disease; Pediatric
    cardiac surgery; Percutaneous
    transluminal coronary angio-
    plasty
Symposia published in 1986, 474–
  475
Syncope from carotid sinus hypersensitivity, 255
Synvinolin, 30–33
Syphilis, diagnosis of, 327

Tachycardia
  inducing cardiomyopathies,
    219–20
  wide complex, 211–12
  See also Supraventricular, tachy-
    cardia
Tetralogy of Fallot, 382–83
  operative repair, 382–83
Thallium imaging
  in acute myocardial infarction,
    142–43
  in coronary artery disease, 49
Thrombolysis, 187–201
Timolol, in acute myocardial
  infarction, 181
Tissue-type plasminogen activator,
  184–87, 457
Tocainide
  in acute myocardial infarction,
    174
  for ventricular arrhythmias,
    232–33

Transplantation
Transposition of great arteries
  (TGA), 383–86
  arrhythmia after Mustard repair,
    383–84
  arterial switch for, 384–85
    pulmonary trunk banding
      after, 385–86
  congenitally corrected, 390–91
  left ventricular function before
    and after repair, 285
  pulmonary trunk banding after,
    385–86
  Senning repair, 384
Tricuspid regurgitation, by
  Doppler, 337
Tricupsid valve atresia, 397–400
Tricyclic antidepressant drugs, 281

Urokinase, in AMI,

Valvular heart disease, 303–50
  aortic regurgitation, 325–29
    ankylosing spondylitis, 328
    coronary artery disease and,
      328
    diagnosis of syphilis, 327
    echocardiography and, 325–26
    exercise and, 326–27
    hydralazine treatment, 328
    Marfan syndrome treatment,
      329
    timing of valve replacement,
      329
  aortic valve stenosis, 315–24
    diastolic filling dynamics,
      322–23
    operative decalcification, 324
    percutaneous transluminal
      valvuloplasty, 323
    severity indications, 315–17
    valve area quantified, 317–22
  calcium deposits determined by
    echocardiography, 338–39
  cardiac valve replacement, 339–
    50
    anticoagulation in pregnancy,
      347–48
    bioprostheses, 339–50, 410–12
    Doppler evaluation of, 339–42
    flow characteristics of
      mechanical, 339
    morphologic studies, 348–50
    performance after, 343
    prosthetic thrombosis, 348
    risk factors after, 342
  infective endocarditis, 329–335
    conduction abnormalities, 333
    fever during therapy, 334